Progressive Care Nursing Certification

PROGRESSIVE CARE NURSING CERTIFICATION

Preparation, Review, and Practice Exams

Thomas S. Ahrens, PhD, RN, CCNS, FAAN
Research Scientist
Barnes–Jewish Hospital
St. Louis, Missouri

Donna Prentice, MSN(R), RN, ACNS-BC, CCRN
Clinical Nurse Specialist
Barnes–Jewish Hospital
St. Louis, Missouri

Ruth M. Kleinpell, PhD, RN, FAAN, FAANP, FCCM
Director, Center for Clinical Research and Scholarship
Rush University Medical Center
Professor, Rush University College of Nursing
Nurse Practitioner, Mercy Hospital & Medical Center
Chicago, Illinois

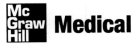 **Medical**

New York Chicago San Francisco Lisbon London Madrid
Mexico City Milan New Delhi San Juan Seoul
Singapore Sydney Toronto

Progressive Care Nursing Certification: Preparation, Review, and Practice Exams

2 3 4 5 6 7 8 9 0 QDB/QDB 15 14 13 12

Set ISBN 978-0-07-176144-4
Set MHID 0-07-176144-6
Book ISBN 978-0-07-176143-7
Book MHID 0-07-176143-8
CD ISBN 978-0-07-176142-0
CD MHID 0-07-176142-X

This book was set in New Baskerville by Glyph International.
The editors were Joseph Morita and Christie Naglieri.
The production supervisor was Catherine Saggese.
Project management was provided by Anupriya Tyagi, Glyph International.
Quad/Graphics was printer and binder.

This book is printed on acid-free paper.

Library of Congress Cataloging-in-Publication Data
Ahrens, Thomas S., author.
    Progressive care nursing certification : preparation, review, and practice exams / Thomas S. Ahrens, PhD, RN, CCNS, FAAN, Research Scientist, Barnes-Jewish Hospital, St. Louis, Missouri, Donna Prentice, RN, APRN, BC, PCCN, Clinical Nurse Specialist, Barnes-Jewish Hospital, St. Louis, Missouri, Ruth M. Kleinpell, PhD, RN, FAAN, FAANP, FCCM, Director, Center for Clinical Research and Scholarship, Rush University Medical Center, Professor, Rush University College of Nursing, Nurse Practitioner, Our Lady of the Resurrection Medical Center, Chicago, Illinois.
        p. ; cm.
    Includes bibliographical references and index.
    ISBN-13: 978-0-07-176144-4 (set)
    ISBN-10: 0-07-176144-6 (set)
    ISBN-13: 978-0-07-176143-7 (book : alk. paper)
    ISBN-10: 0-07-176143-8 (book : alk. paper) [etc.]
    1. Nursing—Examinations, questions, etc.   2. Progressive patient care—Examinations, questions, etc.   I. Prentice, Donna, author.   II. Kleinpell, Ruth M., author.   III. Title.
    [DNLM: 1. Nursing Care—Examination Questions.   2. Progressive Patient Care—Examination Questions.   WY 18.2]
    RT120.P76A37   2011
    610.73076—dc22
                                                                    2010050551

As always, to my ever-tolerant family. I have acquired a nickname of "Vapor" for my tendency to disappear from family events to go and work on projects like this book. Despite this tendency, I am still welcomed when I reappear. Amazing, but something I deeply appreciate. Also, to my new additions since the last book. Now, instead of just Gabriel (my little G man), I also have Sebastian and my darling little Mia. No matter the circumstances, they are always able to make me smile. I am blessed to have such a wonderful family.
Thomas S. Ahrens, PhD, RN, CCNS, FAAN

In loving memory of my dear friend Michael Hunt. I miss your thoughtful and challenging conversations, dry sense of humor, and listening ear. You were a blessing to me and my family that will be forever treasured. For Jesus Christ, the Son of God, who is the entirety of my belief system and my hope. Psalm 28:6-9
Donna Prentice, MSN(R), RN, ACNS-BC, CCRN

To Horace and Horace
Thanks for your ongoing support. My ability to work on projects such as this book is due in part to your understanding and continued encouragement for me to pursue my goals. Love, Ruth
Ruth M. Kleinpell, PhD, RN, FAAN, FAANP, FCCM

Contents

On CD-ROM:
COMPREHENSIVE PRACTICE EXAM—I
COMPREHENSIVE PRACTICE EXAM—II

Martha A. Q. Curley, RN, PhD, FAAN
Director of Critical Care and Cardiovascular
  Nursing Research
Children's Hospital Boston
Boston, Massachusetts

Sharon Manson, RN, MS, ACNP
Manager/Acute Care Nursing Practitioner
Hematology & Stem Cell Transplantation
Rush University Medical Center
Chicago, Illinois

Scott Micek, PharmD
Barnes–Jewish Hospital
St. Louis, Missouri

Lynn Schallom, RN, MSN, CCRN, CCNS
Clinical Nurse Specialist
Barnes–Jewish Hospital
St. Louis, Missouri

Barbara Swanson, PhD, RN, ACRN
Associate Professor
Rush University College of Nursing
Chicago, Illinois

Contributors

Patricia A. Ahrens, RN, TNCC
St. Mary's Health Center
St. Louis, Missouri
Chapter 47: Toxic Emergencies

Mary Kay Bader, RN, MSN, CCNS, FAHA
Neuro/Critical Care CNS
Stroke Fellow, American Heart Association
Mission Hospital
Mission Viejo, California
Chapter 30: Anatomy and Physiology of the Nervous System
Chapter 31: Intracranial Pressure
Chapter 32: Acute Head Injuries and Craniotomies
Chapter 33: Stroke
Chapter 34: The Vertebrae and Spinal Cord
Chapter 35: Encephalopathies and Coma
Chapter 36: Meningitis, Muscular Dystrophy, and Myasthenia Gravis Dystrophy, and Myasthenia Gravis
Chapter 37: Seizures and Status Epilepticus

Eli N. Deal, PharmD, BCPS
Clinical Pharmacist, Internal Medicine
Director, Pharmacotherapy Residency Program
Barnes–Jewish Hospital St. Louis, Missouri
Reviewed Medications for the Entire Book

Robin Gutman, PMHCNS, BS
Barnes–Jewish Hospital
St. Louis, Missouri
Chapter 51: Behavioral and Psychologic Factors in Critical Care

Alexander Johnson RN, MSN, ACNP-BC, CCNS, CCRN
Critical Care Clinical Nurse Specialist
BroMenn Regional Medical Center
Normal, Illinois
Chapter 1: Cardiovascular Anatomy and Physiology
Chapter 2: Diagnosis and Treatment of Cardiovascular Disorders
Chapter 3: The Normal ECG
Chapter 4: The 12-Lead ECG
Chapter 5: Hemodynamic Monitoring
Chapter 6: Acute Coronary Syndrome (Angina Pectoris and Myocardial Infarction)

Chapter 7: Conduction Blocks
Chapter 8: Congestive Heart Failure, Pulmonary Edema, and Hypertensive Crisis
Chapter 9: Cardiogenic Shock
Chapter 10: Hemorrhagic (Hypovolemic) Shock
Chapter 11: Interpreting Dysrhythmias
Chapter 12: Cardiomyopathies and Pericarditis
Chapter 13: Treatment of Cardiac, Valvular and Vascular Insufficiency and Trauma

Ann Petlin, RN, MSN, CCNS, CCRN-CSC, ACNS-BC, PCCN
Clinical Nurse Specialist, Cardiothoracic Surgery
Barnes–Jewish Hospital
St. Louis, Missouri
Reviewed Medications for the Entire Book

Lisa Riggs, RN, MSN, APRN-BC, CCRN
Clinical Nurse Specialist
Mid America Heart Institute of St. Luke's Hospital
Kansas City, Kansas
Chapter 6: Acute Coronary Syndrome (Angina Pectoris and Myocardial Infarction)
Chapter 8: Congestive Heart Failure, Pulmonary Edema, and Hypertensive Crisis

Sharon Ryback, RN, PMHCNS, BC
Barnes–Jewish Hospital
St. Louis, Missouri
Chapter 51: Behavioral and Psychologic Factors in Critical Care

Carrie Sona, RN, MSN, CCRN, CCNS
Clinical Nurse Specialist
Barnes–Jewish Hospital
St. Louis, Missouri
Chapter 49: Burns

Linda Nattkemper York, RN, PhD, PMHCNS, BC, CARN-AP
Barnes–Jewish Hospital
St. Louis, Missouri
Chapter 51: Behavioral and Psychologic Factors in Critical Care

Preface

For those of you taking the PCCN exam, congratulations and good luck. To help you learn the key concepts necessary to pass the exam, you will find the format we have used in the book is one of short, easy to read chapters. Following the PCCN blueprint, we hope these chapters increase your chance of being successful when taking the exam.

We have also placed two practice exams on the accompanying CD. Our goal is to allow you two practice attempts at the exam before taking the real test.

The PCCN exam attempts to reflect what you will see in your practice. While this reflection will vary depending on your clinical practice, the content is something you will generally see in your practice. This is an important point, as the best way to study for the exam is to use the information in this book in your clinical practice. Using the information in your clinical practice makes taking the exam easier, as you already know much of the information tested on the exam.

As always, good luck in taking the exam. Successfully passing the PCCN exam is a major professional event in your career. All the work necessary to pass the exam will seem trivial compared to the pride you will feel after successfully passing the exam.

Thomas S. Ahrens, PhD, RN, CCNS, FAAN
Donna Prentice, MSN(R), RN, ACNS-BC, CCRN
Ruth M. Kleinpell, PhD, RN, FAAN, FAANP, FCCM

Test-Taking Tips

The following are some general test-taking tips. Follow them as you prepare for the examinations in this text and on the PCCN examination. They can make the difference in several points on the examination.

1. Answer all questions. Unanswered questions are counted as incorrect.

2. Be well rested before the examination. Get a good night's sleep before the examination. Do not try to "cram" on the morning of the test: you may confuse yourself if you study right before the test.

3. Have a good but light breakfast. You will be taking the test for perhaps 4 hours. Eat food that is not all carbohydrates so that you can make it through the examination without becoming hungry or getting a headache.

4. Do not change answers unless you are absolutely sure. Many first impressions are accurate.

5. Go through the test and answer all questions. Mark on a piece of scrap paper the questions that are difficult. Then go back and review the difficult questions. Do not be discouraged if there are many hard questions.

6. Do not expect to answer all questions correctly. If you do not know the answer to a question, make a guess and go on. Do not let it bother you that you missed a few questions. You will not have a good perception of how you did until you get the results.

7. Do not let the fact that other people finish early (or that you finish before others) disturb you. People work at different rates without necessarily a difference in results.

8. If you feel thirsty or need to go to the restroom, ask permission from the monitor. Always try to maintain your physiologic status at optimal levels. An aspirin (or similar analgesic) may be in order if a headache develops during the test.

9. Do not try to establish patterns in how the items are written (for example, "Two B's have occurred, now some other choice is likely"). The AACN [K8]Certification Corporation has excellent test-writing mechanisms. Patterns in test answers, if they occur, are coincidental.

I

CARDIOVASCULAR

Thomas S. Ahrens

Cardiovascular Anatomy and Physiology

EDITORS' NOTE

Although basic anatomy is not commonly addressed in the Progressive Care Certified Nurse (PCCN) exam, an understanding of the principles of anatomy may help your perception of more specific questions regarding cardiovascular concepts. The following chapter is a brief review of key anatomic and physiologic cardiovascular concepts that should prove useful in preparing for the test. This chapter also addresses background information on cardiovascular concepts sometimes found on the PCCN exam. If you do not have a strong background in anatomy and physiology, study this section closely. You may want to review the cardiovascular sections of physiology textbooks as well.

The PCCN exam places most emphasis on the cardiovascular component, with approximately 20% of the test questions being in this content area. While many nurses are relatively strong in cardiovascular concepts, do not take this part of the exam lightly. The better you perform in any one area, the greater your chances of overall success on the exam.

NORMAL LOCATION AND SIZE OF THE HEART

The heart lies in the mediastinum, above the diaphragm, surrounded on both sides by the lungs. If one looks at a frontal (anterior) view, the heart resembles a triangle (Fig. 1-1). The base of the heart is parallel to the right edge of the sternum, whereas the lower right point of the triangle represents the apex of the heart. The apex is usually at the left midclavicular line at the fifth intercostal space. The average adult heart is about 5 in. long and $3^1/_2$ in. wide, which is about the size of an average man's clenched fist. The heart weighs about 2 g for each pound of ideal body weight.

NORMAL ANATOMY OF THE HEART

The heart is supported by a fibrous skeleton (Fig. 1-2) composed of dense connective tissue. This skeleton connects the four valve rings (annuli) of the heart: the tricuspid, mitral, pulmonic, and aortic valves. Attached to the superior (top) surface of this skeleton are the right and left atria, the pulmonary artery, and the aorta. Attached to the inferior (lower) surface of the skeleton are the right and left ventricles, and the mitral and tricuspid valve cusps.

The heart can be studied as two parallel pumps: the right pump (right atrium and ventricle) and the left pump (left atrium and ventricle). Each pump receives blood into its atrium. The blood flows from the atria through a one-way valve into the ventricles. From each ventricle, blood is ejected into a circulatory system. The right ventricle ejects blood into the pulmonary circulation, while the left ventricle ejects blood into the systemic circulation. Although there are differences between the right and left sides of the heart, the gross anatomy of each side is similar. Structural features of each chamber are discussed below.

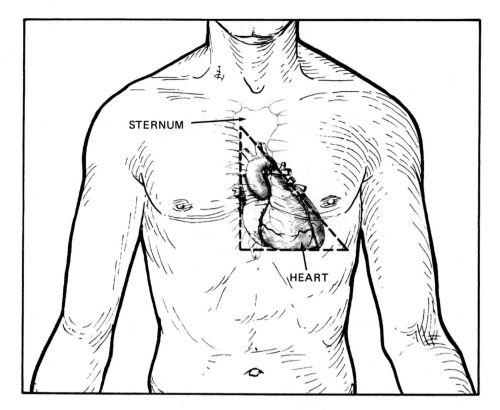

Figure 1-1. Frontal view of the heart.

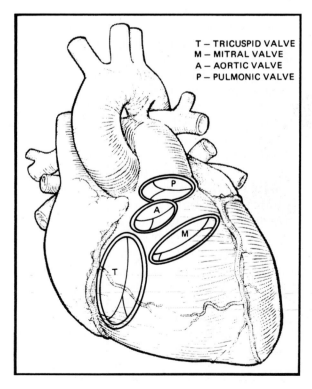

T – TRICUSPID VALVE
M – MITRAL VALVE
A – AORTIC VALVE
P – PULMONIC VALVE

Figure 1-2. Fibrous skeleton of the heart (frontal view).

STRUCTURE OF THE HEART WALL

The heart is enclosed in a fibrous sac called the pericardium. The pericardium is composed of two layers: the fibrous and parietal pericardia. The fibrous pericardium is the outer layer that helps support the heart. The parietal pericardium, the inside layer, is a smooth fibrous membrane.

Next to the parietal serous layer of the pericardium is a visceral layer, which is actually the outer heart surface. It is most often termed the epicardium. Between the epicardium and the parietal pericardium is 10 to 20 mL of fluid, which prevents friction during the heart's contraction and relaxation.

The myocardium, or muscle mass of the heart, is composed of cardiac muscle, which has characteristics of both smooth and skeletal muscles. The endocardium is the inner surface of the heart wall. It is a membranous covering that lines all of the heart's chambers and the valves.

Papillary muscles originate in the ventricular endocardium and attach to chordae tendineae (Fig. 1-3). The chordae tendineae attach to the inferior

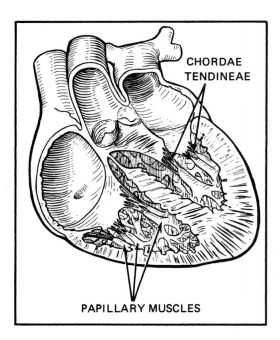

Figure 1-3. Papillary muscles and chordae tendineae.

surface of the tricuspid and mitral valve cusps, enabling the valves to open and close. The papillary muscles are in parallel alignment to the ventricular wall.

CARDIAC MUSCLE CELLS

The information in this section regarding cellular aspects of cardiac muscle anatomy and physiology is not likely to be on the PCCN exam. Questions about this area are rare. However, the concepts addressed in this section form the basis for understanding myocardial dysfunction and pharmacologic intervention. Read this section to become familiar with the concepts but not necessarily to memorize specific details.

The sarcomere (Fig. 1-4) is the contracting unit of the myocardium. The outer covering of the sarcomere is the sarcolemma, which surrounds the muscle fiber. The sarcolemma covers a muscle fiber that is composed of thick and thin fibers, which are often collectively called myofibrils. Sarcomeres are separated from each other by a thickening of the sarcolemma at the ends of the sarcomere. These thickened ends, called intercalated discs, are actively involved in cardiac contraction. Each sarcomere has a centrally placed nucleus surrounded by sarcoplasma.

The sarcolemma invaginates into the sarcomere at regular intervals, resulting in a vertical penetration through the muscle fibrils; thus it comes into

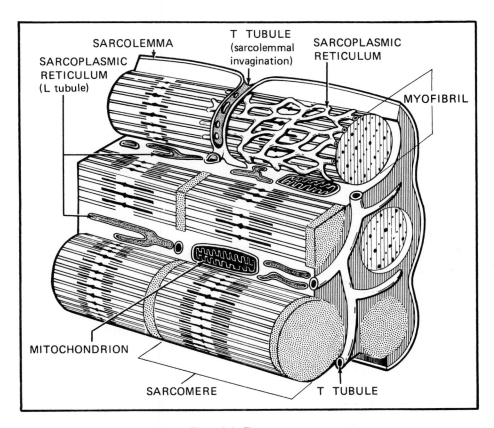

Figure 1-4. The sarcomere.

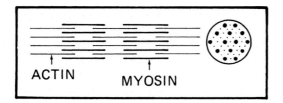

Figure 1-5. Arrangement of myosin and actin myofibrils.

contact with both the thick and thin fibrils. These invaginations form the T tubules. Closely related to but not continuous with the T-tubule system is the sarcoplasmic reticulum. The sarcoplasmic reticulum (containing calcium ions) is an intracellular network of channels surrounding the myofibrils. These channels comprise the longitudinal (L-tubule) system of the myofibrils.

Myofibrils are thick and thin parts of the muscle fiber. Thick fibrils are myosin filaments. They have regularly placed projections that form calcium gates to the thick myofibrils. The thin myofibrils are actin. The myosin and actin myofibrils are arranged in specific parallel and hexagonal patterns (Fig. 1-5). This arrangement of fibers forms a syncytium that causes all of the fibers to depolarize when even one fiber is depolarized. This is known as the "all or none" principle—all fibers depolarize or no fibers depolarize. Troponin and tropomyosin are regulatory proteins attached to or affecting actin. These thick and thin myofibrils slide back and forth over each other, resulting in contraction and relaxation of the sarcomeres and, thus, causing the heart to contract and relax.

The study of the cardiac cycle's physiology examines the means by which the heart pumps blood and the various mechanisms that control the heart pump. Before looking at the heart as a whole, let us examine the contraction of a single sarcomere.

Contraction of the Sarcomere

The sarcomeres are much like striated muscles, but they have more mitochondria than striated or smooth muscles. The mitochondria provide the energy that sarcomeres need to contract. This energy is released by converting adenosine triphosphate (ATP) into adenosine diphosphate (ADP). In addition, the mitochondria are crucial in the storing of energy through the formation of ATP from ADP. The adding of a phosphate molecule to ADP to form ATP is called phosphorylation. This formation of ADP from ATP normally takes place in the presence of oxygen (aerobic metabolism) and is referred to as oxidative phosphorylation. Energy can be produced without oxygen (anaerobic metabolism), but not as efficiently as during aerobic metabolism. Cardiac muscle cells are highly dependent on constant blood flow to maintain adequate supplies of oxygen for the formation of ATP.

In the sarcomere, thick (myosin) and thin (actin) fibrils are arranged side by side in parallel rows. The myosin fibrils have projections that make contact with actin at specific points. These contact points are referred to as calcium gates (Fig. 1-6). During cardiac contraction, the myosin and actin

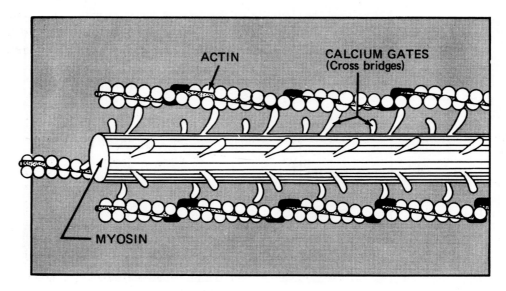

Figure 1-6. Myosin and actin fibrils with calcium gates.

slide together and overlap to as great an extent as possible (Fig. 1-7). (In the normal resting state, there is some overlapping of the myosin and actin fibrils.) Troponin and tropomyosin are protein rods interwoven around the actin fibril, having a regulatory effect upon the actin and its ability to connect with the calcium gates in the presence of calcium ions.

At the start of cellular excitation leading to a contraction, calcium ions (Ca^{2+}) attach to troponin molecules around the actin fibril. This enables the projections (calcium gates) of the myosin fibril to attach to the actin. These projections twist around, causing a sliding of the fibers over each other. The calcium is removed from the calcium gates by calcium pumps located throughout the sarcoplasmic reticulum. As soon as the calcium is removed, the myosin and actin fibers slide back to their original positions. This process is repeated, causing the cardiac cell to contract and relax.

It is important to remember that calcium initiates and regulates the sarcomere's depolarization and repolarization. The role of calcium in the contraction and relaxation of the cardiac muscle cell serves as the basis for several cardiac therapies, including the use of calcium channel blocking agents and the potential inotropic (strength) value in administering calcium. Even though calcium ions initiate the sliding movement of the fibrils, calcium alone is not able to cause the contraction. In addition to the presence of calcium, an exchange of ions (creating electrical energy) must occur during phases of depolarization and repolarization. This ionic exchange is mainly between sodium and potassium, and creates an ionic action potential. The exchange of chemical elements occurs across the semipermeable cell membrane in three ways: filtration, osmosis, and diffusion (active or passive).

Action Potential of the Cardiac Cell

There are five phases of activity during the cardiac cell cycle; each phase is described below. The exchange and concentration of ions differ in each phase. Mainly four ions are involved: sodium (Na^+), potassium (K^+), calcium (Ca^{2+}), and chloride (Cl^-). Normally, there is more sodium, calcium, and chloride outside the cell and more potassium inside it. Since all ions have an electrical charge, an electrical gradient is established. When a state of ionic electrical neutrality exists, the cell membrane is relatively impermeable—a period known as the resting potential. The presence of an electrical and chemical (ion) gradient plus membrane selectively establishes an action potential consisting of five phases: 0 through 4.

Phase 0

As a result of the presence of sodium and potassium outside and inside the cell, respectively, there is an electronegative gradient. A depolarizing stimulus is caused by efflux of potassium from the cell, increasing the cell permeability for sodium. Calcium ions in the T- and L-tubule systems of the sarcomere are at Ca^{2+} gates on the cell membrane and "open" the gates for the influx of sodium. When this gradient reaches about −90 mV inside the cell, there is a rapid increase of the action potential (zero in Fig. 1-8). The result of the depolarization stimulus is an increase in the cell's permeability to sodium. As the sodium threshold (the point at which sodium moves most freely) is reached (about −55 mV), sodium rushes into the cell and depolarizes it. Actually, more sodium rushes in than the amount required to reach electrical neutrality (zero). The cell becomes electropositive at about +20 to +30 mV, causing a spike on the action potential diagram.

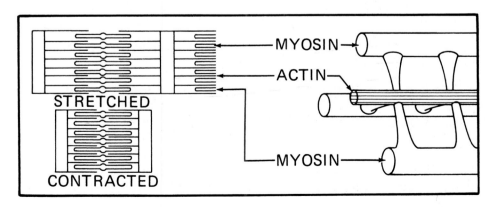

Figure 1-7. Contraction of the myosin and actin fibrils.

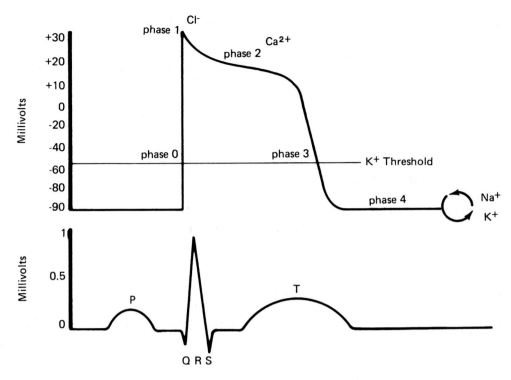

Figure 1-8. Phases of the cardiac potential and ion movement correlated with the ECG tracing.

Phase 1

This is the spike phase of positive electrical charge. There is a brief period of rapid repolarization (tip of spike to phase 1 in Fig. 1-8), which is probably due to a flow of chloride ions into the cell.

Phase 2

This is a plateau phase of repolarization. Calcium entering the cell and potassium leaving the cell balance each other, so there is no net electrical change; thus a flat line (plateau) appears. Sodium entry into the cell is almost completely inactivated. A slow movement on calcium into the cell begins (phase 2 in Fig. 1-8). Also, a small amount of potassium begins leaving the cell at this point.

Phase 3

This is a rapid decline phase of repolarization (phase 3 in Fig. 1-8). Potassium loss from the cell is greatest in this phase. This potassium loss returns the cell to electronegativity. Sodium and calcium currents are completely inactivated.

Phase 4

This is the resting interval between action potentials (phase 4 in Fig. 1-8). The sodium/potassium pumps (diffusely spread throughout the sarcomere) are the most active here in effecting an exchange of position of potassium for sodium across the cell membrane. Potassium continues to leave the cell, and when electronegativity reaches -90 mV, phase 0 starts again if a stimulus occurs.

HEART CHAMBERS

There are four chambers in the heart (Fig. 1-9). The atria are superior to the ventricles and are separated from the ventricles by valves. The right atrium and ventricle are separated from the left atrium and ventricle by the atrial and ventricular septa.

Right Atrium

The right atrium is a thin-walled chamber exposed to low blood pressures. Systemic venous blood from the head, neck, and thorax enters the right atrium from the superior vena cava. Systemic venous blood from the remainder of the body enters from the inferior vena cava. Venous blood from the heart enters the right atrium through the thebesian veins, which drain into the coronary sinus. The coronary sinus is located on the medial right atrial wall just about the tricuspid valve.

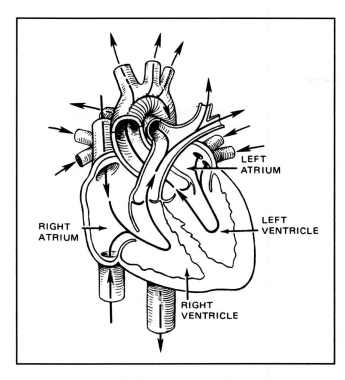

Figure 1-9. The four chambers of the heart.

Right Ventricle

The right ventricle is the pump for the right heart. The right ventricle contracts to pump venous blood into the pulmonary artery and to the lungs. The lungs are normally a low-pressure system. The right ventricle is shaped and functions like a bellows to propel blood out during contraction.

Left Atrium

The left atrium, just like the right one, is thin-walled. Blood flowing passively from the low–lung pressure area does not stress the walls of the left atrium. The left atrium receives oxygenated blood from the four pulmonary veins.

Left Ventricle

The left ventricle is the major pump for the entire body. As such, it must have thick, strong walls. To overcome the high pressure of the systemic circulation, the left ventricle is shaped like a cylinder. As it contracts (starting from the apex), it also narrows somewhat. This cylindrical shape provides a physical force strong enough to propel blood into the aorta and to overcome the high systemic pressure (resulting from the requirement to pump the blood to distant body areas).

HEART VALVES

There are two types of valves in the heart: the atrioventricular and the semilunar valves. All valves in the heart are unidirectional unless they are diseased or dysfunctional. Normally, the valves provide very little resistance to cardiac contractions. If the valves become narrow (stenotic) or allow blood to flow past when they should be closed (regurgitation), the work of the heart will substantially increase.

Atrioventricular Valves

The atrioventricular (AV) valves of the heart are the tricuspid and the mitral valves. These allow blood to flow from the atria into the ventricles during atrial contraction and ventricular diastole. Mnemonics may help you remember which valve is on which side of the heart. Consider the following: "L" and "M" come together in the alphabet and in the heart. The left heart contains the mitral valve. Likewise, "R" and "T" are close in the alphabet. The right heart contains the tricuspid valve. Both the mitral and the tricuspid valves have two large opposing leaflets and small intermediary leaflets at each end.

Mitral Valve

The mitral valve's two large leaflets are not quite equal in size (Fig. 1-10). The chordae tendineae from adjacent leaflets are inserted on the same papillary muscles. This physical feature helps to ensure complete closure of the valve. When the mitral valve is open, the valve, chordae tendineae, and papillary

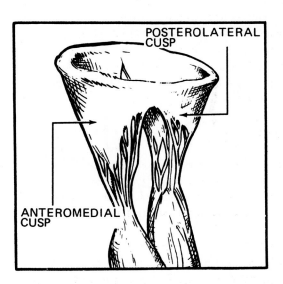

Figure 1-10. Side view of the mitral valve.

muscle look like a funnel. Of all the valves, the mitral is most commonly involved in clinical conditions of valvular dysfunction. Mitral regurgitation is the most common clinical valvular disturbance. Clinically, mitral regurgitation may be insignificant (subclinical) or represent a life-threatening situation (papillary muscle rupture). The key factor influencing the significance of any valvular disturbance is the effect on stroke volume (amount of blood the heart pumps with each contraction).

Tricuspid Valve

The tricuspid valve differs from the mitral valve in that it has three leaflets, and it has three papillary muscles instead of two. Otherwise, the structures and functions of the two valves are similar. Tricuspid dysfunction is not as much of a clinical problem as is mitral dysfunction.

Semilunar (Pulmonic and Aortic) Valves

The semilunar valves (Fig. 1-11) of the heart are the aortic and pulmonary valves. Each has three symmetrical valve cusps to provide for complete opening without stretching the valve. The pulmonary valve is located between the right ventricle and the pulmonary artery. The aortic valve is located between the left ventricle and the aorta.

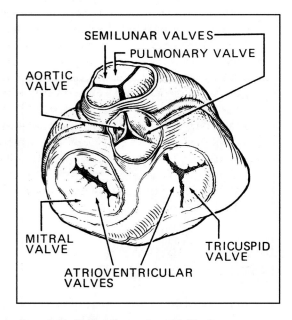

Figure 1-11. The semilunar valves and AV valves (posterior view).

Pulmonary valve dysfunction will potentially affect the performance of the right ventricle. Aortic valve disturbance can affect the performance of the left ventricle.

Physical Assessment of the Cardiac Valves

Cardiac valves can be assessed to some extent through auscultation. Heart sounds can be identified partially based on specific valve functioning. The heart normally generates two sounds; referred to as S_1 and S_2. S_1 is the sound generated through the closure of the mitral (M_1) and tricuspid (T_1) valves. M_1 is best heard at the fifth intercostal space (ICS) in the left midclavicular line. T_1 is best heard at the fourth ICS at the left sternal border. S_1 is produced during ventricular contraction. S_1 can be identified by listening (it normally is the loudest of the two cardiac sounds at the fourth ICS, left sternal border or the fifth ICS, left midclavicular line) or by comparing the sounds to the electrocardiogram (ECG). The S_1 sound occurs immediately after the QRS complex (which indicates ventricular depolarization and contraction).

S_2 is produced by the closure of the aortic (A_2) and pulmonic (P_2) valves. A_2 is best heard at the second ICS, just to the right of the sternum. The P_2 sound is heard best at the second ICS, just to the left of the sternum. S_2 can also be identified by listening (it is loudest in the locations described above) or by comparing it to the ECG. Normally, the S_2 sound occurs during diastole (when aortic and pulmonary blood pressures are higher than ventricular pressures, forcing the aortic and pulmonary valves to close). The S_2 sound normally appears during the T wave or slightly before the QRS complex.

Abnormal Heart Sounds

Heart valves normally produce sound during closure. There are four common abnormal situations when other sounds might develop. These are valve regurgitation, valvular stenosis, ventricular or atrial failure, and disturbances of electrical conduction.

Valve Regurgitation. When a valve becomes regurgitant (sometimes referred to as insufficient), blood flows past the valve, which is normally closed. This produces a sound usually described as a murmur. Murmurs may be described in several ways, such as blowing and swishing. Murmurs are graded in degree from I to VI. A grade I murmur (written as I/VI) is a very soft sound. A grade VI murmur (written as VI/VI) is so prominent that it can be heard with the stethoscope held about 1 in. from the chest wall. The other grades of murmurs are subjectively described as between I and VI. It is frequently up to the clinician to grade a murmur since there are no clear objective criteria for doing this.

Mitral and tricuspid regurgitation will produce a murmur that occurs during systole (normally the mitral and tricuspid valves close during systole). Aortic and pulmonic regurgitation will produce a diastolic murmur.

Valvular Stenosis. A stenosis of a valve produces a murmur that may sound like a regurgitant murmur. However, the reasons for the murmur are different. A mitral or tricuspid stenosis produces a murmur during diastole (normally atrial contraction does not meet resistance to pushing blood past the mitral or tricuspid valve). An aortic or pulmonic stenosis can produce a systolic murmur. Valves can be dysfunctional in isolation (such as a mitral regurgitation) or in multiples. The clinician attempts to identify the cause of the murmur through auscultation and clinical history.

Ventricular or Atrial Failure. During ventricular failure, an increased pressure builds in the ventricles and atrium. After systole, when blood enters the ventricles from the atrium, the high atrial pressure may force blood into the ventricles with considerable force. This increased flow of blood into the ventricles may produce a sound: the S_3 sound. The S_3 sound occurs immediately after the S_2 sound and can be found after the T wave on the ECG. S_3 sounds are not always abnormal but should be considered significant, particularly in the presence of tachycardia. The combination of a tachycardia and S_3 produces a characteristic "gallop" sound associated with left ventricular (congestive heart) failure.

Another sound associated with high pressures is the S_4. It is thought to be an atrial sound associated with high atrial pressures. It can be found immediately before the QRS complex and after the P wave when compared with an ECG tracing.

Electrical Conduction Defects. When there is an electrical conduction defect, such as a bundle branch block, the potential exists for the valves to fail to function in unison. When this happens, a split in the heart sound will occur. For example, a right bundle branch block causes a delay in right ventricular contraction. The result is that the pulmonic valve closes slightly after the aortic valve. The S_2 sound now becomes softer and produces two sounds instead of one. The S_2 can aid in the diagnosis of a right bundle branch block.

Pulsus Paradoxus and Change in Heart Sounds

Heart sounds can be diminished in intensity if air (as in chronic obstructive pulmonary disease) or fluid (pericardial effusion or tamponade) is between the heart and the stethoscope. In tamponade, fluid fills the pericardial sac and limits sound transmission. In addition, the increased fluid restricts ventricular expansion and can dangerously drop the cardiac output. If tamponade occurs, the inability of the ventricle to distend will produce diminished heart sounds, equalizing chamber pressures (e.g., central venous [right atrial] and pulmonary capillary "wedge" [left ventricular end-diastolic] pressures begin to equalize), venous distention develops, and pulsus paradoxus may occur. Pulsus paradoxus is the decrease of blood pressure during inspiration. A decrease in systolic blood pressure during inspiration of more than 10 mm Hg is characteristic of pulsus paradoxus. The blood pressure decreases because of the increase in blood entering the atrium during inspiration, further increasing the pericardial pressure. The added pericardial pressure further decreases stroke volume and systolic blood pressure.

Heart sounds can be useful clinical parameters, but a clinician requires frequent practice in order to become proficient in recognizing them. More accurate tests are replacing the clinical use of heart sounds. If valve dysfunction is thought to exist, echocardiography is the test of choice. If conduction defects exist, electrocardiography is more accurate than echocardiography in detecting abnormalities. For the purpose of the PCCN test, the basic information provided above will help to identify the essential information. Be prepared for questions in which a heart sound is given and you must then identify a clinical condition. However, be aware of the more accurate methods for assessing cardiac function, as they may also be addressed on the test.

NORMAL CONDUCTION SYSTEM OF THE HEART

The conduction of an electrical impulse normally follows an orderly, repetitive pattern from the right atrium, through the ventricles, and into the

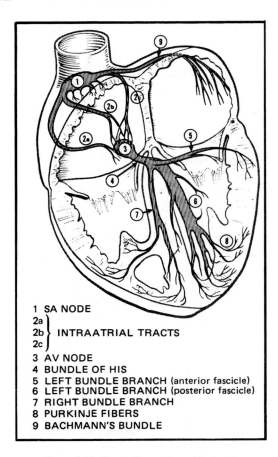

1 SA NODE
2a ⎫
2b ⎬ INTRAATRIAL TRACTS
2c ⎭
3 AV NODE
4 BUNDLE OF HIS
5 LEFT BUNDLE BRANCH (anterior fascicle)
6 LEFT BUNDLE BRANCH (posterior fascicle)
7 RIGHT BUNDLE BRANCH
8 PURKINJE FIBERS
9 BACHMANN'S BUNDLE

Figure 1-12. Conduction system of the heart.

myocardium, where the impulse usually results in ventricular contraction (Fig. 1-12).

The sinoatrial (SA) node is at the junction of the superior vena cava and the right atrium. The SA node is a group of specialized heart cells that are self-excitatory. All self-excitatory cells have automaticity; that is, if the cells can excite themselves, they require no stimulus and may excite themselves at will. This is termed inherent automaticity or spontaneous depolarization. The SA node excites itself faster than any other cardiac cells under normal conditions. For this reason, the SA node becomes the heart's normal pacemaker. Once the impulse originates in the SA node, it spreads through the atria along three paths, called internodal tracts. The impulse continues from the internodal tracts into the AV junction. The AV node is located at the superior end of the junctional tissue, near the tricuspid valve ring just above the ventricular septum. There is a slight pause in the impulse at the upper portion of the AV node to allow for completion of atrial contraction. The impulse traverses the AV node and the junctional tissue, and then reaches the bundle of His. The bundle of His

carries the impulse to the bundle branches. The bundle of His divides into right and left bundle branches.

The left bundle branch continues along the ventricular septum, dividing into two subdivisions called fascicles. The anterior fascicle excites the anterior and superior surfaces of the left ventricle. The posterior fascicle excites the posterior and inferior surfaces of the left ventricle. The right bundle branch continues as a single branch to innervate the right ventricle. Having passed through the bundle of His and the bundle branches, the impulse arrives at the Purkinje's fibers, which spread into the ventricular myocardium. The impulse spread is usually followed by ventricular contraction, and thus the cycle is repeated.

Disturbances in this conduction system are reviewed as to the specific resulting dysrhythmias. The current PCCN format requires a good understanding of the electrical system of the heart and the ability to interpret dysrhythmias and 12-lead ECGs. Whereas specific sections are provided on dysrhythmias and 12-lead analysis, it is important to understand the basic anatomy and physiology of the electrical conduction system.

CIRCULATORY SYSTEMS OF THE BODY

Circulatory paths can be remembered by the mnemonic, "a" for *artery* means "a" for *away*. All arteries carry blood, either oxygenated or deoxygenated (pulmonary), away from the heart. Conversely, all veins carry blood, either oxygenated or deoxygenated, to the heart.

There are two circulatory systems in the body, the pulmonary and the systemic. The heart must pump blood through these two systems in the amount needed by the body to maintain optimal function. In addition, the coronary circulation (a branch of the systemic circulation), the pulmonary circulation, and the systemic circulation have some features that are helpful to note for the purpose of the PCCN exam.

Pulmonary Circulation

The pulmonary system is unique in that it is the only system (excluding the fetal) in which the pulmonary artery carries unoxygenated blood away from the heart to the lungs, and the four pulmonary veins carry oxygenated blood from the lungs to the left atrium. The right ventricle sends venous blood into the main pulmonary artery, which divides into the right and left pulmonary arteries. These arteries follow the normal blood vessel path; that is, arteries to arterioles to capillaries (where the blood becomes oxygenated) to venules to veins.

Systemic Circulation

The aorta is the only artery into which the left ventricle normally ejects blood; it arches over the pulmonary artery. The aorta gives off many branches as it traverses down the body to bifurcate into the iliac arteries. In the capillaries, the blood surrenders oxygen and picks up carbon dioxide. The inferior and superior venae cavae are the final veins returning blood to the right atrium.

Coronary Circulation

The coronary circulatory system begins with the inflow of oxygenated blood into the coronary arteries. The openings of these arteries are located near the cusps of the aortic valve. These arteries fill during ventricular diastole.

The right coronary artery supplies the posterior and inferior myocardia with oxygenated blood. The left coronary artery starts at the valve cusp as the left main coronary artery and bifurcates to form the left anterior descending (LAD) and the circumflex arteries. The LAD artery supplies the anterior and septal myocardium. The circumflex artery supplies the lateral myocardium. These arteries then follow the normal sequence of becoming arterioles, capillaries, venules, and veins as they course through the myocardium. The veins empty into thebesian veins, which in turn empty into the coronary sinus. Blood from the coronary sinus joins the venous blood in the right atrium.

Autonomic Regulation of Peripheral Vessels

The sympathetic nervous system has an adrenergic effect on peripheral vessels. The norepinephrine released by the sympathetic system causes vasoconstriction. This vasoconstriction prevents pooling of blood in the peripheral vessels and augments the return of blood to the heart.

The parasympathetic nervous system has a cholinergic effect upon peripheral vessels. Acetylcholine is released by the parasympathetic nervous system. This causes a vasodilatation of peripheral vessels. With dilation, more blood can remain in the peripheral vessels, and less blood is returned to the heart.

Baroreceptor Control

Baroreceptors are also called pressoreceptors or stretch receptors since these areas respond to a stretching of arterial and venous vessel walls. These receptors are specialized cells located in the aortic arch, carotid sinus, atria, venae cavae, and pulmonary arteries. These receptor sites are responsive to mean arterial pressure greater than 60 mm Hg. When stimulated by an elevated pressure, these receptors send signals to the medulla oblongata in the brain. The medulla then inhibits sympathetic nervous system activity, which allows the vagus nerve of the parasympathetic nervous system to assume control. This results in vasodilatation of peripheral vessels and a decreased heart rate. Under normal circumstances, this will allow the blood pressure to return to normal.

Conversely, if pressure is low, vagal tone is decreased, which allows the sympathetic nervous system to assume control. This results in vasoconstriction of the peripheral vessels and an increased heart rate. Under normal circumstances, this will allow the blood pressure to return to normal.

Vasomotor Center of Regulation

There are two areas of vasomotor control in the medulla oblongata: a vasoconstrictor area and a vasodilator area. The vasomotor center responds to baroreceptors and chemoreceptors in the aortic arch and carotid sinus.

If the vasoconstrictor area is stimulated, normally an increased heart rate, stroke volume, and cardiac output will result because of peripheral vasoconstriction. As the peripheral vessels constrict, more blood is forced from these vessels and returned to the heart. This normally restores arterial blood pressure.

If the vasodilator area is stimulated (by inhibition of the vasoconstrictor area), a decrease in stroke volume and cardiac output will normally occur. The vasodilatation allows for more blood to remain in peripheral vessels; therefore less blood is returned to the heart. The normal end result will be a decrease in blood pressure. This partially explains the bradycardia seen in patients who are hypertensive.

Chemoreceptors are activated by decreased oxygen pressures, an increased carbon dioxide level, and/or a decreased pH. Once activated, the chemoreceptors stimulate the vasoconstrictor area. The events that normally occur with such stimulation are then set into action.

HEART RATE

The other regulator of cardiac output, heart rate, can be used as a guide to therapy and assessment. The heart rate is regulated by the autonomic nervous system through sympathetic (adrenergic) and parasympathetic (cholinergic) mechanisms. Sympathetic regulation occurs through alpha and beta receptors located in the cardiovascular system. There are two types of alpha and beta cells: alpha$_1$ and alpha$_2$, and beta$_1$ and beta$_2$. Parasympathetic effect is primarily through the vagus nerve.

When a bradycardia exists, treatment is based on the factors that control the heart rate. For example, parasympathetic stimulation has a stronger effect on the heart than does sympathetic stimulation. The stronger parasympathetic effect is the reason atropine is the first drug given to treat a bradycardia.

The heart rate is a valuable diagnostic tool in that it is the first compensatory response to a decrease in stroke volume. A sinus tachycardia frequently heralds a decrease in stroke volume. The other reason an increase in the heart rate may occur is an increase in metabolic rate. This requires an increase in cardiac output, which is generally met by increasing both heart rate and stroke volume.

Heart rate elevations—for example, sinus tachycardia—by themselves are not generally dangerous. Although the increase in heart rate will increase myocardial oxygen consumption (MVo$_2$), the reason for the development of the tachycardia is more important. A clinical clue to investigate is the origin of a sinus tachycardia, followed by treating the cause of the tachycardia rather than the tachycardia itself.

RELATIONSHIP OF BLOOD FLOW AND PRESSURE IN THE CARDIAC CYCLE

The pressure of a fluid in a chamber depends on the size of the chamber, the amount of fluid, the distensibility of the chamber, and whether the chamber is open or closed.

The atria (both right and left) are open chambers. The venae cavae in the right atrium and the pulmonary veins in the left atrium are always open.

Thus, pressures in these chambers will remain low unless something occludes the openings or prevents them from emptying.

The anatomic structure of the right ventricle contributes to its low pressure. The right ventricle normally empties into a low-pressure system, the lungs.

The left ventricle has a high pressure. Its anatomic structure contributes to the high pressure. It empties into a high-pressure, closed system, the aorta. Trace the flow of blood through the chambers and examine its relationship to the cardiac valves and the chamber pressures. These relationships are shown in Fig. 1-13.

Atrial Pressure Curve

Throughout diastole, pressure slowly increases in the atria because of the influx of blood. The volume of blood increases in relation to the chamber size (resulting in a V wave on the atrial waveform). With atrial contraction (first curve on the atrial line in Fig. 1-13), there is a sudden increase in pressure (producing an A wave in the atrial waveform) since the contraction decreases the size of the atrium. During atrial contraction, pressure is greater in the atrium than in the ventricle. This higher pressure causes the AV valves to open. Atrial blood flows through the open AV valves into the ventricles.

As the ventricles begin the systolic phase, pressure in the ventricles increases, resulting in closure of the AV valves. The increase in ventricular pressure is so sudden that the AV valves bulge into the atria,

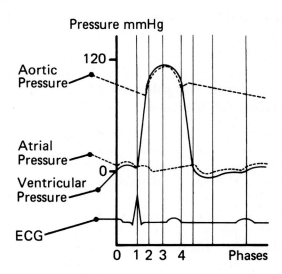

Figure 1-13. Blood flow and pressure during the cardiac cycle.

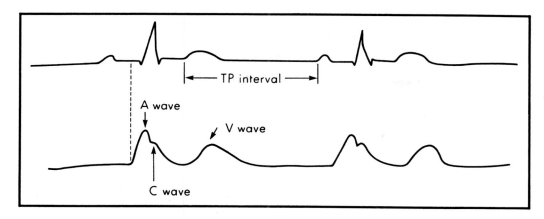

Figure 1-14. Normal atrial waveforms.

increasing the intra-atrial pressure (second curve on atrial pressure wave in Fig. 1-13). Following this second curve, there is a sharp fall in atrial pressure. Gradually, the atrial pressure rises again during the next period of diastole, and the cycle is repeated.

The normal atrial pressures generate three waves: A, C, and V (Fig. 1-14). The A wave is the result of atrial contraction and can be found in the PR interval. The importance of the A wave is that the mean of the A wave is the parameter used to estimate the central venous pressure (CVP).

The C wave is due to closure of the tricuspid and mitral valves. The V wave is due to atrial filling and the bulging of the tricuspid and mitral valves into the atrium. Large V waves can develop with noncompliant atria and mitral or tricuspid regurgitation.

Ventricular Pressure Curve

During diastole, the ventricular pressure is less than the atrial pressure. Just before atrial systole occurs, the AV valves open and blood flows into the ventricles. As soon as the ventricles fill, the blood flow reverses and closes the AV valves. At this point, the ventricles become closed chambers. The ventricle walls contract against the volume of blood in the ventricle. Since the ventricle is a closed chamber, pressure rises rapidly. Aortic pressure during diastole falls to about 80 mm Hg. The period during which ventricular pressure builds from near zero to 80 mm Hg is termed the isometric contraction phase (ventricle curve between lines 1 and 2 in Fig. 1-13). The left ventricle continues to contract strongly, and the pressure rises to about 110 mm Hg. Since left ventricular pressure exceeds the aortic pressure of 80 mm Hg, the aortic valve is forced open, and blood is ejected into the aorta. These same mechanisms occur concurrently in the right ventricle, only under much lower pressures. This is called the rapid ejection phase (ventricle curve between lines 2 and 3 in Fig. 1-13). Pressure begins to drop in the ventricle because blood is being ejected faster than the ventricle is contracting. This is called the reduced ejection phase (ventricular curve between lines 3 and 4 in Fig. 1-13). Ventricular contraction ceases, and the ventricle relaxes. Since the ventricular pressure has dropped rapidly, the blood flow starts to reverse at about 80 mm Hg in the aorta. This backward flow closes the aortic valve. The ventricle again becomes a closed chamber, but since no blood is entering, the pressure does not rise. The pressure in the ventricle continues to fall until it is less than the atrial pressure. Then the cycle begins again.

2

Diagnosis and Treatment of Cardiovascular Disorders

INVASIVE AND NONINVASIVE DIAGNOSTIC TESTS

EDITORS' NOTE

There is no section specifically on testing in the Progressive Care Certified Nurse (PCCN) exam. However, several questions, either directly or indirectly, address cardiovascular assessment via diagnostic tests. In this short section, cardiac diagnostic tests are categorized according to what they do and when they are indicated. Depending on the importance of the test, they will also be covered in chapters on specific cardiac conditions later in this book. This section should help you familiarize yourself with the tests that may be on the exam.

Cardiac Isoenzyme and Protein Level

Following trauma or hypoxia, enzymes and proteins leak from damaged cells. These isoenzymes and proteins are used in the identification of myocardial injury, most commonly myocardial infarction (MI). Any myocardial injury, however—including that due to cardiopulmonary resuscitation, cardiac contusion, and cardiac surgery—will elevate cardiac enzymes and proteins. Some tests are better than others at avoiding confounding factors. The most common cardiac enzymes and proteins are listed in Table 2-1.

Electrocardiography

The electrocardiogram (ECG) is the most commonly used noninvasive diagnostic test for patients with known or suspected cardiac disease. The ECG is a graphic tracing of the electrical forces produced by the heart. A 12-lead ECG provides information beyond the bedside monitor. The bedside monitor is primarily used to assess heart rate, rhythm, and life-threatening dysrhythmias. The 12-lead ECG provides more information in terms of myocardial injury and ischemia, conduction disturbances, axis orientation, and heart size.

It is important to note that, although the ECG's simplicity makes it very useful, it is of limited accuracy and should be used in conjunction with other information, such as physical assessment and laboratory tests. The ECG is not simple to interpret despite its simplicity of use. Many factors alter the ECG's appearance and many of these factors are not clinically significant. However, it is essential for the progressive care nurse to be able to identify important changes on the ECG since many times it is the bedside nurse who is responsible for interpreting the ECG.

Echocardiography

Echocardiography (echo) is excellent at identifying structural changes in the heart. Echocardiography uses pulses of reflected ultrasound to evaluate cardiac structure and function. There are different types of echocardiography, including two-dimensional and transesophageal techniques. Transesophageal echocardiography is more specific but requires the patient to swallow a device resembling a nasogastric tube.

TABLE 2-1. COMMON CARDIAC ENZYME AND PROTEIN DETERMINATIONS USED IN DIAGNOSING CARDIAC INJURY

Cardiac Test	Purpose
Creatine phosphokinase (CPK)	Nonspecific muscle enzyme found in muscle and heart tissue. Some studies have indicated that the greater the rise in the CPK, the greater the damage to the heart. This test is less useful when muscle damage is also present.
CPK-MB	A more specific cardiac muscle enzyme. The most common test used in diagnosing myocardial injury. Highly specific for cardiac injury, although it can also rise with muscle damage.
Lactic dehydrogenase (LDH)	A nonspecific muscle enzyme whose chief value in cardiac diagnostics is its slow rise and persistent elevation. It is used to detect MIs that may be more than 24-h old.
Subforms of CPK-MB	Cardiac isoenzyme subforms ($CPK\text{-}MB_1$ and $CPK\text{-}MB_2$) may be the fastest changing of myocardial enzymes. Evidence exists that MIs can be identified within 2 h of occurrence if these forms are measured and the short-lived $CPK\text{-}MB_2$ is found to exceed $CPK\text{-}MB_1$ ($CPK\text{-}MB_2 > CPK\text{-}MB_1$)
Troponin I	A very specific cardiac muscle protein, one of the first of a new generation of diagnostic tests for cardiac assessment. It rises rapidly, like CPK-MB, but stays elevated for about 8 days.
Myoglobin	A very specific cardiac muscle protein which elevates and returns to normal rapidly. May be useful in rapid detection, with a higher precision than before, of myocardial injury.

MI, myocardial infarction.

Echocardiography can detect valve disturbances, septal defects, the presence of pericardial fluid, and abnormalities of ventricular muscle movement. In conditions such as MI and cardiac contusion, it can detect what part of the heart is damaged by noting dysfunctional movement in the muscle of the heart. It is an essential aspect of identifying disturbances in physical properties of the heart. Since it is noninvasive, many cardiologists consider it one of the diagnostic tests of choice.

Radionuclide Imaging

Radionuclide imaging detects pathologic cardiac conditions through the external detection of photons emitted from the body after the administration of radioisotopes. This is useful in detecting abnormalities in left ventricular wall motion as well as ventricular size, volume, and ejection fraction. Radionuclide imaging is increasingly used to detect disturbances in cell function and blood flow.

The thallium scan is a radionuclide imaging technique used to evaluate regional myocardial perfusion and viability. Thallium scans can be performed with the patient at rest or during exercise. For those patients unable to exercise, dobutamine and dipyridamole thallium scanning are used to increase coronary blood flow in place of exercise.

Positron emission tomography (PET) is a sophisticated imaging technique that measures specific radioisotopes injected into the body via the blood. PET scans may be used to determine the exact part of the heart that is threatened by a loss of oxygen. It is capable of distinguishing dysfunctional but viable myocardium from areas of infarction.

Cardiac Catheterization

Cardiac catheterization involves the insertion of catheters into cardiac chambers and blood vessels to measure intracardiac pressures, oxygen saturation, and coronary blood flow. Angiography, a part of the cardiac catheterization procedure, is used specifically to examine the blood vessels by injecting measurable contrast material. Coronary angiography generally involves the injection of a radiopaque contrast medium into the chambers of the heart, coronary arteries, and great vessels. The passage of the contrast dye is followed and filmed as the heart beats spontaneously. The moving pictures of the coronary circulation are called cineangiograms.

Cardiac catheterization is usually performed to evaluate the presence and severity of coronary artery atherosclerosis. In anticipation of cardiac surgery, virtually all patients undergo cardiac catheterization. Cardiac catheterization is also evolving into a variety of treatments, including percutaneous transluminal coronary angioplasty and intracoronary stent placement.

Electrophysiologic Studies

Electrophysiologic studies (EPSs) are used to assess the conduction of electricity through the heart, which it can do with much more specificity than the surface ECG. EPSs provide definitive diagnostic information on cardiac dysrhythmias, such as premature ventricular contractions (PVCs), and help direct proper therapies. The results of EPSs are similar to those of cardiac catheterization. Intracardiac catheters placed under fluoroscopic guidance are used to record intracardiac electrical activity. They are often used to provoke cardiac dysrhythmias in a controlled, treatment-ready setting. Treatment plans for various dysrhythmias often emerge from the results of EPSs. Many hospitals are not equipped to perform EPSs; therefore, those patients needing such studies must be referred to more specialized settings.

PHARMACOLOGIC TREATMENT

EDITORS' NOTE

You can expect several questions, perhaps as many as 10, that directly or indirectly address pharmacologic treatments for abnormal hemodynamics or dysrhythmias. It is not necessary or desirable to review all therapies while preparing for the PCCN exam. However, it is critical to understand the most common therapies and how they work. The focus of this section is essential pharmacologic therapy used in the treatment of abnormal hemodynamics. More specific therapies, such as thrombolytics and antidysrhythmics, are covered in other chapters. If you have a good understanding of this section, you should be well prepared for the PCCN exam questions on this content.

Treatment of abnormal hemodynamics centers on improving either cardiac output or systemic vascular resistance (SVR). In the treatment of inadequate cardiac output, the components of stroke volume (preload, afterload, and contractility) are the most commonly manipulated parameters. A large number of cardiac therapies are available to treat hemodynamic abnormalities.

Treatment of Low Cardiac Output States

Treatment of conditions that cause low stroke volume and low cardiac output usually centers on the left ventricle. Normally, low cardiac output is caused by weakening of the left ventricle (e.g., due to heart failure [HF], MI, or cardiomyopathy) or inadequate blood volume (hypovolemia). If the problem is a weak left ventricle, therapies that might be used include: (1) reducing preload, (2) reducing afterload, and (3) increasing contractility. There are also a few physical interventions, such as allowing the patient to sit up or attempting to reduce his or her anxiety, as well as mechanical support of the heart with intra-aortic balloon pumps and ventricular-assist devices. Most therapies, however, focus on pharmacologic support. It is this treatment modality that is most important for the bedside clinician to understand.

Improving the Strength of the Heart

In the patient presenting with symptoms of left ventricular dysfunction, relief is obtained by improving the strength of the heart. This is also referred to as inotropic therapy. Inotropic therapy increases the strength of the cardiac contraction. As a consequence of the improved strength, an increase in ejection fraction, stroke volume, cardiac output, and, ideally, tissue oxygenation (e.g., improved SvO_2 and lactate) occur.

Several inotropes are available (Table 2-2). These include dobutamine, dopamine, milrinone, epinephrine, and digoxin. The inotrope most commonly used is dobutamine. Dobutamine acts by stimulating beta cells of the sympathetic nervous system, which in turn strengthens contraction (positive inotropic response) and makes the heart beat faster (positive chronotropic response). Since beta stimulation also causes smooth muscle relaxation, blood

TABLE 2-2. COMMON INOTROPIC (CONTRACTILITY) DRUGS

Drug	Dose	Onset	Route
Dobutamine	2.5–10 mcg/kg/min	1–2 min	IV
Dopamine	2–10 mcg/kg/min	<5 min	IV
Milrinone	Loading 50 mcg/kg over 10 min Maintenance is 0.375–0.75 mcg/kg/min	2 min	IV
Digoxin	Loading 10–15 mcg/kg in divided doses over 12–24 h q 6–8 h (doses reduced in renal dysfunction)	5–30 min	IV

Digoxin	Loading 0.5 mg × 1 then 0.25 mg q 6 h until desired
	    effect or total digitalizing dosage is achieved
	    (doses reduced in renal dysfunction)
	    Maintenance 0.125–0.25 mg/day
		1–2 h	PO

IV, intravenous; PO, by mouth.

vessels dilate. This results in a drop in preload (central venous pressure) and afterload.

Better contractility agents, like levosimendan, are still being investigated. However, the disadvantage to the inotropes is the lack of evidence to support their effect on long-term survival. In addition, they increase myocardial oxygen consumption at a time when the heart may be starved for oxygen. Owing to these concerns, inotropes are likely to be more limited in their application.

Dopamine is also used, particularly in moderate dosages (2–10 mcg/kg/min). However, dopamine stimulates alpha cells of the sympathetic nervous system, causing vasoconstriction (increased SVR). This vasoconstriction might increase the blood pressure, but it also causes an increase in myocardial work.

There are times when sympathetic stimulation cannot provide any more improvement in contractility. At this time, drugs having different mechanisms of action, such as the phosphodiesterase inhibitor milrinone, might be used. This drug increases the availability of intracellular calcium and the strength of the heart.

Digitalis preparations such as digoxin are not used in acute situations. These drugs might be used in chronic ventricular dysfunction but not in acute failure.

Improving Cardiac Strength Through Preload Reduction. The strength of the heart might be improved if overstretched myocardial muscle fibers can be allowed to shrink back to normal. Preload reduction can accomplish this goal. Preload reduction is done through vasodilation or with diuretics.

Diuretics are commonly used for preload reduction, mainly because they help reduce the excess fluid in the circulatory system that results from renal compensation for decreased blood flow through the kidneys. Many types of diuretics are available (Table 2-3). All diuretics work by blocking reabsorption of sodium and water. They usually produce a rapid increase in urine output. How effective the diuretic is depends on the improvement in cardiac performance.

Preload reduction can also occur with vasodilation. Drugs such as nitroglycerin, diltiazem, and morphine can reduce preload through vasodilation (Table 2-4). Vasodilation causes an "internal phlebotomy" by reducing the amount of blood returning to the heart.

Increasing Cardiac Strength Through Afterload Reduction. One of the best methods for improving cardiac performance is to reduce the work that the heart must do to eject blood. This can be accomplished by afterload reduction, which can be achieved with many different drugs (Table 2-5). However, only a few of these drugs are commonly used in critical care.

The use of afterload reducers is common in two situations: during hypertensive episodes and when the cardiac output is low and the SVR is high. The principles of their use are similar in both situations.

While potentially dangerous, the most common drug to reduce resistance is nitroprusside. Nitroprusside acts quickly and is effective only with continuous administration. Once stopped, its effect will wear off in minutes. It is very effective at reducing resistance and is frequently used in ICUs. Nitroprusside use has two disadvantages. First, it breaks down into cyanide. Cyanide levels, therefore, may need to be monitored daily in patients on

TABLE 2-3. DIURETICS

Drug	Dose	Onset	Route
Mannitol (osmotic diuretic)	12.5–200 g/day	Within minutes	IVP (filter) or IV drip
Spironolactone (K⁺- sparing class)	25–200 mg/day	24–48 h	PO
Chlorothiazide (thiazide class)	500–2000 mg/day	1–2 h	PO/IV
Hydrochlorothiazide (thiazide class)	25–200 mg/day	2 h	PO
Metolazone (nonthiazide)	2.5–20 mg/day	1 h	PO
Furosemide (loop diuretic)	20–600 mg/day	1 h	PO
Furosemide (loop diuretic)	≥20 mg/day	5 min	IV
Ethacrynic acid (loop diuretic)	25–400 mg/day	30 min	PO
Ethacrynic acid (loop diuretic)	50–100 mg/day	5 min	IV
Bumetanide (loop diuretic)	0.5–10 mg/day	30 min	PO
Bumetanide (loop diuretic)	0.5–10 mg/day	Within minutes	IV
Acetazolamide	250–375 mg/day	1 h	PO/IV

IV, intravenous; PO, by mouth.

TABLE 2-4. VASODILATORS

Drug	Dose	Onset	Route
Nitroglycerin (nitrate vasodilator)	5–400 mcg/min. Titrate to desired effect; at high dose becomes afterload-reducing agent	1–2 min	IV
Nitroglycerin	0.15–0.6 mg q 5 min × 3	1–3 min	SL
Diltiazem (calcium channel blocker)	20 mg (average) bolus over 2 min. May repeat with 25-mg bolus then start drip	1–2 min	IV
Diltiazem (calcium channel blocker)	Tablets: 120–360 mg total daily dose in 3–4 divided doses Sustained release: 120–360 mg/day in 1–2 divided doses	30–60 min	PO
Nifedipine (calcium channel blocker)	Capsules: 30–180 mg total daily dose in 3–4 divided doses Sustained release: 30–120 mg/day in once-daily dosing	Capsules: 5–10 min Sustained release: 20 min	PO
Nesiritide (b-type natriuretic peptide)	0.01–0.03 mcg/kg/min	15 min	IV

IV, intravenous; PO, by mouth; SL, sublingual.

nitroprusside. Second, it acts as a nonselective arterial dilator. This dilation can open flow into areas that do not need more oxygen. However, as more flow enters these areas, some areas that need more oxygen (ischemic myocardium) might have flow diverted from them. This is called the "coronary steal" phenomenon. Risks associated with nitroprusside limit its use to ICUs, therefore it will probably not appear on PCCN exam.

In order to avoid the problems with nitroprusside, other afterload reducers, such as calcium channel blockers, beta-blocking agents, and natriuretic peptides (e.g., nesiritide) are used. The advantage of agents like natriuretic peptides is that they do not directly reduce cardiac contractility. Calcium channel blockers and beta blockers reduce afterload, but they unfortunately also tend to weaken the heart. If calcium channel blockers (e.g., nicardipine) or beta blockers (e.g., metoprolol, labetalol) are used, their effect on both SVR and cardiac output must be monitored.

There are other afterload reducers, most notably the angiotensin-converting enzyme (ACE) inhibitors. ACE inhibitors are most often used in the management of nonacute forms of cardiac failure because they do not activate compensating neurohumoral responses as do other afterload reducers. This makes them attractive for long-term use in such situations as HF. They tend to reduce SVR without increasing cardiac output. The net effect is a substantial reduction in myocardial oxygen consumption.

Management of Hypovolemia

When hypovolemia is present, the circulating blood volume must be replenished by one of three therapies: blood (e.g., whole blood, packed cells), crystalloids (normal saline, lactated Ringer's solution), and

colloids (hetastarch, albumin). The choice of therapy depends on the clinical situation. General guidelines for fluid replacement are as follows:

1. Blood is used when the patient is actively bleeding, in the presence of acute coronary syndrome, and/or when the hemoglobin levels are in the range of 7–8 g/dL or less. Blood is the only fluid replacement that actually carries oxygen.
2. Crystalloids are used when volume depletion does not have to be corrected rapidly, when depletion of more than vascular volume is suspected, or when hypovolemia is suspected but is not a clear diagnosis.
3. Colloids are used when rapid volume expansion is necessary but the use of blood is not indicated or blood is not available.

Considerable controversy exists regarding the proper fluid replacement therapy. Generally, crystalloids are the first agent used in suspected hypovolemia (Table 2-6). They are inexpensive and do not cause any allergic reactions. However, they take longer to expand the vascular volume than either colloids or blood.

Treatment of Low Systemic Vascular Resistance

Many hemodynamic problems are a result of disturbances of blood flow. In sepsis, one of the most common of these disturbances, SVR is abnormally low. Other conditions can cause this situation as well, including hepatic disease and neurogenic shock.

TABLE 2-5. AFTERLOAD REDUCERS

Direct Arterial Dilator	Dose	Onset	Route
Hydralazine	10–40 mg	10–20 min	IV, IM
Diazoxide	50–150 mg	1–2 min	IV
Nitroglycerin (nitrate vasodilator)	5–160 mcg/min; titrate to desired effect	1–2 min	IV
Nitroglycerin (SL)	0.15–0.6 mg q 5 min × 3	1–3 min	SL
Nitroglycerin (transdermal)	0.2–0.8 mg/h patch qd	<30 min	Topical
IMDUR	30–240 mg daily	1 h	PO
Alpha Inhibitors	**Dose**	**Onset**	**Route**
Prazosin	1–20 mg total daily dose in 2–3 divided doses	30 min–3 h	PO
Phentolamine	0.1–2 mg/min	Immediate	IV
Clonidine	0.1–2.4 mg total daily dose in 1–2 divided doses	30–60 min	PO
Methyldopa	250 mg–3 g total daily dose in 2–4 divided doses	2 h	PO
Calcium Channel Blockers	**Route**	**Onset**	**Route**
Diltiazem	20 mg (average) bolus over 2 min; may repeat with 25-mg bolus then start drip	1–2 min	IV
Diltiazem	Tablets: 120–360 mg total daily dose in 3–4 divided doses Sustained release: 120–360 mg/day in 1–2 divided doses	30–60 min	PO
Nifedipine	Capsules: 30–180 mg total daily dose in 3–4 divided doses	Capsules: 5–10 min	PO
	Sustained release: 30–120 mg/day in once-daily dosing	Sustained release: 20 min	SL
Nicardipine	5 mg/h; maximum dose 15 mg/h	1–5 min	IV
Nicardipine	20–60 mg bid–tid		PO
ACE Inhibitors	**Route**	**Onset**	**Route**
Captopril	25–450 mg total daily dose in 2–3 divided doses	15–30 min	PO
Enalapril	2.5–40 mg qd	1 h	PO
Enalaprilat	1.25–5 mg q 6 h	15 min	IVP
Lisinopril	10–40 mg qd	1 h	PO
Beta Blockers	**Route**	**Onset**	**Route**
Atenolol	50–200 mg qd		PO
Carvedilol	6.25–25 mg bid		PO
Metoprolol	100–450 mg total daily dose in 4 divided doses		PO
Metoprolol	5 mg q 2 min × 3 (for a total dose of 15 mg)		IV
Propranolol	120–240 mg in divided doses		PO
Esmolol	50–300 mcg/kg/min		IV
Labetolol	200–2400 mg total daily dose in 2–3 divided doses	2–4 h	PO
Labetalol	0.25 mg/kg q 10 min initially to a total dose of 50–300 mg	5 min	IV
Angiotensin Receptor Blockers (ARBs)	**Route**	**Onset**	**Route**
Losartan	25–100 mg/day		PO

ACE, angiotensin-converting enzyme; IM, intramuscular; IV, intravenous; IVP, intravenous push; PO, by mouth; SL, sublingual.

TABLE 2-6. VOLUME EXPANDERS

Agent	Dose	Onset	Route
Hetastarch	100–500 mL; maximum 150 mL/day;	30 min	IV
Albumin	25 g initially; maximum 250 g/48 h	Varies	IV
Crystalloids	100–1000 mL/5–30 min	30 min	IV
Normal saline	NA	NA	IV
Lactated Ringer's solution	NA	NA	IV

IV, intravenous.

The key to all treatment is reversal of the underlying problem. For example, in sepsis, antibiotics might be the primary treatment, and hemodynamic interventions are viewed primarily as supportive therapies.

The primary hemodynamic therapies are aimed at achieving three goals: (1) maintaining circulating blood volume with volume expansion, (2) increasing blood flow with inotropic therapy, and (3) maintaining blood flow with agents to increase the SVR.

Maintaining blood flow with volume expansion and inotropic therapy has already been discussed. Maintaining blood flow with agents (vasopressors) to increase the SVR is done with one of four agents (Table 2-7), although vasopressors other than dopamine are unlikely to appear on the PCCN. All of these agents work by stimulating the alpha$_1$ cells of the sympathetic nervous system. These drugs produce vasoconstriction and some also increase the cardiac output. These are potent drugs which should elevate blood pressure and blood flow. However, they must be used with caution because they might elevate the SVR and blood pressure but not increase tissue oxygenation.

Alpha stimulants cause marked vasoconstriction. These drugs are so potent that they are given centrally to avoid the tissue damage that would result in the event of infiltration during peripheral intravenous administration.

Specific Cardiovascular Drugs

Drugs specific to clinical conditions are discussed in the chapters about those conditions. For example, thrombolytics are presented in the chapter on acute coronary syndrome (Chapter 6) and antidysrhythmics are covered in that on dysrhythmias (Chapter 11). This section is designed as a general review of treatment of hemodynamic disturbances. For more information on specific drug therapy, locate the specific condition of interest.

IMPLICATIONS OF CARDIOVASCULAR DYSFUNCTION ON OTHER ORGAN SYSTEMS

EDITORS' NOTE

As it fails, the cardiovascular system will affect every other organ system. Most of these effects are covered in the following chapters on specific organ systems. It is not likely that the PCCN exam will address the specific effects of cardiovascular dysfunction on other organs directly. More likely, the exam will include a few questions that integrate the cardiovascular system into the dysfunction of other systems. Read this short section to familiarize yourself with the general effects of the cardiovascular system on other organs. In order to simplify the contents of this section, all pertinent information is listed in the tables.

In assessing the effect of cardiovascular dysfunction on other organs, it is helpful to understand the blood flow from each ventricle, since the effects of dysfunction are different in each ventricle. For

TABLE 2-7. COMMON VASOPRESSORS

Drug	Dose	Onset	Route
Dopamine	10–20 mcg/kg/min	<5 min	IV
Norepinephrine	2–10 mcg/min 1–20 mcg/min to effect	1–2 min	IV

TABLE 2-8. LEFT VENTRICULAR DYSFUNCTION: HEMODYNAMIC AND SYSTEMIC EFFECTS

Increased preload	Reduced subendocardial perfusion
	Decreased renal perfusion
	Antidiuretic and aldosterone released, causing sodium and fluid retention
	Increased blood volume
	Fluid overload
	Increased beta natriuretic peptide (BNP)
Increased afterload	Catecholamines and angiotensin II released, causing vasoconstriction via the renin-angiotensin-aldosterone compensatory mechanism
	Impaired vascular smooth muscle relaxation
	Increased systemic vascular resistance
Impaired contractility	Decreased cardiac output due to reduced left ventricular reserve
	Decreased skeletal muscle blood flow
	Decreased exercise capacity
	Poor forward blood flow
	Increased backward pressure into the pulmonary vasculature

TABLE 2-9. RIGHT VENTRICULAR DYSFUNCTION: HEMODYNAMIC AND SYSTEMIC EFFECTS

Increased preload	Passive organ congestion
	Hepatic engorgement
	Hepatojugular reflux
	Coagulopathies
	Elevated liver enzymes
	Gastric congestion
	Dependent, peripheral edema
	Distended neck veins
	Decreased cardiac output due to the reduced forward flow from the right ventricle (see Table 2–8)

example, left ventricular dysfunction results in a failure to move blood to the tissues adequately. This threatens every organ's ability to maintain its normal metabolic activity. Since any threat to circulation threatens oxygen delivery, all tissues are at risk when left ventricular function is disturbed. In addition, a back-up of blood into the lungs will eventually occur, causing pulmonary symptoms such as orthopnea (Table 2-8).

Right ventricular dysfunction results in a loss of blood flow through the lungs and a back-up of blood into the venous system, causing symptoms such as venous engorgement (Table 2-9).

Since any organ can be affected, symptoms of dysfunction may be found in any organ. Table 2-10 shows the effects of ventricular dysfunction on each organ.

TABLE 2-10. END-ORGAN EFFECTS OF VENTRICULAR DYSFUNCTION

Left Ventricular Failure	Right Ventricular Failure	Organ System	Effect	Clinical Presentation
+	+	Central nervous system	Reduced cerebral perfusion due to decreased cardiac output	Altered level of consciousness Disorientation Confusion Lethargy Anxiety
			Decreased skeletal muscle perfusion	Insomnia Dizziness/syncope Fatigue Decreased exercise capacity
+	+	Renal system	Reduced renal perfusion, causing Na+ retention and fluid accumulation	Fluid overload Increased SVR Oliguria during day Nocturia Metabolic acidosis Weight gain Peripheral edema Hyponatremia Hypokalemia due to diuretic therapy Dark, concentrated urine
	+	Hepatic system	Passive congestion and reduced perfusion of liver due to elevated systemic venous pressure cause liver damage and dysfunction and deficiencies in coagulation factors	Hepatomegaly Abdominal distention Hepatojugular reflex Elevated liver enzymes (SGOT, SGPT, LDH, GGT, lipase, etc.) Elevated PT, PTT, INR

(Continued)

TABLE 2-10. END-ORGAN EFFECTS OF VENTRICULAR DYSFUNCTION (*CONTINUED*)

Left Ventricular Failure	Right Ventricular Failure	Organ System	Effect	Clinical Presentation
	+	Gastrointestinal system	Passive congestion of gut slows due to visceral edema	Nausea/vomiting Anorexia Ascites Nutritional deficiencies Poor oral medication absorption Cachexia
+		Pulmonary system	Backward pressure due to poor left ventricular systolic function, causing pulmonary edema	Gravity-dependent crackles Wheezes Orthopnea Dyspnea on exertion Paroxysmal nocturnal dyspnea Low Pao_2/Sao_2/pH Use of accessory muscles Cheyne-Stokes respirations Productive cough of blood-tinged, frothy sputum
+		Cardiovascular system	Fluid overload of left ventricular	S_3 and/or S_4 Systolic murmur of mitral regurgitation Stretching of myocardium and valvular radius PMI shifts to the left
			Poor left ventricular contractility	Pulsus alternans Decreased pulse pressure Cold/discolored extremities Cool, clammy skin Decreased capillary refill Diaphoresis
+	+		Reduced subendocardial perfusion	Ischemic symptoms Dysrhythmias Atrial or ventricular bundle branch block
	+		Fluid overload	Jugular vein distention Pulsus paradoxus Pedal edema

GGT, gamma-glutamyl transferase; INR, international ratio; LDH, lactate dehydrogenase; PT, prothrombin time; PTT, partial thromboplastin time; PMI, point of maximal impulse; Pao_2, arterial oxygen pressure; Sao_2, arterial oxygen saturation; SGOT, serum glutamate oxaloacetate transaminase (aspartate aminotransferase); SGPT, serum glutamate pyruvate transaminase (alanine aminotransferase).

3

The Normal ECG

EDITORS' NOTE

Generally, the PCCN exam requires interpretation of fewer than three rhythm strips, but it may also have a few questions regarding 12-lead ECG analysis. However, there may or may not be rhythm strips or 12-lead ECGs actually to interpret (e.g., ischemia, injury, and effects of major electrolytes like potassium). If you understand the major dysrhythmias and key concepts of 12-lead ECGs, you will be fine. The PCCN is not a test on ECGs or 12 leads but more of how they relate to given clinical conditions.

In this chapter, reviews of normal and preferred ECG leads as well as the normal components of ECG waves are provided. Review this chapter carefully if ECG monitoring is not one of your strengths. However, if you have a basic understanding of dysrhythmias, lead placement, and identifying injury and ischemia, this chapter will not add much in your PCCN preparation.

COMPONENTS OF THE NORMAL ECG

The electrocardiograph is a machine that records the electrical activity of the heart on special paper. The result is an electrocardiogram (ECG or EKG). The electrical activity measured by the ECG is the electrical potential between two points on the body, a positive pole and a negative pole. When one is monitoring patients in critical care, all monitoring leads have one negative and one positive pole. For example, in lead I, the right arm is negative and the left arm is positive. Electrical activity in the heart is monitored by these two poles. Electrical activity that is directed toward the positive pole results in an upright deflection. Activity heading toward the negative pole is upside down. The sum of all cardiac electrical activity (referred to as cardiac vectors) is generally in a direction that is inferior and to the left. The leftward direction of cardiac electrical activity is primarily due to the size and, therefore, electrical activity of the left ventricle.

The 12-lead ECG is the graphic recording of the electrical output of the heart from 12 different positions. A 12-lead ECG can be diagnostic in drug toxicity, conduction disturbances, electrolyte imbalances, ischemia, and infarction and can aid in determining the size of the heart chambers and axis orientation of the heart.

Cardiac monitoring uses rhythm strips to assess heart rate, rhythm, and dysrhythmias. Rhythm strips may be run on any one of the 12 leads used in a 12-lead ECG and several other special leads.

The most common leads used to monitor patients are leads II and V_1. Lead II is a common lead, although it is highly limited in the information it can reveal to the clinician. Lead II has a negative pole attached to an electrode placed on the upper chest near the right arm and a positive pole attached to an electrode placed on the lower left side of the chest. Lead II normally sees electrical activity in the heart in an upright ECG pattern since its positive electrode is on the left side of the body. Lead II is especially useful in assessing P waves and QRS complexes that have a small amplitude. It is not, however, the ideal monitoring lead. V_1 is a better routine monitoring lead. MCL_1 is modified chest lead I. It is the bipolar equivalent of V_1 on the 12-lead ECG.

V_1 is an excellent monitoring lead, perhaps the best of the 6 common chest leads of the 12-lead ECG. In V_1, the positive electrode is attached to an electrode placed to the right of the sternum at the fourth

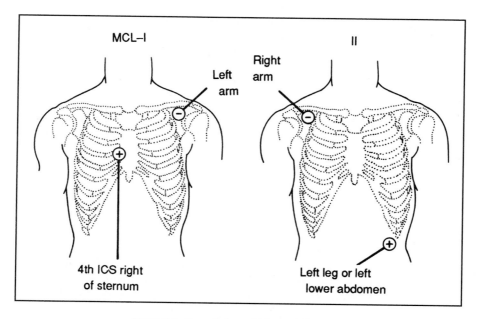

Figure 3-1. Normal placement for leads V₁ and II.

intercostal space (Fig. 3-1). Since the V₁ positive electrode is placed to the right of the sternum, it views the cardiac electrical activity as heading away from it and, therefore, sees the QRS complex as primarily upside down. The V (vector) leads are technically called unipolar leads since the negative pole is the computer-calculated center of all the ECG leads and only the positive electrode is physically visible.

V₁ gives more information on conduction defects, such as right and left bundle branch blocks, than do other routine monitoring leads. As such, it is the routine lead employed to identify most dysrhythmias, particularly aberrant atrial premature contractions, from premature ventricular contractions. The one situation for which V₁ is not as useful is with newer monitoring systems that employ ST-segment analysis. ST-segment analysis operates better when large R waves are sensed. If large R waves are desired, lead II, V₅, or V₆ is employed.

In monitoring dysrhythmias, develop the practice of using multiple leads. Use of a single lead for all situations limits your ability to interpret complex dysrhythmias.

A key ingredient to accurate dysrhythmia analysis is the correct application of lead placement. Although the PCCN exam generally does not ask specific questions on lead placement, such questions are possible. More importantly, accurate lead placement has an effect on correct rhythm and 12-lead analysis. Studies have indicated significant changes in QRS morphology with incorrect lead placement.

ECG Paper

The PCCN exam will not ask questions about the ECG paper. However, you must know the time grids within the ECG paper to make interpretations of dysrhythmias and 12-lead analysis.

The ECG paper has a series of horizontal lines exactly 1 mm apart (Fig. 3-2). The horizontal lines represent voltage (or amplitude). ECG paper also has vertical lines that represent time. Each vertical line is 0.04 s apart. To help in measuring waveforms, every fifth line is darker than the other lines, both horizontally and vertically. The intersection of these lines produces both small boxes (the lighter lines) and large boxes (the darker, bolder lines). Horizontally, each small box represents 1 mm (0.1 mV) and each large box represents 5 mm (0.5 mV). (Note that each large box is made up of five small boxes.) Vertically, each small box represents 0.04 s and each large box represents 0.20 s with a printer paper speed of 25 mm/s. Because of the design of ECG paper, one can measure the duration of impulses (wavelengths) and the amplitude (height) of impulses. All waves will be either isoelectric (no net electrical activity, or flat), positively deflected (upright, toward the positive pole), or negatively deflected (downward, toward the negative pole).

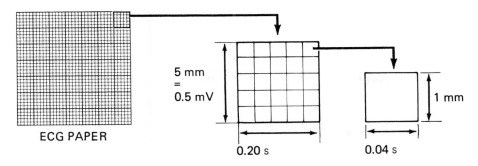

Figure 3-2. ECG paper.

COMPONENTS OF A CARDIAC CYCLE

Before a rhythm strip can be labeled, a systematic analysis of each portion of the strip and the relation of each wave to the electrical activity in the cardiac cycle is made. The interpretations will be made using lead II or V_1 in this text. It is conventional to label the components of the cardiac cycle P, QRS, and T. (There is no reason why these specific letters were chosen.)

There are three prominent deflections in the ECG: the P wave, the QRS complex, and the T wave (Fig. 3-3).

P Wave

This represents the generation of an electrical impulse and depolarization of the atria (Fig. 3-4). The P wave is important in determining whether the impulse started in the sinoatrial (SA) node or elsewhere in the atrium.

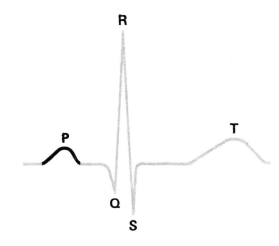

Figure 3-4. The P wave.

QRS Complex

The QRS complex is composed of three separate waveforms, which represent ventricular depolarization (Fig. 3-5). Multiple variations exist in the shape of the QRS complex. A Q wave is the first negative deflection and may or may not be present. A large Q wave may be indicative of myocardial death. To be clinically significant, the Q wave should be greater than 0.04 s and the depth should be greater than one-third the height of the R wave.

The R wave is the first positive deflection in the complex. The R wave is usually large in leads where the positive electrode is on the left (I, II, III, aVL, aVF, V_5, V_6) and small in leads where the positive electrode is on the right (V_1, V_2, V_3, aVR).

The S wave is the negative deflection following the R wave. The S wave can be useful in interpreting terminal electrical activity in the heart. The S wave is large in leads where the positive electrode is on the right and small in leads where the positive electrode is on the left.

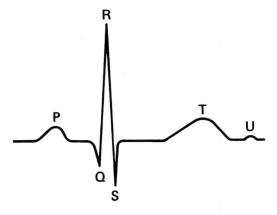

Figure 3-3. The normal PQRST deflections, lead II.

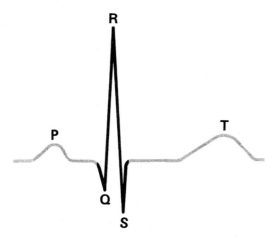

Figure 3-5. The QRS complex.

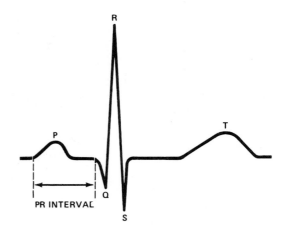

Figure 3-7. The PR interval.

T Wave

The T wave is the third major deflection in the ECG (Fig. 3-6). It represents repolarization of the ventricles. In most lead II of a healthy heart, the T wave is positively deflected. In ischemia or infarction, the T wave may be inverted.

Intervals and Segments

There are four other intervals and segments of a rhythm strip and an ECG that must be identified: the PR and QT intervals and the ST and PR segments.

PR Interval

The PR interval (Fig. 3-7) represents the time for the electrical impulse to spread from the atrium to the atrioventricular (AV) node and His bundle. It is measured from the beginning of the P wave to the beginning of the QRS complex. Normally, this interval is 0.12 to 0.20 s.

ST Segment

The ST segment (Fig. 3-8) represents the time from complete depolarization of the ventricles to the beginning of repolarization (recovery) of the ventricles. In a healthy heart, the ST segment is flat or isoelectric. Since no net electrical activity is present during the recovery phase of the cardiac cycle, the wave is not deflected in either direction. In myocardial injury, the segment may be elevated. In ischemia, the ST segment is depressed.

PR Segment

This segment (Fig. 3-9) represents the normal delay in the conduction of the electrical impulse in the AV node. It is normally isoelectric and is measured from the end of the P wave to the beginning of the R wave.

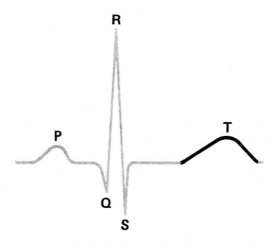

Figure 3-6. The T wave.

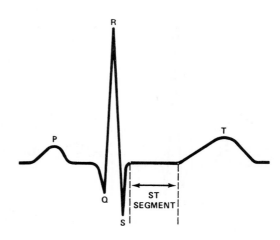

Figure 3-8. The ST segment.

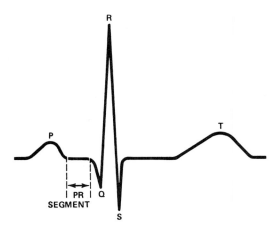

Figure 3-9. The PR segment.

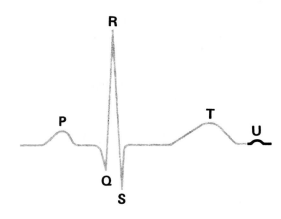

Figure 3-11. The U wave.

Duration of the PR segment varies. Clinically, the PR segment is not usually addressed.

QT Interval

This interval (Fig. 3-10) represents the total period of time required for depolarization and repolarization (recovery) of the ventricles. It is measured from the beginning of the QRS complex to the end of the T wave. It is normally less than 0.40 s but is dependent on heart rate, sex, age, and other factors. A QT interval that is corrected for heart rate is called the QT_c.

Occasionally, another wave is seen after the T wave and before the next P wave. This is called a U wave (Fig. 3-11). The U wave may represent repolarization of the Purkinje fibers or hypokalemia. It may or may not be seen.

INTERPRETATION OF A RHYTHM STRIP

Five basic steps are followed in analyzing a rhythm strip (or an ECG) to aid in the interpretation and identification of a rhythm. Each step should be followed in sequence. Eventually this will become a habit and will enable the clinician to identify a strip correctly, accurately, and quickly.

Step 1

Determine the rates at which the atria and the ventricles are depolarizing. These rates may not be the same. To count the rate of the atria, count the number of P waves present in the 6-s rhythm strip and multiply by 10. (Each mark at the top edge of the ECG paper represents 3 s, and each inch of the ECG paper equals 1 s.) This gives the atrial rate per minute.

Count the number of QRS complexes in a 6-s strip and multiply by 10. This gives the ventricular rate per minute. For the purpose of the PCCN, this is all that is needed.

For regular rhythms, another method may be used. Find the peak of one QRS complex that lands on a heavy dark line. Then find the next QRS complex. The rate is as follows: If the QRS complexes are separated by one large block (five small blocks), the rate is 300. If there are two blocks, the rate is 150; three blocks, 100; four blocks, 75; five blocks, 60. The rate becomes less accurate after this.

Step 2

Determine whether the rhythm is regular or irregular. The most accurate method is to measure the

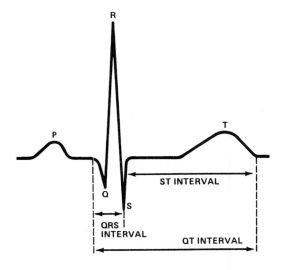

Figure 3-10. The QRS, ST, and QT intervals.

interval from one R wave to the next. (Set one point of the cardiac calipers on the tip of the first R wave and the other point on the tip of the next R wave.) Then move the cardiac calipers from R to R. If the measurement is the same (or varies less than 0.04 s between beats), the rhythm is regular. If the intervals vary by more than 0.04 s, the rhythm is irregular. Often one can tell by simply looking at the strip that the rhythm is irregular. However, if it looks regular, it is best to measure the R to R intervals to be certain.

Step 3

Analyze the P waves. A P wave should precede every QRS complex. All of the P waves should be identical in shape. The normal P wave is fairly sharply curved, less than 3 mm in height, and less than 0.1 s in width in lead II. If the P wave is abnormally shaped or varies in shape from wave to wave, the stimulus may have arisen from somewhere in the atrium other than in the SA node. Almost all impulses that originate in the SA node will meet the "normal" shape and size previously stated if heart function is normal. A biphasic P (a single P wave moves above and below the baseline) may indicate left atrial enlargement; a peaked P may indicate right atrial enlargement, and both of these P waves originate in the SA node. If there is no P wave or if the P wave does not precede the QRS complex, the impulse did not originate in the SA node.

Step 4

Measure the PR interval. This is done from the beginning of the P wave to the beginning of the QRS complex. It should be between 0.10 and 0.20 s. Intervals outside this range indicate a conduction disturbance between the atria and the ventricles.

Step 5

Measure the width of the QRS complex. This is done from the beginning of the Q (if present, otherwise the R) to the end of the S wave. The normal duration is 0.06 to 0.12 s. A QRS measurement of greater than 0.12 s indicates an intraventricular conduction abnormality.

Figure 3-12 is a 6-s lead II rhythm strip. Let us analyze this rhythm strip by applying the five steps just mentioned.

- Step 1: The atrial rate is 80 (eight P waves in 6 s). The ventricular rate is 80 (eight R waves in 6 s). The heart rate is 80.
- Step 2: There is less than a 0.04-s variation from R wave to R wave, so the rhythm is regular.
- Step 3: The P waves are all the same shape, size (in height), and duration. Each P wave appears immediately before a QRS complex. These factors indicate that the impulse starts in the SA node.
- Step 4: The PR interval is about 0.16 s. This is within the normal duration range, indicating normal conduction of the impulse from the SA node to the AV node.
- Step 5: Each QRS complex is less than 0.10 s in duration, which is normal.
- Interpretation of the strip: Normal sinus rhythm.

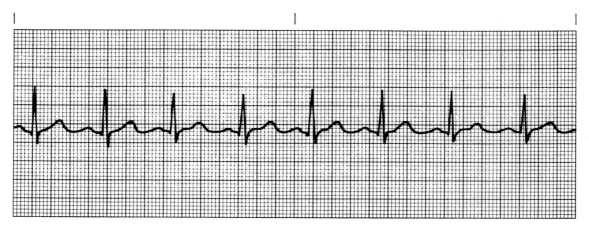

Figure 3-12. Lead II normal sinus rhythm.

The 12-Lead ECG

EDITORS' NOTE

The PCCN exam can include questions that require an understanding of the 12-lead electrocardiogram (ECG). The most important questions to answer relate to the acute coronary syndrome, where ischemia or injury may be present. This should be the most important part of preparing for the PCCN exam in regards to 12-lead interpretation. Other typical questions involving the 12-lead ECG usually focus on conditions such as left and right ventricular hypertrophy, left and right bundle branch blocks, differentiating aberrant atrial premature contractions from premature ventricular contractions (PVCs), and identifying myocardial infarction patterns. This chapter provides the information necessary to interpret these conditions. However, keep in mind the number of questions regarding a 12-lead ECG will be limited. Often it is not the interpretation of the 12-lead ECG which is key to a question, but what does an abnormal component of the 12-lead ECG indicate. For example, you may be told that the ST segment is elevated in certain leads and you need to apply that information to a scenario.

The 12 monitoring leads used to assess myocardial conduction patterns are listed in Table 4-1. In assessing patterns of injury, hypertrophy, or axis deviations, it is essential to note the views of the heart from different leads. Whenever available, a prior 12-lead ECG can help interpret questionable results.

ISCHEMIA

EDITORS' NOTE

The most important aspects of the ECG to understand have to do with identifying myocardial ischemia and injury. Your understanding of how to identify evidence of infarction or ischemia on an ECG will be tested on the PCCN exam. However, these concepts are not as difficult as they sometimes seem. This is particularly true of trying to identify whether a patient might be having a myocardial infarction.

In reviewing the 12-lead ECG for infarction and ischemic injury patterns, keep in mind that the ECG is not foolproof. In a small but substantial percentage of patients who have a myocardial infarction (MI), the ECG will show no evidence of damage. Changes in serum cardiac biomarkers are more accurate, but they take longer to determine. The speed with which an ECG can be obtained is the primary reason why it still has clinical value.

The first step in identifying an MI is to look at the ST segment. It is one of the first parts of the ECG to change with MI. Typically, if MI is occurring, the ST segment will be elevated (Fig. 4-1). Elevation of the ST segment is a strong warning sign of cardiac injury. The ST segment may be depressed if only ischemia of the heart exists (Fig. 4-2). To identify changes in the ST segment, examine where the ST segment is 0.08 s (two small blocks) from the end of the QRS (Fig. 4-3).

The ST segment in the area opposite the MI might show depression, which is a concept referred to as reciprocal change (Fig. 4-4). Whether these changes indicate ischemia in the area or just repolarization abnormalities due to the MI is controversial. Currently, it is believed that the ST changes opposite the MI are relatively benign.

The T wave may also indicate cardiac ischemia and may change before the ST segment does. It usually becomes inverted with cardiac ischemia (Fig. 4-5).

TABLE 4-1. 12-LEAD ECG LEADS

Lead	View of the Heart
I	Lateral wall
II	Inferior wall
III	Inferior wall
aVR (augmented vector of the right)	
aVL (augmented vector of the left)	Lateral wall
aVF (augmented vector of the foot)	Inferior wall
V_1	Ventricular septum
V_2	Anterior wall
V_3	Anterior wall
V_4	Anterior wall
V_5	Lateral wall
V_6	Lateral wall

TABLE 4-2. PARTS OF THE HEART

Location of Injury	Leads
Anterior/septal MI	V_1–V_4
Lateral MI	I, aVL, V_5, V_6
Inferior MI	II, III, aVF
Posterior MI	V_1, V_2
Right ventricular MI	V_3R, V_4R, V_5R, V_6R

Q-wave formation is the primary indication that a patient has had an MI. Q waves are negative deflections in front of R waves (Fig. 4-6). They are considered significant if they are wide (>0.04 s) and large (greater than one-third the height of the R wave). Q waves indicate cardiac muscle death. Because they take about 24 h to form, if a Q wave is present, one can estimate that the MI occurred at least 1 day earlier. From a nursing perspective, we would want to determine whether cardiac damage occurred before the muscle actually died. To do this, we look for ST-segment changes before the formation of a Q wave. If the Q wave is present, you know that the MI is too old for some treatments, such as thrombolysis.

In reading a 12-lead ECG, it is necessary to identify the location of any injury. The heart is normally divided into four parts, each identified with different ECG leads (Table 4-2).

Anterior MIs are usually the most dangerous because of the amount of muscle damaged and the

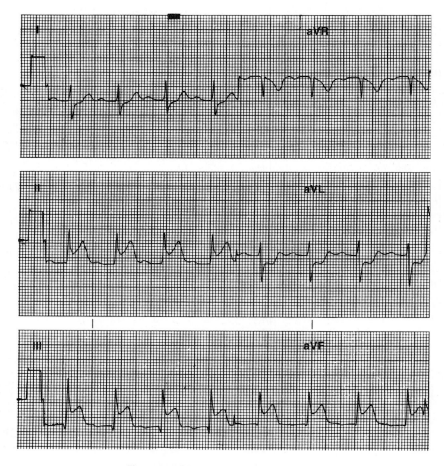

Figure 4-1. ST-segment elevation during MI.

are the second most dangerous type. They frequently produce dysrhythmias, such as second-degree heart block. Inferior MIs are associated with obstruction of the right coronary artery. Inferior MIs are also commonly associated with right ventricular (RV) MIs. RV MIs are identified by using right-sided precordial chest leads, specifically V_3R to V_6R. Posterior MIs are difficult to see with the normal ECG. When the V_1 and V_2 leads are used to examine the back of the heart, the criteria for cardiac death are usually reversed. Instead of having a Q wave indicate an MI, the presence of a large R wave in V_1 and V_2 (the mirror test) might indicate a posterior MI. A posterior MI can be the result of obstruction of either the circumflex or the right coronary artery.

Injury Patterns

The more areas of the heart that are damaged, the more dangerous the MI becomes. For example, an anterior/lateral MI is more dangerous than either one individually. Common patterns include anterior/lateral, inferior/posterior, and anterior/septal.

AXIS DEVIATION

EDITORS' NOTE

....

It is necessary to understand the axis of the heart in order to interpret a 12-lead ECG. However, it is unlikely that the PCCN exam will have a question regarding axis deviation. To be safe, however, this section is included. Read this section if you want to be thoroughly prepared for the exam and feel that you know most areas well enough to allow for some more in-depth reading.

....

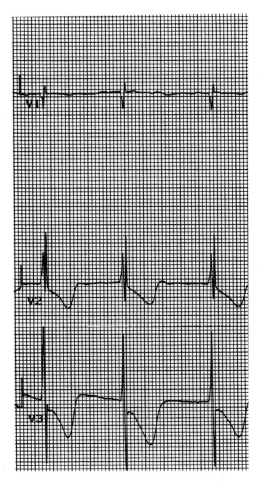

Figure 4-2. ST-segment depression during myocardial ischemia.

injury to the ventricular conduction system. This usually represents obstruction of the left anterior descending (LAD) artery. Lateral MIs might accompany anterior MIs or occur alone. Lateral MIs usually occur with obstruction of the circumflex artery. Inferior MIs

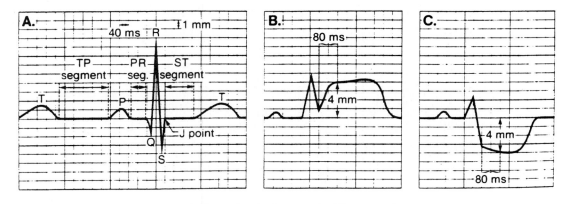

Figure 4-3. Correct location for measuring ST-segment changes.

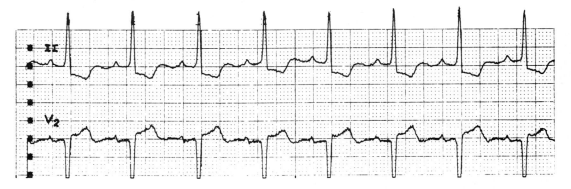

Figure 4-4. Reciprocal changes in the ECG during MI.

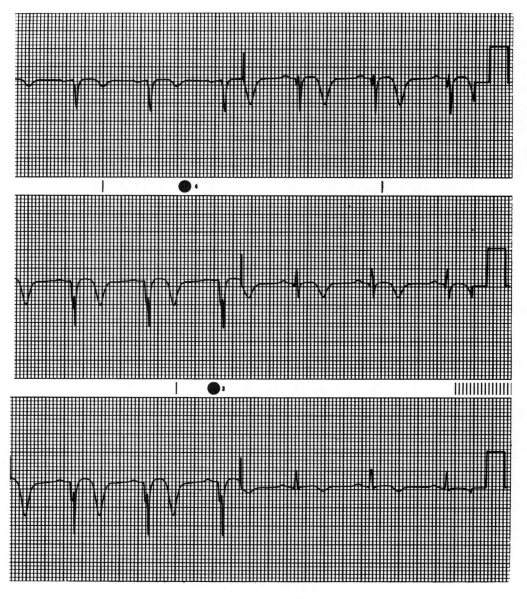

Figure 4-5. T-wave inversion with myocardial ischemia.

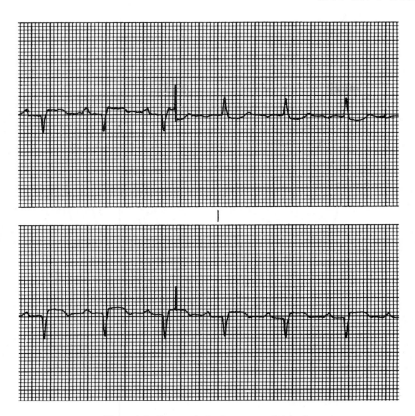

Figure 4-6. Q waves indicating myocardial death.

Axis calculation refers to identifying the source of major electrical activity in the heart. This is done by using vectors. A vector is a quantity that has magnitude and direction. Cardiac vectors represent electrical activity and force and are identified by arrows. If a cardiac vector is headed toward a positive lead on an ECG, it is represented by an upright arrow. If it is headed away from the positive electrode, it is viewed as negative. Normally, the mean cardiac vector is directed inferiorly and to the left (Fig. 4-7). If all the electrical activity in the heart were averaged, the net direction of electrical impulses would be toward the area of largest muscle concentration—that is, the left ventricle.

Vectors are usually represented on a circular diagram known as the hexaxial reference system (Fig. 4-8). As Fig. 4-8 shows, the circle is divided into 30-degree segments. Each lead is represented, separated by 30-degree increments. The axis is indicated by the number to which the major cardiac vector is pointing.

The axis can deviate. Typically these deviations are classified as right axis deviation, left axis deviation, and extreme right axis deviation (Fig. 4-9) (or

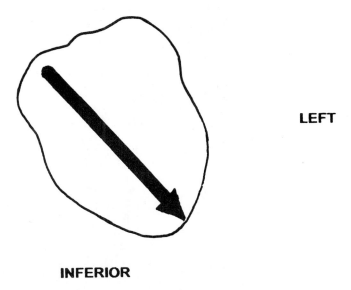

LEFT

INFERIOR

Figure 4-7. Representation of the mean cardiac vector.

indeterminate). Causes for these changes are listed in Table 4-3.

Determining if an axis is normal or abnormal can be done by examining the largest QRS complex

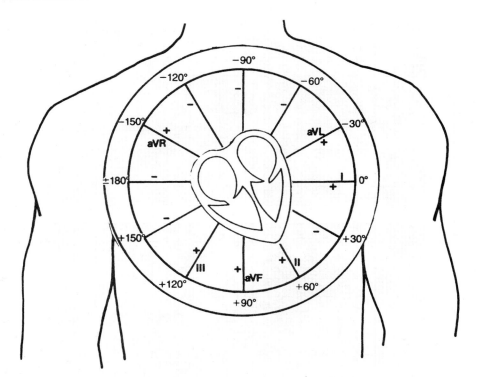

Figure 4-8. Geometric circle for vector measurement.

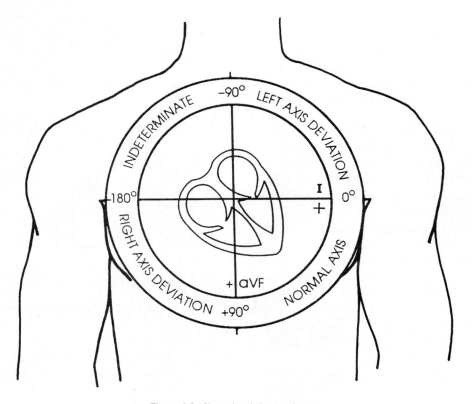

Figure 4-9. Normal and abnormal axes.

TABLE 4-3. COMMON CAUSES FOR AXIS DEVIATIONS

Left axis deviation	Anterior hemiblock
	Left ventricular hypertrophy
	PVCs
Right axis deviation	Posterior hemiblock
	Right ventricular hypertrophy
Extreme right axis deviation	PVCs

PVCs, premature ventricular contractionms.

in the frontal plane leads—that is, I, II, III, aVR, aVL, and aVF. The largest QRS complex results when the cardiac vector heads directly toward or away from the positive electrode.

Using Fig. 4-10 as an example, we can calculate the axis as follows: Note the locations of the positive and negative electrodes in each lead. Then observe the QRS complex in the 12-lead ECG. Note that lead III has the largest deflection. This means the vector is 90 degrees. In Fig. 4-11, aVL has the largest QRS. This means the vector is −30 degrees (330 degrees).

This is a very brief explanation of axis calculation. For simple ECG interpretation and for the purposes of preparing for the PCCN exam, this should be all you need to know.

BUNDLE BRANCH BLOCKS

EDITORS' NOTE

Bundle branch blocks may be on the PCCN exam. It is possible that at least two questions addressing this area might be included. It is helpful to have a basic understanding of this topic.

Interpreting bundle branch blocks focuses on identifying changes in the QRS complex. Normally, the QRS complex in the frontal plane (I, II, III, aVL, aVF) has small Q and S waves. V_1 has a small R wave

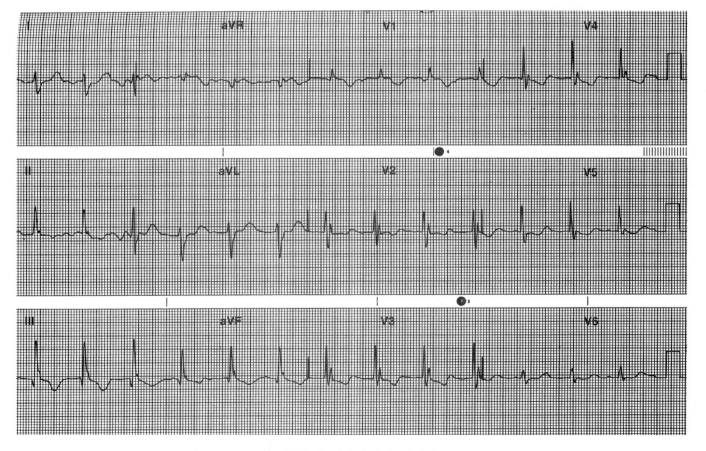

Figure 4-10. Sample lead III axis calculation.

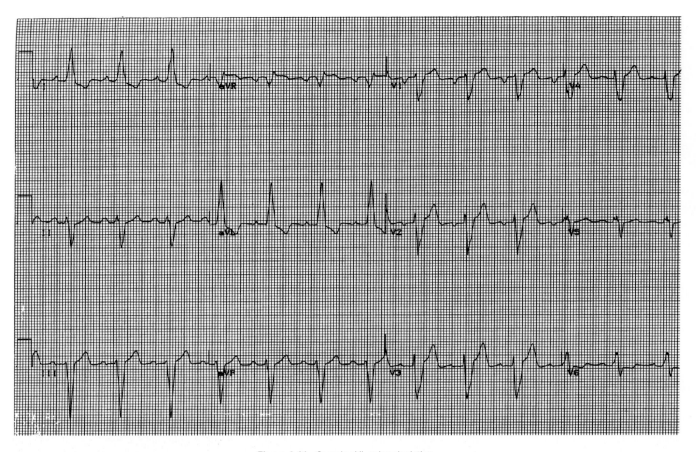

Figure 4-11. Sample aVL axis calculation.

and a large S wave. Conduction blocks can change this appearance. Bundle branch blocks are usually preceded by normal P waves and PR intervals. The primary difference is seen in the QRS complexes. However, these changes may only occur in certain ECG leads. This is why it is important to monitor leads correctly.

To understand conduction blocks, it is important to understand how the ventricles depolarize. Normally, the ventricles depolarize in the following manner: As the impulse spreads from the bundle of His, the left bundle depolarizes slightly ahead of the right. This causes the ventricular septum to be depolarized in a left-to-right direction. Leads with a positive electrode on the right side of the heart view this depolarization wave (vector) as coming toward it, creating an R wave (Fig. 4-12). Leads with a positive electrode on the left side of the heart view this wave as heading away from it, creating a Q wave.

As the impulse spreads to the rest of the heart, the main depolarization wave is directed inferiorly and to the left (Fig. 4-13). This is due to the influence of the large left ventricle related to the size of the right ventricle. Depolarization in this manner creates an S wave for right-sided leads and an R wave for left-sided leads.

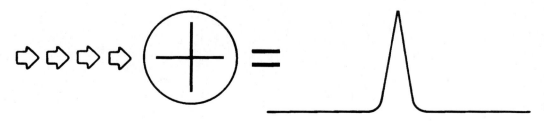

Figure 4-12. Depolarization occurring toward the positive electrode.

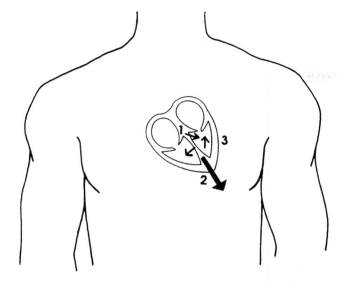

Figure 4-13. Ventricular depolarization vectors.

With conduction disturbances, these normal depolarization waves can be altered. Understanding the changes in depolarization waves is the key to interpreting conduction defects.

Right Bundle Branch Block

A right bundle branch block (RBBB) has two common characteristics, a triphasic pattern (rSR′) in lead V_1 and a deep S wave in lead I (Fig. 4-14). Since the right bundle is blocked, a delayed rightward vector is created. This causes a third wave heading toward the positive electrode in V_1, resulting in a triphasic pattern. It simultaneously produces a wave headed away from the positive electrode in lead I. This causes a deep S wave in lead I. It will also cause a deep S wave in other lateral leads, such as V_6.

An RBBB might have a widening of the QRS but usually by no more than 0.14 s. P waves are usually visible in front of the rSR′ pattern, although they might be lost in the preceding T wave. Variations of the rSR′ pattern are occasionally found; however, the PCCN exam is not likely to cover complex variations from these common conduction patterns.

Left Bundle Branch Block

A left bundle branch block (LBBB) also has two common characteristics, a QS wave in lead V_1 and a wide, notched R wave in leads I and V_6 (Fig. 4-15).

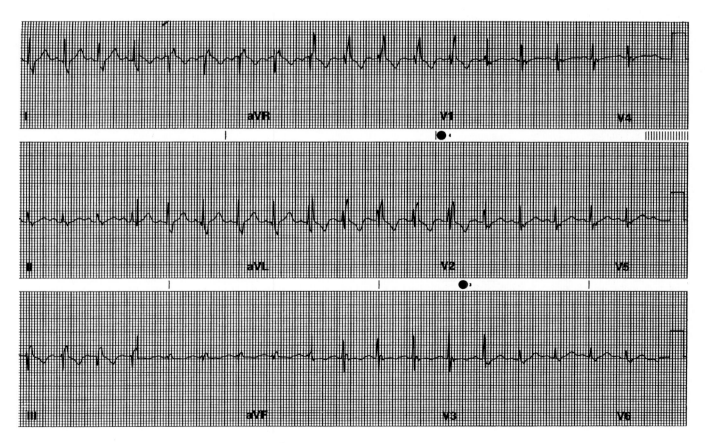

Figure 4-14. RBBB characteristics.

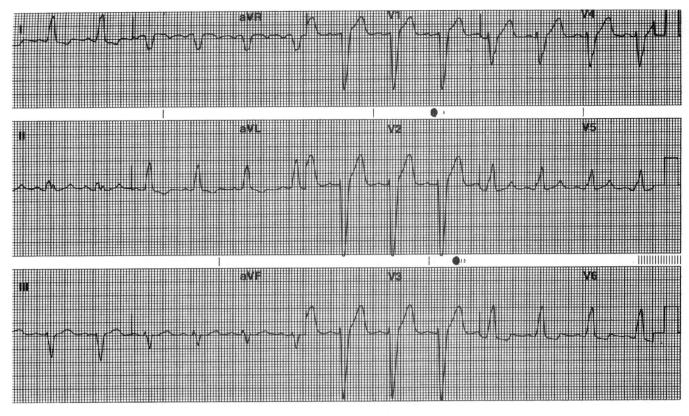

Figure 4-15. LBBB characteristics.

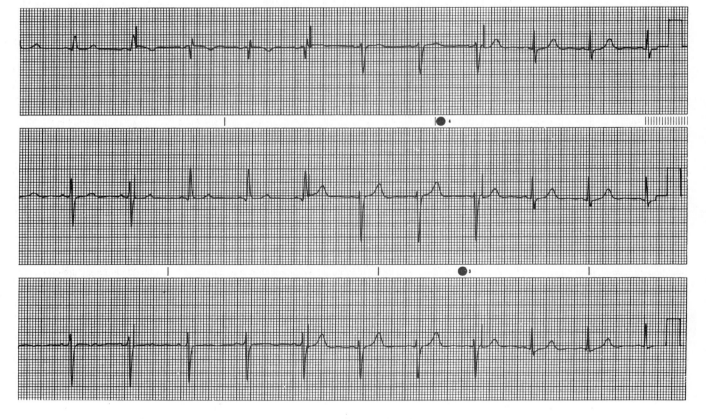

Figure 4-16. Anterior hemiblock characteristics.

With an LBBB, the normal initial septal depolarization is altered. The first vector created is from the right bundle, creating a rightward-directed depolarization wave. This is seen by right-sided chest leads (like V_1) as headed away from it, creating a Q wave. Left-sided chest leads see this as an R wave (lead I).

LBBBs are almost always wide (>0.12 s) and frequently notched. P waves are usually visible but can be lost in the preceding T wave. As with RBBBs, there are some variations from these patterns, but they are not as common.

Anterior Hemiblocks

An anterior hemiblock occurs when the anterior portion of the left bundle is obstructed (Fig. 4-16). The result is a shift in axis forces to the left (usually greater than −60 degrees). This left axis deviation also causes leads II, III, and aVF to become inverted.

Small Q waves may be noted in leads I and aVL. There may or may not be a prolongation of the QRS complex.

Posterior Hemiblocks

A posterior hemiblock occurs when the posterior portion of the left bundle is obstructed. The result is a shift in the axis to the right. The vector in this direction causes large R waves in II, III, and aVF (Fig. 4-17). Small R waves with deep S waves are present in I and aVL. There may or may not be a prolongation of the QRS.

LEFT AND RIGHT VENTRICULAR HYPERTROPHY

Left ventricular hypertrophy (LVH) causes more electrical forces to be generated on the left side of the heart. This can understandably lead to left axis

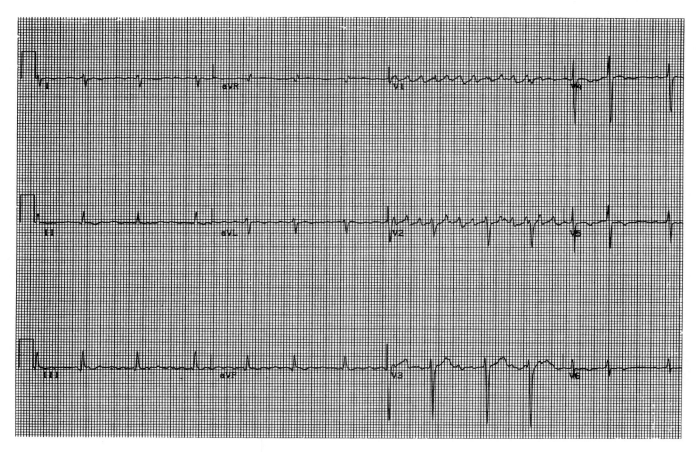

Figure 4-17. Posterior hemiblock characteristics.

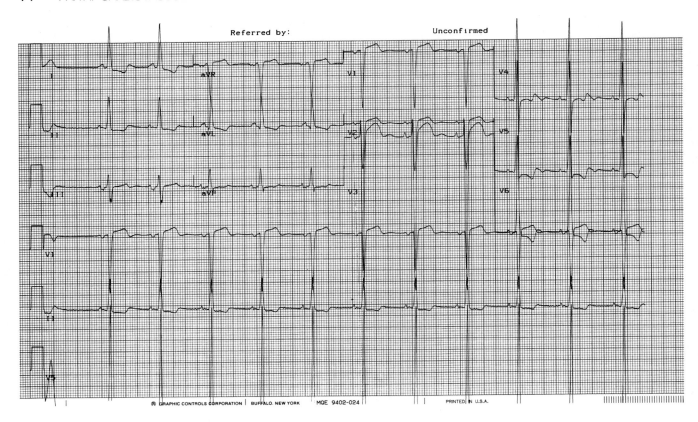

Figure 4-18. Left ventricular hypertrophy.

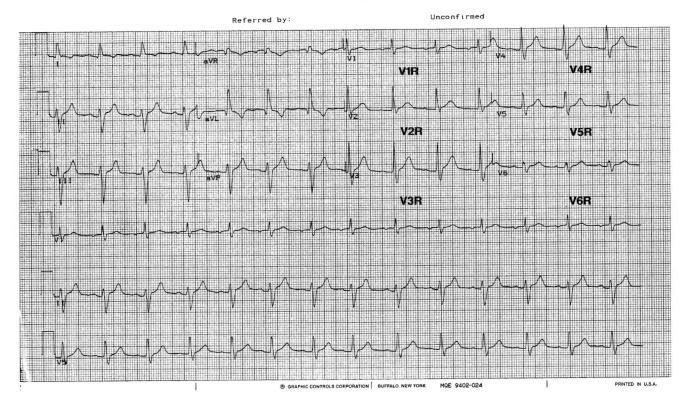

Figure 4-19. Right precordial leads.

TABLE 4-4. CRITERIA FOR LEFT AND RIGHT VENTRICULAR HYPERTROPHY

Condition	Leads and Criteria
Left ventricular hypertrophy	S wave in V_1 + R wave in V_5 >35 mm
	$R_1 + S_3$ >26 mm
Right ventricular hypertrophy	V_3R and V_1 and V_2, R > S V_4R, R:S ratio >1:1

deviation. The leads viewing the heart on the left side (such as V_5 and V_6) will reflect the increased electrical activity by having large R waves. Leads on the right side show large S waves, the opposite of large R waves. The most common criterion for diagnosing LVH is a combination of right and left precordial chest leads. For example, if the height of the R wave in V_5 combined with the depth of the S wave in V_1 exceeds 35 mm, the voltage criterion for LVH is present (Fig. 4-18).

Right ventricular hypertrophy (RVH) is better noted from right precordial leads. Leads V_3R and V_4R are better able to pick out changes in right ventricular size through the presence of large R waves (R:S ratio >1:1). Figure 4-19 illustrates right precordial leads. In addition to possible right axis deviation, the best criteria for RVH include a large R wave in V_1 and V_2 and a deep S in V_5 and V_6. Table 4-4 lists criteria for left and right ventricular hypertrophy.

SUMMARY

If you understand the concepts briefly presented in this chapter, you should do well on the PCCN 12-lead questions. It is more likely that questions will be oriented toward infarction and ischemia, although an occasional question on other areas may appear. However, if they do appear, there will not be many of them.

5

Hemodynamic Monitoring

EDITORS' NOTE

The purpose of this chapter is to review the concepts associated with hemodynamic monitoring, discuss the technology utilized in hemodynamic monitoring, and present methods for interpreting hemodynamic parameters. It is essential that nurses who are planning to take the PCCN exam understand the content of this chapter. There will be several questions taken directly from material covered here. Normally, the questions focus on interpreting hemodynamic data. There will be few if any questions on hemodynamic technology. However, to be safe, key concepts in hemodynamic monitoring, in terms of both interpretation and technology, are presented. There is also a good website, www.pacep.org, that could be helpful in reviewing these concepts.

MONITORING HEMODYNAMIC DATA

Hemodynamic monitoring of critical care patients is commonly used, particularly in cases involving shock states. The technology has changed substantially over the past decade, with less use of flow-directed pulmonary artery catheters (also commonly called Swan-Ganz catheters). Many hospitals are using other technologies, including esophageal and surface Doppler, bioimpedance, pulse contour, and exhaled CO_2. Triple-lumen oximetry is also becoming popular. However, the PCCN will focus on the concepts of hemodynamic monitoring more than the technology. This chapter will prepare you for the exam regardless of the technology being used. Do not focus on learning the technologies.

Cardiac Output, Stroke Volume, and Tissue Oxygenation

The key parameters obtained from hemodynamic monitoring are measures of tissue oxygenation (SvO_2 or $ScvO_2$), cardiac output, and stroke volume. Tissue oxygenation is assessed first as a rule, since the purpose of blood flow is to provide adequate nutrients, such as oxygen, to the tissues. Blood flow parameters are assessed next. If these parameters are adequate, tissue oxygenation is generally adequate; if they are abnormal, a threat to tissue oxygenation may exist. However, stroke volume changes before other parameters, even tissue oxygenation. It is important always to measure stroke volume first and realize that all treatments for the heart focus on improving stroke volume first. In the past, only a pulmonary artery catheter could provide stroke volume during routine bedside monitoring. Now, a number of techniques are available. One technique, the esophageal Doppler, has nine randomized controlled trials demonstrating a reduction in the length of stay in the hospital when it is used to guide stroke volume optimization. The PCCN has not yet emphasized stroke volume as much as needed, but it should become standard practice before long.

Oxygenation and Hemodynamics

It is critical to understand that the human cardiopulmonary system exists only to provide nutrients to the tissues, with the primary nutrient being oxygen. Hence, hemodynamics need to be viewed in terms of the adequacy of tissue oxygenation.

Several parameters reflect tissue oxygenation (Table 5-1). However, the most helpful in terms of real-time monitoring is the mixed venous oxyhemoglobin (SvO_2) measurement. SvO_2 are values obtained from the pulmonary artery. $ScvO_2$ (central

TABLE 5-1. MEASURES OF TISSUE OXYGENATION

Parameter	Normal Level	Consider Intervention
SvO_2	60%–75%	<60% or >75%
$ScvO_2$	70%–80%	<70% or >85%
StO_2	75%–85%	<70% or >90%
Lactate	1–2 mmol/L	2 mmol + pH <7.25
		>4 mmol is a medical emergency

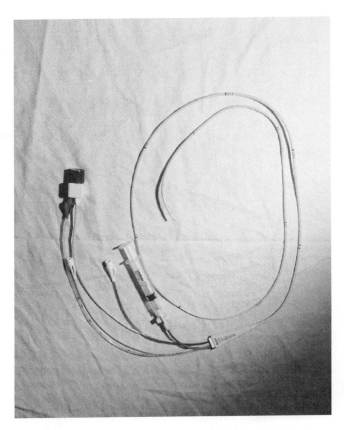

Figure 5-1. Flow-directed pulmonary artery catheter and triple-lumen oximeter.

venous oxygen saturation) values are obtained from the right atrium, as with a triple-lumen oximeter. Both can be used, although the $ScvO_2$ is normally slightly higher than the SvO_2 owing to more mixing of blood from the coronary sinus, inferior and superior vena cava. There are two ways to measure venous oxyhemoglobins:

1. Sampled directly from the distal port of the pulmonary artery catheter or right atrium. When measuring the SvO_2 in the pulmonary artery, draw the sample slowly so as not to aspirate pulmonary capillary blood (producing an arterial-like blood sample).

2. Continuously measured via fiberoptics in the pulmonary artery catheter or triple-lumen oximeter (Fig. 5-1). This technique has the obvious advantage of providing a continuous reading of SvO_2, or $ScvO_2$, avoiding the expense of blood gases and loss of blood as well as the risk of exposure of the nurse to blood.

The value of measuring SvO_2 and $ScvO_2$ centers on the concept that the amount of oxygen returning to the lungs is an accurate reflection of tissue oxygenation. Consider that oxygen is normally removed from hemoglobin as it passes through the capillary bed. Normally, about 25% of the oxygen in hemoglobin is removed. This means the amount of oxygen returning to the lungs still attached to hemoglobin should be about 75%. The oxygen that is in hemoglobin is the only oxygen reserve in the body. If the tissues are deprived of oxygen, either by too little delivery of oxygen (oxygen delivery, DO_2) or an increase in oxygen demand (oxygen consumption, VO_2), the tissues will extract more oxygen from hemoglobin. This extraction occurs as the tissue PO_2 falls, creating an increased oxygen tension gradient between the tissues and blood. In clinical situations,

SvO_2 levels (the amount of oxygen still in hemoglobin when it returns to the lungs) are generally at least 60%. If they drop below this level, a potential threat to tissue oxygenation has to be considered.

Deciding when a hemodynamic parameter, such as cardiac output or blood pressure, has changed in a clinically significant manner is one of the most important responsibilities facing the bedside clinician. The use of SvO_2 monitoring makes the decision-making process easier.

StO_2 (Tissue Oxygenation)

A new parameter, tissue oxygen saturation (StO_2), may be a new method of estimating oxygen extraction. Placed on the thenar aspect of the thumb, it detects oxyhemoglobin in the microcirculation. In theory, as oxygen transport falls and the tissues extract more oxygen, the hand would show changes even before central organs, perhaps even before SvO_2 or $ScvO_2$. As such, StO_2 could become a new monitor. Research in how to best use the technology is still developing.

Lactate Values

Lactate levels are another indicator of tissue oxygenation. Normal levels are 1 to 2 mmol. If the lactate level is increasing, anaerobic metabolism is possibly present. If lactate levels are increasing, monitor for the presence of a metabolic acidosis. Since lactate levels can increase without producing hypoxia if a metabolic acidosis is not present, it is important to monitor both lactate and parameters such as bicarbonate, pH, and base excess. For example, if a lactate level is 4.4 mmol with a pH of 7.30 and a bicarbonate (HCO_3^-) level of 18 (which is low), then hypoxia of the tissues might be present.

Lactate levels do not change as rapidly as SvO_2 or $ScvO_2$ levels, making drug titration a little more difficult if lactate levels are used. Normally, lactate levels are drawn (either arterial or venous samples) once or twice a shift, using SvO_2 as a guide to show whether therapy has improved tissue oxygenation and lactates to confirm the improvement.

Cardiac Output and Index

Normal hemodynamic parameters are given in Table 5-2. Normal cardiac output is usually in the range of 4 to 8 L/min. The cardiac index, which is an adjustment of cardiac output based on the size of the person, is another commonly used descriptor of blood flow. A normal cardiac index is 2.5 to 4.0 L/min/m^2. Levels below 2.2 L/min/m^2 indicate a threat to tissue oxygenation and require that consideration be given to beginning treatment.

Generally, the cardiac index is a better parameter to use than the cardiac output. Some patients tolerate a low cardiac index without clinical problems. It is more useful to track trends in the cardiac index than to monitor single data points since temporary changes in values may not be clinically significant. By

monitoring both cardiac index and tissue oxygenation parameters—such as mixed venous oxyhemoglobin (SvO_2)—together, the clinician can increase the accuracy with which a clinically dangerous event can be identified.

Cardiac output is determined by two factors: heart rate and stroke volume. It is essential to understand heart rate and stroke volume in order to know how to treat abnormal cardiac output. Abnormal cardiac output is most commonly related to a problem with stroke volume.

Stroke Volume, Stroke Index, and Ejection Fraction

Stroke volume is defined as the amount of blood ejected with each heartbeat. The stroke index, like the cardiac index, is a more useful measure that individualizes the stroke volume based on the patient's size.

The ejection fraction is defined as the amount of blood pumped with each contraction in relation to the amount of blood available to be pumped. For example, assume the left ventricular (LV) end-diastolic volume (LVEDV), the amount of blood left in the heart just before contraction, is about 100 mL and that the stroke volume is 80 mL. Since 80 mL of the possible 100 mL in the ventricle is ejected, the ejection fraction is 80%. A normal ejection fraction is usually 60% or more.

In any condition in which the heart begins to malfunction, the stroke volume/index will decline; however, in certain circumstances, such as LV failure and sepsis, the stroke volume may not initially decline because of the heart's compensatory mechanisms. If a patient with coronary artery disease begins to have LV dysfunction, the left ventricle will dilate, causing the LVEDV to increase. Although the increase in LVEDV might prevent a drop in stroke volume, dysfunction can still be detected by observing a drop in the ejection fraction. For example, assume a patient starts with the following:

LVEDV	90 mL
Stroke volume	65 mL
Ejection fraction	72% (65/90)

Over time, the same patient begins to have LV dysfunction with dilation of the left ventricle. Although the heart muscle begins to weaken, the stroke volume is maintained by the increase in LVEDV:

LVEDV	150 mL
Stroke volume	65 mL
Ejection fraction	43% (65/150)

TABLE 5-2. NORMAL HEMODYNAMIC PARAMETERS

Parameter	Normal Level	Consider Intervention
Stroke volume	50–100 mL/beat	<50 mL
Stroke index	25–45 mL/m^2	<25 mL
Cardiac output	4–8 L/min	<4 L/min
Cardiac index	2.5–4 L/min/m^2	<2.2 L/min/m^2
Ejection fraction	>60%	<40%
Wedge pressure (PCWP or PAOP)	8–12 mm Hg	<8 (hypovolemia)[a] >18 (LV failure)[a]
Central venous pressure	2–5 mm Hg	<2 (hypovolemia)[a] <10 (RV failure)

[a]If stroke volume is low.
LV, left ventricle; PCWP, pulmonary capillary wedge pressure; PAOP, pulmonary artery occlusive pressure; RV, right ventricle.

Notice that the stroke volume is maintained but the ejection fraction falls and LVEDV rises, reflecting early LV dysfunction. Because changes in the ejection fraction (and end-diastolic volumes) can provide early warning of ventricular dysfunction, they are ideal monitoring parameters. Unfortunately, monitoring of these parameters is not routinely available because of limitations in technology.

The stroke volume or index thus becomes the single most important piece of information regarding cardiac function in the absence of ejection fraction monitoring. The stroke volume is extremely important because it will typically fall once blood volume becomes too low (hypovolemia) or the left ventricle becomes too weak (LV dysfunction) to eject blood. In some cases, as with exercise or in clinical conditions such as sepsis, the stroke volume can be increased; however, low stroke volume is more commonly found during hemodynamic monitoring. For the diagnosis of hypovolemia or LV dysfunction to be made, there generally must be a reduced stroke volume.

Regulation of Stroke Volume

Three factors regulate stroke volume: preload, afterload, and contractility. Definitions of preload, afterload, and contractility are presented in Table 5-3. Preload is concerned with factors that affect the stretch of myocardial muscle, including the pressure and volume in the ventricle as well as the compliance (ability to stretch) of the muscle.

TABLE 5-3. DETERMINANTS OF STROKE VOLUME

Preload	Amount of stretch in a muscle just before contraction	Estimated by the PCWP for LV assessment and by the CVP for RV assessment Also estimated by FTc and SVV
Afterload	Resistance a muscle faces as it attempts to contract	Estimated by the SVR for LV resistance by the PVR for RV resistance
Contractility	Strength of the muscle contraction	Estimated by SV and PCWP or CVP. If the stroke volume is low and the PCWP or CVP is high, then the heart is assumed to be weakened Can also be estimated by ejection fraction and peak velocity

CVP, central venous pressure; FTc, flow time; LV, left ventricle; PAOP, pulmonary artery occlusive pressure; PCWP, pulmonary capillary wedge pressure; PVR, pulmonary vascular resistance; RV, right ventricle; SV, stroke volume; SVR, systemic vascular resistance; SVV, stroke volume variation.

According to Starling's law, the more a muscle stretches, the more forceful the contraction. If the muscle stretches too much, however, the contraction becomes weaker. It is difficult to measure preload in clinical practice, and so we estimate it from the ventricular filling pressure. If the ventricular filling pressure increases beyond normal (normal LV diastolic filling pressure is about 8 to 12 mm Hg), it is assumed that the left ventricle is weakening. If the pressure exceeds 18 mm Hg, the ventricle is assumed to be near failure level (the point where the muscle is stretching excessively). Conversely, when the ventricular filling pressure is too low (<8 mm Hg), it is assumed that the blood volume is low (hypovolemia).

This estimate is frequently inaccurate, since pressure alone does not determine preload. However, the assumption used to estimate preload is important to understand since it is widely used in critical care. To increase the accuracy of assessments based on pressure alone, pressure measurements should always be compared with the stroke volume or stroke index. As the filling pressures elevate, they should decrease the stroke index if they are clinically significant. If the filling pressures are low, the stroke index must be low as well before hypovolemia can be assumed to exist. It is essential to combine the stroke index with the filling pressure in order to avoid misinterpreting the filling pressure.

Newer Measures

New technologies, like the esophageal and surface Doppler, give indications of cardiac strength through peak velocity measurements (normal 50 to 120 cm/s). These technologies also give indications of volume status through systolic flow time (FTc) (i.e. time spent in systole), with normal levels of 330 to 360 mm/sec. If a patient has a low PV, then left ventricular weakness is present. If the flow time is low, then hypovolemia is suspected.

Stroke Volume Variation

In patients on mechanical ventilation, fluctuations in stroke volume during mechanical ventilation might indicate volume status. For example, if the change in stroke volume is greater than 10% during mechanical ventilation, hypovolemia might be present.

Heart Rate

The heart rate must be evaluated in order to detect early changes in hemodynamics. Since cardiac output is a product of stroke volume multiplied by heart rate, any change in stroke volume will normally produce a change in the heart rate. If the stroke volume is elevated, the heart rate may decrease (as seen in adaptation to exercise). The exception to this guideline is during an increase in metabolic rate, in which both the stroke volume and the heart rate increase.

If the stroke volume falls, the heart rate normally increases; thus evaluation of tachycardias becomes an essential component of hemodynamic monitoring. Generally, bradycardia and tachycardia are significant because they may reflect a potentially dangerous interference in cardiac output. Bradycardia that develops suddenly is almost always reflective of a threat to cardiac output. Tachycardia, a more common clinical situation, may also indicate a threat to cardiac output.

Sinus tachycardia develops for three reasons:

1. An increase in metabolic rate (as with a temperature elevation)
2. A psychological factor (anxiety, fear)
3. A reduction in stroke volume

All three factors need to be considered in evaluating a rapid heart rate. For example, if a patient has a heart rate of 120 beats per minute, the clinician must rule out a fever or anxiety or pain before assuming that the heart rate is increased due to a reduced stroke volume.

If the heart rate is increased and a raised metabolic rate or a psychological factor does not appear to be the cause, then a low stroke volume is suspected and an investigation into its cause is necessary. The two most common reasons for a low stroke volume are hypovolemia and LV dysfunction. Both causes of low stroke volume can produce an increased heart rate if no abnormality exists in regulation of the heart rate (such as autonomic nervous system dysfunction or the use of drugs that interfere with the sympathetic or parasympathetic nervous system).

An increased heart rate can compensate for a decrease in stroke volume, although this compensation is limited. The faster the heart rate, the less time there is for ventricular filling. Because an increased heart rate reduces diastolic filling time, the potential exists eventually to reduce the stroke volume. There is no specific heart rate at which diastolic filling is reduced so severely that stroke volume decreases. However, it should be remembered that as the heart rate increases, stroke volumes can be negatively affected.

Another important concept regarding heart rate has to do with the effect it has on myocardial oxygen consumption (MVo_2). The higher the heart rate, the more likely it is that the heart will consume more oxygen. Typically, the MVo_2 can only be estimated because direct measurement is not easy. Since heart rate is not the only determinant of oxygen consumption (contractility and vascular resistance are also determinants), heart rate alone will not predict MVo_2. Keeping heart rates as low as possible, particularly in patients with altered myocardial blood flow, is one way of protecting myocardial function.

Hemodynamic Pressures

Hemodynamic pressures are among the most common parameters monitored in critical care. Blood pressure, central venous pressure (CVP), and pulmonary artery and pulmonary capillary wedge pressures ([PCWP]/pulmonary artery occlusive pressure [PAOP]) are sometimes monitored in the care of critically ill patients. New, less invasive parameters are increasingly being used with a reduced emphasis on use of cardiac pressures. Although it is important to be able to apply the significance of cardiac pressures to patient conditions in critical care, it is unlikely that values such as the CVP and PCWP will appear on the PCCN.

Interpreting Arterial Pressures

The arterial pressure is among the most commonly used parameters to assess the adequacy of blood flow to the tissues. Although the blood pressure is often misleading, it is still one of the most commonly used parameters in hemodynamic monitoring. Whereas the role of blood pressure in patient assessment needs serious review based on its inaccuracy, the measurement of blood pressure is still a standard of care. Blood pressure is determined by two factors: cardiac output and systemic vascular resistance (SVR). This fact is critical to the interpretation of blood pressure. Blood pressure will not reflect early clinical changes in hemodynamics because of a compensatory mechanism by which cardiac output and SVR interact to maintain adequate blood pressure. Although this interaction is not always predictable, it works as follows: If the cardiac output decreases, the SVR will increase just enough to overcome the fall in cardiac output and maintain blood pressure at near normal levels (Table 5-4). Conversely, if the SVR falls, the cardiac output will increase to offset the fall in SVR.

In addition, the cardiac output is maintained by the heart rate and stroke volume. The two interact to keep the cardiac output normal. If the stroke volume begins to fall because of loss of volume (hypovolemia) or dysfunction (LV failure), the heart rate will increase

TABLE 5-4. REGULATION OF BLOOD PRESSURE

Cardiac Output	Systemic Vascular Resistance	Blood Pressure
Normal	Normal	Normal
Decreased	Increased	Remains near normal
Increased	Decreased	Remains near normal
Increased	Increased	Rapidly elevates
Decreased	Decreased	Rapidly falls

to offset this decrease in stroke volume. The net effect will be to maintain the cardiac output at near normal levels. If the cardiac output does not change, there will be no change in the blood pressure.

The key point to these interactions is that the blood pressure cannot signal early clinical changes. If a patient begins to bleed postoperatively, the blood pressure will generally not reflect this event until it becomes so severe that an increase in the heart rate and SVR no longer compensates. This is also the case for patients who have congestive heart failure or myocardial infarction.

Blood pressure is typically defined as normal if it falls within the following parameters: systolic 90 to 140 mm Hg, diastolic 60 to 90 mm Hg, mean 65 to 110 mm Hg. Blood pressure is considered normal if two problems can be ruled out: hypotension, which is associated with inadequate blood flow to the tissues, and hypertension, which is associated with excessive pressure and damage to the peripheral circulation.

Hypotension is probably present if there is evidence of deficits in tissue oxygenation. Blood pressure, therefore, must be assessed along with measures of tissue oxygenation, such as SvO_2 and lactate levels. The implication of the interaction between tissue oxygenation and blood pressure is that blood pressure cannot be viewed in isolation.

Hypertension is more difficult to identify since there are fewer clinical parameters to indicate when peripheral circulatory changes are occurring. However, pressure alone is an important determinant of circulatory damage. As such, it is a little more reliable as a parameter in hypertension than in hypotension. Studies of hypertension-induced injury have not shown clearly what blood pressure produces actual injury. As a guideline, however, a systolic blood pressure of 140 mm Hg or greater is considered potentially injurious to the circulation.

Interpreting Pulmonary Artery Pressures

Pulmonary artery and cardiac pressures are typically obtained from a flow-directed catheter inserted into a major vein and directed into the heart and pulmonary artery (Figs. 5-2 and 5-3). Since the pulmonary vasculature is normally a low-resistance system, the pulmonary artery blood pressure is generally approximately 25/10 mm Hg. If the pressure in the pulmonary vasculature rises, the capillary hydrostatic pressure exceeds capillary osmotic pressure and fluid is forced out of the vessels. Interstitial and alveolar flooding can then occur, with resulting interference in oxygen and carbon dioxide exchange.

The pulmonary artery pressures can be helpful in diagnosing many clinical conditions. Pulmonary artery pressure greater than 35/20 mm Hg is considered pulmonary hypertension. Application of pulmonary artery pressure values are unlikely to appear on the PCCN exam.

Interpreting the Central Venous Pressure

The determination of intracardiac pressure frequently centers on measurement of atrial pressure. Atrial pressure is used to estimate ventricular end-diastolic pressures. Ventricular end-diastolic pressure is potentially useful, since it partially reflects preload. Right atrial pressure is also referred to as the central venous pressure (CVP); left atrial pressure is referred to as the pulmonary capillary wedge pressure (PCWP) (also called pulmonary artery occlusive pressure [PAOP]).

The CVP is an estimate of right ventricular (RV) end-diastolic pressure (RVEDP) and is used to assess the performance of the right ventricle. The guidelines for interpreting the CVP have traditionally been relatively simple. The CVP is normally between 2 and 6 mm Hg. However, current guidelines are to keep the CVP between 8 and 12 mm Hg to avoid hypovolemia, and perhaps greater than 12 mm Hg if the patient is on mechanical ventilation. If the CVP is low, hypovolemia is assumed to exist. If the CVP is normal, normovolemia is present. If the CVP is high, RV dysfunction and fluid overload may be present. Although an understanding of how to apply these cardiac pressures is valuable when caring for critical care patients, questions regarding pressure values will probably not appear on the PCCN exam. However, the best way to interpret pressure values is to compare them to another parameter, such as the stroke index. If both the CVP and the stroke index are low, then hypovolemia is likely. However, if the CVP is low and the stroke index is normal, then hypovolemia may not be present. The opposite is also true; that is, if the CVP is high and the stroke index is low, RV dysfunction is probable. However, if

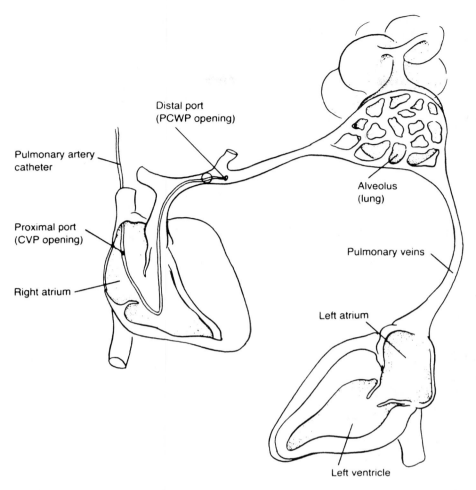

Figure 5-2. Pulmonary artery catheter in place within the pulmonary artery. (Adapted from Ahrens, T. S. [1992]. *Hemodynamic Waveform Recognition.* Philadelphia: Saunders. With permission.)

the CVP is high and the stroke index is normal, then RV dysfunction may not be present (or clinically significant). Perhaps the most difficult part of interpreting pressures is that normal pressures do not indicate normal cardiac functioning. The significance of cardiac pressure trending over time is also far more valuable than point-in-time readings.

Although the CVP is useful in assessing RV function, the assessment of LV function is generally more important. If the left ventricle dysfunctions (such as with myocardial infarction or cardiomyopathies), then a threat to tissue oxygenation and survival may exist.

The CVP is commonly used to fluid volume status, despite evidence suggesting that it is almost worthless. A far more accurate assessment of volume response is to measure stroke volume and observe how it changes with fluid administration or other therapies.

Interpreting the Pulmonary Capillary Wedge Pressure

Assessment of LV preload is commonly performed by obtaining the PCWP. The use of the PCWP to estimate left ventricular end-diastolic pressure (LVEDP) is based on the assumption that a measurement from an obstructed pulmonary capillary will reflect an uninterrupted flow of blood to the left atrium since there are no valves in the pulmonary arterial system. A second assumption is that when the mitral valve is open, left atrial pressure reflects LVEDP. As long as these assumptions are accurate, the use of the PCWP to estimate LVEDP is acceptable. The guidelines for interpreting the PCWP are relatively simple and similar to those of CVP interpretation. Normal PCWP is about 8 to 12 mm Hg. If the PCWP is low, hypovolemia is assumed to be present. If the PCWP is normal, normovolemia is present. If the PCWP is high,

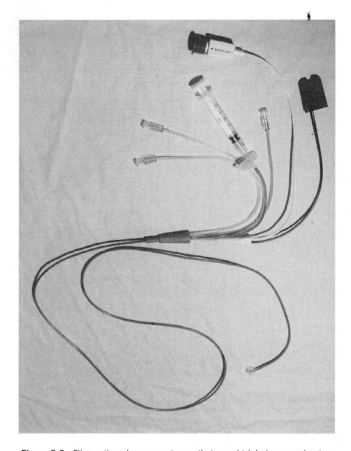

Figure 5-3. Fiberoptic pulmonary artery catheter and triple-lumen oximeter.

LV dysfunction is present. However, PCWP interpretation has the same limitations as CVP interpretation, plus a few more. As with the CVP, the PCWP should not be interpreted in isolation. In analyzing the PCWP, always use the stroke index to help interpret the value. If the PCWP is low and the stroke index is low, hypovolemia is probable. If the PCWP is low and the stroke index is normal, hypovolemia is not likely. Use care when interpreting high PCWP values as well. If the PCWP is high and the stroke index is low, LV dysfunction is probable. However, if the PCWP is high and the stroke index is normal, LV dysfunction may not be present (or clinically significant).

Systemic and Pulmonary Vascular Resistance

One of the most common derived parameters is vascular resistance (Table 5-5). Vascular resistance is frequently assumed to represent afterload, or the resistance the ventricles face during ejection of blood. It is important to keep in mind that afterload is not measured by vascular resistance alone. Afterload is

also influenced by blood viscosity and valvular resistance. While these values can change, vascular resistance can be used to estimate afterload since viscosity and valvular resistance tend to change less often than blood vessel resistance.

In clinical practice, this formula is:

$$SVR = \frac{Mean\ arterial\ pressure - right\ atrial\ pressure}{Cardiac\ output}$$

The value obtained from this formula is then multiplied by a factor of 80 to generate a value measured in dynes/s/cm^5.

Two types of vascular resistance are commonly measured, systemic and pulmonary. Systemic vascular resistance (SVR) reflects LV afterload, whereas pulmonary vascular resistance (PVR) reflects RV afterload.

Normal SVR is about 900 to 1300 dynes/s/cm^5. If the SVR is elevated, the left ventricle will face increased resistance to the ejection of blood. The SVR commonly rises for two reasons. It can increase in response to primary systemic hypertension or secondary systemic hypertension (peripheral vascular disease) or to compensate for a low cardiac output, as would occur in shock states. It is important for the clinician to know why the SVR is elevated. If the SVR is elevated because of systemic hypertension, afterload-reducing agents are a critical part of the therapy. However, if the SVR is elevated in compensation for low cardiac output, therapy is directed at improving the cardiac output more than reducing SVR.

If the SVR is low, the left ventricle meets with lower resistance to the ejection of blood. Generally, the SVR does not lower except as a pathologic response to inflammation. The SVR can also be reduced in hepatic disease (because of increased

TABLE 5-5. NORMAL DERIVED HEMODYNAMIC PARAMETERS

Parameter	Normal Level	Consider Intervention
Mean arterial pressure (MAP)	65–110 mm Hg	<65 mm Hg
Mean pulmonary arterial pressure (MPAP)	15–25 mm Hg	>25 mm Hg
Systemic vascular resistance (SVR)	900–1300 dynes/s/cm^5	<800 dynes/s/cm^5 >1500 dynes/s/cm^5
Pulmonary vascular resistance (PVR)[a]	40–150 dynes/s/cm^5	>200 dynes/s/cm^5

[a]Where MAP = [(2 × DBP) + SBP]/3; MPAP = [(2 × DPAP) + SPAP]/3; SVR = [MAP − CVP × 80]/CO; PVR = [MPAP − PCWP × 80]/CO, where DBP/SBP = diastolic/systolic blood pressure, DPAP/SPAP = diastolic/systolic pulmonary artery pressure, and CO = cardiac output.

collateral circulation) or neurogenic-induced central vasodilation. If the SVR is reduced, attempts to increase the resistance center on vasopressors. More important to consider, though, is the treatment of the underlying condition. If the underlying condition is not treated, the use of vasopressors will provide only short-term success.

Pulmonary vascular resistance reflects the work the right ventricle faces as it attempts to contract. The PVR is normally between 40 and 150 dynes/s/cm^5. The PVR rises for one of three reasons: (1) primary pulmonary hypertension; (2) secondary active pulmonary hypertension; or (3) secondary passive pulmonary hypertension. In primary pulmonary hypertension, the cause is unknown and the PVR is markedly elevated. No known cure exists for this condition, although lung transplantation and use of prostacyclins and vasodilators may help alleviate symptoms and prolong life. In secondary active pulmonary hypertension, a cause is known but the condition is not very responsive to treatment. For example, chronic obstructive pulmonary disease or pulmonary emboli can cause this type of pulmonary hypertension. Secondary passive pulmonary hypertension is the result of LV dysfunction. In this case, the pulmonary arterial pressure decreases as LV function improves. It is the most responsive pulmonary hypertension in terms of treatment. Also, this form of pulmonary hypertension can be identified by noting the close correlation between the PCWP and the pulmonary artery diastolic pressure (normally the pulmonary artery diastolic pressure is slightly higher than the PCWP).

INTERPRETING HEMODYNAMIC WAVEFORMS

EDITORS' NOTE

....

Reading hemodynamic waveforms is the key to obtaining the pressures used in hemodynamic monitoring. Learning how to read waveforms is very easy, however there are unlikely to be any questions that address this content on the PCCN exam.

....

6

Acute Coronary Syndrome (Angina Pectoris and Myocardial Infarction)

EDITORS' NOTE

The PCCN exam can be expected to contain many questions on assessing and treating coronary artery disease. This chapter provides brief but key concepts in the area of coronary artery disease. Expect several questions in the PCCN exam on the assessment, diagnosis, and treatment of angina and myocardial infarction.

Acute coronary syndrome (ACS) describes a continuum of coronary artery disease (CAD). Acute coronary heart disease encompasses partial loss of myocardial blood and ischemia (angina) to complete occlusion of the coronary artery without collateral circulation resulting in myocardial infarction (MI). MIs are subdivided into ST-segment elevation myocardial infarctions (STEMI) and non–ST-segment elevation myocardial infarctions (NSTEMI). This chapter emphasizes the key features of the origin, symptomatology, and medical and nursing interventions associated with ACS. Angina (including coronary artery vasospasm and unstable angina) and MI are common test items on the PCCN exam.

The chapter starts with a brief section on the pathophysiology of ACS. However, most of the chapter is centered on the diagnosis and treatment of ACS. The chapter is sequentially focused, beginning with a patient with chest pain or being admitted with suspected ACS. This approach allows for differentiating angina, unstable angina, NSTEMI, and STEMI, along with the differences in their treatment.

PATHOPHYSIOLOGY

The PCCN exam will not ask many questions on the pathophysiology of ACS. However, it is important to understand a few key concepts. These should prepare you for the exam as well as for clinical practice.

Plaque (atheroma) rupture with the precipitation of vasospasm and clot formation is the likely precipitating event in myocardial ischemia and ACS. A combination of chronic lipid accumulation and acute endothelial injury with subsequent thrombosis formation probably forms the basis for plaque formation and eventual obstruction of blood flow.

There is increasing evidence for the role of inflammation in the generation of the obstruction. The inflammation may be subclinical and initially unrelated to the plaque. Markers of inflammation, such as C-reactive protein, are increasingly being seen as suggestive of CAD. A normal level of C-reactive protein is 0.03 to 1.1 mg/dL. Such inflammation is likely in the coronary artery rather than from any ischemic area.

Over time, atherosclerotic lesions (atheromata) form. These lesions are asymmetric, isolated thickenings in the coronary arteries (as well as other arteries throughout the body). They form in the intima, the innermost lining of the heart. The atheroma consists of several different types of cells, including endothelial, smooth muscle, and inflammatory cells. The atheroma is preceded by a fatty deposit, which is composed of lipid cells beneath the endothelium. Why such an atheroma develops is still under investigation. Young people can have atheromas that are asymptomatic or disappear. However, in patients with ACS, the atheroma interferes with blood flow. In the past, it was thought that the atheroma caused severe narrowing of the coronary artery, which caused the symptoms of ACS. Such narrowing is not likely the only cause, owing to the development of collateral circulation as the plaque extends. Recent research suggests that it is not always the degree of narrowing as much as it is the degree to which the atheroma or plaque is activated, resulting in plaque rupture or endothelial rupture.

Activation of an atheroma or plaque may be initiated by the rupture of a thin plaque or by an inflammatory response. The activation may be the result of hemodynamic flow or shear factors. This process takes place over time, but for unclear reasons, the plaque will elicit an inflammatory response. That is, the inflammatory macrophages, T cells, and mast cells will help cause a clot to form at the site of the plaque.

After an MI, ventricular remodeling occurs. This includes changes in the size, shape, and thickness of the ventricle, which can occur in both the infarcted and noninfarcted areas.

RISK FACTORS

There are some relatively well-known risk factors for the development of ACS. These can be divided into unalterable and alterable risk factors. For example, unalterable risk factors include:

1. A hereditary predisposition to the development of atherosclerosis.
2. Age, since ACS is more prevalent in older persons than in younger persons.
3. Gender appears to be a factor in the development of atherosclerosis, since the condition develops earlier in men than in women. However, recent evidence suggests incidence of myocardial disease in postmenopausal women begins to approach that in men.

Medically Alterable Risk Factors

1. Hypertension has been shown to be related to the development of atherosclerosis. Close medical treatment of hypertension may slow the development of atherosclerosis.
2. Diabetics develop atherosclerosis more often than nondiabetics. Close medical treatment and control of diabetes may reduce the atherosclerotic process.

3. Hyperlipidemia may have an important bearing on the development and/or progression of atherosclerosis. The presence of low-density lipoproteins appears to be a precursor to the development of atherosclerosis. Medical treatment of hyperlipidemia will help slow the atherosclerotic process.

Personal Alterable Risk Factors

The following can be altered by the individual to decrease the possibility or progression of atherosclerosis:

1. Weight control can be beneficial in reducing the risk of CAD.
2. Cigarette smokers have a higher incidence of heart disease than do nonsmokers. Elimination of smoking will reduce the risk of MI.
3. Sedentary lifestyles predispose to the development of atherosclerosis. Exercising three to four times per week for 30 min or activity that pushes the heart rate into the target zone or aerobic exercise will reduce the rate of CAD.
4. Moderate alcohol intake may reduce the risk of CAD. However, the limitation to moderate intake is difficult for many people, and the risk of alcoholism may outweigh the benefit.

If an individual is sufficiently motivated, the four risk factors mentioned earlier can be incorporated into a personal lifestyle.

PROGNOSIS

One cannot change some risk factors; however, one can alter other risk factors with medical treatment, and one can eliminate some risk factors if so motivated. If risk factors are not modified, atherosclerosis may progress from the development of angina and ischemia to MI, congestive heart failure, or sudden death. Despite the prognosis with alterable risk factors, coronary atherosclerosis is still one of the leading causes of death in the United States.

IDENTIFICATION OF ACS AND ITS TREATMENT

In this section, an easy-to-follow guideline for the treatment of ACS is presented (Figs. 6-1 and 6-2). The guideline walks through the diagnosis and

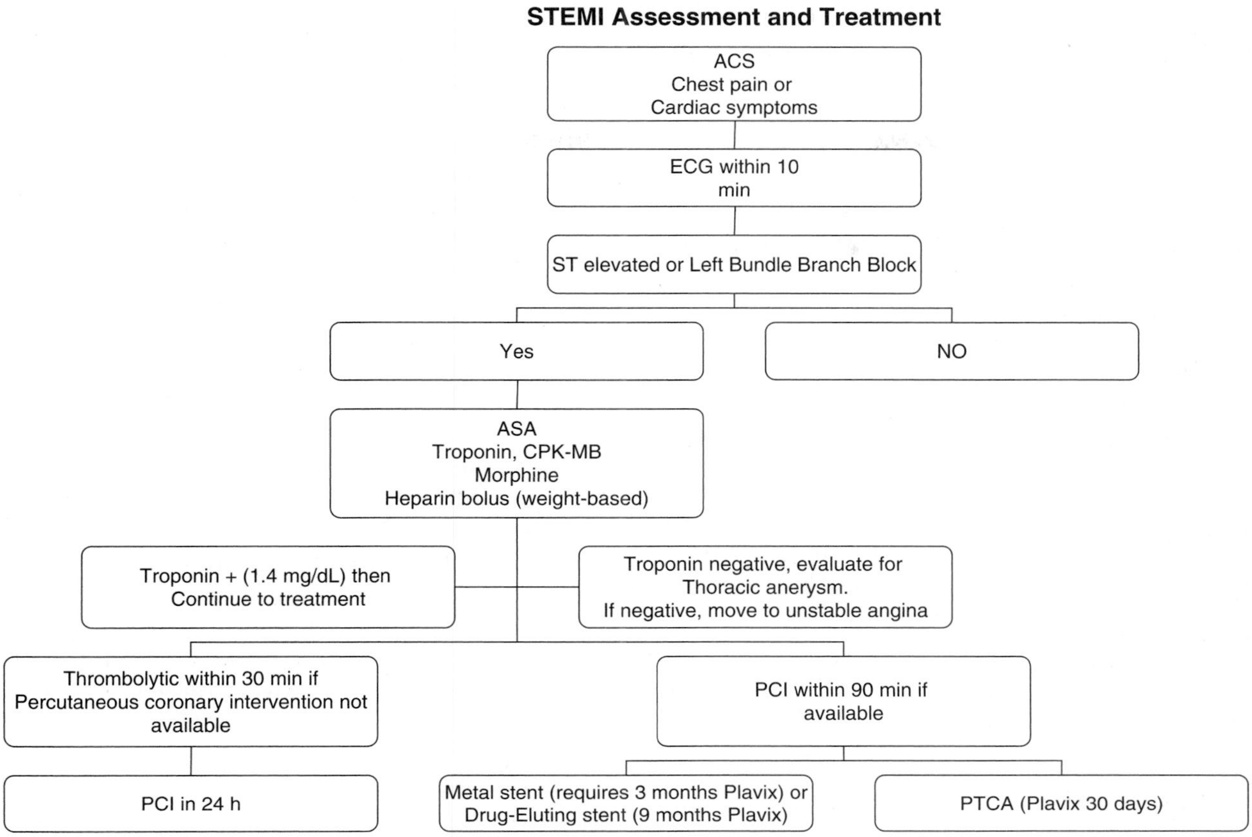

STEMI Assessment and Treatment

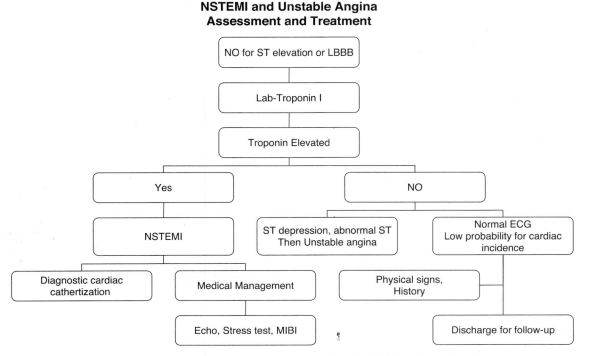

Figure 6-1. Algorithm to assess and treat ST-elevation MI (STEMI).

NSTEMI and Unstable Angina
Assessment and Treatment

Figure 6-2. Algorithm to assess and treat non–ST-elevation MI (NSTEMI) and unstable angina.

treatment of a patient with symptoms of cardiac disease.

The following sections provide a brief overview of MI and angina. The guidelines presented in Figs. 6-1 and 6-2 contain much of what the PCCN will likely expect you to know. These next sections provide additional background information that should help strengthen your overall knowledge of ACS.

ANGINA PECTORIS

Angina can result from a reduced blood flow, low oxygen content, or myocardial oxygen demand in excess of supply. No or minimal injury to the myocardial muscle occurs during most types of angina. Autopsy results of patients with angina have demonstrated frequent total occlusion of coronary vessels with subsequent development of extensive collateral circulation. The development of collateral circulation can allow maintenance of coronary perfusion and no permanent injury to the myocardium even when cardiac catheterization results indicate total occlusion. Differing types of lesions are noted during cardiac catheterization (Fig. 6-3).

Causes of reduced blood flow to the myocardium include atherosclerosis, valvular dysfunction, hypotension, and coronary vasospasm. Low oxygen content can also precipitate anginal episodes. Causes of low oxygen content include reduced hemoglobin and low oxygen pressure/saturation (PaO_2/SaO_2) levels. Causes of excessive oxygen demand relative to

perfusion include hypertension, exercise, and increased metabolic rate. Many predisposing factors can precipitate reduced blood flow, decreased oxygen content, or increased myocardial oxygen demand.

The occurrence of angina is variable, depending substantially on the degree of collateral circulation that has developed. Angina can be suddenly precipitated by any event that increases oxygen demand (such as anxiety, stress, eating, or exercise) or reduces blood flow (smoking).

CLINICAL PRESENTATION

Pain is the primary symptom of angina. It may be described as burning, squeezing in a tight band, or as extreme heaviness or pressure on the lower sternum. It may radiate to the neck, jaws, shoulders, arms, and stomach. Atypical symptoms often found in African Americans and women are fatigue, shortness of breath, indigestion-type symptoms, and shoulder/back discomfort. Characteristically, the pain begins after eating or physical activity and subsides with rest. The pain usually lasts 1 to 4 min, but it may require as long as 10 min to subside completely. Anginal pain should always last less than 30 min. Pain for more than 30 min suggests MI and the need for immediate treatment. Not all CAD will present with anginal symptoms. Some patients can have evidence of ischemia without symptoms. This possibility of ischemia without pain serves as a clue in the education of patients with angina and MI. Frequent evaluation of cardiac status, as with exercise testing, can enable the clinician to detect symptoms early rather than waiting for an anginal episode to indicate ischemia.

DIAGNOSIS

Diagnosis of angina is based on history and electrocardiographic (ECG) findings. Cardiac markers are usually normal. The 12-lead ECG usually has depressed ST segments over the affected area. ST-segment elevation (Prinzmetal's angina) can occur but is less common.

TREATMENT

The pathology of angina is plaque formation without rupture, leading to narrowing of the coronary artery and diminished blood flow. The goal is to dilate the vessels so as to increase the size of the

Variation in Lesions

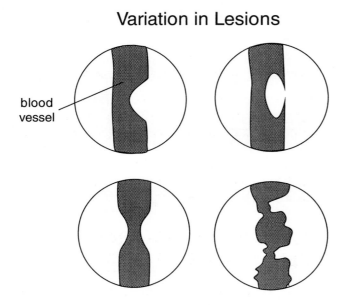

blood vessel

Figure 6-3. Different types of lesions noted during cardiac catheterization.

arterial lumen, decrease oxygen demand, and increase oxygen availability. Vasodilators, such as sublingual nitroglycerin, usually relieve the angina within 0.5 min. Nitroglycerin taken before an activity may prevent an attack. Changing one's lifestyle to eliminate the alterable risk factors may help to decrease the severity and frequency of attacks. If the anginal attacks increase in frequency or intensity (crescendo angina), stress testing and/or cardiac catheterization to determine the extent of the disease is indicated. Nitrates and beta blockers may be used alone or in combination to resolve anginal episodes. The patient may be a candidate for angioplasty or coronary artery bypass surgery, which will stop the angina and decrease the risk of MI. The patient is advised to exercise within the limits of pain and obtain adequate rest. Coronary artery bypass grafting (CABG) is the treatment for failure of medical intervention. CABG has demonstrated the potential for alleviating symptoms of angina, although it does not necessarily prolong life.

UNSTABLE ANGINA

The pathology of unstable angina (UA) includes plaque formation with rupture and platelet activation, hence varying degrees of blood supply and unpredictable discomfort. The platelet activation is the rationale for the American College of Cardiology's (ACC) recommendation for **glycoprotein IIb/IIIa inhibitors** (GP IIb/IIIa) with presentation of UA.

There are several variations of angina, the most prevalent being UA. It differs from stable angina in that it is more easily initiated. UA may involve crescendo angina, may occur at rest, and is characterized by increasing severity. Clinically, the patient may complain that it takes less activity to stimulate an anginal episode and that the severity of symptoms is increasing.

Treatment of UA usually requires additional medical therapy. Beta blockers (e.g., metoprolol) are helpful in reducing myocardial oxygen consumption. Calcium channel blockers (e.g., nifedipine) may be useful in reducing afterload and myocardial oxygen use.

Another type of angina is Prinzmetal's variant angina (PVA). The origin of PVA is thought to be both coronary vasospasm and stenosis. The patient presents with symptoms most often including pain at rest and other symptoms of angina. Patients tend to be younger women who do not have the usual cardiac risk factors (except for smoking). The attacks can be triggered by drinking iced liquids, alcohol,

cocaine, nicotine, and other factors. The attacks tend to fall into a circadian rhythm, often occurring early in the morning and during the menstrual cycle. Calcium channel blockers have a potential benefit due to their ability to relieve or prevent vasospasm.

The ECG shows reversible ST-segment elevation rather than depression. Dysrhythmias may occur with this form of angina, often with marked ST-segment elevation (>4 mm). Sudden cardiac death is markedly more likely with dysrhythmias caused by PVA.

The pathogenesis of PVA is not well understood. Activation of the autonomic nervous system (alpha-adrenergic receptors) seems to be a major factor. Precipitating events are those that stimulate alpha-adrenergic receptors (e.g., acetylcholine) and blocked by alpha-receptor blockers (e.g., atropine, prazosin and clonidine). Autonomic nervous system involvement is supported by the fact that surgical sympathetic denervation has been effective in patients unresponsive to medical therapy.

PVA is diagnosed by 24-h Holter monitoring (to find episodes of symptoms associated with ST-segment elevation) and sympathetic stimulation with ergonovine. Exercise testing and coronary angiography are of little value in the diagnosis of PVA.

Calcium channel blockers have a positive effect in reducing the anginal episode, as do nitrates. Diltiazem, nifedipine, and verapamil are effective in reducing episodes of PVA. An alpha antagonist blocker like prazosin may be useful if nitrates and calcium channel blockers are not effective.

Beta blockers and high-dose aspirin may aggravate PVA. If medical therapy fails, both UA and PVA may require CABG, angioplasty, or stent placement. With treatment and smoking cessation, prognosis with PVA is usually good.

Coronary Artery Vasospasm

Coronary artery vasospasm, a form of variant angina, is a transient narrowing of a large coronary artery. The origins are unclear but could include sympathetic stimulation, prostaglandin mediation, or pharmacologic stimulation. Treatment is similar to that for angina, with more emphasis on calcium channel blockers as well as nitroglycerin.

ACUTE MYOCARDIAL INFARCTION (STEMI AND NSTEMI)

Myocardial infarction is the actual necrosis, or death, of myocardial tissue because of reduced

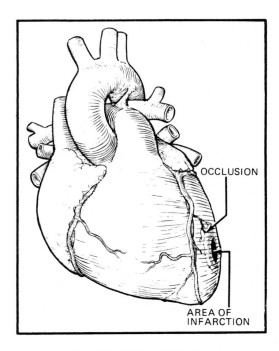

Figure 6-4. Myocardial infarction.

blood supply (loss of oxygen) to a specific area of the heart (Fig. 6-4).

ETIOLOGY

In most MIs, atherosclerotic heart disease is present. The remaining cases of MI are likely due to coronary artery spasm in which the artery constricts enough to prevent blood from reaching the myocardium.

Most MIs have been demonstrated to be the result of the formation of a coronary thrombus on top of an atherosclerotic plaque. The rapid identification of MI is crucial to treatment. Within 6 h of onset, myocardial muscle generally becomes irreversibly damaged. Although this time period can vary and some tissue can be salvaged later, the earlier the treatment, the more likely the recovery.

DIAGNOSIS AND CLINICAL PRESENTATION

Chest pain—with nausea (and maybe vomiting), diaphoresis, and weakness—is the most common symptom of an MI. The pain of an infarct differs from that of angina. With an MI, the chest pain is constant, severe, and not relieved by nitroglycerin. The location of the pain is similar to that of anginal pain. It is, however, not relieved with rest or lying down. The duration of pain exceeds 30 min, without relief. In fact, it often occurs at rest without a clear precipitating event. As the pain, nausea, weakness, and diaphoresis continue, the patient becomes dyspneic and often becomes extremely apprehensive, often developing a sense of impending doom.

However, MIs may present without any symptoms or with only mild signs, such as indigestion. These "silent" MIs are extremely difficult to treat, since the signs are not severe enough to prompt a visit to the hospital or physician.

The 12-lead ECG reveals initial T-wave inversion, followed quickly by ST-segment elevation in the affected area. Q-wave formation, indicating cellular death, occurs after 24 h and is considered more diagnostic of MI. Areas of the heart and their corresponding ECG leads for MI interpretation are presented in Table 6-1. Figure 6-5 gives an example of MI of the anterior septal region; Fig. 6-6 gives an example of an inferior MI.

Abnormalities in serum cardiac markers are the best diagnostic criteria for MI, specifically troponin I (cTnI). The troponin complex consists of three subunits, TnT, TnI, and TnC. Normally, troponin levels are not detectable in blood assays. cTnI levels above 1.4 mg/dL are considered diagnostic of MI, although even lower levels are now being identified as being consistent with MIs. cTnI levels have replaced creatine phosphokinase (CPK) isoenzymes as the main biomarkers for MIs. cTnI remains elevated for more than 8 days, and may remain high even longer with decreased renal excretion. If a patient has had a recent MI, the troponin level will not indicate how recent the event was. This is why some centers still use CPK isoenzymes, including the subset of MB bands. The CPK-MB band is specific for cardiac muscle. If the CPK-MB band rises above 12 IU, MI can be diagnosed (Table 6-2). CPK isoenzymes rise within hours of injury, peaking within 24 h, and returning to normal within a few days.

TABLE 6-1. AREAS OF THE HEART AND THEIR CORRESPONDING ECG LEADS FOR INTERPRETATION OF MI

Location	ECG Location	ECG Changes
Anterior	$V_2–V_4$	Q waves, ST-segment elevation
Inferior	II, III, aVF	Q waves, ST-segment elevation
Lateral	I, aVL, V_5, V_6	Q waves, ST-segment elevation
Right ventricular	$V_3R–V_6R$	ST-segment elevation
Posterior	V_1, V_2	Large R wave
Septal	V_1	Q waves, ST-segment elevation

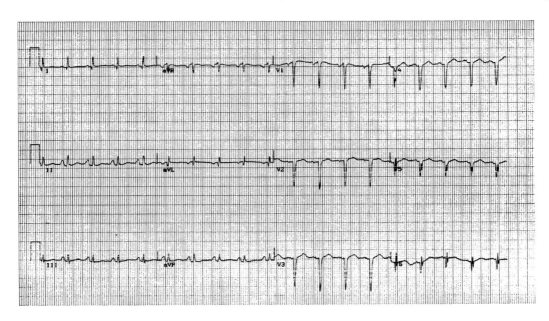

Figure 6-5. Anterior septal myocardial infarction.

Other diagnostic tests include the use of echocardiography and radionuclide imaging. Echocardiography reveals MIs by identifying defects in regional wall motion. Negative results also help rule out MIs.

LOCATION OF INFARCTION

Occlusions of the right coronary artery results in an inferior MI. Inferior MIs have a lower mortality rate than anterior MIs. Symptoms associated with an inferior MI include more mild AV node dysrhythmias, such as first- and second-degree type I blocks. Approximately 30% of inferior MIs include right ventricular (RV) infarction. Symptoms of RV infarction include hypotension from a decrease in the preload available to the LV because of decreased RV emptying.

Occlusion of the left anterior descending coronary artery results in an anterior MI. Anterior MIs

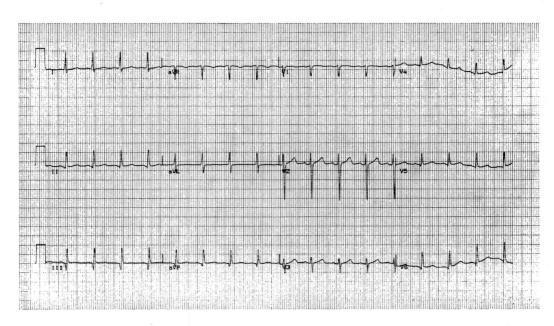

Figure 6-6. Inferior myocardial infarction.

TABLE 6-2. SERUM CARDIAC MARKERS AND PROTEINS USED IN THE DIAGNOSIS OF MYOCARDIAL INFARCTION

CPK	30–200 IU	Not specific by itself for MI; the size of MI is referenced to the degree of total CPK elevation (i.e., the higher the CPK, the greater the size of the MI)
CPK-MB	<5 ng/mL	>8 ng/mL suggests MI
Troponin I	<0.15, normal; >0.4–1.4, cardiac injury likely; >1.4 ng/mL suggests MI; elevates within 4 h of MI and remains elevated for up to 5–10 days	

CPK, creatine phosphokinase; CPK-MB, CPK MB band.

have a higher mortality rate and are associated with more serious dysrhythmias. Rhythm disturbances are more likely to include second- and third-degree blocks. Anterior MIs are also most likely responsible for diminished ejection fraction and symptoms of heart failure.

Less serious MIs are lateral and posterior, each with lower mortality rates than inferior or anterior MIs. More dangerous MIs are those that affect multiple regions, such as anterolateral MIs. When more than 40% of the left ventricle is acutely damaged, mortality is extremely high.

RV MIs are less common but are associated with obstruction of the right coronary or left circumflex artery. Mortality is lower with RV MIs. Diagnosis is made from the ECG, indicating a posterior MI pattern (large R waves in V_1 and V_2) and ST-segment elevation in the right precordial leads (e.g., V_4R and V_6R).

Symptoms include elevated central venous pressure (CVP) despite normal pulmonary artery occlusive pressure (PAOP). Venous congestion, the result of the high CVP from RV failure, is the primary symptom. Treatment centers on maintaining CVP values higher than normal, up to 25 mm Hg, in order to improve blood flow through the right ventricle. In severe RV failure, less blood is pumped into the lungs, and a drop in PAOP results.

TREATMENT AND COMPLICATIONS

Figures 6-1 and 6-2 provide a simple overview of treatment for STEMI and NSTEMI. Immediate reperfusion is the main goal in treating an MI. Table 6-3 is a summary of key treatments in ACS. Reperfusion can be either in the cardiac catheterization lab or via a thrombolytic drug. In the cath lab, a stent will be placed (perhaps a drug-eluting stent [DES]), which reduces the rate of reocclusion) to reestablish reperfusion.

TABLE 6-3. THROMBOLYTIC AND OTHER THERAPIES USED IN TREATING ACS

Drug Class	Examples of Drugs	Dose and Route
Antiplatelet	Clopidogrel	300–600 mg PO loading with 75 mg daily thereafter
	Prasugrel	60 mg PO loading dose, followed by 10 mg PO daily thereafter (5 mg PO daily if weight is less than 60 kg)
	Aspirin	160–325 mg PO
Antithrombin	Direct thrombin inhibitors	
	Bivalirudin	0.75 mg/kg IV bolus, followed by continuous infusion
Anticoagulants	Unfractionated heparin	Weight-based IV bolus (~5000 U) and infusion titrated to achieve aPTT value of 1.5–3.0 times baseline
	Enoxaparin	1 mg/kg SQ q 12 h
	Fondaparinux	2.5 mg SQ qd
Thrombolytics	Alteplase	Weight >67 kg: 15-mg IV bolus followed by 50 mg infusion over 30 min, then 35 mg infusion over the following 60 min for a total of 100 mg over 120 min
		Weight <67 kg: 15-mg IV bolus followed by 0.75–mg/kg infusion over 30 min (not to exceed 50 mg), then 0.5–mg/kg infusion over the following 60 min (not to exceed 35 mg)
	Reteplase	10 U IV over 2 min followed in 30 min by a second injection of 10 U IV over 2 min
	Tenectaplase	Weight-based IV injection: range of 30–50 mg. Do not exceed 50 mg
GP IIb/IIIa inhibitors: all have reduced dosages with renal impairment	Abciximab	0.25-mg/kg IV bolus followed by 0.125 mcg/kg/min for 12 h
	Eptifibatide	180-mg IV bolus (repeat 180-mg IV bolus after 10 min for PCI patients) followed by 2 mcg/kg/min for 18 h
	Tirofiban	0.4 mcg/kg/min for 30 min, then infusion of 0.1 mcg/kg/min for 12–24 h
Beta blocker	Metoprolol	5 mg IV initially

aPTT, activated partial thromboplastin; GP IIb/IIIa; IV, intravenous; PCI, percutaneous coronary intervention; PO, by mouth; SQ, subcutaneous.

Pain relief is a prime objective and is usually accomplished with intravenous analgesics such as morphine sulfate. Vasodilators, such as nitroglycerin, may be used but may also produce unwanted hypotension and may not relieve pain.

Thrombolytic Therapy

If the patient cannot get to a cath lab within 90 min, thrombolysis is the treatment of choice. Thrombolytics require clear evidence of MI before they are administered. Usually at least ST-segment elevation or a new left bundle branch block is required for treatment.

Nursing care of the patient with thrombolytic therapy centers on reducing potential episodes of bleeding. Only those arterial punctures and venipunctures that are absolutely necessary should be performed. Finger oximetry should be employed, for example, rather than drawing blood gases to obtain a PaO_2 level. If venipuncture must be performed, extra time must be spent holding the site to achieve hemostasis. Bed rest or fall precautions are necessary in patients with high risks of bleeding. Avoidance of automated blood pressure cuffs is encouraged owing to severe bruising from the high cuff pressures associated with automated systems.

It is important to assess the patient for signs of bleeding. Hypotension, tachycardia, or specific organ changes (i.e., reduced level of consciousness) are indicators of possible bleeding.

Reperfusion dysrhythmias are common. Bradycardias are frequently seen after infusion of thrombolytic agents. Ventricular tachycardias are also common.

Cardiac catheterization is performed as soon as possible; perhaps even during the acute MI episode. Percutaneous coronary intervention (PCI) is indicated for patients who present with symptom onset of less than 12 h, evidence of cardiogenic shock, or hemodynamic or electrical instability. Stent placement, angioplasty, atherectomy, thrombectomy, or surgery (CABG) may be performed at this time.

Intracoronary Stent Placement

Stent placement has become the treatment of choice in reperfusion. A stent is a device that holds open the coronary artery where narrowing has occurred. The design of stents is continuing to evolve. A balloon is used to open the stainless steel stent, which remains in place after the balloon is deflated (Fig. 6-7).

The most common problem following stent placement is the development of reocclusion due to

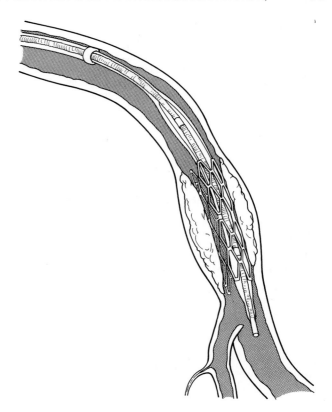

Figure 6-7. Stent inflated by a balloon.

endothelial overgrowth. This complication has been markedly reduced by the DES, which decreases and/or prevents endothelial overgrowth. This has made the DES the preferred stent. Reocclusion due to platelet activation and aggregation also results in reocclusion of the stented vessel; therefore, antiplatelet therapy is necessary following stent placement. Clopidogrel and prasugrel, antiplatelet agents, are used following stent placement in addition to life-long aspirin therapy. The duration of dual antiplatelet therapy is evolving. The DES requires dual antiplatelet therapy at least 12 months, while bare metal stents require therapy with clopidogrel for a shorter time. The patient's ability to use clopidogrel for an extended period of time can be a determining factor for the use of angioplasty, bare metal stents, or DES. The role of newer antiplatelet agents such as ticagrelor or cangrelor has not yet been well delineated.

ANGIOPLASTY

Angioplasty is the dilatation of a stenotic coronary artery through the insertion of a catheter into the artery. This technique has markedly declined in use

TABLE 6-4. CRITERIA FOR ANGIOPLASTY IN MI PATIENTS

Clear Criteria

PCI should be performed in new onset LBBB or ST elevation if symptom onset <12 h earlier and PCI can be performed in ≤90 min by a skilled individual (who has performed more than 75 PCI procedures per year) in a facility that performs more than 200 PCIs per year.

Other indications:
   Cardiogenic shock, age <75 years
   Myocardial failure (e.g., Killip's class III or IV)
   Prior Q wave in another region of the heart
   Patient is not a candidate for thrombolytic therapy

Uncertain Criteria

Clinical appearance of MI but not clear based on ECG

Patient presents >12 h after onset of symptoms

Prior CABG

Cardiogenic shock, age >75 years

CABG, caronary artery bypass grafting; LBBB, left bundle branch block; PCI, percutaneous coronary intervention.

since the development of the DES. Once the catheter is inserted, the stenotic area (identified by cardiac catheterization) is compressed by expanding a balloon at the end of the catheter. Angioplasty has the benefit of avoiding CABG while maintaining good results in expanding the stenotic area.

Several criteria for stent placement or angioplasty must be met (Table 6-4): one-vessel CAD, stable angina of less than 1 year, no prior MI, a lesion that is easy to reach (proximal), and discrete, and normal LV function. A patient meeting these criteria is a candidate for CABG if necessary.

Nursing care of the patient treated with a stent or angioplasty includes care of the cardiac catheterization insertion site (rest and site compression) and observation for signs of reocclusion (dysrhythmias). If the stenosis recurs, chest pain or symptoms of decreased cardiac output may occur.

Atherectomy and Thrombectomy

Atherectomy is removal of the atherosclerotic plaque by excision. Thrombectomy is aspiration of the clot.

Medical Therapy

If cardiac support is necessary, dobutamine and milrinone are positive inotropic (strengthening) therapies that may be used in states of low cardiac output. Dopamine is reserved for episodes of hypotension or at low doses (<5 mcg/kg/min). If medical support is not adequate, intra-aortic balloon pumping has

been demonstrated effectively to increase hemodynamic performance.

Vasodilators, such as nitroglycerin or nitroprusside, may be cautiously employed in an attempt to reduce preload and afterload. Continuous hemodynamic monitoring is necessary to manipulate accurately many of the cardiac medications. It is critical to reduce myocardial work in order to avoid episodes of congestive heart failure. The use of angiotensin-converting enzyme (ACE) inhibitors (enalapril) has become a key aspect of post-MI treatment because of their ability to reduce afterload (systemic vascular resistance) without increasing cardiac output. Other therapies, such as beta blockers (labetalol), may also be used. However, beta blockers should be used with caution in patients who already have cardiovascular shock. Beta blockers have negative inotropic (weakening) effects on the heart. However, their effect in reducing myocardial oxygen consumption usually offsets the negative effects on the heart; therefore, they are commonly used in treating an MI.

Early initiation of statins also improves cardiovascular outcomes. Life-long therapy is also necessary. These drugs have given strong indications that they can restrict the development of atherosclerosis. Statins are 3-hydroxy-3-methylglutaryl coenzyme A (HMG CoA) reductase inhibitors. By blocking the conversion of HMG CoA mevalonate kinase, they inhibit hepatic cholesterol synthesis, thus decreasing the amount of low-density lipoprotein. In addition to their impact on lipid synthesis, statins have been shown to have anti-inflammatory effects as well as stabilization of athersclerotic plaques.

Continuous cardiac monitoring is used to provide for the early identification of and intervention in dysrhythmias. If the patient survives the initial infarction and subsequently dies, death is usually due to a shock syndrome. Dysrhythmias of all types, including conduction disturbances, occur.

Oxygen therapy is usually started to ensure that the myocardium receives enough oxygen for its needs. An intravenous line is started for use in emergency situations. Food, usually low in sodium, is given as tolerated.

Hemodynamic monitoring must be continuous for early intervention in congestive heart failure, ventricular failure with pulmonary edema, and cardiogenic shock. Bed rest and emotional support are necessary to help heal the injured myocardium. Use of platelet inhibitors to decrease clotting is part of standard therapy. Currently, low-dose aspirin (81 mg) appears adequate to avoid early reocclusion.

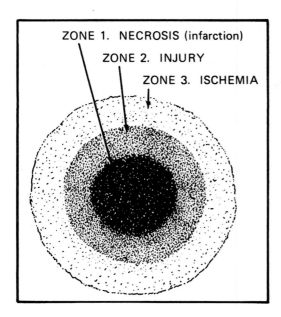

ZONE 1. NECROSIS (infarction)

ZONE 2. INJURY

ZONE 3. ISCHEMIA

Figure 6-8. The development of scar tissue following myocardial infarction.

Long-term immobility may result in venous pooling, with an increased risk of thromboembolism. Passive and active range-of-motion exercises and support hose help reduce this risk.

Less common but equally lethal complications of an MI include pericarditis, papillary muscle rupture, ventricular aneurysm, and ventricular rupture. These complications are generally seen 5 to 10 days following the acute infarction event. Sudden death commonly occurs with the last three of these complications.

Recovery

Recovery begins as soon as myocardial injury and necrosis stop. Scar tissue develops (Fig. 6-8) at the necrotic area. This process takes 6 to 8 weeks to complete.

Emotional support of the patient and family is a key factor in recovery. Cardiac patients often feel that their active and productive lives are over. It is not uncommon to see the patient and family members going through the stages of grief following an MI. Symptoms of depression must, therefore, be identified early in the course and the patient referred for treatment. Recent data point to the recurrence of a CV event and mortality at 1 to 5 years, with associated depression. The nurse plays an essential role in educating the patient and family as to lifestyle changes and the elimination of alterable risk factors, thus helping both the patient and family to work through this difficult process.

References

Krumholz H, Anderson J, Brooks N, Fesmire F, Lambrew C, Landrum M, et al. (2006). ACC/AHA clinical performance measures for adults with ST-elevation and non-ST-elevation myocardial infarction: a report of the American college of cardiology/American heart association task force on performance measures (writing committee to develop performance measures on ST-elevation and non-ST-elevation myocardial infarction. *J. Am. Coll. Cardiol, 47,*236-265.

Conduction Blocks

Conduction blocks can be expected to be tested with one to four questions. Often, the PCCN exam will not ask directly about conduction blocks but will put them in a situation. If you have an actual electrocardiographic (ECG) strip with a conduction block, there is likely to be only one test item. However, because conduction blocks are at times confusing, read the following material thoroughly.

FIRST-DEGREE BLOCK

Etiology

First-degree atrioventricular (AV) junctional block may be caused by heart disease (coronary artery disease [CAD]), acute myocardial infarction (MI), AV node ischemia, and drugs that act at the AV node (e.g., digitalis). The AV node delays the progression of the impulse from the sinoatrial (SA) node for an abnormal length of time (Fig. 7-1).

Identifying Characteristics

The rate is normal; the rhythm is regular; P waves are normal; and the PR interval is prolonged beyond 0.20 s. The QRS complex is normal and conduction is normal except for the prolonged delay at the AV node.

Risk

First-degree block is not a serious dysrhythmia in itself. It may progress to a second-degree type I block and less commonly to a second-degree type II or third-degree block.

Treatment

If the PR interval is less than 0.25 s and it does not increase, no treatment may be required. The length of the PR interval is not as significant as the effect on stroke volume and heart rate. No treatment is indicated unless a bradycardia results.

Nursing Intervention

Document the dysrhythmia with a rhythm strip. Monitor the patient closely for progression to a slower heart rate or a worsening block. If progression develops, document with a rhythm strip and notify the physician immediately.

SECOND-DEGREE BLOCK TYPE I AND TYPE II

The terms *Mobitz' type I block* and *Wenckebach's block* (named after cardiac physiologists of the early twentieth century) are sometimes used instead of type I. the term *Mobitz' II* is also used in place of type II. These terms are not used in this section, although it is helpful to remember that you may see them on the exam or in clinical practice.

Both type I and type II are AV junctional blocks. The AV node delays the progression of the SA node impulse for longer than normal. The AV node actually halts progression of some SA node impulses, which never reach the ventricular conduction system. The characteristics, treatment, and prognosis for these two forms of second-degree AV block differ.

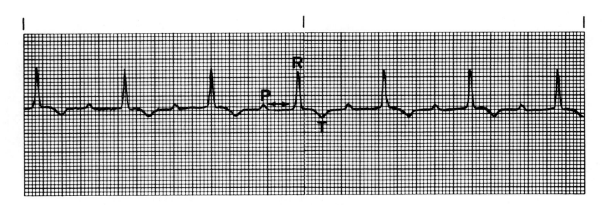

Figure 7-1. First-degree AV heart block.

The type I form of second-degree block is considered first.

Second-Degree Type I

Etiology
Conduction arises normally from the SA node and progresses to the AV node. With each succeeding impulse, it becomes more difficult for the AV node to conduct the impulse. Eventually, one impulse is not conducted and a QRS complex does not occur. The progression then begins again. Ischemia or injury to the AV node is the cause of this progression (Fig. 7-2).

Identifying Characteristics
The following are the key components of second-degree type I heart block:

1. A progressive prolongation of the PR interval
2. An increment of conduction delay that is greatest between the first and second sinus beats in each cycle

3. A progressive decrease in succeeding increments of delay
4. A progressive shortening of the PR interval before each pause
5. A pause in the ventricular rhythm that is less than twice the PP interval or sinus cycle length

Risk
Second-degree type I is often a temporary block following an acute MI. It may, however, progress to a complete (third-degree) block. For this reason, second-degree type I is considered a potentially dangerous dysrhythmia, although by itself it usually does not produce a clinical problem.

Treatment
Frequently no treatment is indicated. If the ventricular rate is slow, atropine may increase AV conduction. Epinephrine may be used to increase the rate of the SA node and thus the overall rate. On occasions, an external pacemaker or temporary transvenous pacemaker may be inserted.

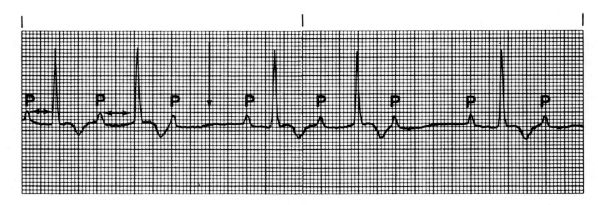

Figure 7-2. Second-degree AV block type I (Wenckebach's or Mobitz' I).

Nursing Intervention

Document the dysrhythmia with a rhythm strip. Monitor the patient, although this dysrhythmia is normally not clinically significant. If the ventricular rate slows enough to produce symptoms, document it with a rhythm strip and notify the physician.

Second-Degree Type II

Etiology

An impulse originates in the SA node and progresses normally to the AV node. Below the AV node in the common bundle or bundle branches, impulses are blocked on a regular basis, with every second, third, or fourth impulse not being conducted. In this block, a QRS complex is regularly missing. More than one P wave is present for every QRS complex. This dysrhythmia is due to disease of the AV node, the AV junctional tissue, or the His-Purkinje system (Fig. 7-3).

Identifying Characteristics

The atrial rate may be normal. The ventricular rate is usually one-half or one-third of the atrial rate (referred to as 2:1 or 3:1 block). At times, the block rate may be even greater than 3:1. The ventricular rate depends on the frequency of the block. (In 4:1 block, there are four atrial beats to every one QRS complex.) The atrial rhythm is regular. Ventricular rhythm is regular or irregular but slow. P waves are normal. The PR interval is constant. The QRS complex may be normal or widened. Conduction is normal in the atria and may be abnormal in the ventricles.

Risk

Type II block is unpredictable and may suddenly advance to complete heart block or ventricular standstill; this is especially common after inferior infarction and is a dangerous warning dysrhythmia.

Treatment

If the ventricular response is slow, atropine or epinephrine may be tried. Because the condition is so unpredictable, a temporary pacemaker is often the treatment of choice. A permanent pacemaker is frequently necessary.

Nursing Intervention

Document the dysrhythmia with a rhythm strip. Determine the width of the QRS complex. Monitor the patient closely for a widening of the QRS complex. The width of the QRS complex indicates the location in the conduction system of the block. The wider the complex, the lower in the bundle branch system the block will be. Document the widening, if it occurs, with a rhythm strip, notify the physician immediately, and prepare for the insertion of a transvenous pacemaker or use of an external pacemaker. Assess the patient frequently for hemodynamic compromise if the ventricular response is slow (3:1 and 4:1 block).

Although type I and II heart blocks are differentiated by the changes in the PR interval, another feature is important to bear in mind with these two types of dysrhythmias. Consider that the right coronary artery is responsible for feeding the AV node in most of the population. In addition, the right coronary artery supplies the inferior region of the left ventricle. Therefore, in inferior MIs, a common dysrhythmia is AV block, specifically type I block. Clinically this is relevant, since type I blocks may appear like type II blocks (i.e., in 2:1 patterns). Although these 2:1 blocks are generally less dangerous because the bundle branches remain intact. If a pacemaker is required, a temporary one will usually suffice.

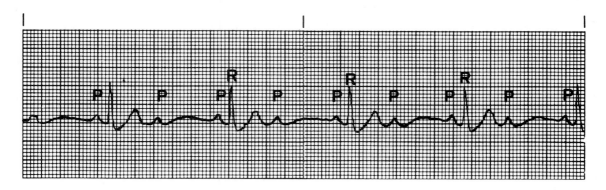

Figure 7-3. Second-degree AV block type II.

Anterior MIs are different, however, in their effect of producing type II blocks. An anterior MI is usually the result of obstruction of the left anterior descending (LAD) artery. This artery also feeds the left and right bundle branches. In the presence of an anterior MI, a type II block may also appear in a 2:1 pattern. This pattern is more dangerous with an anterior MI, since the block is due to loss of ventricular conduction system, i.e., the left and/or right bundle system. Type II blocks in the presence of an anterior MI require more attention. Pacemakers for this dysrhythmia must usually be permanent.

THIRD-DEGREE BLOCK— COMPLETE HEART BLOCK
Etiology

Ischemia or injury to the AV node, junctional tissue, or His-Purkinje tissue is the cause of complete heart block. The ischemia may be secondary to CAD, acute MI, drug use (e.g., digitalis toxicity), systemic disease, or electrolyte imbalances (especially in renal patients) (Fig. 7-4).

Identifying Characteristics

Atrial rates are faster than ventricular rates. P waves are not conducted. The ventricular rate is 30 to 40 (unless there is a junctional escape mechanism). The rhythm is regular for both the atria and the ventricles even though they are depolarizing completely independently of one another. P waves are normal and not associated with a QRS complex. The PR interval is not constant. QRS complexes are close to normal if they arise near the AV node. The QRS complex may be wide and bizarre if the impulse arises from the ventricles. There is no AV conduction.

The atrial pacemaker controls the atria, and the ventricular pacemaker controls the ventricles.

Risk

The main danger of third-degree heart block is the possibility that bradycardia will produce a decrease in cardiac output, leading to hypotension and myocardial ischemia. The loss of AV synchrony in third-degree block is a key reason for the decrease in cardiac output. Third-degree heart block is a potentially lethal dysrhythmia.

Treatment

Immediate pacemaker insertion is the treatment of choice. A temporary or transcutaneous pacemaker may be tried initially until the presence of the block has been determined to be permanent. Complete heart block may be temporary after MI, and pacing should be available for several days after the return of a normal sinus rhythm.

Nursing Intervention

Document the dysrhythmia with a rhythm strip and notify the physician immediately. Monitor the patient for signs of ventricular failure and hypotension. Hemodynamic status is compromised by the slow ventricular rate, and circulatory collapse is not uncommon.

ATRIOVENTRICULAR DISSOCIATION

Many conditions can be termed AV dissociation. Ventricular tachycardia and conduction defects where the atrial and ventricular rhythms do not

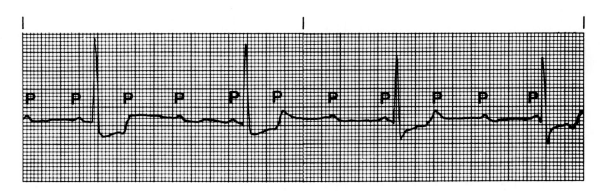

Figure 7-4. Third-degree (complete) AV block.

match can all be examples of AV dissociation. Some clinicians make the mistake of using the term *third-degree block* synonymously with *AV dissociation*; however, third-degree block is only one form of AV dissociation.

Etiology

The many causes of AV dissociation include anesthesia, medications, infections, acute MI, and ischemic heart disease (Fig. 7-5).

Identifying Characteristics

The PR interval is inconsistent since the atrial and ventricular pacemakers are independent of one another. The P wave, usually normal in form, may vary slightly in measurements. The P wave may fall immediately before, during, or after a QRS complex during the absolute refractory period of the ventricles (the period in which they cannot depolarize). The QRS complex may be normal or abnormal depending on whether the ventricular pacemaker is at or below the bundle of His.

Risk

Atrioventricular dissociation by itself is significant since atrial and ventricular contractions are not in synchrony. The loss of synchrony can produce a substantial reduction in cardiac output. However, rather than treat AV dissociation, the underlying rhythm producing AV dissociation should be addressed.

Treatment

Treatment is dependent on the underlying rhythm and the effect on hemodynamics. Treatments range from pacemakers for bradycardias to antidysrhythmics for ventricular tachycardia.

Nursing Intervention

Monitor the patient closely for signs of cardiac decompensation and progression of the dysrhythmia. Document the dysrhythmia with a rhythm strip and notify the physician.

BUNDLE BRANCH BLOCKS

EDITORS' NOTE

The PCCN exam can have one to four questions on cardiac conduction defects. This section provides an overview of how these conduction problems are read.

For more information on bundle branch blocks, see the complete review in Chap. 4.

Bundle branch blocks (BBBs) are also termed intraventricular conduction defects. There may be a right or left BBB. In addition, the left bundle has two divisions, referred to as fascicles. These fascicles may also become blocked. Obstructions of the fascicles are termed hemiblocks. There may be a left anterior hemiblock of the anterior fascicle of the left bundle branch or there may be a left posterior hemiblock of the posterior fascicle of the left bundle branch. Trifascicular blocks involve both left bundle fascicles and the right bundle branch. Bifascicular blocks usually involve the right bundle branch and one fascicle

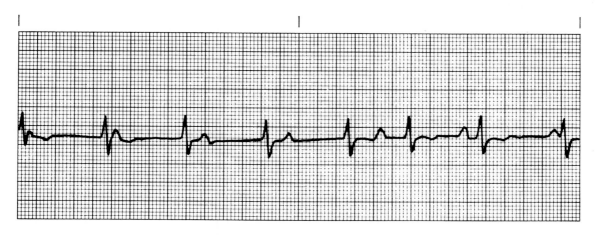

Figure 7-5. One type of AV dissociation.

TABLE 7-1. CRITERIA FOR VENTRICULAR CONDUCTION DEFECTS

Condition	Lead	QRS Appearance
Right bundle branch block	V₁	rSR′
	I and V₆	Deep S wave
Left bundle branch block	I and V₆	Wide QRS (>0.12)
	I and V₆	Notched QRS
	V₁	QS wave
Anterior hemiblock	I, aVF	Left axis >30 degrees
	I, aVL	Initial Q wave
	II, III, aVF	Small R wave, deep S wave
Posterior hemiblock	I	Large S wave
		Right axis
	I, aVL	Initial R wave
	II, III, aVF	Large R wave

of the left bundle branch or both fascicles of the left branch. BBBs may be suspected by observing a rhythm strip (due to a wide QRS or abnormal QRS configuration) but *cannot* be diagnosed by a rhythm strip. A 12-lead ECG is necessary to diagnose a BBB.

Criteria for diagnosing conduction defects are listed in Table 7-1. It is useful to identify conduction defects for several reasons, ranging from identifying areas of disease in the heart to assessing the significance of injury patterns. In addition, it is helpful to interpret conduction defects, particularly right BBBs, in differentiating atrial premature contractions with aberrant conduction from premature ventricular contractions.

Etiology

Several different factors may cause a BBB. For example, an acute MI may cause ischemia in the intraventricular conduction system. This is probably the most common cause. However, other factors, such as chronic degeneration with fibrous scarring, may permanently block the bundle branches, or such blocks may be congenital or rate-dependent (i.e., they appear only at certain heart rates).

Identifying Characteristics

Rate is usually normal, although it may vary if the BBB varies. Rhythm is regular. P waves may be normal. The PR interval is normal. The QRS complex is wide (>0.12 s) and may be notched depending on the lead viewed.

Risk

The development of BBBs indicates marked ischemia of the intraventricular conduction system,

and BBBs are potentially more dangerous than AV blocks, since these blocks are subjunctional. The involvement of more than one fascicle often progresses to complete heart block. In these instances, the prognosis is poor.

Treatment

It is not uncommon for the BBB to cause no symptoms. Because of the lack of symptoms, most BBBs require no direct treatment. Many patients tolerate conduction defects such as BBBs for long periods of time without developing any problems. The potential danger of the BBB, however, is that it can deteriorate into a more severe obstruction, such as complete heart block. In this case, the treatment is focused on improving the heart rate, as with atropine or a pacemaker.

Nursing Intervention

The primary consideration is to identify the conduction defect and document the type of block. Notify the physician if the block is new. Monitor the rhythm and be aware of the potential for a bradycardia, such as complete heart block, to develop.

PACEMAKERS

There are many pathologic states that may be most efficiently treated by the use of an artificial pacemaker. Pacemakers may be particularly useful in the treatment of symptomatic bradycardias that have not responded to atropine or epinephrine.

Definition

A pacemaker is a system consisting of a lead and a pulse generator. The generator is capable of producing repeated, timed bursts of electrical current for a prolonged period of time. The bursts of electrical current are of sufficient magnitude to initiate depolarization of the heart.

Modes of Pacing

For the purposes of the PCCN, pacemakers do not have to be understood in great depth. There have been remarkable advances in pacemakers, ranging from very simple ones to complex pacemaker/defibrillators. This section focuses on what you need to know for the exam and most critical care situations.

There are two modes of pacing. Temporary pacing is the mode used mainly to manage emergencies such as acute heart block and cardiac arrest. There are two types of temporary pacemakers: transvenous or transthoracic and transcutaneous (external). In the transvenous or transthoracic mode, the lead is inserted into the right atrium or ventricle. The pulse generator is external. Insertion routes include the transvenous (brachial via cutdown), subclavian, femoral, or jugular (via percutaneous entry), post-surgery (endocardial), and transthoracic (needle through chest into heart muscle). The power supply for temporary pacing is an external battery (the pulse generator). For a specific insertion procedure, the nurse is referred to his or her institution's policy.

Transcutaneous cardiac pacing has gained increasing acceptance. The transcutaneous method is based on sending direct current transcutaneously between electrodes placed on the skin. The advantages of transcutaneous pacing are the ease of use (it can be applied in a'matter of minutes) and the fact that no invasive equipment is necessary. The benefit of pacing is obtained through this method without the difficulty of inserting the transvenous or transthoracic pacing mode.

In the transcutaneous mode of pacing, the nurse must be aware of the potential for some discomfort to the patient because of the electrical stimulation, which will cause superficial as well as cardiac muscle contraction. Some conscious patients, particularly if the milliampere setting (determining how much energy is given) is high, may complain of pain on stimulation. Sedatives or analgesics may be required.

Permanent pacing with a fully implantable system is a second mode of pacing the heart. The pulse generator, which is implanted into the patient, contains the circuit for the specific pacing mode selected and a battery that provides energy to the circuit. The components are encased in a nonconductive plastic material that does not react with body tissue.

Indications for Pacing

The major indication for pacing is the development of second-degree type II or third-degree heart block. Pacemakers can be used for any bradycardia that is producing hypotension or signs of reduced cardiac output.

Chronic heart block of varied degrees may be treated by pacing if the patient has syncopal episodes, congestive heart failure, convulsions, or evidence of cerebral dysfunction.

Intermittent complete heart block (third degree) is often treated with a pacemaker. Usually there is evidence of block in one or two of the three bundle branches (fascicles). Thus, these patients rely solely on the third fascicle, which may become dysfunctional at any time.

Complete heart block that develops in conjunction with an acute MI may be an indication for pacing. If the infarction is anterior, the involved artery is usually the LAD. This results in ischemia or necrosis of part of the ventricular septum with damage to the intraventricular conduction system below the His bundle. These patients may die despite the insertion of a pacemaker because of the extent of myocardial damage. If the infarction is posterior or inferior, the artery involved is usually the right coronary (90% of the time) or the circumflex (10% of the time). The area of damage is the AV node area. Types I and II may be indications for pacing. Type I may progress into a type II (2:1) or higher block. Type II, because it occurs below the AV node, often progresses into third-degree heart block. A block that develops after infarction is usually transient and responds to atropine or a brief period of time with a temporary pacemaker.

Conduction defects may occur after a cardiac surgical procedure. For this reason, most cardiac surgeries (e.g., coronary artery bypass grafting) include the use of pacing wires attached to the epicardium for postoperative management. Some centers also use a pacing port through a pulmonary artery catheter.

Pacemakers may be used in other rhythm disturbances if bradycardia is a component of the dysrhythmia. Sick sinus syndrome indicates dysfunction of the SA node. This may occur as sinus bradycardia, sinus arrest, and/or brady-tachy syndromes.

Pacemakers may also be used to treat tachydysrhythmias, such as atrial or ventricular tachycardia. In these rhythms, the pacemaker rate is increased to a level higher than the tachycardia. Once the pacemaker is controlling the rate, the rate is slowed to a more acceptable level.

A pacemaker may be used as a diagnostic aid to evaluate SA node and AV node function. They may be used to eliminate multiple ectopic foci by overriding the rate of the foci, or they may be used to abolish reentry phenomena by delivering a premature stimulus that breaks the reentry pattern.

Types of Pacing Modes

There are several types of pacing modes. These are categorized according to the Inter-Society

TABLE 7-2. FIVE-POSITION PACEMAKER CODE[a]

I. Chamber Paced	II. Chamber Sensed	III. Mode of Response	IV. Programmability	V. Tachyrhythmia Functions
V = ventricle	V = ventricle	I = inhibited	P = programmable rate and/or output	B = burst
A = atrium	A = atrium	T = triggered		N = normal rate completion
D = atrium and ventricle	D = atrium and ventricle	D = atrial triggered and ventricular inhibited	M = multiprogrammability	S = scanning
O = none	O = none		O = none	E = external
		O = none	C = programmable with telemetry	

[a]Based on the Inter-Society Commission on Heart Disease (ICHD) nomenclature.

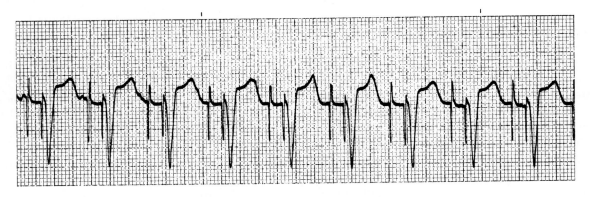

Figure 7-6. Normal pacemaker (DVI) electrical pattern.

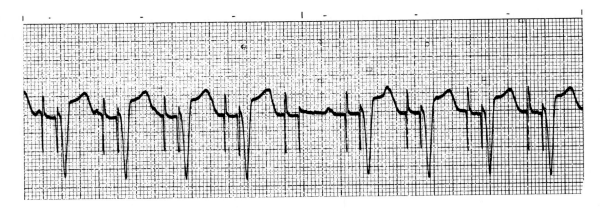

Figure 7-7. Failure of pacemaker to capture.

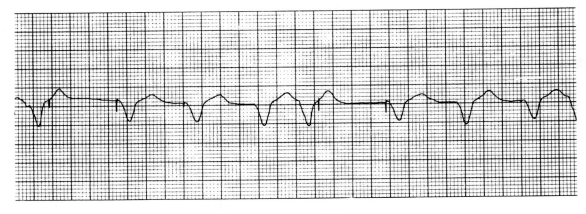

Figure 7-8. Failure of pacemaker to sense.

Commission on Heart Disease (ICHD) nomenclature given in Table 7-2. There are two codes, a simplified three-letter code and a more comprehensive five-letter code. Table 7-2 contains the five-letter code. In the PCCN exam, only a few pacing modes may be addressed. As a rule, the PCCN exam requires you to remember only the simpler three-letter code.

The major concept to remember is that the pacemaker electrically paces a cardiac chamber (the first letter), senses an electrical impulse in a cardiac chamber (the second letter), and discharges the impulse in either a triggered or inhibited manner (the third letter). In critical care, the inhibited manner is almost always used.

If a patient had a transvenous pacemaker inserted that would pace and sense only in the ventricle, the ICHD description would be a VVI. If the pacemaker paced both atrium and ventricle but sensed only in the ventricle, the pacemaker would be a DVI (AV sequential) pacemaker.

Nursing Care

The patient with a temporary pacemaker will need documentation as to the effectiveness of rhythm capture and sensing. The electrical signal indicating that a pacemaker impulse has occurred should be evident only immediately prior to capturing a paced beat (Fig. 7-6). If a pacemaker signal is present and the heart is not in a refractory mode, a captured beat should follow. If no beat occurs, this would be called failure to capture (Fig. 7-7). Failure to sense would be a paced beat or pacemaker artifact occurring too soon after a spontaneous beat. The spontaneous beat should inhibit the next paced impulse; if it does not, failure to sense is present (Fig. 7-8). Notify the physician if either of these conditions occurs more than once.

Care of the pacemaker insertion site is the same as for any central intravenous catheter. It is important to explain the purpose and duration of the pacemaker carefully in order to avoid causing the patient unnecessary anxiety.

8

Heart Failure: Congestive Heart Failure, Pulmonary Edema, and Hypertensive Crisis

EDITORS' NOTE

The assessment of abnormal hemodynamics, particularly in regard to left and right ventricular failure, is a common topic for questions in the PCCN exam. However, the focus of the exam is on acute heart failure rather than the management of chronic heart failure. This chapter reviews the major concepts normally employed in the assessment of acute ventricular failure as well as its diagnosis and associated interventions. Expect several questions on the PCCN exam from this content area.

It is important to understand advances in the understanding of heart failure (HF) in the course of studying conditions such as HF, pulmonary edema, and hypertensive crisis. The management of these conditions begins long before intensive care unit (ICU) admission. However, in order to understand hospital treatment of HF (comprising congestive HF, pulmonary edema, and hypertensive crisis), it is helpful to understand the process of HF in general. An overview of HF, along with contributing factors such as hypertension, will provide a better understanding of the assessment and treatment of HF overall.

Before discussing the specific clinical conditions of HF, pulmonary edema, and hypertension, we will review the factors that regulate cardiac output (i.e., preload, afterload, and contractility). Ventricular failure can be assessed and treated by regulating these three components. Although

ventricular failure can be assessed by noting each component of cardiac output, each ventricle is assessed slightly differently. For example, preload of the left ventricle is hard to assess without a pulmonary artery occlusive (or wedge) pressure (PAOP), while preload of the right ventricle is assessed by the central venous pressure (CVP). Other factors used to differentiate left and right ventricular influences are listed in Table 8-1.

The specific pressures frequently used in the assessment of ventricular preload are listed in Table 8-2. Although these guidelines are general examples, the PCCN exam is likely to utilize values such as these when clinical scenarios are provided in situations describing ventricular failure. More sophisticated measures to estimate cardiac performance, such as echocardiography, are available. However, the basic guidelines listed in Tables 8-1 and 8-2 are useful in assessing cardiac performance in most clinical practice settings. Because of the common application of these concepts, it is helpful to understand their role in clinical assessment.

HEART FAILURE

Heart failure is the inability of the heart to pump blood through the systemic circulation in an amount sufficient to meet the body's needs. HF normally refers to biventricular failure, although it is important to understand that each ventricle can fail independently of the other. Left ventricular (LV) failure is a common precursor to right ventricular (RV) failure and can precede RV dysfunction. RV failure is

TABLE 8-1. METHODS TO ASSESS LEFT AND RIGHT VENTRICULAR PERFORMANCE

Parameter	Right Ventricle	Left Ventricle
Preload	CVP	Improved breathing
Afterload	PVR	SVR
Contractility	Ejection fraction, peak velocity	Ejection fraction, peak velocity

CVP, central venous pressure; PVR, pulmonary vascular resistance; SVR, systemic vascular resistance.

frequently associated with lung disease or dysfunction, or it may be the result of ischemia of the right-sided coronary circulation. RV failure will produce LV hypovolemia by failing to move blood through the lungs.

Chronic HF (CHF) is categorized in stages: A through D (Table 8-3). Management of HF is summarized in Table 8-4. CHF is the gradual inability of the heart to pump sufficient blood to meet the body's demands. CHF can become acute without an obvious cause or may be precipitated by an acute ischemic cardiac event. The presence of RV failure in the face of LV failure usually indicates a more advanced disease state and worse prognosis.

Etiology

Unless specified otherwise, assume that the term *heart failure* implies biventricular failure. Signs and symptoms of HF result from the failure of both ventricles. However, even though signs and symptoms of HF are biventricular in nature, the origin of the failure is usually the left ventricle. Factors commonly influencing the development of LV dysfunction and eventually causing HF are listed in Table 8-5.

LV pump failure usually occurs before RV pump failure. The LV myocardium weakens to the extent that it cannot eject blood in the normal amount. This reduces the cardiac output secondary to a reduction in stroke volume. Before stroke volume decreases, however, two changes in myocardial

TABLE 8-2. USE OF THE CENTRAL VENOUS PRESSURE (CVP)

Value	Stroke Index	Condition Indicated
CVP		
0–5	<25–45	Normal or hypovolemia
5–10	25–45	Beginning failure or fluid overload
>10	<25	RV failure

RV, right ventricular.

TABLE 8-3. STAGES OF THE EVOLUTION AND PROGRESSION OF CHF

Stage	Definition	Examples
A	High risk of HF but no structural heart disease or signs of failure	Hypertension, coronary artery disease, diabetes, family history of cardiomyopathy
B	Structural heart disease but no signs of failure	Prior MI, systolic dysfunction, valvular heart disease, RV hypertrophy
C	Structural heart disease and signs of failure (either in the past or currently)	Symptoms include dyspnea, fatigue, exercise intolerance, orthopnea
D	Refractory HF despite maximal medical therapy	

MI, Myocardial infarction; RV, right ventricular.

function may take place. First, if the failure is slow, the left ventricle enlarges in both capacity (measured by end-diastolic volume [EDV]) and muscle size. This is called ventricular remodeling. The ventricle changes in shape as well, becoming more spherical. This change in shape makes it less effective at pumping blood and leads to worsening cardiac function. As the remodeling continues, the second problem develops; i.e., the ability of the heart to eject blood (measured by stroke volume and ejection fraction [EF]) is reduced. This reduction is initially offset by factors such as increased EDV (ventricular stretch), but it is just a temporary solution.

The factors that produce the change in the shape of the heart are partially modifiable. Neurohumoral factors that contribute to this change include the release of sympathetic stimulants, activation of the renin-angiotensin-aldosterone system (RAAS), and secretion of vasopressin. Although these neurohumoral factors initially are designed to help the injured or failing heart, they eventually contribute to HF. For example, the sympathetic stimulants (e.g., norepinephrine, dopamine) help to increase cardiac output by their positive inotropic effects. They also produce vasoconstriction, as will angiotensin II and vasopressin. Aldosterone increases sodium and water retention in an attempt to maintain cardiac output. However, all these factors will eventually contribute to worsening cardiac performance.

The body will try to compensate for these effects by releasing substances like natriuretic peptides (NPs). These peptides are naturally occurring proteins that produce vasodilation and increase urine output. There are several types of NPs, including atrial (ANP), brain (BNP), and C

TABLE 8-4. MOST COMMON TREATMENTS OF HF

Category	Dose	Action	Adverse Events, Monitoring, and Special Instructions
Acute and Chronic Management			
ACE inhibitors:			
Lisinopril	Initial dose, 2.5–5.0 mg PO qd; target dose, 20–40 mg PO qd	Afterload reducer, blocks RAAS	Observe for hypotension, renal dysfunction, angioedema
Enalapril	Initial dose, 2.5–5.0 mg PO bid; target dose, 10–20 mg PO bid		
Captopril	Initial dose, 6.25–12.5 mg PO tid; target dose, 50 mg PO tid		
Beta blockers:			
Metoprolol	Initial dose, 12.5–25.0 mg PO qd (succinate form) or 6.25–12.5 mg PO bid–qid (tartrate form); target dose, 100–200 mg PO qd (succinate form)	Beta blockade (and with carvedilol, alpha blockade)	
Carvedilol	Initial dose, 3.125 mg PO bid; target dose, 25–50 mg PO bid	The result is vasodilation (reducing work of the ventricle) and reduced myocardial work (slows the heart and weakens contractility)	
Bisoprolol	Initial dose, 1.25 mg PO qd; target dose, 10 mg PO qd		
Nitrates:			
Isosorbide dinitrate	Initial dose, 10 mg PO tid–qid; target dose up to 40 mg PO qid	Promote venous dilation, producing a drop in venous return and CVP	Hypotension, headache; avoid around the clock administration to allow for a nitrate-free period
Diuretics:			
Aldosterone antagonists, spironolactone	25 mg PO qd	Inhibit aldosterone release, promoting diuresis	Renal dysfunction, hyperkalemia
Eplerenone	Initial dose, 25 mg PO qd; target dose, 50 mg PO qd		
Furosemide	20–40 mg PO, up to 320 mg bid	Inhibit Na reabsorption, promoting diuresis	Hyponatremia, electrolyte losses, and renal dysfunction
Torsemide	Initial dose 5–10 mg; up to 40 mg per dose		
Bumetanide	2.5–5.0 mg PO qd		
Metolazone	10 mg qd		
Inotropic Agents:			
Digoxin	0.125 mg PO qd, 0.25 mg PO qd	Acts as a positive inotrope, increasing contractility	Cardiac arrhythmias
Primarily Acute Management			
Inotropes:			
Dobutamine	1–20 mcg/kg/min	Sympathetic stimulant (beta); increases contractility and stroke volume, cardiac output	Cardiac arrhythmias
Milrinone	0.05 mg/kg IV over 10 min, then 0.375–0.75 mcg/kg/min	Phosphodiesterase inhibitor, acts by increasing intracellular calcium; results is improved contractility, stroke volume, and cardiac output	
Afterload reducers:			
Nitroglycerin	10–100 mcg/min	All will reduce afterload (SVR) through differing mechanisms	
Hydralazine	10–40 mg IM, 5–20 mg IV	Smooth muscle relaxant	
Natriuretic	Bolus of 2 mcg/kg; infusion of 0.01 mcg/kg/min		
Peptides (e.g., nesiritide)		Smooth muscle relaxant, decreases sympathetic stimulation, promotes diuresis and vasodilation	

ACE, angiotensin-converting enzyme; CVP, central venous pressure; IM, intramuscular, IV, intravenous; PO, by mouth; RAAS, renin-angiotensin-aldosterone system; SVR, systemic vascular resistance.

TABLE 8-5. CONDITIONS THAT CONTRIBUTE TO DEVELOPMENT OF HF

Systemic hypertension	Atrial and ventricular tachydysrhythmias	Worsening ischemic heart disease; e.g., MI, angina
Mitral regurgitation	Cardiomyopathy	Aortic stenosis
Obesity	Hyperthyroidism	Worsening bundle branch block (especially left bundle branch block)
Infections, such as pneumonia	Treatment of arthritis, with either nonsteroidal anti-inflammatory drugs or high dosages of aspirin	Untreated anemia

MI, myocardial infarction.

TABLE 8-6. SYMPTOMS OF SYSTOLIC AND DIASTOLIC HF

	Systolic Failure	Diastolic Failure
Stroke volume	Reduced	Reduced
Ejection fraction	Reduced	Normal
Age	All ages, 50–70 years common	More common in age >70 years
Sex	More common in men	More common in women
Heart sounds	S_3	S_4
Heart cavity size	Enlarged	Often normal

type. ANP is located in atrial storage granules, while BNP is located in both the atria and ventricles (despite the term *brain natriuretic peptide*). The NPs are elevated in HF. BNP is useful as a clinical tool in the diagnosis of HF. Although there are different testing methods to measure BNP, one common method used at the point of care has demonstrated that a value of 100 pg/mL is strongly suggestive that a patient has HF. Some investigators have suggested that an elevated BNP is among the most accurate methods of identifying CHF.

As this process progresses, HF develops. A weakened LV is signaled by a loss of strength; for example, in ejection fraction. Normally, about 70% of the EDV is ejected with each beat. The amount of blood thus ejected is the stroke volume. The amount of blood ejected (stroke volume [SV]) in comparison with the EDV is termed the ejection fraction (SV/EDV = EF). As the contractile ability of the heart worsens, the ejection fraction falls. As the ejection fraction decreases to less than 40%, exercise limitations become evident and progress to interfere with activities of daily living. Newer technologies, like esophageal Dopplers, measure contractility by different techniques (e.g., peak velocity). The PCCN exam is unlikely to include these new technologies.

If the left ventricle cannot pump all the blood it receives from the atrium, a build-up of blood and pressure occurs in the left atrium. As the pressure in the left atrium increases, it becomes more difficult for blood to enter the atrium from the pulmonary veins. As the blood in the pulmonary veins becomes unable to flow into the left atrium, it backs up in the lung vessels. When pressure in the pulmonary capillaries exceeds 18 to 25 mm Hg, fluid from the capillaries leaks into the interstitial spaces. Once this

leakage of fluid into the pulmonary interstitial space exceeds the ability of the pulmonary lymphatics to drain the fluid, pulmonary edema begins to develop.

HF can be categorized into two types: systolic and diastolic dysfunction. Symptoms differentiating these types of HF are listed in Table 8-6 and summarized below.

Systolic Dysfunction

Systolic dysfunction is characterized by a decrease in muscle strength. Forward blood flow falls, producing systemic hypoperfusion. Stroke volume and ejection fraction also fall. Systolic dysfunction also causes pulmonary congestion, but it is more dangerous because of the potential to decrease forward blood flow.

Diastolic Dysfunction

Diastolic dysfunction is the inability of the ventricle to fully relax. The result is increasing pressure and volume in the ventricle. This produces pulmonary congestion as pressures "back-up" the pulmonary veins. In diastolic dysfunction, the strength of the heart is often normal (e.g., ejection fraction and peak velocity are within normal levels). Stroke volume is gradually reduced owing to the limitation in ventricular chamber size.

In both types of HF, pulmonary compliance can compensate for some increases in pressure as the heart becomes dysfunctional. Since the lung vasculature is distensible, it can accept a moderate amount of increased pressure and volume. However, without intervention, the pressure in the pulmonary capillaries increases to the point that the right ventricle cannot eject its blood into the lungs for oxygenation. As the backflow pressure increases, the right ventricle fails and the CVP increases. Then blood from the right atrium cannot drain completely, and consequently the right atrium cannot accommodate all of the blood entering from the venae cavae. Since venous blood flow to the heart is impeded, venous pooling and eventual organ congestion with venous blood occur.

Left Versus Right Heart Failure

Right HF is most commonly caused by left HF and then by all the factors that cause left HF. Right HF may also be caused by isolated right coronary ischemia, pulmonary emboli, essential pulmonary hypertension, and chronic obstructive pulmonary disease.

Left HF alone can occur from the same factors that cause HF. Since left HF occurs before right HF in these cases, initial symptoms of left HF differ from those of HF. Because of the potential for left heart before right HF, measures that formerly were used to estimate left heart function by right-sided measures (such as CVP) have been demonstrated to be inaccurate.

Clinical Presentation

Symptoms of left and right ventricular failure are presented in Table 8-7.

Complications

The major complications of HF are the progression of failure and loss of cardiac output and oxygen delivery. In addition, progression of cardiac failure can lead to the development of lethal dysrhythmias. It is also important to keep in mind that therapies to treat HF may cause drug toxicity (including oxygen toxicity) and fluid and electrolyte imbalances.

Treatment and Nursing Intervention

The goal of treating HF is to improve ventricular function and prevent the progression to right HF.

TABLE 8-7. SYMPTOMS OF LEFT AND RIGHT VENTRICULAR FAILURE

Left Ventricle	Right Ventricle
Orthopnea	Distended neck veins
Dyspnea of exertion	Dependent edema
Crackles	Hepatic engorgement
Low Pao_2/Sao_2/Spo_2	Hepatojugular reflux
S_3, S_4	
Systolic murmur	

There are three methods of treatment (inotropes, reduction of afterload, and reduction of preload) which are based on the factors regulating stroke volume.

Inotropes

The first method of treatment is to improve the contractility of the ventricle. Depending on the severity of the problem, different agents may be attempted. For example, in mild HF, preload and afterload reducers would be initiated. In severe HF, inotropes would be added. Improving contractility can occur with positive inotropic agents such as dobutamine and milrinone. Within the limits of Starling's law and balancing the good (improved cardiac output, stroke volume) against the bad (increased myocardial oxygen consumption), this method of treatment can be useful in the short term. However, long-term use has been shown to worsen mortality and is considered palliative. In theory, these agents are good treatments because of their ability to directly improve stroke volume, ejection fraction, and cardiac output. However, inotropes come with a cost—that is, increased myocardial oxygen consumption at a time when oxygenation of the heart is threatened. Digitalis preparations, such as digoxin, have been used in the chronic control of HF. Their role in acute HF is less clear.

Part of the less than optimal effectiveness of inotropes (especially dobutamine) may involve "downregulation," which refers to the lack of responsiveness of cardiac muscle to sympathetic stimulation. In chronic HF, sympathetic stimulation has been occurring for a long time. This chronic stimulation leads eventually to failure of the cardiac muscle to respond to further stimulation. Because of the failure of long-term oral inotropes in the presence of HF, the current therapy emphasizes manipulation of preload and afterload to improve contractility.

Downregulation and the increased oxygen demand of inotropes has made biventricular pacing a more common treatment for poor contractility. One required indication for biventricular pacing is evidence of a bundle branch block (BBB). The dysynchrony of right and left ventricular contraction in a BBB compounds the pump failure. When the right and left ventricles contract at the same time, the septum is stable. When the right and left ventricles contract one after the other in a BBB, the septum moves back and forth, causing less efficient ejection of blood from the ventricles. Biventricular pacing restores synchronized ventricular contraction, thus maximizing the efficiency of ventricular contraction and increasing cardiac output.

Reduction of Afterload

Afterload is the resistance of the blood, valves, and blood vessels that the left ventricle must overcome to eject blood. A decrease in any of these factors will decrease afterload. Reduction in afterload (estimated by the SVR) eases the work of the left ventricle. Reduced work may allow for improved contractility, thereby increasing stroke volume and cardiac output. Afterload agents include vasodilators of several different pharmacologic types, including nitroprusside, angiotensin-converting enzyme (ACE) inhibitors (captopril and enalapril), calcium channel blockers (nifedipine and nicardipine), and many other agents. Common agents used to reduce afterload in HF are included in Table 8-8. The intra-aortic balloon pump (IABP) is a nonpharmacologic afterload reducer.

Reduction of Preload

If the volume of blood entering the left atrium can be lowered, stress on the left ventricle is reduced. Diuretic therapy (as with furosemide and thiazides), venodilators (with nitroglycerin), and fluid and sodium restriction are examples of treatment of preload. Examples of diuretics used in the treatment of HF are listed in Table 8-9.

Close monitoring of the patient and his or her response to these treatments is very important in the early detection of a deteriorating state requiring more aggressive therapy.

High-Output Failure

Some conditions are associated with high cardiac output. When associated with symptoms of HF, these conditions are called high-output failure. Table 8-10 lists conditions commonly associated with high-output failure. Treatment of high-output failure is based on relieving the underlying condition, such as excess catecholamines and thyroid dysfunction.

PULMONARY EDEMA

Pulmonary edema is the most serious progression of HF. It may occur when pressure in the pulmonary vasculature exceeds 18 to 25 mm Hg. This results in the extravasation of fluid from pulmonary capillaries into interstitial tissue and intra-alveolar spaces. The intrapulmonary shunt worsens, as is evident by the need for high oxygen requirements (increased FiO_2) and worsening intrapulmonary shunts (e.g., PaO_2/FiO_2 ratios worsen).

Etiology

Acute pulmonary edema is usually the result of LV failure, although noncardiac forms of pulmonary edema (e.g., adult respiratory distress syndrome) exist. Symptoms of HF are exacerbated in pulmonary edema. Dyspnea and orthopnea become markedly pronounced; crackles may be heard throughout the lungs and be accompanied by blood-tinged, frothy sputum. Hypoxemia will worsen as lung function deteriorates from the increased fluid. Restlessness and anxiety precede a changing level of consciousness as cerebral oxygenation falls.

Radiographic Changes

Changes due to pulmonary edema occur on radiographs in stages equal to the progression and/or

TABLE 8-8. AFTERLOAD REDUCERS—CATEGORIES OF AGENTS

Calcium Channel Blockers	Beta Blockers	ACE Inhibitors	Direct Arterial and Venous Dilators	ARBs
Nifedipine	Metoprolol,	Benazepril	Olmesartan	
Verapamil	Bisoprolol, and Carvediolol are preferred in HF	Captopril	Nitroglycerin	Valsartan
Nicardipine		Enalapril		Losartan
Diltiazem (use not recommended in systolic HF)	Propanolol, Timololol	Fosinopril		Telmisartain
Verapamil (use not recommended in systolic HF)	Atenolol, Pindolol, Labetalol	Lisinopril		Candesartan
Isradipine		Moexipril		
Amlodipine		Quinapril		
Nimodipine		Perindopril		
Felodipine		Ramipril		
		Trandolapril		

HF, heart failure; ACE, angiotensin-converting enzyme; ARBs, angiotensin receptor blockers.

TABLE 8-9. PRELOAD REDUCERS

Diuretics			
Loop	**Thiazides**	**Potassium-Sparing**	**Vasodilators**
Bumetanide		Amiloride	Nitroglycerin
	Chlorothiazide	Spironolactone	
Ethacrynic acid	Chlorthalidone	Triamterene	
	Hydrochlorothiazide	Eplerenone	
Furosemide	Metolazone		

severity of the pulmonary edema. The first change is an enlargement of the pulmonary veins. As interstitial edema occurs, the vessels become poorly outlined and foggy. This is frequently referred to as hilar haze. As intra-alveolar edema develops, the radiograph shows a density in the inner middle zone. This gives the appearance of a "bat wing" or "butterfly" at the hilum.

Treatment and Nursing Intervention

The treatment for pulmonary edema is the same as for HF, with a few exceptions. The goal of therapy is to resolve the pulmonary edema by improving cardiac function, which will improve renal function while supporting respiratory needs. The goal is to decrease preload, decrease afterload, and increase contractility.

Preload is reduced by diuretic therapy. For example, furosemide (Lasix) has been a mainstay in the management of pulmonary edema for decades. Pulmonary edema responds well to furosemide, possibly because of its vasodilatory effect as much as its diuretic action. Anxiety is best treated by improving cardiac function and providing constant reassurance to the patient that treatments are being given. Some clinicians still use analgesics such as morphine sulfate, which is given intravenously to both relieve anxiety and cause vasodilation, resulting in a reduced afterload. At times, patients with a history of long-standing use of diuretics are refractory to the diuretic effects and it becomes difficult to decrease the preload. Ultrafiltration via dialysis or renal replacement therapy can be considered for fluid removal. Newer modalities of mechanical fluid removal are also being developed.

TABLE 8-10. CAUSES OF HIGH CARDIAC-OUTPUT FAILURE

Hyperthyroidism	Thiamine deficiency
Severe anemia	Paget's disease
Arteriovenous fistula	

Cardiac function can be immediately supported with inotropes (e.g., dobutamine). If no response from dobutamine is seen, milrinone can be given. It is important to monitor the patient's response to make sure that the benefit to inotropes is worth the cost. If hypotension exists, middose vasopressors (e.g., dopamine, norepinephrine) may be given. However, it is advisable to use as minimal a dose as possible and titrate to tissue oxygenation endpoints (e.g., SvO_2 or $ScvO_2$).

Normally, hypoxemia is treated, but not in isolation. Improving arterial oxygenation is important, but not at the expense of tissue oxygenation (a danger in using any positive-pressure therapy, such as mechanical ventilation or positive end-expiratory pressure [PEEP] or biphasic positive airway pressure [BIPAP]). Hypoxemia can be treated by increasing the fraction of inspired oxygen (FiO_2). Oxygen therapy is usually administered by a high-flow face mask system, with oxygen concentrations over 50% being required. The addition of continuous positive airway pressure (CPAP) or intubation and implementation of PEEP or BIPAP may be necessary for patients whose hypoxemia (PaO_2 levels below 60 mm Hg) does not respond to oxygen therapy. PEEP or BIPAP can decrease preload by compressing the inferior vena cava. However, when positive pressure is applied, care must be taken to avoid a decrease in cardiac output.

Nursing intervention focuses on monitoring significant changes in preload, afterload, and contractility. If the preload (PAOP) changes, the nurse must observe whether other parameters (e.g., stroke volume, cardiac output, and SvO_2) have changed. Trends in data analysis are more important than absolute numbers. It is very important to monitor treatments over several readings as opposed to a single data to ensure the accurate assessment of clinical conditions.

Emotional support of the patient with pulmonary edema is made difficult by the patient's fear of shortness of breath. It is important to decrease this fear concurrently with providing treatment.

HYPERTENSIVE CRISIS

Hypertension is not a disease but rather the symptom of a disease. Guidelines from the National Heart, Lung and Blood Institute (NHLBI) changes the former blood pressure definitions to the following: normal, <120/<80 mm Hg; prehypertension, 120 to 139/80 to 89 mm Hg; stage 1 hypertension, 140 to 159/90 to 99 mm Hg; stage 2 hypertension, ≥160/≥100 mm Hg. Primary hypertension (idiopathic, or of unknown cause) is common in the general population, with up to 30% of the population being affected. Hypertensive crises, however, occur only in a small percentage of the hypertensive population.

Mean arterial pressure (MAP) is routinely lower in normal populations (MAP of between 60 and 90 mm Hg) than in chronic hypertensive patients (MAP commonly between 120 and 160). The fact that hypertensive patients have higher mean pressures is important when therapeutic endpoints are identified. The patient with chronic hypertension may tolerate a higher MAP, and rapid reduction to normal levels is generally not necessary.

The severity of the hypertensive disturbance can be identified according to the guidelines of the Joint National Committee on Detection, Evaluation and Treatment of High Blood Pressure, published yearly. Emergencies are blood pressure levels that need treatment within 1 h; urgencies are blood pressure levels that need treatment within 1 day. The characteristics of emergencies are listed in Table 8-11.

Etiology

Hypertension may be classified by etiology:

1. Unknown origin accounts for 90% of all cases of hypertension identified. This is termed essential hypertension.
2. Adrenal origin results from a tumor (pheochromocytoma) secreting epinephrine and norepinephrine, Cushing's disease, or a brain tumor.
3. Renal origin is due either to an interruption of blood supply or to a disease state of the kidney itself (e.g., pyelonephritis).
4. Cardiovascular hypertension can be in response to either HF or myocardial ischemia or it may act as their cause. Postoperative hypertension is common, particularly early in coronary artery bypass grafting (CABG) recovery. The postoperative hypertension is probably due to excess catecholamine release.
5. The origin of obstetric hypertension is unclear, but the condition usually presents in the second trimester of pregnancy.
6. Medications that cause vasoconstriction.
7. Lack of compliance with medical therapy in "known" hypertension or inadequate treatment of such hypertension. Also, certain drugs may cause hypertension.

Clinical Presentation

The most common symptom is severe headache accompanied by nausea, vomiting, restlessness, and mental confusion, which may rapidly advance to coma and/or convulsions. Signs of a specific organ injury may be present. For example, myocardial ischemia, cerebral vascular accident, hematuria, or retinopathy may become evident. Sudden elevations in blood pressure are more likely to present with symptoms than are gradual elevations.

Treatment

Treatment of hypertensive crisis centers around the reduction of blood pressure to safe levels without producing a subsequent hypotension. Remember, hypotensive symptoms can appear at higher than expected pressures in the patient with chronic hypertension. Gradual reduction of the MAP to 110 to 115 mm Hg is acceptable; then, if the patient is showing no symptoms of hypotensive

TABLE 8-11. CHARACTERISTICS OF EMERGENCY HYPERTENSION

Diastolic blood pressure >120 mm Hg
Presence of one of the following:
    Acute aortic dissection
    LV failure with or without pulmonary edema
    Myocardial ischemia
    Acute renal failure
    Cerebrovascular or subarachnoid bleed
    Hypertensive encephalopathy
    Head injuries
    Grade 3–4 Keith-Wagener-Barker retinopathy
    Toxemia of pregnancy
    Burns
    Medication interaction
    Pheochromocytoma crisis

LV, left ventricular.

TABLE 8-12. MEDICATIONS TO TREAT HYPERTENSIVE EMERGENCIES

Agent	Dose	Onset of Action	Actions and Precautions
Intravenous Medications			
Nitroglycerin	5–100 mcg as IV infusion	2–5 min/5–10 min	Action: Venodilation Side effects: Headache, tachycardia, vomiting, flushing, methemoglobinemia; requires special delivery system due to drug binding to IV tubing
Nicardipine	5–15 mg/h IV infusion	1–5 min/15–30 min, but may exceed 12 h after prolonged infusion	Action: Calcium channel blockade Side effects: Tachycardia, nausea, vomiting, headache, increased intracranial pressure; hypotension may be protracted after prolonged infusion
Clevidipine	1–2 mg/h IV infusion; doses usually <16 mg/h	2–4 min	
Hydralazine	5–20 mg as IV bolus or 10–40 mg IM; repeat every 4–6 h	10 min IV/ >1 h (IV) 20–30 min IM/ 4–6 h (IM)	Action: Direct vascular smooth muscle relaxation Side effects: Tachycardia, headache, vomiting, aggravation of angina pectoris, sodium and water retention, and increased intracranial pressure
Fenoldopam mesylate	0.1–0.3 mcg/kg/min IV infusion	<5 min/30 min	Action: Peripheral dopamine$_1$ receptor antagonism Side effects: Headache, tachycardia, flushing, local phlebitis, dizziness
Esmolol	500 mcg/kg bolus injection IV or 50–100 mcg/kg/min by infusion. May repeat bolus after 5 min or increase infusion rate to 300 mcg/kg/min	1–5 min/15–30 min	Action: Beta blockade Side effects: First-degree heart block, congestive HF, asthma
Labetalol	20–40 mg as IV bolus every 10 min; up to 2 mg/min as IV infusion	5–10 min/2–6 h	Action: Beta blockade Side effects: Bronchoconstriction, heart block, orthostatic hypotension, bradycardia
Enalaprilat	0.625–1.25 mg every 6 h IV	Within 30 min/12–24 h	Action: ACE inhibition Side effects: Renal dysfunction, hyperkalemia hypotension
Phentolamine	5–10 mg as IV bolus	1–2 min/10–30 min	Action: Alpha-adrenergic blockade. Used primarily in pheochromocytoma Side effects: Tachycardia, orthostatic hypotension
Oral Agents			
Captopril	6.25–25 mg PO, repeat as needed; SL, 25 mg	15–30 min/6–8 h SL 10–20 min/2–6 h	Action: ACE inhibition Side effects: Hypotension, coughing, renal dysfunction, angioedema
Clonidine	0.1–0.2 mg PO, repeat hourly as required to total dose of 0.6 mg	30–60 min/8–16 h	Action: alpha-adrenergic agonism Side effects: Hypotension, drowsiness, light-headedness, dry mouth
Labetalol	200–400 mg PO, repeat every 2–3 h	1–2 h/2–12 h	Action: Beta blockade Side effects: Bronchoconstriction, heart block, orthostatic hypotension
Amlodipine	5–10 mg PO	Daily	Action: Calcium channel blocker Side effects: Hypotension, headache
Prazosin	1–2 mg PO, repeat hourly as needed	1–2 h/8–12 h	Action: Alpha-adrenergic blockade Side effects: Syncope (first dose), palpitations, tachycardia, orthostatic hypotension

ACE, angiotensin-converting enzyme; IM, intamuscular; IV, intravenous; PO, by mouth; SL, sublingual.

effects, further reductions to about 85 mm Hg are generally safe. Therapeutic modalities to achieve the MAP reduction generally involve a rapidly acting agent initially, with conversion to an oral agent as soon as possible. A diuretic is frequently added to counter potential water and sodium disturbances resulting from normal renal mechanisms to compensate for the hypertension. Examples of rapidly acting and oral maintenance agents are listed in Table 8-12.

9

Cardiogenic Shock

EDITORS' NOTE

Expect a few questions addressing the assessment and treatment of cardiogenic shock. This is a condition that will quickly be moved to an intensive care unit setting. However, an understanding of hemodynamic monitoring will substantially assist in answering these questions. Invasive parameters like those obtained from a pulmonary artery catheter will not be on the PCCN exam. Many of the principles of treating cardiogenic shock are covered in the earlier discussion of the treatment of heart failure in Chapter 8.

ETIOLOGY

Cardiogenic shock produces the same cellular disruption of oxygen as does hypovolemic shock, but for different reasons. In cardiogenic shock, mortality is high. As with hypovolemic shock, mean arterial pressure (MAP) is <60 mm Hg. Tissue oxygenation parameters, like the $ScvO_2$ level, are abnormally low: <0.60. Preload is elevated, characterized by a central venous pressure (CVP) of >8 mm Hg. Because the left ventricle is unable to maintain the forward flow of blood, pressure builds in the ventricle, causing an increased left ventricular (LV) end-diastolic pressure (preload). Two primary manifestations of the reduced cardiac output are seen. The most dangerous is the development of systemic hypotension. In addition, pulmonary congestion secondary to the increased preload will occur, with a resulting increase in the intrapulmonary shunt (decrease in arterial oxygen pressure [PaO_2] and saturation [SaO_2] levels).

COMPENSATION MECHANISMS

Cardiogenic shock produces compensatory mechanisms—aimed to maintain tissue perfusion—similar to those for hypovolemic shock. Two of these key mechanisms are as follows:

1. Sympathetic stimulation. Release of sympathetic stimulants such as epinephrine, norepinephrine, and dopamine, which act to increase heart rate, improve contractility, and cause vasoconstriction to increase blood pressure. Epinephrine has a mild vasoconstrictive effect, although it is predominately a beta stimulant, resulting in improved cardiac output and slight vasodilation. Norepinephrine, which has a strong vasoconstrictive effect, is released, with a resultant mild increase in heart rate, strength, and impulse transmission. The increased contractility and heart rate serve to increase the cardiac output. The increased vasoconstriction acts to maintain perfusion pressures and improve core organ blood flow.
2. Activation of the renin-angiotensin-aldosterone system (RAAS), promoting vasoconstriction and sodium and water retention. This mechanism acts to increase an already normal or elevated total vascular volume compartment. This mechanism, like sympathetic stimulation, is designed to help maintain blood flow but can actually make the situation worse.

IDENTIFYING CHARACTERISTICS

The patient in cardiogenic shock will present with the symptoms listed in Table 9-1. In addition, the patient may present with hyperventilation brought

TABLE 9-1. SYMPTOMS OF HYPOVOLEMIC AND CARDIOGENIC SHOCK

Symptoms	Hypovolemic	Cardiogenic
Common		
Blood pressure	Low	Low
Pulse	Tachycardia	Tachycardia
Urine output	Low (<0.5 mL/kg/hour)	Low
Level of consciousness	Altered	Altered
Skin	Cool, clammy	Cool, clammy
Pulse quality	Weak	Weak
Differentiating		
Pao_2	Normal	Low
Sao_2	Normal	Low
Cyanosis	Absent	May be present
a/A ratio	Normal	Low
PAOP	Low (<10)	High (>18)
Orthopnea	Minimal	Present
Crackles	Minimal	Present
Dependent edema	Absent	Present

PAOP, Pulmonary occlusive pressure.

on in an attempt to compensate for a lactic acidosis. The nurse should attempt to identify any potential risk factors that might help to identify the type of shock involved.

TREATMENT

In a patient who presents with cardiogenic shock, myocardial function must be improved as rapidly as possible. Much of the current treatment centers on pharmacologic or mechanical support of the heart.

Pharmacologic Treatment

Improving Cardiac Output/Contractility or the Use of Inotropes
Improvement in cardiac output is most often achieved with the use of dobutamine, although milrinone and mid-dose dopamine may also be used. New agents such as levosimendan are promising but are not the standard of care as yet. Improving contractility comes with a price. Although the potential exists to increase cardiac output, there is a resultant increase in myocardial oxygen consumption. Inotropes should be used with caution and only after less dangerous treatments have been tried first (e.g., preload reduction).

Improving Cardiac Output/ Preload Reduction
Diuretics and vasodilators (nitroglycerin, diltiazem) may be employed. The use of a pulmonary artery catheter may facilitate assessment of the effectiveness of these agents. The goal of preload reduction is to reduce the stretch of ventricular muscle and improve myocardial contractility while reducing pulmonary congestion.

Improving Blood Pressure
In the patient with severe hypotension, vasoconstrictors such as norepinephrine, phenylephrine, or dopamine may be employed. Vasopressin, another vasoconstrictor, is not used in cardiogenic shock (as there is no evidence for the deficiency of endogenous vasopressin). Use of these drugs is not without risk because of the increased myocardial oxygen consumption associated with their vasoconstrictive properties. Although a general understanding of these agents is helpful, they are not likely to appear on the PCCN exam. The hope is that the improvement in blood pressure is accompanied by an improved myocardial blood flow and, therefore, may offset the increased myocardial oxygen consumption. However, an improved blood pressure does not always improve blood flow. Use of oxygenation parameters, such as venous oxygen saturation (SvO_2) values and lactate levels, will help determine whether an improvement in blood pressure has improved blood flow.

Adjuncts to Pharmacologic Support

If the cardiogenic shock is due to a recent MI, cardiac catheterization for stent placement and/or thrombolytic therapy may also be employed. The goal is to reestablish perfusion in the fastest, most effective manner. If stent placement can occur quickly, it is preferred. In the absence of rapid stent placement, thrombolysis may be preferred.

Use of mechanical support of the heart for the patient with cardiogenic shock is increasingly common. Such support ranges from intra-aortic balloon pumping to ventricular-assist devices; however, these modalities will not appear on the PCCN exam.

Protecting Ventilation

Intubation and aggressive oxygen therapy are frequently necessary in the treatment of cardiogenic shock. Positive end-expiratory pressure (PEEP) should be used cautiously, and the nurse should monitor changes in cardiac output if PEEP is employed.

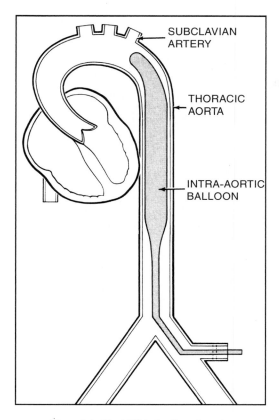

Figure 9-1. The IABP in the thoracic aorta.

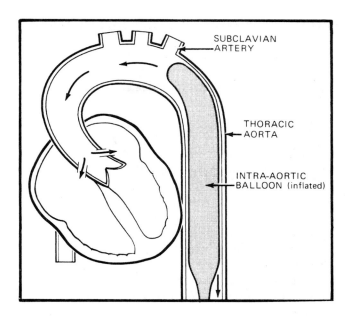

Figure 9-2. The IABP inflated during ventricular diastole.

measure, if the pH is below 7.20, bicarbonate administration to maintain pH levels above 7.20 may buy time in reestablishing blood flow. Monitoring the SvO_2 (return to normal of >60% to 70%) will aid in treating tissue hypoxia.

Treating Lactic Acidosis

Lactic acidosis will resolve if perfusion is reestablished. In the case of severe disturbances in systemic pH (<7.20), small doses of sodium bicarbonate may be necessary. Despite the controversy over this

Intra-Aortic Balloon Pump

Use of the aortic counterpulsation balloon, or the intra-aortic balloon pump (IABP), is increasingly available. The IABP reduces afterload of the left ventricle and increases blood flow into the coronary

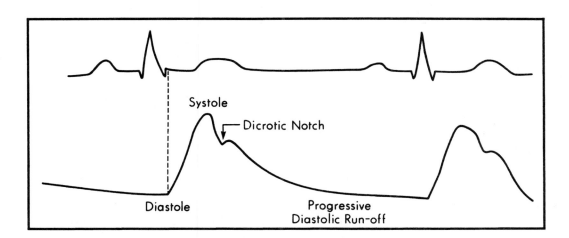

Figure 9-3. Normal arterial waveform.

arteries, which makes it useful in treating refractive cardiac failure and cardiogenic shock. The IABP may be used as a supplement to medical treatment for cardiogenic shock or as a cardiac augmentation mechanism when surgery is imminent. IABP content will not be covered on the PCCN exam.

Principles of the IABP

The IABP decreases strain on the left ventricle by lowering afterload in the aorta. With a reduced afterload, the ventricle does not have to contract as forcibly to expel its blood into the aorta (Fig 9-1).

During ventricular diastole, the balloon inflates to improve coronary blood flow. Blood is forced back into the coronary arteries with proper inflation (Fig. 9-2). The correct point for inflation is frequently near the dicrotic notch. Closure of the aortic valve is the event that produces the dicrotic notch on the arterial wave (Fig. 9-3). As discussed earlier, prior to ventricular systole (Fig. 9-4), the balloon deflates, decreasing the aortic afterload.

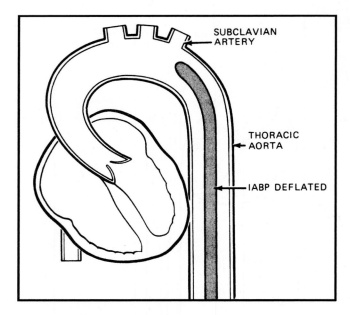

Figure 9-4. The IABP deflated prior to ventricular systole.

10

Hemorrhagic (Hypovolemic) Shock

EDITORS' NOTE

The PCCN exam is likely to include several questions that test your knowledge of treatment of the major forms of shock. In this chapter, a simple approach to understanding hypovolemic shock is presented. This approach should provide you with the information necessary to successfully answer questions on the concept of hypovolemic shock. Table 10-1 presents a simple guide to identifying hypovolemia. If you follow it, you will be able to recognize any case of hypovolemia on the PCCN exam.

This section presents a brief review of the physiology of microcirculatory compensation in shock. This compensation is not restricted to hypovolemia but occurs in all forms of shock.

Hypovolemic shock, caused by a loss of circulating blood volume, presents with a loss of blood flow to the tissues. Although this loss of blood volume is commonly associated with bleeding, it also is commonly accompanied by early sepsis. Sepsis presents in a phasic manner, with early phases presenting with low cardiac outputs while the later phase presents with a hyperdynamic state with high cardiac outputs. In this chapter, the emphasis is placed on identifying hypovolemia and early sepsis. The hemodynamic changes associated with the hyperdynamic state of sepsis are discussed in Chap. 5.

The PCCN exam can be anticipated to contain questions on each type of shock. The review presented here is designed to build on previous chapters and improve your ability to recognize and differentiate the conditions that produce hypovolemia.

Hypovolemic shock occurs when there is a threat to tissue oxygenation secondary to a loss of cardiac output and stroke volume. The threat to tissue oxygenation is accompanied by several clinical factors, including a low SvO_2 (<60%) or low $ScvO_2$ (<70%), high lactate (>4 mmol), and low mean arterial pressure (MAP) (<60 mm Hg). Perhaps most importantly, hypovolemia is accompanied by a low stroke volume (normal varies, but <50 mL is usually abnormally low). Stroke volume can also be interpreted with Doppler values (a low flow time [FTc] of <330 m/s) or pulse contour devices showing a stroke volume variation of >10%. An easier way to see if a patient is hypovolemic is to give fluids and see if the stroke volume increases by >10%. If it does, an additional fluid bolus should be given. Fluid should be administered until no further increase in stroke volume is seen.

Hypovolemic shock is characterized by loss of blood volume due to active bleeding, chronic loss of vascular volume, or capillary (endothelial wall) leakage.

The causes of the loss of blood volume are wide ranging and include trauma, postoperative bleeding, and third spacing of fluid. Specific causes of hypovolemic shock are listed in Table 10-2. Both medical and surgical units are likely to see hypovolemic shock. Loss of vascular volume—due to bleeding, dehydration, or capillary leakage—is the most common cause of loss of blood flow, making this the most common reason for hypotension. When a patient is admitted with hypotension of unknown origin, hypovolemia must be suspected and treated before other forms of therapy are instituted.

ETIOLOGY

The loss of circulating blood volume leads to a reduction in preload (stretch of the ventricular muscle) and eventually a reduction in stroke volume and cardiac output. The loss of stroke volume can be

TABLE 10-1. HYPOVOLEMIA: EASY REVIEW AND APPLICATION

Presents with a threat to tissue oxygenation
Svo_2 or $Scvo_2$ is low (<60% or <70%, respectively)
Lactate is elevated (>4 mmol)
Cardiac output is low
Heart pumps <4 L/min
Cardiac index is low (<2.5 mL/m^2)
Stroke volume is low (<50 mL)
Stroke index is low (<25 mL/m^2)
Cardiac filling pressures are low or normal
CVP is <6

CVP, central venous pressure.

compensated for by an increase in heart rate. Such an increase in heart rate can be substantial enough to prevent a reduction in blood pressure. Because of the compensating increase in heart rate, the early phases of hypovolemic shock may not be reflected in blood pressure changes.

As the increase in heart rate fails to compensate for the loss of stroke volume and cardiac output falls, SVR increases as a second compensatory mechanism. Again, the blood pressure does not change markedly until the SVR can no longer regulate the blood pressure. At the same time that heart rate and SVR are compensating for loss of stroke volume, microcirculatory changes are occurring in an attempt to maintain organ blood flow.

Physiology of the Microcirculation

EDITORS' NOTE

It is unlikely that this content will be directly addressed on the PCCN exam. However, this information is good background material for understanding how blood flow is regulated at the tissue level. These mechanisms occur in all forms of initial compensation to loss of blood flow—for example, all initial stages of shock. Septic shock is a little different because of its phasic nature. However, early sepsis is likely to be governed by these factors as well.

The microcirculation of blood vessels acts to regulate the blood supply to the tissues (Fig. 10-1). The components of the microcirculation are capillaries, which form the vascular system between arterioles and venules. The arterioles bifurcate at points called metarterioles or precapillary arterioles. Smooth muscle cells cover the metarterioles at the bifurcation but disappear as each metarteriole becomes a true capillary.

At the point of metarteriole bifurcation into true capillaries, there is a muscle sphincter. This precapillary sphincter acts as an autoregulatory system, dilating to allow increased perfusion when blood pressure is low or constricting when blood pressure is increased to adjust to the metabolic needs of the tissues in normal states.

The precapillary sphincter constricts in cases of shock and sympathetic nervous system stimulation to maintain perfusion of the vital organs. This constriction directs the available blood from nonessential tissues, such as the stomach, to vital organs, especially the heart and brain. This is the first major compensatory mechanism to be activated with the onset of shock.

Many chemical and humoral factors alter the regulation of the microcirculatory system. Neurochemical controls provide a negative feedback response that results in adaptive responses to maintain cellular oxygenation. If the shock is mild and/or

TABLE 10-2. CAUSES OF HYPOVOLEMIC AND CARDIOGENIC SHOCK

Hypovolemic	Cardiogenic
Trauma	Myocardial infarction
Postoperative bleeding	Atrial tachydysrhythmias (atrial tachycardia, flutter, fibrillation)
Gastrointestinal bleeding	Ventricular tachycardia, fibrillation
Burns	Congestive heart failure
Capillary leak syndromes	Papillary muscle rupture
	Septal or ventricular wall rupture
	Tension pneumothorax
	Pericardial tamponade

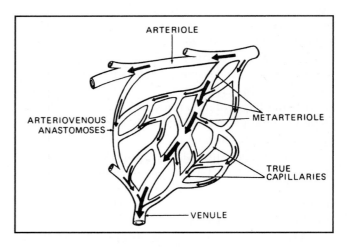

Figure 10-1. Microcirculation.

slow in developing, the negative feedback of the microcirculatory system will reverse the shock state. If the shock is severe or rapid in developing, this negative feedback of the microcirculatory system may not reverse the shock state. Failure to restore a hemostatic state allows a positive feedback system to develop. In this vicious cycle of positive feedback, inadequate tissue perfusion leads to a deterioration in cardiovascular function, which decreases tissue perfusion even more. Consequently, in these instances, the shock state precipitates an even more severe shock state, leading to death if not reversed.

The release of catecholamines (epinephrine and norepinephrine) in early shock results in vasoconstriction of the microcirculatory vessels at the precapillary sphincter level. The precapillary sphincter constricts in an attempt to increase venous return to the heart (by preventing blood flow in unnecessary tissues), which in turn improves cardiac output and tissue perfusion (Table 10-3).

The hemodynamic mechanism to resolve shock is movement of fluid from the interstitial space into the vascular tree, causing an increase in plasma volume. This fluid shift occurs because a change in the hydrostatic pressure in the capillaries alters fluid exchange across the capillary membrane. With increased fluid shifting into the vascular tree, the plasma is diluted, decreasing plasma oncotic pressure and fostering more fluid movement into capillary beds. After hemorrhage, the liver immediately synthesizes new proteins to replace the lost plasma proteins in an attempt to force the fluid shift from the interstitium to the vascular tree and thus maintain adequate intravascular volume.

The renin-angiotensin-aldosterone cascade is activated by decreased renal blood flow. The renin is acted upon in several stages to convert it to angiotensin II. Angiotensin II is one of the most potent vasoconstrictors known. It augments the blood pressure and ideally increases blood flow in the process. Angiotensin II and the catecholamines (epinephrine and norepinephrine) increase vasoconstriction in all organs except the brain and heart. At the same time, aldosterone secretion is stimulated by angiotensin II. Aldosterone increases sodium retention by the kidneys, thereby increasing water reabsorption in the convoluted tubular system of the nephron. This additional retention of water helps increase intravascular volume.

A low cardiac output, secondary to hypovolemia, stimulates the neurohypophysis to increase the release of the antidiuretic hormone (ADH). ADH promotes water reabsorption through its actions on the convoluted tubules and collecting ducts of the kidneys. ADH also has a vasoconstricting effect that further increases arterial pressure. Because of this action, ADH is sometimes called vasopressin.

Symptoms of Hypovolemia

Chronic hypovolemia can manifest itself physically in many ways. Acute hypovolemia, however, may be difficult to detect until hypotension develops. Shock states will all produce common changes, such as tachycardia, hypotension, changes in level of consciousness, and reduction in urine output. SvO_2 and lactates will be abnormal in hypovolemia as well as cardiogenic and septic shock. However, one method for improving the specificity of physical symptoms of hypovolemia is to apply the concept of preload. Preload (pulmonary artery wedge pressure [PAWP] or pulmonary artery occlusive pressure [PAOP]) and the central venous pressure (CVP) in hypovolemia are low or normal, differentiating hypovolemic shock from heart failure (HF) and cardiogenic shock. The low preload does not produce any of the symptoms of pulmonary or vascular congestion seen in HF and cardiogenic shock. Specific symptoms of hypovolemic shock are given in Table 10-1.

Orthostatic blood pressure changes can indicate hypovolemia, although these changes are often inaccurate. These changes, which are measured by changing the patient's position from supine to sitting, are defined by an increased heart rate (more than 10 beats per minute) and a fall in systolic (<25 mm Hg) and diastolic blood pressures (<10 mm Hg).

Since initial symptoms of any shock are minimal, observation to detect subtle changes is important.

TABLE 10-3. REGULATION OF THE MICROCIRCULATORY SYSTEM

Chemical	C	D	Humoral	C	D
Hypoxemia		+	Catecholamines		
Hydrogen		+	Epinephrine	+	+
Potassium		+	Norepinephrine	+	
Hypercapnea	+		Dopamine	+	+
Hyperosmolarity	+		Amines		
			Serotonin	+	+
			Acetylcholine		+
			Histamine		+
			Polypeptides		
			Angiotensin	+	
			Kinins	+	
			Vasopressin		+

C, vasoconstriction; D, vasodilatation.

A gradually increasing heart rate coupled with a downward trend in blood pressure may be a clue to impending hypovolemia. Early intervention can result in a much more favorable outcome. If intervention is delayed, enough cellular damage may occur that the shock becomes irreversible. Measurement of oxygenation will give an idea of the severity of the shock state. Lactate levels, for example, have been correlated with survival in patients with hemorrhagic shock. If lactate levels exceed 4 mmol/L and are associated with a decrease in pH, the likelihood of survival drops markedly. Lactate levels are easy to obtain, from either a venous or arterial sample. Lactate will increase if the hypovolemia is producing systemic reductions to oxygen delivery to the tissues.

Systemic signs of hypovolemia include a possible decrease in urine output (<30 mL/h or <0.5 mL/kg/h), change in level of consciousness (LOC) or behavior (cerebral ischemia may develop when the cerebral perfusion pressure drops below 60 mm Hg), increase in respiratory rate, and change in pulse quality. These symptoms are highly variable in the initial stages of shock. As shock progresses, severe depression in LOC, cool clammy skin, oliguria, hypotension, and tachycardia are common.

COMPLICATIONS

Sustained hypoperfusion due to hypovolemia will lead to impaired organ function and eventually cell death. It is possible that apoptosis (preprogrammed cell death) may be stimulated by hypoperfusion. Hypovolemia requires rapid treatment to avoid a potentially harmful or even fatal outcome.

TREATMENT

The primary focus in hypovolemic shock is the replacement of lost vascular volume. The treatment modalities for the correction of hypovolemic shock are controversial, centering on which type of plasma expander, crystalloid or colloid infusion, should be used.

Often, whole blood and a crystalloid solution (e.g., normal saline or lactated Ringer's solution) is used to provide a balance between the infusion of red blood cells, electrolytes, and fluid that would affect all three compartments (intravascular, intracellular, and extracellular). Interstitial and intracellular compartments are not replenished by blood or other colloidal agents. Blood administration increases vascular volume, osmotic pressure, and oxygen-carrying capacity.

Colloidal therapy is based on the administration of fluids that contain high molecular weight solutes, such as albumin or a glucose polymer (hetastarch). The proponents of colloidal agents claim that increasing the colloid osmotic pressure in the vascular tree will either "pull" interstitial fluids back into the vascular system or at least provide for rapid volume expansion since fluid will not leak out of the vascular compartment. Many authorities believe that acute hypovolemia can best be managed with the use of colloidal agents; others feel that there is a greater risk of overtransfusion with colloids, which remain in the intact vascular tree, than with crystalloids, which can be absorbed into intracellular and interstitial spaces.

Recent research suggests that crystalloids, like normal saline, have the same impact on patient outcome as colloids, such as albumin. This research suggests that initial therapies to treat hypovolemia should start with normal saline. In addition, the optimal method to administer the saline is to have a goal (the concept of goal-directed therapy). The best criterion to use in determining how much fluid to give is the SvO_2 level. Although normal saline can be administered at an estimated volume (e.g., 20 mL/kg), the exact amount that should be given is not known. That is why it is best to administer fluids until the SvO_2 level returns to normal (e.g., 70%).

Blood

The administration of blood is controversial. Unless the patient is actively bleeding and the hemoglobin is <7 g/dL, blood should be given with caution. Recent research indicates that the administration of blood has been associated with activation of the recipient's immune system. Nosocomial infections increase with the administration of blood and, as a result, outcomes are adversely affected. If blood is given, a better endpoint is tissue oxygenation (e.g., SvO_2) rather than an arbitrary hemoglobin value.

NURSING INTERVENTION

Monitoring hemodynamic parameters of hypovolemic shock usually involves measuring the SvO_2 or the $ScvO_2$. The CVP or pulmonary artery catheter may be used. Newer hemodynamic technologies, such as esophageal Dopplers, bioimpedance, pulse contour, exhaled CO_2, and capnography are also emerging as methods to guide the effectiveness of treatment by better monitoring of stroke volume or index.

Older treatments for hypovolemia may still be used, although the research on their impact on outcome is not clear. Patients traditionally have been placed in the Trendelenburg position or positioned with use of "shock blocks." Research indicates that a supine position or elevation of only the legs provides adequate circulation to the brain. In cases of severe shock, a supine position with legs elevated 20 to 30 degrees by pillows may increase venous return. Whether this helps improve survival is not known. If a concurrent head injury exists, the head of the bed may be placed in a slightly upright position.

Cardiovascular status, in addition to hemodynamic status, is continuously monitored for signs of dysrhythmias. Dysrhythmias due to electrolyte disturbance are common with massive blood transfusions and with inadequate vascular volume.

Vasomotor tone is normally controlled by constriction secondary to sympathetic and catecholamine factors. Sympathetic stimulants such as norepinephrine (Levophed) and dopamine may have to be administered to maintain blood pressure after volume resuscitation has been completed.

Acid-base disturbances may be severe, and mixed metabolic and respiratory acidosis is common. Respiratory acidosis is corrected by adequate ventilation. Metabolic acidosis may be corrected by reversing decreased organ blood flow. If the pH is severely reduced (i.e., <7.20), sodium bicarbonate ($NaHCO_3$) may be used to raise the pH to tolerable levels (<7.20). An initial loading dose for sodium bicarbonate is 1 mEq/kg of body weight. Additional doses depend on the arterial blood gas values. The use of sodium bicarbonate remains controversial, however, and changes in the guidelines for its application may alter the above recommendations.

Renal function is monitored hourly, usually with an indwelling Foley catheter. Severe or sustained hypovolemia may result in acute tubular necrosis, although prerenal azotemia is the first renal response. The blood urea nitrogen (BUN) may rise disproportionately to the creatinine, creating an increased BUN/creatinine ratio (>15:1).

Nutritional support is essential, since a shock state rapidly depletes glucose storage with a resulting negative nitrogen balance, and protein catabolism increases acidotic states. Enteral feeding is preferred.

Emotional support consists of reassurance and explanation of procedures. Families may be provided with information by way of brochures or websites that will help explain medical conditions in an easy to understand manner (e.g., www.ICU-USA.com and the National Library of Medicine). Short, brief comments regarding the patient's condition and the use of monitoring equipment will help to decrease anxiety. Explanations to the patient and family members about the patient's current status and nursing procedures usually serve to console them.

11

Interpreting Dysrhythmias

EDITORS' NOTE

The PCCN exam can be expected to directly address either the interpretation or treatment of sinus and atrial dysrhythmias. There are only a few questions on the PCCN exam that will ask you to interpret dysrhythmias. However, there may be several questions where dysrhythmias are a part of the test question. The most likely dysrhythmias are atrial tachycardia, flutter, and fibrillation. The most important concepts in this area are the correct interpretation of dysrhythmias and the treatment each would require. Most of this information is included in a basic electrographic (ECG) course. However, if the interpretation of dysrhythmia is not a strength for you, review this chapter carefully.

All dysrhythmias are caused by a disturbance in the formation of the cardiac impulse or a disturbance in its conduction. The classification of dysrhythmias is shown in Table 11-1.

Every dysrhythmia has specific identifying characteristics. The first four dysrhythmias discussed in this chapter originate in the sinoatrial (SA) node. The next six dysrhythmias originate in the atrium but not in the SA node. The final eight dysrhythmias originate from electrical impulses initiated in the junctional tissue around the atrioventricular (AV) node. (*Note:* All rhythm strips are 6 s, lead II.)

SINOATRIAL NODE DYSRHYTHMIAS

Sinus Arrhythmia (or Sinus Dysrhythmia)

Etiology

Variations of impulse formation in the SA node are caused by the vagus nerve and changes in venous return to the heart. This results in an irregular rhythm with alternating fast and slow rates (Fig. 11-1).

Identifying Characteristics

The rate varies; it is usually between 60 and 100 beats per minute. The rate increases with inspiration and decreases with expiration. Both atrial and ventricular rhythms are regularly irregular if the variation is due to a regular breathing pattern. The P waves are normal and the PR interval is within normal limits. The QRS complex is normal. The difference between normal sinus rhythm and sinus arrhythmia is seen in the variation in the RR intervals. In sinus arrhythmia, the variation is at least 0.04 s between the shortest and longest RR intervals. The variation in normal sinus rhythm is less than 0.04 s.

Risk

There is no risk for the patient because this dysrhythmia is a normal variant and causes no hemodynamic compromise.

Treatment

No treatment is needed.

Nursing Intervention

Document the dysrhythmia with a rhythm strip. This interpretation can be substantiated if the patient holds his or her breath and the rate stabilizes.

Sinus Bradycardia

Etiology

Parasympathetic (vagal) control over the SA node due to ischemia, pain, drugs, sleep, or athletic conditioning decreases the formation of electrical impulses (Fig. 11-2).

TABLE 11-1. CLASSIFICATION OF DYSRHYTHMIAS

Dysrhythmias due to Disorders in Impulse Foundation or Accessory Pathway	Dysrhythmias due to Conduction Disturbances
SA node dysrhythmias	SA block
Sinus tachycardia	AV blocks
Sinus bradycardia	First-degree AV block
Sinus arrhythmia	Second-degree type I AV block
Wandering pacemaker	Second-degree type II AV block
SA arrest	Third-degree (complete) AV block
Atrial dysrhythmias	Intraventricular blocks
Premature atrial contractions	Left bundle branch blocks
Paroxysmal atrial tachycardia	Right bundle branch blocks
Atrial flutter	Bilateral bundle branch blocks
Atrial fibrillation	
AV nodal area (junctional) dysrhythmias	
Premature junctional contractions	
Junctional escape rhythm	
Paroxysmal junctional tachycardia	
Junctional tachycardia	
Ventricular dysrhythmias	
Premature ventricular contractions	
Ventricular tachycardia	
Ventricular fibrillation	
Ventricular asystole	

Identifying Characteristics

The rate is less than 60 but usually more than 40. Both atrial and ventricular rhythms are usually regular. P waves are normal. The PR interval is within the upper limits or is slightly prolonged. The QRS complex is normal. Conduction is normal.

Risk

This dysrhythmia may lead to syncopal attacks, angina, premature beats, ventricular tachycardia, heart failure (HF), and cardiac arrest. It is a serious warning dysrhythmia if the rate is low (about 40) and accompanied by hypotension (blood pressure below 90/60 mm Hg). Sinus bradycardia is generally benign but should be assessed for its effect on hemodynamics.

Treatment

No treatment may be necessary if the rate is close to 60 or if the patient is asymptomatic. If the rate is low and/or the patient is symptomatic, first try to find out whether there is a reversible cause, such as hypoxemia. Give supplemental oxygen if the pulse oximeter is low. If more severe symptoms are present (e.g., hypotension or signs of HF), intravenous atropine is the drug of choice to increase the heart rate. An external or temporary pacemaker may be required if pharmacologic management is unsuccessful.

Nursing Intervention

Document the dysrhythmia with a rhythm strip. Monitor and document the effectiveness of drug therapy. Do not administer drugs, such as digitalis or

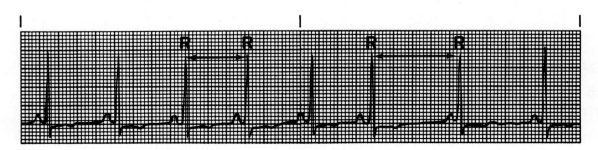

Figure 11-1. Sinus arrhythmia.

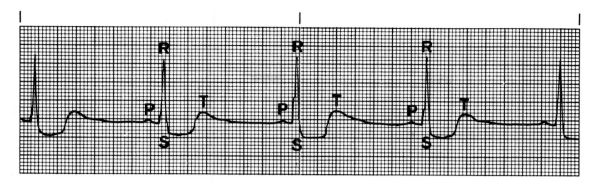

Figure 11-2. Sinus bradycardia.

beta blockers, that may further slow the heart rate. Be especially alert for premature ventricular contractions (PVCs). If PVCs occur, obtain a rhythm strip and notify the physician; do not treat with lidocaine or other agents that may eliminate the PVCs. PVCs associated with a bradycardia are generally treated with atropine or another therapy to remove the cause of the bradycardia. As the heart rate increases, the PVCs usually disappear.

Sinus Tachycardia

Etiology

Cardiac decompensation (heart failure [HF]) is the most serious cause of sinus tachycardia. The increase in heart rate during HF is a compensatory response due to a reduced stroke volume. Sinus tachycardia may also be caused by any factor that stimulates the sympathetic nervous system, such as anxiety, exertion (physical), and fever (Fig. 11-3).

Identifying Characteristics

The rate is greater than 100 and is usually between 100 and 160. Both atrial and ventricular rhythms are regular. The P wave is normal but may be difficult to identify because of the rapid rate. (*Note:* Look for the P wave superimposed on the T wave with fast rates.) The PR interval is usually at the lower limits of normal.

Risk

Regardless of the etiology, prolonged sinus tachycardia may precipitate HF in patients with borderline cardiac function. The ability to tolerate a prolonged sinus tachycardia is dependent on the patient's underlying cardiac function.

Treatment

Effective treatment depends on controlling the underlying cause. Normally, sinus tachycardia does not in itself require treatment. In case of a persistent sinus tachycardia that is compromising cardiac output, pharmacologic treatment may be required, with drugs such as calcium channel blockers (e.g., verapamil), beta blockers (e.g., esmolol, diltiazem), or adenosine or digitalis preparations (e.g., digoxin). Normally, however, resolving the cause will be the focus of treatment for sinus tachycardia.

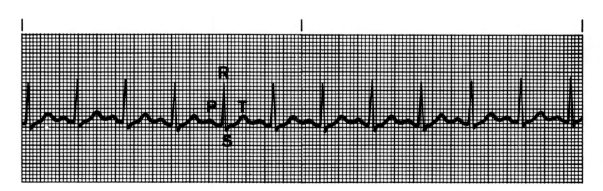

Figure 11-3. Sinus tachycardia.

Nursing Intervention

Document the dysrhythmia with a rhythm strip. Monitor the patient for signs of left ventricular (LV) failure (restlessness, orthopnea, cough, shortness of breath). Attempts to calm the patient and to decrease the patient's stress may be helpful.

Sinus Pause/Arrest, Sinoatrial Block

Etiology

These more complex atrial dysrhythmias will rarely be on the PCCN exam. Therefore, this information is more supplemental than essential. Ischemic injury to the SA node is the most common and important cause of SA block. There is a technical but not a clinical difference between sinus pause/arrest and SA block. In the pause/arrest, the SA node does not form an electrical impulse. In SA block, the node initiates an impulse, but it is prevented from leaving the node and thus cannot be visualized. Regardless of this difference, the end result is that no impulse stimulates the atria or the ventricles. The terms *pause* and *block* are often used interchangeably. Sinus disease, vagal effect, digitalis toxicity, and sympathetic stimulation may be causes of SA block (Fig. 11-4).

Identifying Characteristics

The rate is usually slower than normal. Rhythm (both atrial and ventricular) is generally regular except for the arrest/block complex. P waves are absent in arrest and block for a specific time. Otherwise, P waves are normal. The PR interval is absent in the arrest/block complex. The QRS complex may be normal or abnormal in arrest depending on the escape site. No QRS complexes are seen during the block. Conduction depends on the escape site in arrest and is absent in sinus block for that specific interval.

Risk

The greatest risk is that both sinus pause/arrest and sinus block may proceed to a reduced cardiac output if the arrest or block is frequent. If the arrest or block is infrequent and self-limiting, it is not dangerous.

Treatment

If the arrest or block is rare, it does not require treatment. If the arrest is frequent, treatment is essential. If drugs are the underlying cause, they should be evaluated and stopped. Atropine and epinephrine may be effective at increasing the heart rate. If these are not

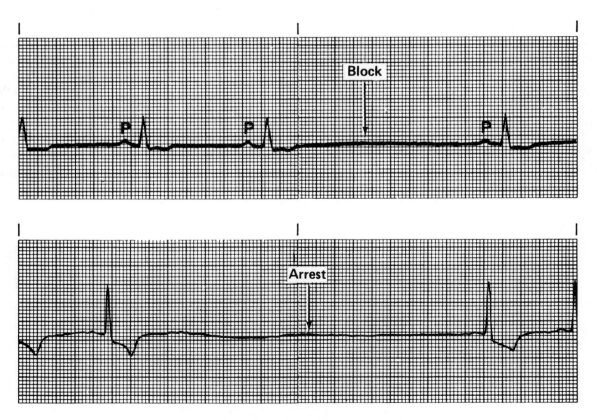

Figure 11-4. SA arrest or block.

effective and the patient is symptomatic, an external pacemaker could be applied initially, but long-term treatment will require a permanent pacemaker.

Nursing Intervention

Document the dysrhythmia with a rhythm strip. If a drug is the possible underlying cause, withhold the drug until it is reordered. Monitor the patient closely to determine whether the frequency of arrest or block is increasing. If it is, document with rhythm strips and notify the physician; a pacemaker may be indicated.

ATRIAL DYSRHYTHMIAS

Paroxysmal Atrial Tachycardia

Etiology

The term *paroxysmal atrial tachycardia* (PAT) describes several causes for a rapid atrial heart rate (Fig. 11-5). Another term, *paroxysmal supraventricular tachycardia* (PSVT or just SVT), is also used to describe this rhythm. In PAT, excessive sympathetic stimulation or abnormal conduction situations are present. Abnormal conduction situations include AV nodal reentry problems or the presence of accessory pathways.

Identifying Characteristics

Three characteristics are associated with PAT:

1. It starts suddenly.
2. It ends abruptly.
3. The ventricles respond either to every impulse created by the focus (1:1 conduction) or to most impulses, creating a rapid ventricular response.

Both atrial and ventricular rates are usually between 150 and 250. The rhythm is regular. P waves are present but may be very difficult to identify. The P wave will not have the normal, smooth, rounded shape of a sinus P wave, since this impulse originates in the atrium. The PR interval varies. It may be within normal limits and is frequently greater than might be expected for the rate. However, in some accessory pathway situations, the PR interval may be shortened. The QRS complex is usually normal. Once again, however, if the problem is due to an accessory pathway, an initial distortion in the QRS complex may be present. This distortion is sometimes seen as a delta wave, causing a slurring of the upstroke on the R wave of the QRS complex.

Risk

PAT frequently stops spontaneously. If it does not, the rapid rate may lead to myocardial ischemia and eventually cardiac decompensation. If PAT occurs after a myocardial infarction (MI) or in a patient with limited cardiac function, it may lead to increased myocardial ischemia and injury and LV failure.

Treatment

Vagal stimulation and other vagal maneuvers, such as coughing and pressure on the eyes, may terminate the dysrhythmia. Having the patient perform a Valsalva maneuver stimulates the vagus nerve. If this fails to terminate the rhythm, carotid massage by the doctor (or nurse if allowed) often terminates PAT. If this fails and the patient is asymptomatic, drug therapy may be tried. Beta blockers such as esmolol or digoxin, calcium channel blockers (verapamil or diltiazem), or adenosine given intravenously may terminate PAT. If the patient is symptomatic (complains of angina and becomes diaphoretic,

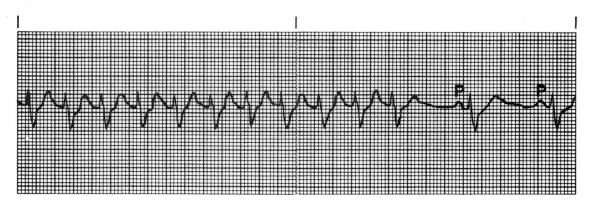

Figure 11-5. Paroxysmal atrial tachycardia.

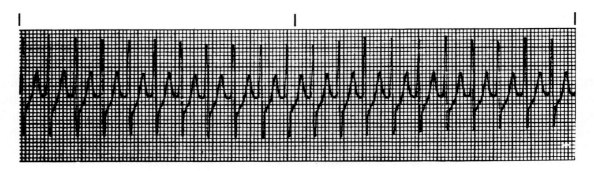

Figure 11-6. Atrial tachycardia.

short of breath, and hypotensive), synchronized cardioversion may be used immediately. Cardioversion usually terminates PAT.

Surgical interventions and radiofrequency ablation are increasingly seen as options for the patient with PAT. In order to cut the accessory pathway surgically (or eliminate the path with radiofrequency ablation), extensive electrical mapping of the heart in an electrophysiology lab in order to locate the origin of the abnormal pathway is required.

Nursing Intervention

Document the dysrhythmia with a rhythm strip. Assess and monitor the patient for signs of ischemia and decompensation. Medicate as ordered by the physician. Be prepared for synchronized cardioversion.

Atrial Tachycardia

The impulse of atrial tachycardia originates in the atrium. The rate of atrial tachycardia is constant. The difference between PAT and atrial tachycardia is only that PAT starts and stops suddenly. Atrial

tachycardia is a constant rhythm, not irregular. All other parameters of PAT apply to atrial tachycardia (Fig. 11-6).

Premature Atrial Contractions

Premature atrial contractions (PACs) are also called atrial premature beats.

Etiology

On occasion, an irritable focus in the atrium or an impulse through an accessory pathway causes an unexpected complex initiating depolarization. The irritable focus does not become the heart's pacemaker except for this single beat (Fig. 11-7).

Identifying Characteristics

The underlying rate is usually normal. The rhythm has an occasional irregularity due to the premature nature of the beat and a brief pause after the premature beat. The P wave is abnormally shaped for the premature beat only. The PR interval is usually prolonged but may be normal or shortened. The QRS complex is normal. PACs may be blocked or may

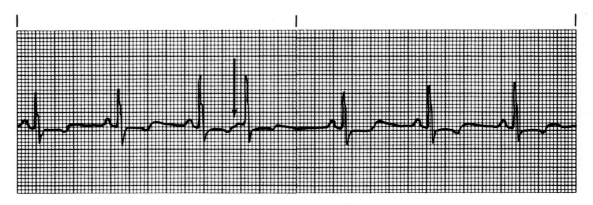

Figure 11-7. Premature atrial contraction.

have an aberrant (abnormal or wide QRS) conduction. Conduction below the atria (junctional and ventricular) is usually normal.

Risk
If PACs occur infrequently, there is no risk. If they occur six or more times per minute, they indicate atrial flutter, atrial fibrillation, or atrial tachycardia.

Treatment
PACs of fewer than six per minute do not need treatment. There is no specific number that dictates when treatment is needed. Those PACs that require treatment are more likely those causing symptoms that disrupt normal activities. Common treatments for PACs include digitalis, calcium channel blockers, and beta blockers.

Nursing Intervention
Document the dysrhythmia with a rhythm strip. Monitor the patient for increasing frequency of PACs. More frequent PACs may cause anxiety, some hemodynamic compromise, hypotension, and dyspnea. Document an increase in frequency with rhythm strips and notify the physician of the increase.

Wandering Atrial Pacemaker

Etiology
Various foci within the atrium or from the AV node supersede the SA node as the pacemaker for a variable number of beats (Fig. 11-8).

Identifying Characteristics
Rate is usually normal but may be slow. Rhythm is frequently regular. P waves are abnormal, and they change in size, shape, and deflection. The PR interval may vary or may be constant. The QRS complex is normal. Conduction is abnormal in the atrium and

sometimes in the AV node. Below the AV node, conduction is normal.

Risk
Generally there is no risk. The presence of a wandering atrial pacemaker is normally insignificant, although it may indicate the presence of SA disease.

Treatment
Usually no treatment is necessary. If the rhythm produced symptoms, the symptoms would be treated. For example, a bradycardia could be treated with atropine.

Nursing Intervention
Document the dysrhythmia with a rhythm strip. Monitor for an unacceptably low ventricular rate (below 50 beats per minute) and treat as necessary.

Atrial Flutter

Etiology
An irritable atrial focus or accessory pathway may supersede the SA node and produce atrial flutter. This is a fairly common dysrhythmia in atherosclerotic heart disease and some congenital heart diseases (Fig. 11-9).

Identifying Characteristics
The atrial rate is rapid, usually 250 to 350 beats per minute. Atrial rhythm is regular, and ventricular rhythm varies with the number of impulses transmitted through the AV node. The P wave is replaced by a flutter wave (F wave). Flutter waves have no isoelectric interval between the waves. The PR interval is usually prolonged, although it is difficult to measure from a rhythm strip. The QRS complex is usually normal. Conduction is abnormal in the atria, and the AV node normally blocks many of the F waves.

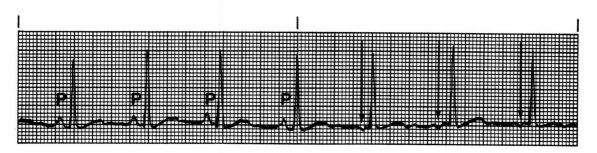

Figure 11-8. Wandering atrial pacemaker.

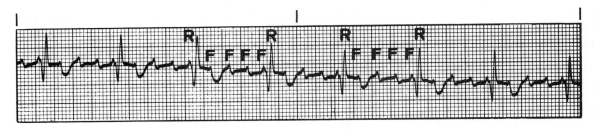

Figure 11-9. Atrial flutter.

Risk

Heart failure (formerly referred to as congestive heart failure) may occur quickly if the patient has limited cardiac function and the AV node conducts almost all of the F waves. There is the possibility of severe hemodynamic compromise. If the ventricular response is rapid, there is insufficient filling time for the ventricle. The rapid rate can cause a reduction in cardiac output. Rapid response of the ventricle increases myocardial oxygen demand, which cannot be met due to the decreased cardiac output. If severe, the hemodynamic compromise may lead to HF.

Treatment

Digitalis preparations may be used in treating this dysrhythmia if the ventricular response is not fast (e.g., <150). If the ventricular response is rapid, synchronized cardioversion with low voltage is the preferred treatment. If the rhythm is unclear, adenosine can be given in an attempt to slow the rhythm somewhat so that a better diagnosis can be made.

Nursing Intervention

Document the dysrhythmia with a rhythm strip. Monitor the patient closely for signs of hemodynamic compromise. The physician should be notified when this dysrhythmia develops. If adenosine is used, the patient should be warned about a potentially negative feeling as the drug is administered. The feeling will be temporary.

Atrial Fibrillation

Etiology

Many irritable foci develop in the atrium to such a degree that normal atrial contraction becomes impossible. This condition may be caused by rheumatic heart disease, coronary disease, hypertension, thyrotoxicosis, and congenital heart disease (Fig. 11-10).

Identifying Characteristics

The atrial rate is not measurable but is probably greater than 300. At such a high atrial rate, the AV node cannot accept all the stimuli it receives. Consequently, the atrial and ventricular rates are markedly different. The atrial and ventricular rhythms are irregular. P waves are nonexistent and are replaced by fibrillatory waves. There is no true PR interval. The QRS complex may be normal or abnormal. Ventricular response may be slow, normal, or

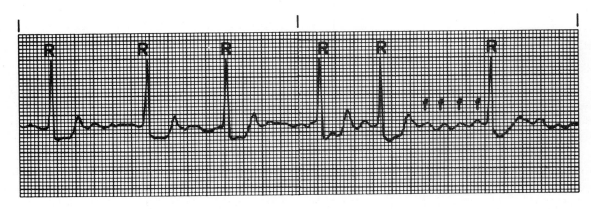

Figure 11-10. Atrial fibrillation.

very rapid. Conduction is abnormal in both the atria and the AV node. The number of impulses that the AV node transmits determines the degree of AV block.

Risk

There may be a rapid development of HF. Atrial thrombi may form, leading to embolization. Marked hemodynamic disturbance is common if the rhythm is of recent onset. Angina and increased myocardial ischemia may occur.

Treatment

If the dysrhythmia is not causing hemodynamic compromise, digitalis preparations (digoxin) are commonly employed. Other antidysrhythmics, such as dihydropyradine calcium channel blockers (verapamil and diltiazem) and beta blockers can also be used. If hemodynamic compromise develops, synchronized cardioversion is essential to reduce and control the ventricular response provided that the dysrhythmia has not been present for 48 h or more. After 48 h, the risk that an atrial thrombus will develop contraindicates the use of cardioversion to terminate the dysrhythmia since it may produce embolization. If concerns exist for atrial thrombus or cardioembolic phenomenon, acute anticoagulation with heparin or related medications is indicated. Anticoagulation for long-term atrial fibrillation, including warfarin or aspirin, is common. Ablation is also an option if drug therapy is to be avoided.

If there is hemodynamic compromise within the first 48 h, synchronized cardioversion is essential to reduce and control a rapid ventricular response. This is considered an acute form of atrial fibrillation.

A chronic form of atrial fibrillation is considered to exist if there is no hemodynamic compromise, if the dysrhythmia has been present for more than 48 h, and if the patient is asymptomatic and has a ventricular response of greater than 50 but less than 100 complexes per minute. In these instances, treatment may not be needed.

Nursing Intervention

Document the dysrhythmia with a rhythm strip. Notify the physician if atrial fibrillation develops suddenly. Monitor the patient carefully for hemodynamic compromise and embolization. Contact the physician if a rapid ventricular response develops or if an unacceptably low ventricular response develops (less than 50 beats per minute).

ATRIOVENTRICULAR NODE AND VENTRICULAR DYSRHYTHMIAS

EDITORS' NOTE

The most common dysrhythmias likely to be addressed on the PCCN exam involve disturbances of the AV node (junctional rhythms and conduction blocks) and ventricular ectopy (premature ventricular contractions, ventricular tachycardia, and fibrillation). This section contains information that addresses several questions from the exam. Each of these areas can also be expected to contain information addressed on the PCCN exam. Once again, if dysrhythmias are not a strength for you, review this chapter carefully.

It was once thought that the AV node itself could initiate impulses. Such rhythms were termed nodal rhythms. Research has shown that the AV node itself does not initiate an electrical impulse but that an electrical impulse is initiated in the junctional tissue around the AV node. This finding has resulted in changing the term *nodal rhythm* to the more accurate term of *junctional rhythm*.

Junctional Rhythm

Etiology

This dysrhythmia is often due to an acute MI, an SA block, digitalis toxicity, or treatment with drugs that slow the atrial rate (e.g., digitalis and procainamide) (Fig. 11-11).

Identifying Characteristics

The rate is usually 40 to 60 beats per minute. The rhythm is usually regular. P waves are abnormal in shape and size and may precede or follow the QRS complex or be buried in it. If seen, the P wave is usually inverted (negatively deflected). This inversion is caused by the electrical impulse originating in junctional tissue and moving both down into the ventricles (a normal path) and back up into the atrium (retrograde movement, an abnormal path). The PR interval, if present, is less than 0.10 s and often is not measurable. The QRS complex is normal unless a P wave is buried in it. Conduction to the atria is abnormal owing to its retrograde depolarization of the atria.

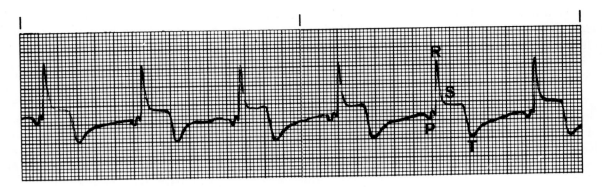

Figure 11-11. Junctional rhythm.

Risk

The junctional impulse formation is slow. The junctional rhythm is normally a protective rhythm, taking over as the pacemaker of the heart when the SA node slows to rates below 40 to 60 beats per minute. Hemodynamic balance may be compromised by a slow ventricular rate, leading to poor cardiac output and perhaps ventricular failure.

Treatment

Medications that increase the heart rate, such as atropine, would be considered if the bradycardia were associated with hypotension or HF. If medications fail to work, pacemakers can be used to override the slow rate. If drug toxicity is the underlying cause, the drug should be stopped immediately.

Nursing Intervention

Document the dysrhythmia with a rhythm strip. Monitor the patient closely. PVCs may occur and do not respond well to lidocaine or other ventricular antidysrhythmic agents since the PVCs are usually a result of decreased cardiac output. Increasing the heart rate is a more effective method of eliminating the PVCs. Monitor for signs of hemodynamic compromise. Notify the physician immediately if compromise occurs.

Premature Junctional Contraction

Etiology

An irritable focus in the junctional tissue initiates an impulse early. The impulse depolarizes the ventricles normally and the atria in a retrograde fashion. Coronary artery disease (CAD), acute MI, and digitalis toxicity are frequent causes. Any factor that increases junctional ischemia may produce a premature junctional contraction (PJC) (Fig. 11-12).

Identifying Characteristics

The underlying rate may be normal or slow. The rhythm is regular except for the premature (early) beat. P waves are abnormal, inverted, and may precede, follow, or be buried in the QRS complex of the PJC. The PR interval varies with the position of the pacemaker and is frequently not measurable. The QRS complex is normal unless the P wave is buried in it or aberration occurs. Conduction is normal

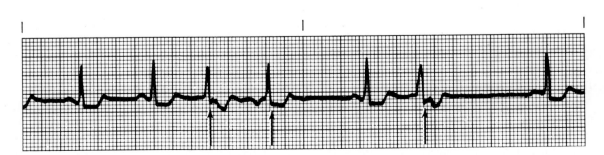

Figure 11-12. Premature junctional contraction.

through the ventricles and retrograde through the atria.

Risk

PJCs may lead to a supraventricular tachycardia if frequent. If rare, PJCs do not pose a threat for the patient.

Treatment

If PJCs are infrequent or the patient is asymptomatic, no treatment is necessary. If frequent, PJCs may be controlled by digitalis preparations or other atrial antidysrhythmics such as pronestyl.

Nursing Intervention

Document the dysrhythmia with a rhythm strip (to justify junctional origin rather than ventricular origin). Monitor the patient for increasing frequency of PJCs and notify the physician if the frequency does increase.

Paroxysmal Junctional Tachycardia

Etiology

Paroxysmal junctional tachycardia (PJT) is probably similar to PAT in both origin and in treatment. The cause may be disease of the AV node or abnormal pathways, either anatomic or physiologic (Fig. 11-13).

Identifying Characteristics

The rate is usually 150 to 250 beats per minute. The rhythm is usually regular. P waves are abnormal and inverted, and they may precede, follow, or be buried in the QRS complex. If present, the PR interval is shortened or not measurable. The QRS complex is normal unless the P wave is buried in it or it is aberrantly conducted. Conduction of the QRS may be normal. Atrial conduction is retrograde. PJT may be difficult to distinguish from PAT. These arrhythmias are often called supraventricular tachycardia (SVT).

Risk

The danger associated with PJT is the same as for PAT. The faster the rate, the greater the likelihood of a decreased cardiac output. If the cardiac output is reduced enough, LV failure will result.

Treatment

The treatment is similar to that for PAT.

Nursing Intervention

Document the dysrhythmia with a rhythm strip. Assess the patient for hemodynamic compromise. If compromise occurs, notify the physician and medicate as the situation dictates.

Idioventricular Rhythm

Etiology

In this rhythm, there is no functioning pacemaker above the ventricles. A secondary pacemaker in the ventricles initiates an impulse in order to generate a heart rate. Normally, a ventricular pacemaker is very slow, generally less than 40 beats per minute. The terms *idioventricular pacemaker* (which means unknown ventricular pacemaker) and *ventricular escape rhythm* both apply to this dysrhythmia. All diseases and injuries that cause loss of function from the SA node down are etiologic factors (Fig. 11-14).

Identifying Characteristics

The ventricles initiate a rate at their inherent ability, usually 20 to 40 beats per minute. The rhythm is regular but may slow as a "dying heart syndrome" progresses. There is no P wave. There is no PR interval. The QRS complex is wide and bizarre, measuring 0.12 s or more.

Risk

The imminent danger is ventricular standstill. It is possible that the electrical event is not leading to an

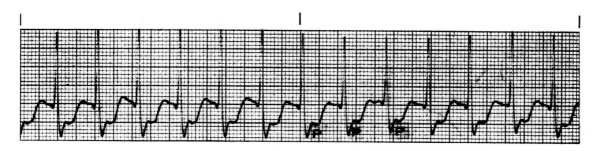

Figure 11-13. Paroxysmal junctional tachycardia.

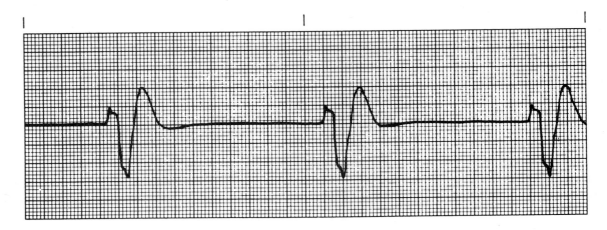

Figure 11-14. Idioventricular rhythm.

effective contraction, which means that electrical mechanical dissociation has developed. This rhythm is normally a protective or compensatory response. It may be the last natural pacemaker in the heart, so treatment becomes urgent.

Treatment
A pacemaker is the only reliable and totally effective form of treatment. In a crisis, until a transvenous or external pacemaker can be applied, atropine or isoproterenol hydrochloride may accelerate the heart rate.

Nursing Intervention
Document the dysrhythmia with a rhythm strip. Notify the physician immediately. Assess and treat the patient continuously for hypotension or signs of HF. Prepare an external pacemaker for use or be prepared to assist in the insertion of a transvenous pacemaker.

Accelerated Idioventricular Rhythm

Etiology
The etiology is the same as for the idioventricular rhythm (Fig. 11-15).

Identifying Characteristics
These are the same as for an idioventricular rhythm with the exception that the rate is usually 60 to 100 beats per minute.

Risk
The immediate risk is that the accelerated focus may cease and the dysrhythmia may convert to an idioventricular rate or cardiac standstill. The accelerated idioventricular rhythm generally poses no danger by itself.

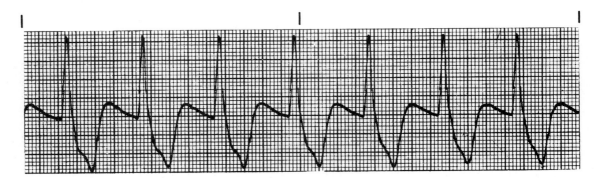

Figure 11-15. Accelerated idioventricular rhythm.

Treatment

No treatment is indicated unless the patient demonstrates signs of hemodynamic compromise. Since the rate is normal, this dysrhythmia may generate an adequate cardiac output.

Nursing Intervention

Monitor the patient for signs of hypotension or HF.

Premature Ventricular Contractions

Premature ventricular contractions (PVCs) are also termed premature ventricular beats (PVBs) or ventricular premature contractions (VPCs).

Etiology

An irritable focus in the ventricle initiates a contraction before the normally expected beat. The irritability may be due to acute MI (most common), atherosclerotic heart disease (ASHD), HF, drug toxicity, hypoxia, electrolytes, acidosis, or bradycardia (Fig. 11-16).

Identifying Characteristics

The rate is variable. Rhythm is irregular because of the premature beat. P waves are present but frequently not visible. P waves are most commonly lost in the QRS complex of the PVC. However, they may be slightly before or after the PVC. The PR interval is not present, since the atrial impulse does not conduct the PVC. The QRS complex is wide and bizarre, exceeding 0.12 s and frequently being greater than 0.14 s. It usually has a compensatory pause that allows the R-R interval to re-establish rhythm following the PVC.

Risk

The danger of a PVC is the possibility of increasing myocardial irritability, leading to an increasing frequency of PVCs. With an increased occurrence of PVCs, ventricular tachycardia and/or ventricular fibrillation may occur. There is an increased potential for problems when any of the following occur:

1. PVCs occur from more than one focus (multiform PVCs).
2. PVCs occur more often than six per minute, including rhythms such as bigeminy (every other beat is a PVC), or short runs of PVCs occur frequently (two to three sequential PVCs) every few beats.
3. There are variable coupling intervals (the period between the beginning of a normal QRS and the beginning of the QRS of the PVC).
4. The PVC occurs on the T wave of the preceding complex (described as the R-on-T phenomenon). If the PVC occurs on the T wave, it may precipitate ventricular fibrillation.

Treatment

Treatment of PVCs depends on their clinical significance. Acute development of PVCs might indicate myocardial ischemia and removing the ischemia would remove the PVCs. If the PVCs are aysmptomatic, obversation might be the best clinical treatment. If elimination of PVCs is desired, agents such as lidocaine and amiodarone can be used. A lidocaine bolus followed by a lidocaine drip is the treatment of choice. (*Note:* If a lidocaine bolus has been given and 10 to 15 min have elapsed, another bolus must be administered before the drip is hung to establish and maintain therapeutic blood levels of the drug.) If hypokalemia is present, potassium may terminate the PVCs. If lidocaine treatment is unsuccessful, procainamide or bretylium may be tried.

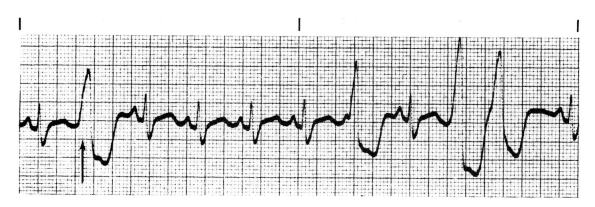

Figure 11-16. Premature ventricular contraction (PVC, PVB, or VPC).

Chronic PVC control is usually managed with oral preparations, such as tocainide or mexiletine. Many agents are available for the control of chronic PVCs. If PVCs are not controlled by conventional therapies, amiodarone may be required. Amiodarone is usually used as an end-stage treatment because of the multiple side effects associated with this agent. However, amiodarone is nevertheless increasingly used since, unlike many other antidysrhythmics, it has not been shown to have a proarrhythmic effect. In the past few years, a trend toward tolerating PVCs, especially in the absence of acute ischemia, is developing.

Nursing Intervention

Document the dysrhythmia with a rhythm strip. Differentiate the PVC from an atrial premature contraction (APC) with aberrant conduction. Monitor the patient closely for increasing frequency of PVCs or the development of multiform PVCs. Bolus with lidocaine or another antidysrhythmic agent and document the effect. Prepare a continuous drip to maintain control over the PVC frequency. Notify the physician. Observe the patient and monitor closely for ventricular tachycardia and ventricular fibrillation.

Differentiating APCs with Aberrant Conduction from PVCs

APCs with abnormal (aberrant) conduction can mimic PVCs. Criteria that help different APCs with aberrant conduction from PVCs have been described in both medical and nursing research articles. Table 11-2 provides the criteria necessary to aid differentiation. The key to identifying an aberrantly conducted APC centers around two features. First, identify any characteristics of an APC that are different from those of a PVC. For example, in Fig. 11-17, note the P wave on the downstroke of the T wave.

TABLE 11-2. DIFFERENTIATING APCs WITH ABERRANT CONDUCTION FROM PVCs

Criteria for PVCs	Criteria for APCs
Extreme right axis	rSR′ in V_1
Rr′ in V_1	Biphasic or triphasic QRS
rS in V_6	Normal axis
Precordial concordance (all V leads show same axis pattern; i.e., upright or inverted)	
Initial R wave >0.03 s	
Beginning of R to nadir (lowest point) of S wave >0.10 s	

APCs, atrial premature contractions; PVCs premature ventricular contractions.

This is suggestive of an APC. Second, note the shape of the QRS complex. The morphology or appearance of the QRS complex is a key factor in differentiating APCs with aberrancy from PVCs. Table 11-2 provides clues to the appearance of the QRS complex in the two dysrhythmias. The PCCN exam frequently has a question, and sometimes a rhythm strip, on differentiating between the two, so it is wise to be familiar with the differences.

Ventricular Tachycardia

Etiology

Advanced irritability of the ventricles allows a ventricular focus to become the heart's pacemaker. The myocardial irritability may be due to ASHD, HF, acute MI, electrolyte imbalance, hypoxia, acidosis, or occasionally drugs (Fig. 11-18).

Identifying Characteristics

The rate is greater than 100; often 120 to 220 beats per minute. The rhythm is regular or only slightly irregular. P waves are usually not discernible, although it is

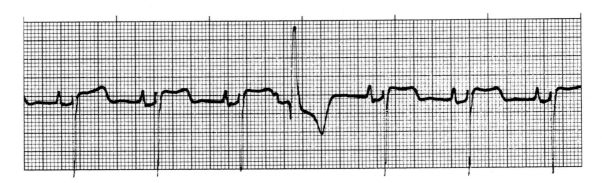

Figure 11-17. Aberrantly conducted APC.

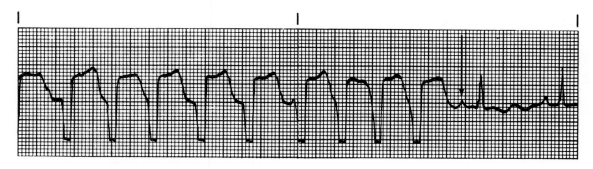

Figure 11-18. Ventricular tachycardia terminating spontaneously.

important to try to identify them. If P waves are present, they will not be related to the QRS complex (AV dissociation exists). There is no measurable PR interval. The QRS complex is wide and bizarre, resembling essentially a salvo (or burst) of PVCs. A ventricular focus initiates ventricular depolarization.

Risk
The risk with ventricular tachycardia is the potential to develop dangerous or lethal reductions in cardiac output.

Treatment
According to the American Heart Association (AHA), there are several types of ventricular tachycardia. Treatment is dependent on the type of ventricular tachycardia. The types of ventricular tachycardia and treatments are listed in Table 11-3.

Nursing Intervention
Document this dysrhythmia with a rhythm strip. If the patient is unconscious, immediate defibrillation and institution of cardiac arrest procedures are essential.

TABLE 11-3. VENTRICULAR TACHYCARDIA CATEGORIES AND TREATMENT

Characteristics	Treatment
No symptoms	Amiodarone
	Lidocaine
	Pronestyl
	Bretylium
Mild symptoms (chest pain, shortness of breath)	Synchronized cardioversion, beginning at 50 J and progressing to 360 J
Serious symptoms (pulmonary edema, hypotension)	Defibrillation, beginning at 50 J and progressing to 360 J (doses vary depending on whether mono or biphasic defibrillation is used)
No pulse	Treat as ventricular fibrillation

Ventricular Fibrillation

Etiology
Owing to extensive ventricular irritability, ventricular fibers fail to depolarize in sequence; instead, they depolarize individually, creating an uncoordinated series of muscle depolarizations. No substantial cardiac output is generated. Ventricular fibrillation may occur after an acute MI. It may, however, occur as a result of ASHD, HF, digitalis or other drug toxicity, and electrolyte imbalance (Fig. 11-19).

Identifying Characteristics
There is no identifiable rate. The rhythm is irregular and not measurable. P waves are replaced by undulating waves as the baseline. The PR interval is nonexistent or not measurable. The QRS complex is an undulating asymmetrical line.

Risk
The development of neurodynamic collapse may occur within seconds, followed by death within 4 to 8 min.

Treatment
Immediate defibrillation is the only possible means of establishing a viable cardiac rhythm. The American Heart Association (AHA) has recommended a series of actions to occur when ventricular fibrillation occurs. The key is rapid defibrillation. Defibrillation energies have undergone a change since the introduction over a decade ago of the biphasic defibrillator. For example, the traditional guidelines of the AHA have advised defibrillating initially at 200 J. If this is unsuccessful (determined by assessing for the return of a pulse), the defibrillation is to be repeated at 300 J. If this effort is still unsuccessful, defibrillation is to be repeated at 360 J.

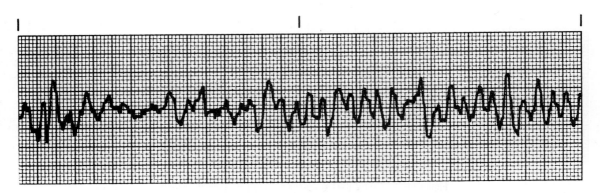

Figure 11-19. Ventricular fibrillation.

Today, use of the biphasic defibrillator has been shown to lead to as good or better outcomes with the application of much less energy (e.g., 150 J three times or 120, 150, and 180 J).

If initial defibrillations are unsuccessful, begin cardiopulmonary resuscitation (CPR) and establish an artificial airway and venous access. Repeat defibrillations after medical therapies (e.g., with amiodarone). The key is successful defibrillation. Without a return to spontaneous circulation within minutes, survival is unlikely. End-tidal CO_2 levels ($PETCO_2$), which are indicators of cardiac output, have been shown to aid identifying which patients will survive. A persistently low $PETCO_2$ level (less than 10) is highly correlated with death.

BIBLIOGRAPHY

Singer, D.E., Albers, G.W., Dalen, J. E., Fang, M. C., Go, A. S., Halperin, J. L., . . . Manning, W. J. (2008). Antithrombotic therapy in atrial fibrillation: American College of Chest Physicians Evidence-Based Clinical Practice Guidelines (8th ed.). *Chest*, 133:546S.

Fuster, V., Ryden, L.E., Cannom, D.S., Crijns, H., Curtis, A., Ellenbogen, K., . . . Wann, S. (2006). ACC/AHA/ESC 2006 Guidelines for the Management of Patients with Atrial Fibrillation A Report of the American College of Cardiology/American Heart Association Task Force on Practice Guidelines and the European Society of Cardiology Committee for Practice Guidelines (Writing Committee to Revise the 2001 Guidelines for the Management of Patients with Atrial Fibrillation). *Journal of the American College of Cardiology*, 48:e149.

12

Cardiomyopathies and Pericarditis

It would be disproportionate to devote many pages to cardiomyopathies when the PCCN exam will have no more than a few questions on this topic. Pericarditis has been removed from the current PCCN exam. Therefore, this chapter is intentionally short, with an emphasis on practical information that will be seen both in practice and on the exam. Much of the information in this chapter is also found in the discussion of heart failure (Chap. 8).

CARDIOMYOPATHIES

Clinical Presentation

In the past, cardiomyopathy was roughly defined as heart muscle disease of unknown etiology. However, that is not true because the origins of some types, such as ischemic cardiomyopathy, are known. Possible origins of cardiomyopathy are listed in Table 12-1. Regardless of the origin, the disease tends to involve most of the muscle of the heart, although some parts of the heart might be more affected than others. This presents a clinical picture whereby the cardiomyopathy can appear differently in different patients. One patient might exhibit more left-sided dysfunction while another might exhibit right-sided dysfunction. Some patients might have systolic ventricular failure, others diastolic dysfunction. The most common presentation appears to be a combination of the above.

All cardiomyopathies will involve increased ventricular pressures by the time such patients present with symptoms.

There are three common presentations of cardiomyopathy: dilated, hypertrophic, and constrictive (Fig. 12-1). The most common is dilated cardiomyopathy. It presents with symptoms resembling those of heart failure (HF) (formerly referred to as congestive heart failure [CHF]). The patient will have a decreased stroke volume and ejection fraction as well as symptoms of pulmonary congestion. Left ventricular (LV) volumes are increased. Eventually, hypotension will occur, with death resulting from severe LV failure. Dilated cardiomyopathy presents with a highly compliant ventricle. This usually means that higher ventricular filling pressures (a pulmonary artery occlusive pressure [PAOP] of 20 mm Hg) can be tolerated relatively easily. Fluid administration in the presence of this PAOP can be employed without a major increase in extravascular lung water. However, the key parameter to monitor is stroke volume (and ideally ejection fraction).

Hypertrophic cardiomyopathy is more of a diastolic dysfunction as a result of the inability of the heart to relax during diastole. Clinical symptoms include pulmonary congestion but close to normal stroke volume and ejection fraction, at least until end stages.

Constrictive cardiomyopathy presents with a very noncompliant ventricular muscle, leading to presentations of HF. Ventricular volumes are decreased, although stroke volume and ejection fraction can be maintained at near normal levels.

TABLE 12-1. POSSIBLE CAUSES OF CARDIOMYOPATHY

Dilated	Idiopathic (unknown)
	Inflammatory/infectious
	Autoimmune disease
	Toxic (drugs, alcohol)
	Hereditary
	Ischemic
	Metabolic (uremia, vitamin deficiency)
	Endocrine (thyroid)
Constrictive	Idiopathic
	Interstitial disease (sarcoidosis)
	Eosinophilic heart disease
	Radiation
	Drug toxicity
Hypertrophic	Idiopathic
	Systemic hypertension

Diagnosis

The only clear diagnostic technique is the use of endomyocardial biopsy. The prognosis for all cardiomyopathy is poor. No curative measures currently exist.

Treatment

Dilated cardiomyopathy is usually treated similarly to HF. Inotropic agents (dobutamine or milrinone in acute cases, digoxin in chronic cases), diuretics, vasodilators (e.g., angiotensin-converting enzyme [ACE] inhibitors, angiotensin II antagonists), and beta blockers are commonly used. Aggressive measures such as cardiomyoplasty and mechanical support devices may be used until heart transplantation is possible.

Treatment of constrictive cardiomyopathy is difficult. The focus is generally on diuretics and afterload reducers in an attempt to improve diastolic function. Although this might help temporarily, eventually systemic hypotension results, with a worsening of clinical symptoms. Treatments tend to be supportive, although if a specific condition is present, such as eosinophilic cardiomyopathy, cytotoxic agents (hydroxyurea), or steroids might be used.

In hypertrophic cardiomyopathy, the focus is on reducing afterload, particularly with beta blockers.

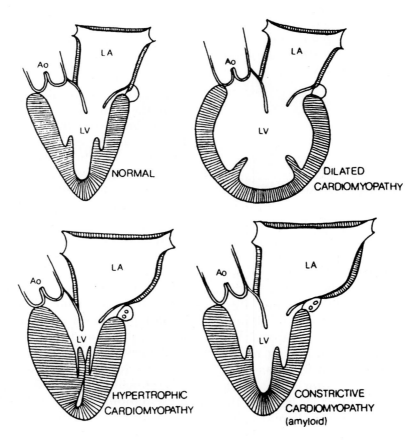

Figure 12-1. Types of cardiomyopathies.

Diuretics and other afterload reducers, such as calcium channel blockers, might be used. If atrial dysrhythmias (such as atrial fibrillation) develop, electrotherapy (cardioversion) or drugs for supraventricular tachycardia would be employed.

PERICARDITIS

Etiology

Pericarditis may be present or may develop in essentially any disease process. It may be viral or bacterial in etiology (most common); have a metabolic cause, as in uremia; or have an unknown cause. It may be secondary to systemic disease or myocardial trauma, or it may follow acute myocardial infarction (MI).

Clinical Presentation

Symptoms vary with the etiology of the pericarditis. Most commonly, pain is present. The pain may mimic an acute MI, angina, or pleurisy. Pain usually increases with deep respiration and when the patient is lying supine. Sitting up and leaning forward usually diminishes the pain. Fever is commonly present because of the infectious or inflammatory process. Pericardial friction rub may be present for only a few days (post-MI) or prolonged for many days (uremia). The pericardial friction rub is a scratchy, superficial sound with three components best heard at the lower left sternum. Classic electrocardiographic (ECG) changes are ST-segment elevation in all leads except aVR.

Complications

Complications of pericarditis include dysrhythmias, tamponade, and restriction of ventricular contraction. Each complication must be treated promptly. Hemodynamic monitoring with a pulmonary artery catheter is useful in the early detection of tamponade. Equalization of pressures in the heart, particularly the central venous pressure (CVP) and PAOP, may signal the presence of tamponade. Auscultation of heart sounds is essential on a regular and frequent schedule, with the clinician attempting to identify whether a muffling of the heart sounds has occurred.

Treatment

Pain relief is essential to promote normal and adequate ventilation. Anti-inflammatory and steroid therapies may be tried. Treatment of the underlying cause is imperative. Antipyretic agents will control the fever if the patient is uncomfortable. Pericardiocentesis or a pericardial window may be performed if there is a possibility of tamponade developing. Anticoagulants are contraindicated in order to avoid an increase in pericardial fluid.

Nursing Intervention

Perform continuous ECG monitoring for signs of dysrhythmias that may indicate the early development of cardiac tamponade. The most dangerous dysrhythmia is electromechanical dissociation (an ECG pattern is present but there is no pulse). Monitoring with a noninvasive Doppler is more sensitive to early changes. The nurse should be prepared to assist with an emergency pericardiocentesis if it becomes warranted. Especially close auscultation of cardiac sounds is imperative for early intervention. Medications to relieve pain and fever are administered as ordered.

Arterial blood gases or pulse oximetry should be monitored at regular intervals to determine ventilatory status and allow early intervention if hypoxemia develops. Emotional support and explanations of the reasons for the close monitoring will help to alleviate some of the patient's anxiety.

Cardiac Tamponade

If fluid accumulates in the pericardial sac, there is a potential for the development of cardiac tamponade. Cardiac tamponade will have a constrictive effect on the heart, producing a condition initially like diastolic dysfunction (the heart cannot relax and fill with blood). This is particularly aggravated on inspiration, where increased RV volume (due to inspiration) increases the pericardial pressure, thus limiting LV expansion and producing a drop in blood pressure during inspiration. The term *pulsus paradoxus*, where the systolic blood pressure decreases by about 20 mm Hg, describes a condition that is commonly seen with cardiac tamponade. Other clinical features include an equalization of left and right filling pressures (the CVP and PAOP are about the same) and pulmonary and venous engorgement.

Treatment involves treating the underlying cause of the fluid or blood in the pericardial sac. Emergent treatment might involve pericardiocentesis.

Treatment of Cardiac, Valvular, and Vascular Insufficiency and Trauma

EDITORS' NOTE

Cardiovascular surgery has assumed a greater role in critical care over the past decade, and the PCCN exam reflects this trend. Expect several questions on cardiovascular surgery, including a few (usually only one or two) on cardiac transplantation. Use this section in conjunction with the preceding chapters in order to be able to apply hemodynamic analysis to the concept of cardiovascular surgery. This will help in understanding the assessment of and need for the surgical treatment of cardiovascular disorders.

CARDIAC, VALVULAR, AND VASCULAR SURGERY

Cardiovascular surgery in the critical care environment can include many procedures, although the key surgical interventions generally center around problems involving the cardiac or vascular circulation. The cardiac disturbances that require emergency surgery include acute coronary artery obstruction, ventricular septal rupture, pericardial tamponade, and papillary muscle rupture. Other than acute coronary artery obstruction, the problems present with symptoms similar to those of cardiogenic shock are not discussed here. Although this section does not specifically address emergent problems except for the acute obstructed artery, the principles discussed cover most essential information related to cardiovascular surgery. This section

does not address all possible surgical interventions but rather focuses on the common major cardiac and vascular surgeries of coronary artery bypass grafting (CABG), vascular aneurysm, and occlusive disease interventions. An introduction to the principles of cardiac transplantation rounds out this section.

Knowledge of these common problems and the associated nursing care will prepare you for most PCCN questions in this area, including emergent surgical procedures. With the greater emphasis on the cardiovascular component of the PCCN exam, an understanding of cardiovascular surgical concepts has increased in importance.

Coronary Artery Bypass Grafting

Coronary artery bypass grafting (CABG) is the technique of using blood vessels obtained from another part of the body to replace obstructed coronary arteries. The internal mammary artery is generally used because of its long-term patency. The saphenous vein is generally harvested because most patients requiring surgical revascularization need three or more bypass grafts. Other alternative conduits include the free radial artery, gastroepiploic artery, and inferior epigastric artery. Nursing care postoperatively differs somewhat for the different types of grafts; with saphenous vein removal, for example, one must care for the wound created by removal of the graft. Otherwise, postoperative care does not markedly change from one type of procedure to another.

TABLE 13-1. INDICATIONS FOR INVASIVE REVASCULARIZATION PROCEDURES

Stable angina refractory to medical therapy and interfering with the patient's ability to function at an acceptable level of activity

Exercise-induced hypotension or ventricular dysrhythmias secondary to myocardial ischemia

Left ventricular dysfunction and clinical evidence of heart failure

Unstable angina

Acute myocardial ischemia or infarction

Determination of the Need for CABG

Indications for surgical revascularization continue to be revised as the roles of less invasive forms of treatment are refined. Coronary stent placement, percutaneous transluminal coronary angioplasty (PTCA), and CABG are the major revascularization therapies. General criteria for invasive revascularization are presented in Table 13-1.

Advances in minimally invasive cardiac surgery have changed how many patients receive surgery—minimally invasive direct coronary artery bypass (MIDCAB) and robotic surgery, in which the major sternal incision is eliminated in favor of a small incision. Off-pump, or "beating heart" CABG, allows the heart to beat during surgery, eliminating the need for the cardiopulmonary bypass machine.

Surgical revascularization remains the treatment of choice in patients with triple-vessel disease with left ventricular (LV) dysfunction or complex lesions and those with greater than 75% stenosis of the left main coronary artery. Other considerations include age, general health status, associated cardiac disease, and comorbid conditions. If there are multiple obstructions in a single artery, making bypass difficult, surgery is generally not indicated or helpful. Pain relief from bypass surgery is individualized, since such surgery is effective primarily if blood flow to viable cardiac muscle is reestablished.

Indications for emergency operation are as follows:

1. Complications of PTCA
2. Ischemia that is uncontrolled by medical therapy
3. Evolving MI

The emergent CABG patient has either unstable hemodynamics (hypotension), unremitting chest pain despite maximal medical treatment, or the potential to become unstable (subjective assessment). Elective surgeries are utilized for those patients with hemodynamic stability and symptoms partially controlled through medical therapy. Unfortunately, surgical revascularization is not curative. Some patients require reoperation because of the progression of coronary artery disease or loss of graft patency. Patients undergoing reoperation have at least double the operative risk because their average age is higher and the atherosclerotic disease is more advanced. Patients undergoing reoperation tend to be more challenging to care for because of these considerations.

Surgical Procedure

The surgical techniques utilized during CABG are unlikely to be covered on the PCCN exam. However, this section contains information that provides a useful background on this surgical procedure.

During CABG, several surgical techniques are employed to improve success rates. The patient is typically cooled to near 28°C to 30°C (to reduce oxygen demand) and is placed on cardiopulmonary bypass (CPB). CPB is a technique for diverting blood from the heart during surgery while simultaneously oxygenating the blood and removing carbon dioxide. During CPB, three maneuvers help achieve safe and successful extracorporeal oxygenation: hemodilution, hypothermia, and anticoagulation. While these techniques help reduce complications, they also form the basis for many of the postoperative observations by the critical care nurse.

Physiologic consequences of CPB include the following:

1. Damage to blood elements (i.e., platelets, red blood cells, white blood cells, and plasma proteins)
2. Incorporation of abnormal substances into the blood (i.e., bubbles, fibrin particles, and platelet aggregates)
3. A systemic inflammatory response, which results in increased capillary permeability and fluid in the interstitial space
4. An initial decrease in systemic vascular resistance, then a progressive increase as hypothermia is induced
5. An increase in circulating catecholamines
6. An increase in venous tone

As fluid leaks from the blood vessels, the nurse should be alert for the need to give volume (either crystalloid or colloid) to maintain fluid status. Patients may gain several pounds following CPB owing to the loss of vascular volume into the interstitial space. Careful observation of urine output to assess vascular volume is helpful. Impaired gas exchange as manifest by low arterial oxygen pressure/saturation (Pao_2/Sao_2) levels also indicates excess capillary leaking. Improved blood gases can indicate clearing of third-space volume.

Postoperative bleeding is usually not due to CPB. Measurement of the partial thromboplastin time will best detect an excessive heparin effect from CPB. Protamine sulfate is given to reverse heparin-induced anticoagulation. Protamine sulfate can cause a severe adverse reaction accompanied by profound vasodilation and hypotension.

Postoperative Measures

The primary postoperative assessments following CABG involve hemodynamic monitoring, pain relief, dysrhythmia control, and recovery from surgical techniques such as CPB. Hemodynamic monitoring centers on maintaining adequate blood pressure, cardiac indices (>2.2 L/min/m^2), and tissue oxygenation (Svo_2 above 0.60). Acceptable blood pressure and cardiac index are achieved through providing sufficient preload (assessed via central venous pressure [CVP] and/or pulmonary artery occlusive pressure [PAOP] monitoring), afterload reduction, and the use of inotropes to enhance contractility and maintain normal stroke volume. As the patient warms postoperatively, vasopressors may initially need to be used to maintain blood pressure. A temporary external pacemaker, antidysrhythmic agents, and sedatives may also be employed to optimize hemodynamic status.

More aggressive measures to maintain cardiac output may be required. This would include the use of artificial devices for mechanical support. Devices that may be utilized include an intra-aortic balloon pump (IABP); ventricular assist devices (VADs) for right, left, or biventricular support; extracorporeal membrane oxygenator (ECMO); and a CPB-portable system. However, few (if any) questions on the PCCN exam cover these aggressive measures at this time.

Problems encountered in the early postoperative period include the following:

1. Bleeding, either from a surgical site or due to a coagulopathy. This may result in cardiac tamponade. Postoperative blood loss should not exceed 300 mL/h in the first several hours. After this time, bleeding should be less than 150 to 200 mL/h. The average blood loss is 1 L total. The physician should be notified when blood loss is excessive. Autotransfusion is typically employed to aid in the replacement of normal blood loss. Autotransfusion is the reinfusion of shed mediastinal blood. In most centers, all mediastinal bloodshed is filtered and returned to the patient.
2. Low cardiac output syndrome, where the stroke volume/index or cardiac index is less low. Postoperative causes of low cardiac index include hypovolemia, elevated systemic vascular resistance (SVR), myocardial dysfunction, cardiac tamponade, and dysrhythmias.
3. Profound hypotension.
4. Hypertension.
5. Electrolyte imbalances (primarily hypokalemia).
6. Dysrhythmias (primarily premature ventricular contractions [PVCs], atrial fibrillation, atrial flutter).
7. Cardiac arrest.

Monitoring of temperatures is typically indicated by pulmonary artery or rectal (or bladder) temperature probes. The patient will attempt to rewarm through shivering; although this reflex is effective, the increase in oxygen consumption is undesirable. The nurse can aid in rewarming the patient through external methods (blankets, radiant lights) and internal methods (warmed blood, warmed inspired gases). Some institutions advocate the administration of paralytic agents to avoid the muscle activity associated with shivering. Avoidance of marked shivering is one key goal of the rewarming therapy.

During rewarming, the patient appears to be hypovolemic as vasodilation occurs. Volume replacement and vasopressors may be required to initially combat the decrease in PAOP, CVP, and SVR.

The nurse must maintain pain reduction while simultaneously allowing for the recovery of ventilatory function. Aggressive pulmonary toilet via suctioning initially and then encouraging coughing will aid in reducing pulmonary complications. The nurse's support in pain reduction and the sensitivity shown for the patient's adjustment to temporary dependence on nursing will help the patient to adapt to the immediate postoperative recovery.

Dysrhythmia control centers on two factors. First, any metabolic disturbance that may precipitate either atrial or ventricular dysrhythmias should be corrected. For example, potassium (K^+) levels should be monitored when dysrhythmias, particularly ventricular ectopy (PVCs), exist. Second, pharmacologic or electrical therapy can be utilized to control dysrhythmias. Pharmacologic treatments are dictated by the type of dysrhythmia. For example, atrial tachycardias are treated with agents such as beta blockers (esmolol), calcium channel blockers (verapamil, diltiazem), adenosine, or a combination of these agents. Electrical cardioversion may also be used. Ventricular tachycardias and PVCs are treated with amiodarone or lidocaine.

Electrical therapy is usually performed through epicardial pacing wires placed on the right atrium and ventricle near the end of the CABG procedure. These pacing wires can be used postoperatively to manage both supraventricular tachycardias and bradycardias. Postoperative bradycardia is the most common indication for the use of the pacing wires. Atrial (for bradycardia) or atrioventricular (AV) sequential (for AV block) pacing is preferable to ventricular pacing because atrial kick accounts for 15% to 30% of cardiac output. Certain dysrhythmias (paroxysmal atrial tachycardia, atrial flutter) may be treated with rapid overdrive pacing. A wide variety of external temporary pacemakers are available.

Complications of Cardiac Surgery

Potential complications of cardiac surgery include hemorrhage, cardiac tamponade, MI, ventricular dysfunction, dysrhythmias, and death. In addition, patients may be predisposed to problems with other organ systems (i.e., neural, pulmonary, renal).

Cardiac tamponade is among the most challenging complications to manage in the postoperative period. This is a condition in which the heart is compressed by blood that has accumulated in the pericardial space or mediastinum. As a result, the heart is unable to fill adequately, causing cardiac output and blood pressure to fall. The usual signs of tamponade are enlargement of the cardiac silhouette on radiograph, equalization of right and left heart filling pressures (CVP), pulsus paradoxus, and acute hypotension. Typically, patients with initially heavy bleeding from chest tubes suddenly stop bleeding and become hypotensive. Temporary measures to support cardiac function include volume administration and inotropic support. Emergent treatment involves reopening of the sternal incision in the ICU and an immediate return to the operating room.

Cardiac Transplantation

Heart transplantation is generally not covered on the PCCN exam. Nonetheless, transplantation may be an option for patients with cardiomyopathy, and you should be familiar with the procedure.

In patients with cardiomyopathies or reduced cardiac function from coronary artery disease, CABG will not improve cardiac performance. Replacement of the heart is indicated in patients with end-stage heart disease untreatable by medical or CABG intervention. Once identified as a candidate for transplantation and if no contraindications to the transplant are present (Table 13-2), the patient is categorized as to severity. The patient typically has less than 1 year of expected survival without transplantation. The time between being placed on the list and undergoing transplantation is highly variable and can serve as a major source of anxiety to the potential recipient.

The success rate for transplantation is very good, with 1-year survival for heart transplantation at 76%; thereafter there is approximately a 4% mortality per year over the subsequent 11 years. However, the shortage of donors means that not all patients who might benefit from transplantation actually undergo the procedure.

The surgical procedure has been improved since the time of the first transplantation in 1966, but the prime difference has been in the area of immunosuppression. Suppression of rejection

---

TABLE 13-2. ELIGIBILITY CRITERIA FOR CARDIAC TRANSPLANTATION

1. End-stage, ischemic, valvular, or congenital heart disease with maximal medical therapy, not amenable to conventional or high-risk surgery
2. New York Heart Association (NYHA) functional class III–IV heart failure with maximal medical therapy
3. Prognosis for 1 year survival, <75%
4. Age, generally <65 years
5. Psychologically stable, compliant, reliable patient able to understand the procedure and risks involved
6. Strong family support system
7. Able to adhere to complex medical regimen
8. Absence of the following contraindicating factors:
   Systemic disease or infection
   Serious, irreversible impairment of hepatic, renal, or pulmonary functions
   Recent cerebrovascular accident or neurologic deficits
   Recent pulmonary embolization or infarction
   Peptic ulcer disease
   Active substance abuse
   Pulmonary vascular resistance greater than 6 Wood units
   Psychologic instability
   Malignancy
9. Relative contraindications:
   Advanced peripheral atherosclerosis
   Diabetes mellitus

through such agents as cyclosporine, azathioprine, and corticosteroids has been the major factor in improving outcome following transplantation.

Postoperative care is similar to that for CABG surgery with the exception of medications for immunosuppression. The electrocardiogram (ECG) has two sinus nodes initially (due to the retention of the recipient sinus node), and the recipient sinus node gives P waves unrelated to the QRS complex. Since the transplanted heart has no innervation from the autonomic nervous system, normal cardiac responses to various reflexes do not occur. In addition, the patient will feel no angina-like pain. Because of the denervation, sympathetic stimulants such as isoproterenol may be necessary to increase heart rate and support cardiac function until the ventricle adjusts to the absence of autonomic innervation.

Valvular Heart Disease

The cardiac valves provide for a unidirectional forward flow of blood through the heart. Dysfunctional cardiac valves are classified as stenotic or incompetent. When a cardiac valve restricts the forward flow of blood, it is referred to as stenotic. If the cardiac valve does not close competently, thereby allowing backward flow of blood, it is known as an incompetent (regurgitant or insufficient) valve.

Valves that are stenotic cause an elevated afterload, subsequently resulting in hypertrophy of the atrium or ventricle, which is contracting against the increased pressure load. Regurgitant valves allow blood to flow back into the preceding heart chamber, thus causing volume overload and dilation of the chamber.

The primary cause of acquired valvular heart disease is rheumatic fever. Other causes include infective endocarditis, degenerative changes of the tissue, trauma, papillary muscle rupture from MI, systemic diseases, and others. The aortic and mitral valves are more commonly affected by acquired valvular heart disease than the tricuspid or pulmonic valves.

Mitral insufficiency allows blood to be ejected back into the left atrium. The patient presents with dyspnea, orthopnea, paroxysmal nocturnal dyspnea, elevated PAOP, pulmonary hypertension, decreased cardiac output, crackles, a holosystolic murmur heard best at the apex, S₃, atrial fibrillation, and signs of right heart failure. The progression of mitral insufficiency is slow, and such patients may remain asymptomatic for years. Postoperative care of patients requiring valvular surgery is similar to the general care of the cardiac surgery patient.

Mitral stenosis is most commonly due to rheumatic fever. The symptoms are produced as the size of the opening decreases. As the opening becomes smaller, developing symptoms include dyspnea on exertion, progressive fatigue, cough, hemoptysis, right heart failure, elevated PAOP, elevated RV pressures, and atrial fibrillation. Medical therapy for mitral stenosis includes treatment for pulmonary edema and anticoagulants for prophylaxis of embolization. However, the definitive treatment for mitral stenosis is surgical intervention.

Aortic insufficiency results in LV overload, causing dilation and hypertrophy of the left ventricle. The presentation of aortic insufficiency includes fatigue, dyspnea, paroxysmal nocturnal dyspnea, orthopnea, angina, widened pulse pressure, S₃, systolic murmur heard best in aortic area and Erb's point, sinus tachycardia, and elevated PAOP. Symptoms of heart failure, hypertension, and dysrhythmias are medically managed.

Aortic stenosis causes an obstruction of the blood from the left ventricle to the systemic circulation during systole. Symptoms of aortic stenosis include syncope, fatigue, palpitations, and angina. As the diseased valve continues to narrow, symptoms of left heart failure develop. Surgical repair is the treatment of choice for patients with aortic disease. However, medical therapy is needed for angina, heart failure, and dysrhythmias.

Vascular Surgery

The two most common problems requiring vascular surgery are aneurysms and occlusions. Aneurysms are more problematic when they occur in major arteries. Occlusions are problematic when they occur in major arteries or veins.

Aneurysms

Aortic Aneurysms. The two common types of aortic aneurysms are thoracic and abdominal. Abdominal aneurysms are more common (65% of aneurysms) than thoracic aneurysms. The aneurysm can typically take on one of two patterns: a weakness and bulging of the entire vessel wall or a weakness within the vessel wall (intimal tear or dissection). It is estimated that 5% of individuals over the age of 60 have an abdominal aortic aneurysm (AAA).

Aortic Dissection. Aortic dissection is potentially life threatening because of the rapid progression of shock, loss of vascular volume, potential bleeding into the pericardial sac (with resultant tamponade), and disruption of the aortic valve with resultant LV failure. Ascending aortic involvement is more difficult to correct surgically than descending aortic dissecting aneurysm because of the proximity of the major cardiac structures.

The origin of aortic dissection is usually hypertension. The presentation is one of hypertension with severe unremitting chest and/or abdominal pain frequently radiating to the back. Immediate surgical treatment is necessary. Medical management with antihypertensives can take place but may be unsuccessful.

Abdominal Aneurysms. Abdominal aneurysms may occasionally be identified by noting a palpable mass on physical examination. Symptoms may include abdominal or back pain with tenderness on palpation.

Diagnosis. The use of computed tomography (CT) and magnetic resonance imaging (MRI) to identify abdominal and thoracic vascular structures is common practice. Routine chest and abdominal radiographs and ultrasound may detect the aneurysm, although the detail is not as great as with CT or MRI. Angiography is a good test to demarcate the boundaries of the blood vessels.

Treatment. Replacement of the aneurysm with a graft is the most common surgical intervention. Figure 13-1 contains an example of the surgical replacement technique. The closer the aneurysm is to the heart, the more difficult the surgery will be. Thoracic aneurysms of the descending aorta and abdominal aneurysms offer the surgeon a better operative field and reduce postoperative complications.

Endovascular surgical grafting techniques have become more commonplace. If effective, this approach will eliminate the need for cross clamping of the aorta and, therefore, decrease most of the complications of major aortic surgery.

Postoperative Considerations. The most serious complication following aortic surgery is MI, accounting for almost half of the postoperative mortality from aortic surgery. Monitoring cardiovascular performance such as cardiac index, stroke index or volume, PAOP, CVP, ST segments, and ECG rhythms is helpful in assessing cardiac performance.

The second most common complication is bleeding, which results from injury or from coagulopathies. The nurse must be aware of symptoms of hypovolemia (Chap. 10), indicating a potential bleed. The presence of a strong pulse on palpation of the femoral artery gives an indication of adequate patency of the aorta.

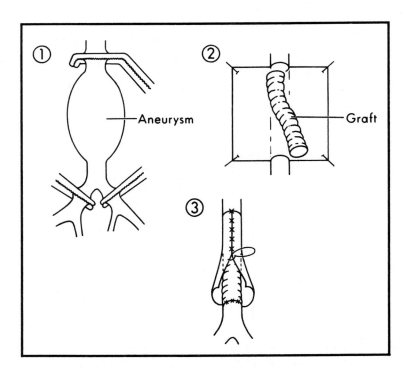

Figure 13-1. Aneurysm graft technique.

Renal failure, the third complication, is especially great in patients with preexisting kidney disease. Acute renal failure is usually caused by periods of prolonged ischemia either from extended aortic cross clamping above the renal arteries; hypotensive episodes before, during, or after surgery; and/or atheroembolization of the renal arteries. Renal function is assessed through the measurement of urine volume, intake and output, and serum and urine creatinine and electrolytes.

Acute limb ischemia is most commonly the result of atheroembolism and can occur in one or both legs. Significant cutaneous ischemia may occur despite maintenance of palpable pedal pulses (blue-toe syndrome, or "trash foot"). Assessment of pulses, skin color, temperature, movement, and sensation should be completed hourly. Pain in an extremity can be a significant indicator of acute ischemia.

Ruptured Abdominal Aortic Aneurysms. At least 50% of patients who experience a ruptured AAA die before reaching the hospital. Although the risk of rupture correlates with aneurysm size, even small aortic aneurysms can rupture. Symptoms most commonly associated with a ruptured AAA are abdominal and back pain, tender abdominal mass, hypotension, and/or shock. These symptoms occur in 50% or less of patients. The location of pain is dependent on the location of the retroperitoneal hematoma.

Mortality with a ruptured AAA ranges from 15% to 88% and is most commonly the result of a delay in operating. The team must be prepared for the massive infusion of fluid and blood products perioperatively. The same complications exist with the ruptured AAA as with elective AAA repair, but they occur with greater frequency. Patients with ruptured AAA repair have a 50% chance of renal failure and a 20% chance of an MI. The patient usually has a longer ventilator course and is more prone to colon ischemia than with elective AAA repair.

Bowel and spinal cord ischemias are less common complications but are associated with a high incidence of morbidity and mortality. Respiratory complications may be avoided through routine postoperative therapy; that is, incentive spirometry, early ambulation, and, if necessary, postural drainage and percussion.

Occlusive Disorders

Obstruction of arterial or venous flow due to atherosclerosis is the most common cardiovascular disturbance. Obstruction can occur anywhere along the major arterial tree; in critical care settings, however, aortofemoral obstructions are most likely to bring the patient to the ICU setting.

Obstruction due to arterial flow usually results in pain on exercise. Lower extremity obstruction is more common than upper extremity obstruction. Pain in the legs on activity due to obstruction is called intermittent claudication. Arterial obstructions are potentially more dangerous because of the loss of oxygen and substrates necessary for the generation of energy. Venous obstructions tend to be more chronic and are less likely to be seen in the critical care setting.

Clinical indications of decreased arterial blood flow include diminished pulses, loss of temperature (cool skin), change in color (cyanosis reflects venous obstruction, pallor reflects arterial obstruction), and diminished sensation. If the obstruction is sudden, severe pain distal to the obstruction is a common symptom.

Assessment of the need for surgery generally includes Doppler ultrasound studies and possibly abdominal aortic ultrasound and CT examinations. Surgery is indicated when the patient has symptoms severe enough to restrict activities of daily living.

Surgical Intervention. The optimal surgical method to relieve obstruction to blood flow depends on the location of the obstruction. Figure 13-2 illustrates the most common types of surgical procedures to bypass obstructions of the aorta and femoral arteries.

Endovascular therapies (balloon angioplasties, atherectomy, and laser angioplasties) can provide effective symptom relief in patients with peripheral vascular disease.

Postoperative Considerations. Assessment of blood flow is an important nursing measure both preoperatively and postoperatively. Blood flow assessment includes pulse quality, capillary refill, and sensation. Pulse presence does not necessarily mean that the graft has good patency. Doppler assessment is a better parameter to measure flow than is palpation.

Loss of flow following surgery can be due to failure of the bypass graft or obstruction as a result of clot formation. In the case of clot formation, there is a danger of potential embolization. In arterial surgery, the emboli will obstruct a site beyond the site of surgery and may result in loss of a portion of the extremity involved. If obstruction is on the venous side, the emboli will result in pulmonary embolization. Symptoms of pulmonary emboli are chest pain, shortness of breath, decreased PaO_2/SaO_2, and elevation of pulmonary artery pressures.

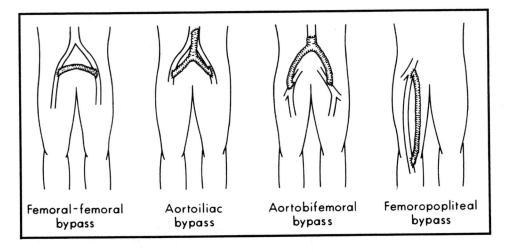

Figure 13-2. Femoral vascular bypass techniques.

CARDIAC TRAUMA

EDITORS' NOTE

Expect about two or less questions on the exam covering cardiac trauma. This section, in conjunction with the previous sections, will enable the clinician to understand the hemodynamic effects of cardiovascular trauma.

Cardiac injuries can be among the most life-threatening traumatic injuries and are second in mortality only to neurologic injuries. Most are the result of motor vehicle crashes and are, therefore, due to blunt trauma. There is an increasing number of chest injuries due to gunshot wounds and stabbings. Injury to the heart and/or great vessels causing disruption of the structures can reduce circulating blood volume and lead to hypovolemia and shock. Direct trauma to the heart muscle, as in myocardial contusion, can lead to a decrease in myocardial contraction, resulting in low cardiac output.

Cardiac Contusion

Cardiac contusion is the most common blunt injury to the heart. It is only rarely fatal. Suspect myocardial contusion if the patient has anterior chest wall trauma and/or fractures of the sternum or ribs. Signs and symptoms are the same as for myocardial ischemia and/or infarction. Specific treatment is to monitor cardiac status with daily ECGs, since some ST- and T-wave changes may not become apparent for up to 48 h. Dysrhythmias are the greatest concern and are treated with standard antidysrhythmic

agents as needed. Isoenzyme level elevations, specifically troponin I (cTnI) or troponin T (cTnT), are perhaps the most accurate indicators of myocardial injury. Two-dimensional echocardiography and/or multigated angiography may be useful in determining abnormalities in ventricular wall movement and ejection fraction. Severe visceral injury may result in delayed cardiac rupture, ventricular septal defect, and ventricular aneurysm, all of which would receive conventional treatment. Symptoms include angina-like chest pain, unexplained tachycardia, and, after some lapse of time, a pericardial friction rub.

Cardiac Rupture

This is a blunt trauma injury and is the most common cause of death. The sequence of frequency of rupture is right ventricle, left ventricle, right atrium, and left atrium. There is no treatment for cardiac rupture other than surgical intervention.

Valvular Injury

This is a blunt trauma injury. The aortic valve is the most commonly injured valve. Signs and symptoms are valve regurgitation and heart failure. Specific treatment could include valve replacement or the normal medical treatment for heart failure.

Cardiac Tamponade

This may result from blunt or penetrating trauma to the pericardium and/or heart. Blood gets into the

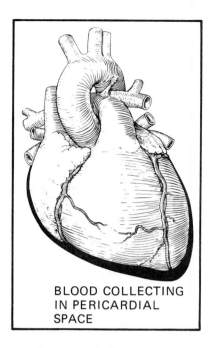

Figure 13-3. Cardiac tamponade.

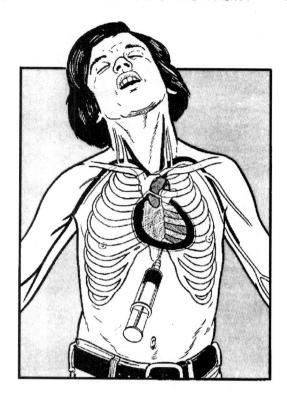

Figure 13-4. Paraxiphoid approach to pericardiocentesis.

pericardial sac but cannot get out. As more blood enters the sac, more pressure is placed against the heart, thus inhibiting or compromising ventricular filling (Fig. 13-3). A subsequent decrease in stroke volume leads to a decrease in cardiac output.

Cardiac tamponade presents with hypotension, muffled or distant heart sounds, and distended neck veins. Additional clues are a falling systolic blood pressure, narrow pulse pressure, pulsus paradoxus (a drop of >20 mm Hg in systolic blood pressure during inspiration), elevated CVP, and various degrees of shock. In a trauma patient, the classic symptoms may be obscured by hypovolemic shock.

Treatment and Nursing Intervention

The objective of treatment is to confirm the diagnosis and relieve the tamponade. This is best accomplished by a pericardiocentesis. Local anesthesia may be achieved with lidocaine. The patient is placed supine with the head elevated at a 45-degree angle. A 16- or 18-gauge 6-in. or longer over-the-needle catheter is attached to a 60-mL syringe. The needle is inserted at a 45-degree angle, lateral to the left side of the xiphoid, 1 to 2 cm inferior to the left of the xiphochondral junction (Fig. 13-4). Blood is aspirated during introduction of the needle. Usually some immediate improvement in cardiac performance is noted upon aspiration of fluid from the pericardial sac. Pericardial blood should not clot.

Rapid clotting of pericardial blood can mean the heart has been entered by the pericardial needle. The underlying cause of the tamponade must be determined. If pericardiocentesis does not relieve the tamponade, thoracotomy for direct repair of the pericardial wound is indicated.

Aortic Rupture

Aortic rupture is the result of a blunt trauma deceleration injury. Although most patients die immediately, 10% to 20% survive to reach a hospital when a tamponade occurs around the rupture. This allows some blood to leave the left ventricle and pass beyond the distal end of the rupture.

Aortic rupture is diagnosed by aortogram. Radiography may reveal a widened mediastinum, which is suggestive of aortic rupture. The aortogram will identify the area of rupture. Figure 13-5 identifies the most common sites of aortic rupture.

Symptoms may include an increased blood pressure and pulse in the upper extremities and a decreased blood pressure and pulse in the lower extremities; the radiograph may show a widened mediastinum. Shortness of breath, weakness, chest or back pain, and varied abnormalities involving the lower extremities may be present.

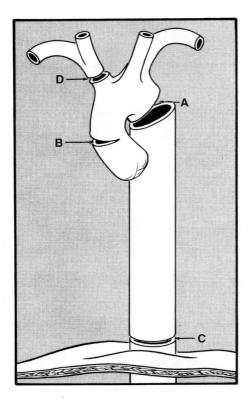

Figure 13-5. Sites of aortic rupture: **(A)** arch of aorta; **(B)** area just above aortic valve; **(C)** end of thoracic aorta; **(D)** subclavian vein. The aortic arch is the most common site; the subclavian vein is the least common.

Treatment and Nursing Intervention

Treatment consists of thoracotomy to repair the rupture. If the thoracotomy cannot be performed immediately, the patient is treated medically as a patient with dissecting aortic aneurysm until surgery.

Nursing interventions include monitoring the respiratory, cardiovascular, neurologic, and renal systems since these suffer first owing to the decreased blood flow. Sodium nitroprusside is usually administered until the patient can be taken to surgery. Nursing care of the patient on ventilatory support and in need of close monitoring before and after surgery applies to the patient with a ruptured aorta.

BIBLIOGRAPHY

Abrams, J. (2005). Clinical practice. Chronic stable angina. *New England Journal of Medicine,16, 352*(24), 2524–2533.

Achar, S. A., Kundu, S., & Norcross, W. A. (2005). Diagnosis of acute coronary syndrome. *American Family Physician, 72*(1), 119–126.

The Albumin Reviewers (Alderson, P., Bunn, F., Lefebvre, C, Li W. P., Li L., Roberts I., Schierhout G.). (2004). Human albumin for resuscitation and volume expansion in critically ill patients. *Cochrane Review, 4,* CD001206.

Boldt, J. (2004). Fluid choice for resuscitation of the trauma patient: A review of the physiological, pharmacological, and clinical evidence. *Canadian Journal of Anesthesiology, 51*(5), 500–513.

Bridges, E. J, & Dukes, S. (2005). Hemodynamic aspects of septic shock. *Critical Care Nurse, 25,* 14–40.

Carter, T., & Ellis, K. (2005). Right ventricular infarction. *Critical Care Nurse, 25,* 52–62.

Cloonan, C. C. "Don't just do something, stand there!": To teach or not to teach, that is the question—intravenous fluid resuscitation training for Combat Lifesavers. *Journal of Trauma, 54*(5 Suppl), S20–S25.

Futterman, L. G, & Lemberg, L. (2003). Diuretics, the most critical therapy in heart failure, yet often neglected in the literature. *American Journal of Critical Care, 12*(4), 376–380.

Futterman, L. G., & Lemberg, L. (2005a). The expanding role of the HMG-CoA reductase inhibitor, the most widely prescribed drug in the world. *American Journal of Critical Care, 14*(6), 555–558.

Futterman, L. G.,& Lemberg, L. (2005b). Atrial fibrillation. *American Journal of Critical Care, 14*(5), 438–440.

Gibler, W. B, Cannon, C. P, Blomkalns, A. L. , Char, D. M., Drew, B. J., Hollander, J. E., . . . Pollack, C. V. (2005). Practical implementation of the Guidelines for Unstable Angina/Non–ST-Segment Elevation Myocardial Infarction in the emergency department. *Annuals of Emergency Medicine, 46*(2), 185–197.

Hollenberg, S. M., Ahrens, T. S, Annane, D., Astiz, M. E., Chalfin, D. B., Dasta, J. F., . . . Zanotti-Cavazzoni, S. (2004). Practice parameters for hemodynamic support of sepsis in adult patients: 2004 update. *Critical Care Medicine, 32*(9), 1928–1948.

Humbert, M., Sitbon, O., & Simonneau, G. (2004). Treatment of primary pulmonary hypertension. *New England Journal of Medicine, 351,* 1425–1436.

Hunt, S. A., Abraham, W. T., Chin, M. H., Feldman A. M., Francis G. S., Ganiats T. G., . . . Riegel B. (2005). ACC/AHA 2005 Guideline Update for the Diagnosis and Management of Chronic Heart Failure in the Adult: A report of the American College of Cardiology/American Heart Association Task Force on Practice Guidelines (Writing Committee to Update the 2001 Guidelines for the Evaluation and Management of Heart Failure): Developed in collaboration with the American College of Chest Physicians and the International Society for Heart and Lung Transplantation: Endorsed by the Heart Rhythm Society. *Circulation, 112*(12), e154–e235.

Jessup, M., & Brozena, S. (2003). Heart failure. *New England Journal of Medicine, 348,* 2007–2018.

Kee, V. R. (2003). Hemodynamic pharmacology of intravenous vasopressors. *Critical Care Nurse, 23,* 79–82.

Keller, K. B., & Lemberg, L. (2004). Prinzmetal's angina. *American Journal of Critical Care, 13*, 350–354.

King, S. B., Smith, S. C., Hirshfeld, J. W., Jr, Jacobs, A. K., Morrison, D. A, Williams, D. O, . . . Yancy, C. W. (2008). 2007 Focused Update of the ACC/AHA/SCAI 2005 Guideline Update for Percutaneous Coronary Intervention: A Report of the American College of Cardiology/American Heart Association Task Force on Practice Guidelines: 2007 Writing Group to Review New Evidence and Update the ACC/AHA/SCAI 2005 Guideline Update for Percutaneous Coronary Intervention, Writing on behalf of the 2005 Writing Committee. *Circulation, 117*, 261.

Page, R. L., Viswanathan, M. N. (2009). Pharmacological therapy for atrial fibrillation: current options and new agents. Expert Opinion on Investigational Drugs, *18*, 417-431.

Prahash, A., Lynch, T. (2004). B-type natriuretic peptide: A diagnostic, prognostic, and therapeutic tool in heart failure. *American Journal of Critical Care, 13*(1), 46–53.

Reid, M. B., & Cottrell, D. (2005). Nursing care of patients receiving intra-aortic balloon counterpulsation. *Critical Care Nurse, 40*, 25–49.

Rhee, P., Koustova, E., & Alam, H. B. (2003). Searching for the optimal resuscitation method: Recommendations for the initial fluid resuscitation of combat casualties. *Journal of Trauma, 54*(5 Suppl), S52–S62.

Roberts, I., Alderson, P., Bunn, F, Chinnock, P., Ker, K., Schierhout, G. (2004). Colloids versus crystalloids for fluid resuscitation in critically ill patients. *Cochrane Reviews, 4*, CD00067.

Smith, S. C., Jr., Feldman, T. E., Hirshfeld, J. W., Jr., Jacobs, A. K., Kern, M. J, King, S. B. 3rd, . . . Riegel, B. (2005). ACC/AHA/SCAI 2005 guideline update for percutaneous coronary intervention—summary article: A report of the American College of Cardiology/American Heart Association Task Force on Practice Guidelines (ACC/AHA/SCAI writing committee to update the 2001 Guidelines for Percutaneous Coronary Intervention). *Catheterization and Cardiovascular Intervention, 67*(1), 87–112.

The SAFE Study Investigators (2004). A comparison of albumin and saline for fluid resuscitation in the intensive care unit. *New England Journal of Medicine, 350*, 2247–2256.

Vincent, J. L., Navickis, R. J., & Wilkes, M. M. (2004). Morbidity in hospitalized patients receiving human albumin: A meta-analysis of randomized, controlled trials. *Critical Care Medicine, 32*, 2029–2038.

Wiegand, D. L. (2003). Advances in cardiac surgery: Valve repair. *Critical Care Nurse, 23*, 72–88.

PART I

Cardiovascular Practice Exam

1. Which of the following statements regarding the coronary sinus is correct?
   (A) It provides arterial blood flow to the lateral LV wall.
   (B) It provides arterial blood flow to the sinus node.
   (C) It is the main venous drainage vessel of the heart.
   (D) It stimulates secretion of the atrial natriuretic factor.

2. Which of the following are atrioventricular (AV) valves?
   (A) Mitral and tricuspid
   (B) Pulmonic and aortic
   (C) Mitral and aortic
   (D) Tricuspid and pulmonic

3. Two circumstances may produce a systolic murmur. One exists when backward flow of blood (regurgitant flow) occurs through a valve that is normally closed during systole. The second exists when blood has difficulty getting past a valve (stenosis) that is normally easily opened. Which two situations may produce a systolic murmur?
   (A) Aortic stenosis and mitral regurgitation
   (B) Pulmonic regurgitation and tricuspid stenosis
   (C) Aortic and tricuspid stenosis
   (D) Pulmonic and mitral regurgitation

4. All of the following but one are considered key treatments in the management of heart failure. Which one is NOT a key treatment in heart failure?
   (A) Angiotensin-converting enzyme (ACE) inhibitors
   (B) Beta blockers
   (C) Diuretics
   (D) Nitroprusside

5. Pericardial tamponade presents with all but one of the following symptoms. Identify the symptom NOT associated with pericardial tamponade.
   (A) Equalization of left and right atrial pressures (CVP and PAOP)
   (B) LV failure without RV involvement
   (C) Hypotension
   (D) Distended neck veins

Questions 6 and 7 refer to the following scenario:

A 62-year-old man is admitted to your unit with the diagnosis of acute subendocardial infarction. At present, he has no chest pain and his vital signs are normal. As you talk with him, he complains of sudden severe shortness of breath. His blood pressure is 80/50 mm Hg, pulse 118, respiratory rate 34. Heart sounds are easily heard but he has a new systolic murmur, grade V/VI, over the left sternal border.

6. Based on the preceding information, which condition is likely to be developing?
   (A) Pericardial tamponade
   (B) Mitral valve rupture
   (C) Ventricular wall rupture
   (D) Aortic valve rupture

7. Which treatment would be indicated for this condition?
   (A) Immediate surgery
   (B) Dopamine, nitroprusside
   (C) Fluid challenges
   (D) Thrombolytic therapy

8. Which of the following cardiac chambers contains deoxygenated blood?
   (A) Right ventricle
   (B) Left ventricle
   (C) Pulmonary veins
   (D) Left atrium

9. Where is the sinoatrial (SA) node located?
   (A) Right atrium
   (B) Left atrium
   (C) Right ventricle
   (D) Superior vena cava

10. What is the preferred first treatment for ventricular fibrillation?
    (A) Nifedipine
    (B) Lidocaine 1 mg/kg
    (C) Synchronized cardioversion, 50 to 100 J
    (D) Defibrillation, 200 to 300 J monophasic or 120 to 200 biphasic

11. Which of the following leads are used in the diagnosis of an inferior MI?
    (A) V_1, V_2, V_3, V_4
    (B) I, aVL
    (C) V_5, V_6
    (D) II, III, aVF

12. Which of the following leads are used in the diagnosis of an anterior MI?
    (A) V_1, V_2, V_3, V_4
    (B) I, aVL
    (C) V_5, V_6
    (D) II, III, aVF

13. Which of the following leads are used in the diagnosis of a lateral MI?
    (A) V_1, V_2, V_3, V_4
    (B) I, aVL, V_5, V_6
    (C) V_2R, V_3R, V_4R
    (D) II, III, aVF

14. Inferior MIs produce conduction defects different from those seen in anterior MIs. Which type of dysrhythmia is more likely to occur in inferior as opposed to anterior MIs?
    (A) Second-degree type I
    (B) Second-degree type II
    (C) Multiform PVCs
    (D) APCs with aberrancy

15. What is the initial treatment of sinus tachycardia?
    (A) Verapamil
    (B) Initially carotid massage, then digoxin
    (C) Esmolol or propranolol
    (D) There is no primary treatment; the source of the tachycardia must be found

Questions 16 and 17 refer to the following scenario:

A 65-year-old man is admitted to your unit with chest pain. The chest pain developed 2 h ago at his home. The pain went away while he rested but then returned. Currently, he has substernal chest pain radiating to the left arm and chin. The pain is the same regardless of position. No change in the pain occurs during inspiration. Vital signs are as follows: blood pressure 132/86 mm Hg, pulse 96, respiratory rate 25. The patient's 12-lead ECG shows depressed ST segments in the inferior leads. Small Q waves, less than one-third the height of the R wave, are present in the inferior leads.

16. Based on the preceding information, which condition is likely to be developing?
    (A) Angina
    (B) Acute MI
    (C) Pericarditis
    (D) Pericardial tamponade

17. What would be the most likely treatment for the condition?
    (A) Nitrates and beta blockers
    (b) Thrombolytic therapy
    (C) Pericardiocentesis
    (D) Aspirin and analgesics

18. Which of the following is an advantage of a transcutaneous pacemaker?
    (A) It is easy to apply.
    (B) It requires lower electrical stimulation to capture the heart rate.
    (C) It requires peripheral intravenous access.
    (D) Electrical stimulation is not perceived by the patient.

19. What is the inherent rate of the AV node area?
    (A) 20 to 40.
    (B) 40 to 60.
    (C) 60 to 80.
    (D) The AV nodal area has no inherent rate.

20. Passage of the electrical impulse through the AV node is represented by which ECG complex?
    (A) PR interval
    (B) QRS complex
    (C) ST segment
    (D) T wave

21. A junctional rhythm has all of the following characteristics but one. Which of the following characteristics is NOT indicative of a junctional rhythm?
    (A) Normal QRS complex
    (B) Wide QRS complex
    (C) Heart rate between 40 and 60 beats per minute
    (D) Absent P waves

22. Which of the following isoenzymes is most diagnostic in identifying MI?

(A) Troponin I (cTnI)
(B) CPK-MB band
(C) Troponin K (cTnK)
(D) CPK-BB band

23. A 51-year-old man is admitted to your unit with the symptoms of crushing chest pain that is unrelieved by nitrates or rest. He has ST segments elevated 3 mm in V_1 through V_4 with ST-segment depression in II, III, and aVF. His blood pressure is 94/64 mm Hg, pulse 110, and respiratory rate 32. Based on this information, which type of MI would most likely be represented by the ECG changes?
(A) Anterior
(B) Inferior
(C) Lateral
(D) Posterior

24. Unstable angina is characterized by all of the following features but one. Which feature does NOT characterize unstable angina?
(A) Increasing frequency of chest pain
(B) Chest pain at rest
(C) Increasing severity of symptoms
(D) Q-wave formation

25. Which type of medication is common in the treatment of unstable angina?
(A) Diuretics
(B) Vasodilators
(C) Beta blockers
(D) Sympathetic stimulants

Questions 26 and 27 refer to the following scenario:

A 59-year-old man is admitted to your unit with the diagnosis "rule out myocardial infarction." He states that at work, 1 h ago, he felt severe chest pain, became cool and clammy, and felt nauseated. He came immediately to the hospital. The ECG indicates ST-segment elevation in leads II, III, and aVF. ST-segment depression exists in V_1 through V_6. He has not responded to nitrates in the emergency department or the ICU. His vital signs are as follows:

Blood pressure	98/68 mm Hg,
Pulse	107,
Respiratory rate	32.

26. Which type of MI is represented by these ECG changes?
(A) Anterior
(B) Inferior
(C) Lateral
(D) Posterior

27. Based on the preceding description, which initial treatment is indicated?
(A) Dobutamine
(B) Thrombolytic therapy
(C) Coronary artery bypass grafting (CABG)
(D) Cardiac catheterization for stent placement

28. Thrombolytic therapy is commonly associated with complications. Which of the following is NOT a complication of thrombolytic therapy?
(A) Bradycardia
(B) Bleeding from venipuncture sites
(C) Ventricular ectopy
(D) Extension of the MI due to embolic phenomena

29. Pulsus paradoxus is utilized to identify which of the following conditions?
(A) Cardiac tamponade
(B) MI
(C) Respiratory failure
(D) Ruptured papillary muscle

30. Orthostatic hypotension results from which of the following conditions?
(A) LV failure
(B) Pulmonary hypertension
(C) Hypovolemia
(D) Portal hypertension

31. Orthostatic hypotension is manifested by which of the following clinical symptoms following a change from lying down to sitting up?
(A) A fall in systolic blood pressure of >25 mm Hg and a decrease in diastolic blood pressure of >10 mm Hg
(B) Systolic blood pressure is unchanged while a decrease in diastolic blood pressure of >10 mm Hg occurs
(C) A decrease in systolic blood pressure while diastolic blood pressure increases slightly
(D) An increase in systolic blood pressure while diastolic blood pressure falls

32. Physical signs associated with CHF include all but one of the following. Identify the one sign that is NOT associated with CHF.
(A) Dependent crackles in the lungs
(B) S_3 heart sound
(C) Dependent edema
(D) Pansystolic murmur

33. A 71-year-old man is admitted with a history of CAD and CHF. He is on the following medications. Which of these medications are not consistent with long-term management of CHF?

(A) Diuretics
(B) Beta blockers
(C) ACE inhibitors
(D) Parasympathetic inhibitors

34. Which of the following would not be an expected treatment in CHF?
(A) Inotrope (e.g., milrinone or dobutamine)
(B) Calcium channel blocker (e.g., nicardipine)
(C) Beta natriuretic peptide (e.g., nesiritide)
(D) Diuretic (e.g., furosemide)

35. Which of the following is NOT an indication for a CABG?
(A) Unstable angina
(B) 90% narrowing of the left anterior descending (LAD) coronary artery
(C) Distal stenosis of the LAD coronary artery
(D) Multiple-vessel stenosis

36. Which of the following is a common sign in cardiac tamponade?
(A) Decreased PAOP
(B) Increased diastolic blood pressure
(C) Pulsus paradoxus
(D) Ejection fraction >75%

37. Which blood vessel is commonly used as the graft vessel in a CABG?
(A) Femoral vein
(B) Axillary artery
(C) A coronary artery that is unobstructed
(D) Internal mammary artery

38. Which of the following is the best method to treat cardiomyopathy?
(A) Heart transplantation
(B) CABG
(C) IABP assistance
(D) Coronary angioplasty

39. What is the most common type of aortic aneurysm?
(A) Ascending thoracic
(B) Descending thoracic
(C) Abdominal
(D) Aortic arch

40. Dissecting aneurysms present with several symptoms. Which of the following is NOT a symptom of a dissecting aortic aneurysm?
(A) Gastrointestinal bleeding
(B) Severe abdominal pain

(C) Pain radiating to the back
(D) Palpable abdominal mass

41. Which of the following is the most common complication causing death following aortic surgery?
(A) Stress ulcers
(B) Acute tubular necrosis (ATN)
(C) Bleeding
(D) MI

42. All of the following but one are symptoms of obstructed arterial flow. Select the one that represents venous, NOT arterial, obstruction.
(A) Pallor of the skin
(B) Cyanosis of the skin
(C) Intermittent claudication
(D) Decreased pulses

43. Which of the following is a common sign of acute arterial obstruction?
(A) Pain distal to the obstruction
(b) Edema distal to the obstruction
(c) Cyanosis distal to the obstruction
(d) Warm skin proximal to the obstruction

44. Deep venous thrombosis can potentially release emboli. Which of the following could result from an embolism originating from a deep venous thrombosis?
(A) Loss of the dorsalis pedis pulse
(B) Loss of pulses in the femoral artery
(C) Superior vena cava syndrome
(D) Pulmonary embolism

45. A 62-year-old man is admitted to your unit postoperatively following abdominal aortic aneurysm repair. Four hours after returning from the operating room, he begins to complain of chest pain and shortness of breath. Breath sounds are equal with inspiratory crackles noted posteriorly. Heart sounds indicate a clear S_1, S_2, and S_3. On the basis of this information, the patient is most likely developing which of the following?
(A) MI
(B) Pulmonary emboli
(C) Tension pneumothorax
(D) Dissecting thoracic aneurysm

PART I

Cardiovascular Practice Exam

Practice Fill-Ins

1. _____
2. _____
3. _____
4. _____
5. _____
6. _____
7. _____
8. _____
9. _____
10. _____
11. _____
12. _____

13. _____
14. _____
15. _____
16. _____
17. _____
18. _____
19. _____
20. _____
21. _____
22. _____
23. _____
24. _____

25. _____
26. _____
27. _____
28. _____
29. _____
30. _____
31. _____
32. _____
33. _____
34. _____
35. _____
36. _____

37. _____
38. _____
39. _____
40. _____
41. _____
42. _____
43. _____
44. _____
45. _____

PART I

Answers

1.	C	13.	B	25.	C	37.	D
2.	A	14.	A	26.	B	38.	A
3.	A	15.	D	27.	D	39.	C
4.	D	16.	A	28.	D	40.	A
5.	B	17.	A	29.	A	41.	D
6.	B	18.	A	30.	C	42.	B
7.	A	19.	B	31.	A	43.	A
8.	A	20.	A	32.	D	44.	D
9.	A	21.	B	33.	D	45.	A
10.	D	22.	A	34.	B		
11.	D	23.	A	35.	C		
12.	A	24.	D	36.	C		

II

PULMONARY

Donna Prentice

14

Pulmonary Anatomy and Physiology

EDITORS' NOTE

The PCCN exam will have a few questions that are directly related to the anatomy of the pulmonary system. However, as you read this chapter, concentrate on understanding the major pulmonary features rather than minute details. Try to understand the anatomy as it relates to clinical application rather than memorizing details of anatomy.

For the PCCN exam, it is crucial to understand concepts in pulmonary physiology as they apply to pulmonary care. Although much of this chapter is explanatory and somewhat theoretical, it is important to be familiar with most of the concepts presented. As you read this chapter, focus on understanding key principles rather than on minute details. This is a long chapter, and it may be useful to read it in sections in order to improve your understanding of the key concepts. You can expect the PCCN exam to include several questions addressing major concepts in pulmonary physiology, so be familiar with the information in this chapter.

The major function of the pulmonary system is the exchange of oxygen and carbon dioxide in the body. The pulmonary anatomy includes the thoracic cage, the muscles of the chest, the upper airway, and the lower airway. A grasp of pulmonary physiology is key to understanding pulmonary disturbances; this topic includes gas exchange principles and the analysis of blood gases.

THORACIC CAGE

The thoracic cage (Fig. 14-1) is the bony frame of the chest. The thorax is shaped like an inverted cone with the apex about 2.5 cm above the clavicles. The clavicles and first ribs form the protective barrier of the superior portion of the thoracic cage. The diaphragm is the inferior portion of the thoracic cage.

The sternum makes up the anterior portion of the thoracic cage and is actually three connected flat bones: the manubrium, the body, and the xiphoid process. Seven pairs of ribs, called the "true ribs," attach to the sternum. The remaining five ribs form the anterior portion of the thoracic cage. Each rib is attached to the rib above it by intercostal muscles and cartilage. The posterior thoracic cage is formed by the vertebrae and 12 pairs of ribs attached to the vertebrae. The ribs are C-shaped and serve as the bony protective sides of the thoracic cage (Fig. 14-2).

MUSCLES OF RESPIRATION

The diaphragm is the major muscle of respiration. On inspiration, the diaphragm contracts (Fig. 14-3), lengthening the chest cavity. The external intercostal muscles contract to raise the ribs, enlarging the diameter of the chest. On expiration, the diaphragm relaxes, becoming dome-shaped and decreasing the size of the thorax (Fig. 14-3).

Expiration is passive, accomplished by relaxation of the diaphragm and external intercostal muscles and the lungs' normal tendency to collapse. Relaxation of the musculature is the major mechanism for exhalation.

The intercostal muscles are composed of two layers: the internal and external intercostals. Changes in the chest muscles alter normal thoracic pressures, affecting ventilation. The internal intercostal muscles pull the ribs down and inward. They are used for forceful expiration, coughing, sneezing, in other stressful states, and in exertional activities.

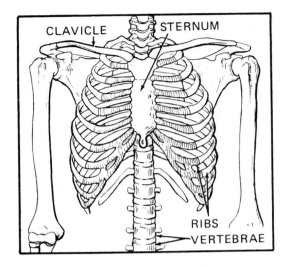

Figure 14-1. Thoracic cage.

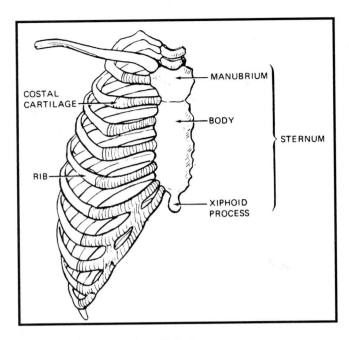

Figure 14-2. Sternum.

The intercostal muscles may facilitate a smooth transition from inspiration to expiration.

In pulmonary distress and/or disease, accessory muscles are used to facilitate inspiration. The accessory muscles of respiration include the scalene, sternocleidomastoid, trapezius, and pectoralis muscles.

MEDIASTINUM

The lung parenchyma and the mediastinum are contained within the bony thoracic cage. The mediastinum is a space midline in the chest and contains the heart, great vessels, trachea, major bronchi,

esophagus, thymus gland, lymphatics, and various nerves (Fig. 14-4).

PLEURA

Each lung lies free in its own pleural cavity except at its single point of attachment, the hilum (Fig. 14-4). The pleural covering of each lung is composed of two layers. The visceral layer is contiguous with the lung

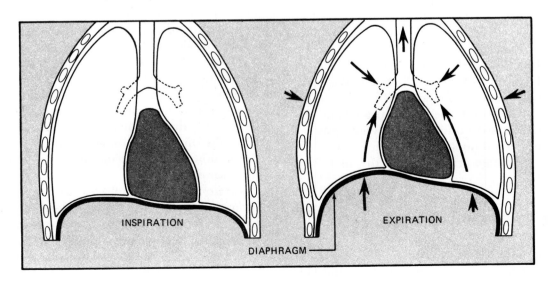

Figure 14-3. Diaphragm on inspiration and expiration.

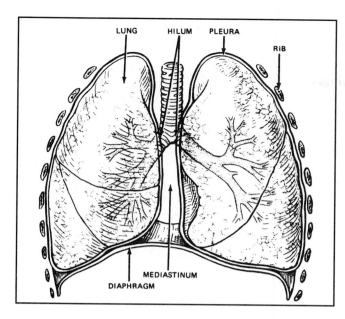

Figure 14-4. Mediastinum and hilum.

and does not have sensory (pain) nerve fibers. The parietal layer is the outer pleural layer that lines the inside of the thoracic cage and contains sensory nerve fibers. The two pleural layers are separated by a small amount of pleural fluid that allows the two surfaces to slide easily over each other during inspiration and expiration. If the pleurae become inflamed, movement is restricted and the resulting irritation causes pleuritic pain. The diaphragm is the inferior border for each pleural space; the chest wall is the lateral border and the mediastinum is the medial border.

LUNG

Each lung is made up of lobes. There are three lobes on the right and two on the left. Each lobe of the lung is separated from the adjacent lobe by fissures. The left lung also has an upper and lower division of its superior lobe, separated by a fissure. This fissure is called the lingula. The area of the lingula is equal to or smaller than that of the middle lobe of the right lung. Each lobe is further divided into segments; 10 in the right lung and 8 in the left lung (Fig. 14-5).

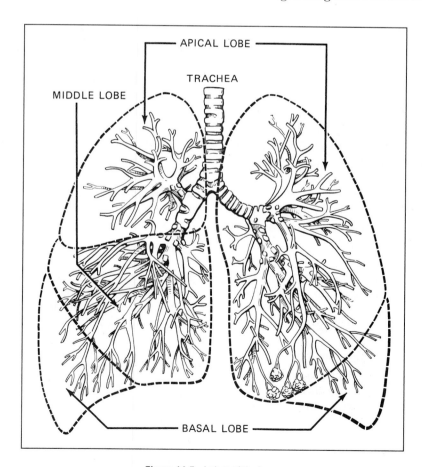

Figure 14-5. Lobes of the lung.

UPPER AIRWAY

The upper airway consists of the mouth, nose and oral pharynx, and larynx. The larynx functions in part as a transitional structure between the upper and lower airways. The purpose of the upper airway is to warm, humidify, and filter the inspired air. This is essential to protect the lower airway and alveoli.

The entire upper airway is lined with a mucous membrane that moisturizes and warms the inspired air by means of the vast blood supply and thick layer of watery mucus produced by serous glands and the thick, tenacious mucus produced by the epithelial goblet cells. The ciliated portions of the upper airway filter pollutants, irritants, and fine particles (1 to 4 μm in size). Such particles come in contact with the respiratory mucosa and are trapped. They are carried to the pharynx by the mucous blanket, where they are swallowed.

Nose

Air normally enters the respiratory system through the nose. The nose has skeletal rigidity, which maintains patency during inspiration. The first two-thirds of the nose are cartilaginous and the last third is bony. The cartilaginous septum, straight at birth, frequently becomes deviated during life and may obstruct airflow. The nasal septum divides the nose into two fossae; the lateral borders are the alae. The openings between the alae and the nasal septum are the nostrils, or nares. The nose has a small inlet and a large outlet, allowing inspired air to have maximum contact with the upper airway mucosa. By sniffing through the nose, inhaled air is directed toward the superior turbinates and olfactory bulb (Fig. 14-6).

The first one-third of the nose is lined with nonciliated squamous epithelium. The remaining two-thirds of the nose are lined with ciliated pseudostratified epithelium. Coarse particles larger than 4 μm are entrapped by nasal hairs. The nasopharynx is lined with ciliated pseudostratified epithelium.

Pharynx

The main function of the pharynx is to collect incoming air from the mouth and nose and project it downward to the trachea. The pharynx is subdivided into the nasopharynx, the oropharynx, and the laryngopharynx (Fig. 14-6). The nasopharynx is the space behind the oral and nasal cavities and above the soft palate; it contains the orifices of the eustachian tubes. The pharyngeal tonsils (adenoids), an important

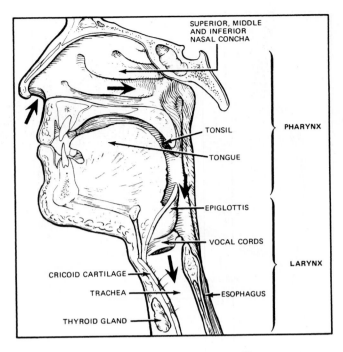

Figure 14-6. Upper airway, pharynx, and larynx.

defense mechanism of the pulmonary system, are located in the superior nasopharynx.

The oropharynx is the area from the soft palate to the base of the tongue. It receives air from the mouth and nose and food from the mouth. The faucial tonsils are located at the anterolateral borders of the oropharynx.

The laryngopharynx is the lower portion of the pharynx, extending from the base of the tongue to the opening of the esophagus. The laryngopharynx contains muscles within its wall, the pharyngeal constrictors, that aid in the mechanism of swallowing.

Larynx

The larynx lies in the anterior portion of the neck, extending from cervical vertebrae C4 to C6 and connecting the upper and lower airway. It aids in speech and is an essential part of the mechanism of coughing. The larynx is composed of cartilage connected by membranes and muscle. The laryngeal mucosa is stratified squamous epithelium above the vocal cords and pseudostratified columnar epithelium below.

The glottis is the opening into the larynx. The epiglottis, a flexible cartilage attached to the thyroid cartilage, helps prevent foreign material from entering the airway by covering the glottis during swallowing. In the adult, the thyroid cartilage (Fig. 14-7) is

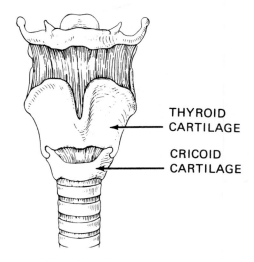

Figure 14-7. Thyroid-cricoid cartilages.

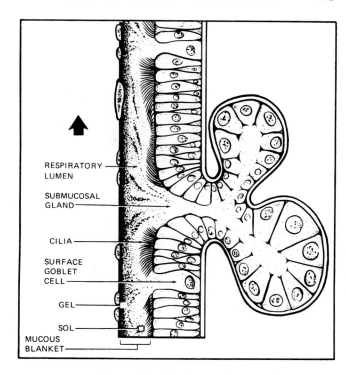

Figure 14-8. Mcociliary escalator.

the narrowest part of the air passage of the larynx. As muscles in the larynx contract, the vocal cords change shape and vibrate. This vibration of the vocal cords produces sound.

The cricoid cartilage is a complete ring located just below the thyroid cartilage, where the vocal cords are located. The cricothyroid membrane is an avascular structure that connects the thyroid and cricoid cartilages. It is through this membrane that an airway may be established in an emergency. In this way, the posterior wall of the larynx and vocal cords are not injured.

LUNG DEFENSE MECHANISMS

The mucociliary escalator is the primary protective mechanism for the entire respiratory system. The entire respiratory tree is lined with varying types of epithelial cells as well as cilia, which are fine, hair-like filaments projecting into the airway lumen. Goblet cells in the epithelium produce watery, thick mucus which covers the inner lumen of the airway. The mucous lining is called the mucous blanket. Various mechanisms move the mucous blanket to the pharynx, where it will be swallowed; to the larynx, where coughing will expel it; and to the nose, where it will be expelled by blowing and sneezing. Cilia lining the larger airways will help to move the mucous blanket up the respiratory tract by the continuous undulating movement of the cilia, referred to as the mucocilary escalator (Fig. 14-8).

The sneeze reflex is a reaction to irritation in the nose. The cough reflex is a reaction to irritation

in the upper airway distal to the nose. Both processes are complex mechanisms that require the integration of increased intrathoracic pressure, complete and tight closure of the epiglottis and vocal cords, and strong contraction of the abdominal musculature, diaphragm, and intercostal muscles.

LOWER AIRWAY

The lower airway consists of two divisions, the tracheobronchial tree and the lung parenchyma. The tracheobronchial tree is a system of progressively narrower conducting tubes providing air passage to the alveoli. The trachea divides into the right and left mainstem bronchi. Further subdivisions include the bronchi, bronchioles, terminal bronchioles, and alveoli.

Trachea

The trachea extends from approximately C6 to the carina, the point of bifurcation of the right and left mainstem bronchi. It is composed of C-shaped cartilaginous rings with a posterior muscle that is membranous and friable. This muscle relaxes on inspiration, increasing the tracheal diameter. On exhalation, the muscle contracts, decreasing the tracheal diameter. Occasionally, the muscle relaxes and

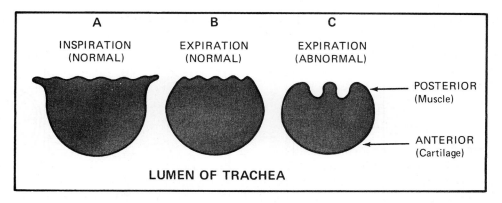

Figure 14-9. Movement of posterior muscles of the trachea.

bows in on exhalation, decreasing the effectiveness of the mucociliary stream in clearing secretions from the lungs (Fig. 14-9).

The trachea divides into the right and left mainstem bronchi at the carina, located at the angle of Louis at the sternomanubrial junction, at about the second intracostal space. The right mainstem bronchus comes off the trachea in almost a straight line, while the left mainstem bronchus comes off the trachea at an angle of approximately 40 degrees. The right mainstem bronchus is wider in diameter than the left. Foreign matter tends to lodge in the right mainstem bronchus because of its size and the angle at which it takes off from the trachea (Fig. 14-10).

The right and left mainstem bronchi separate into 22 divisions before the terminal respiratory

bronchioles. These divisions are cartilaginous; the terminal respiratory bronchioles are small tubes without cartilage. Only smooth muscle surrounds the respiratory epithelium. Contraction of this smooth muscle results in bronchospasm.

The respiratory bronchioles branch into alveolar ducts and then into the alveoli, which make up the lung parenchyma. The alveoli and alveolar ducts have common walls, termed septa, which play an important role in the elastic recoil of the lung. The septal wall is composed of smooth muscle that contracts to narrow the lumen of the alveolar duct.

Alveolar Sacs and Cells

At the terminal end of the tracheobronchial tree are the alveolar sacs. These dead-end structures prevent ambient air from going further. The sacs, made up of 15 to 20 alveoli, each share a common wall with adjacent sacs (Fig. 14-11).

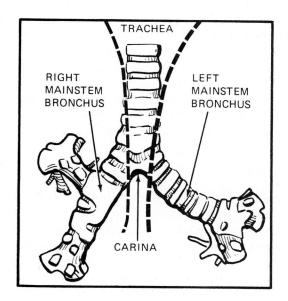

Figure 14-10. Right and left mainstem bronchi.

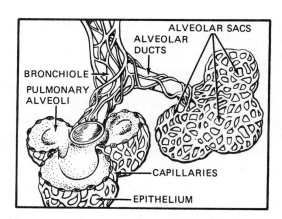

Figure 14-11. Terminal bronchiole and alveolar sac.

The 200 to 600 million alveoli in the normal lung comprise an average total surface area of 40 to 100 m^2; approximately the size of a football field. This surface area is directly related to body length and decreases by about 5% per decade.

Alveolar sacs are lined with epithelium, which is composed of three types of cells. Type I cells are characterized by cytoplasmic extensions and make up most of the lung. Type II alveolar cells are found where one extension interfaces with another; these active metabolic cells contain organelles that synthesize surfactant. Type III alveolar cells are phagocytes that arise from bone marrow or from type II cells.

Pulmonary Surfactant

Alveolar epithelium is lined with a phospholipid protein fluid called surfactant. The phospholipid is insoluble but highly permeable to all gases. The function of surfactant is to reduce the surface tension in the alveoli. Two pathologic states that are complicated by insufficient or absent surfactant are (1) hyaline membrane disease and (2) acute respiratory distress syndrome (ARDS).

Surfactant functions by forming a thin, monomolecular layer at the interface of the air and fluid in the alveoli. Without surfactant, an air-fluid interface would produce surface tension that would collapse the small alveoli. By preventing the development of the air-fluid interface, surfactant decreases the surface tension in the alveoli. Surfactant provides stability to smaller alveoli, which have a greater pressure and tend to collapse. Without the proper amount of surfactant, there is a filtration of fluid from the alveolar wall capillaries into the alveoli, leading to development of pulmonary edema and/or ARDS. In sum, the effects of the loss of surfactant include stiff, less compliant lungs; atelectasis; and fluid-filled alveoli.

The alveoli are where gas exchange occurs. Oxygen diffuses across the alveolar epithelium, the basement membrane, and the small interstitial space and through the capillary membrane, the plasma fluid, and the erythrocyte membrane. At this point, the capillary is so small that the erythrocytes must line up in a single column to move through it. Oxygen diffuses rapidly through the erythrocyte membrane and attaches to the hemoglobin molecule of the erythrocyte. Carbon dioxide molecules diffuse across the alveolar capillary membrane in the opposite direction at a rate 20 times faster than oxygen. The capillary endothelium is very sensitive and is easily damaged by endotoxins, oxygen, and other noxious substances.

PULMONARY CIRCULATION

The lung receives deoxygenated blood from the right side of the heart via the pulmonary artery. The oxygenated blood is returned to the left side of the heart via the pulmonary vein, where it is pumped from the left ventricle through the cardiovascular system.

The lungs' arterial system follows the bronchial tree, bifurcating at each bronchial division and following close to the bronchus and its subdivisions. As the bronchioles become smaller, some arteries fail to bifurcate and nearby arteries send out branches from their stem to provide oxygenated blood to the central part of the alveolar tissue (Fig. 14-12).

Venous blood flows through the capillaries and venules to the periphery of the alveoli and then reenters the venous circulation to be directed back to the right atrium.

The total volume and rate of pulmonary blood circulation is about 5 L/min. Because of gravity, blood flow is greatest to the dependent portions of the lung. Thus, in an erect person, the apex of the lung will have the least circulating blood volume. When the person is lying down, the anterior lung surfaces will have the least circulating blood volume.

The erythrocyte completes the pulmonary circulation very rapidly (within 0.75 s at rest). This rapid circulation helps maintain adequate perfusion. The total volume of blood in the pulmonary arteries, veins, and capillaries is about 500 to 750 mL in the average adult male or about 10% to 15% of the total blood volume, serving as a reservoir in times of increased cardiac output.

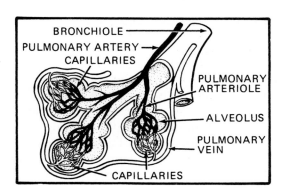

Figure 14-12. Blood flow in the parenchyma.

CONTROL OF VENTILATION

Three major factors control ventilation: neural, central chemical, and peripheral chemical control mechanisms.

Neural Control

The respiratory center is in the medullary portion of the brainstem. Neurons initiate impulses that result in inspiration. An increase in the rate of impulses results in an increase in respiratory rate; an increase in their strength increases tidal volume.

Normally, chemical factors keep the inspiratory and expiratory centers in balance, resulting in normal ventilatory patterns. The inspiratory center is in the dorsal aspect of the medulla oblongata, in close association to the vagus nerve and the glossopharyngeal nerves. There appears to be an inherent automaticity in the electrical impulse release for inspiration. The apneustic center, in the pons, acts to prevent the interruption of these inspiratory impulses.

If the apneustic center takes control over the normally balanced ventilation pattern, apneustic breathing occurs, consisting of slight pauses following some expirations in an otherwise normal breathing pattern.

Expiration control is in the pneumotaxic center, located in the upper pons. The neurons there transmit impulses to limit inspiration. When the pneumotaxic center controls ventilation, there is irregular, deep, shallow breathing with randomly spaced periods of varying lengths of apnea.

The walls of the pulmonary bronchi and bronchioles have stretch receptors that interact with the vagus nerve in what is known as the Hering-Breuer reflex. When they become overstretched, there is a feedback mechanism to the inspiratory center to prevent hyperinflation of the lungs.

Central Chemical Control

The pH of the cerebrospinal fluid (CSF) constitutes the primary control of respiratory center stimulation. A change in the hydrogen ion concentration of the CSF occurs very quickly in relation to arterial carbon dioxide pressure ($PaCO_2$), resulting in the appropriate change in stimulation of the neural respiratory center. Acidosis, or a rise in CSF hydrogen ion concentration, increases stimulation to respiratory centers. Alkalosis, or a drop in CSF hydrogenion concentration, decreases stimulation to neural respiratory centers.

$PaCO_2$ provides the normal neurochemic control of the respiratory cycle because of its effect on the CSF pH. A rise in CSF hydrogen ion concentration will first increase respiratory depth and then the respiratory rate.

Peripheral Chemical Control

Chemoreceptors are located at the bifurcation of the internal and external carotid arteries, carotid bodies, and aortic bodies at the aortic arch. These highly vascular neural bodies are stimulated by any decrease in oxygen supply, such as decreased blood flow, decreased hemoglobin, increased pH, or increased $PaCO_2$. Stimulation of the carotid and/or aortic bodies will increase cerebral cortical activity, resulting in tachycardia, hypertension, and increased respiratory rate, tidal volume, pulmonary resistance, bronchial smooth muscle tone, and adrenal gland secretions.

Factors Affecting Ventilation

Certain drugs depress the respiratory center by decreasing alveolar ventilation or blocking the central respiratory center. Decreased alveolar ventilation is characterized by shallow respirations and a respiratory rate of less than 12 breaths per minute.

Chronic respiratory disease may alter normal respiratory patterns. Patients with chronic CO_2 retention have a constantly elevated $PaCO_2$, thus decreasing the peripheral chemoreceptors' sensitivity to changes in hydrogen ion concentration. A decrease in the level of arterial oxygen pressure (PaO_2) stimulates ventilation. High-flow oxygen therapy may result in apnea, suppressing the hypoxic drive mechanism.

PROCESS OF RESPIRATION

The process of respiration has four phases. Phase I is ventilation, the movement of ambient air into and out of the lungs. Phase II is the diffusion of oxygen and carbon dioxide in the alveoli. Phase III is the delivery of oxygen and removal of carbon dioxide from the cells. Phase IV is the regulation of ventilation.

Phase I: Ventilation

Normal barometric pressure at sea level is 760 mm Hg. For the average healthy person at rest, the intrapleural pressure is slightly subatmospheric at 755 mm Hg. If the pressures were equal, there would be no flow of air into or out of the lung.

As inspiration begins, the thoracic cage increases in size, producing a negative intrapleural pressure compared to the atmosphere and resulting in airflow into the lungs. If one considers atmospheric pressure to be zero (0), then resting intrapleural pressure is −5 and inspiratory intrapleural pressure is −10. As inspiratory muscle activity ends, the normal elastic recoil of the lung decreases the size of the thoracic cage and gas flows out of the lung.

Lung Pressures

The pulmonary system is a low-pressure system. It allows the capillaries to distend easily to accommodate increased volumes from the systemic circulatory system in times of distress and/or exertion. This distensibility helps regulate resistance to blood flow through the pulmonary system. In the normal disease-free lung, the average pulmonary artery systolic pressure is 25 (±2) mm Hg and the average diastolic pressure is 10 (±2) mm Hg. The pressure necessary to move blood from the right heart to the left heart is the left atrial pressure, or the pulmonary capillary wedge pressure or pulmonary artery occlusive pressure (PAOP). The normal left atrial PAOP is 8 to 12 mm Hg. The mean pulmonary artery pressure must always be higher than the left atrial pressure in order to move blood from the right heart through the lungs to the left atrium.

Compliance

Compliance is a measure of the distensibility of the lungs and thorax. Compliance is expressed as change in volume (V) for a change in the intra-alveolar pressure (P). Greater compliance means that there is a larger volume change in the lung for each pressure change. Reduced compliance means that there is less volume change in the lung for each pressure change. In other words, the more pressure needed to change the volume in the lung, the less compliance. The standard measure is units of L/cm H_2O. The normal lung plus thorax compliance of an adult is around 0.1 L/cm H_2O.

Any disease that stiffens the lungs will decrease compliance. Diseases that increase congestion in the lungs—such as atelectasis, pneumonia, or pulmonary edema—result in decreased lung compliance and decreased gas exchange. Space-occupying neoplasms, infections, or increased extravascular lung water also decrease lung compliance (Table 14-1).

Any condition that limits the ability of the bony thorax to expand will also decrease lung compliance. An example of a restrictive cause of decreased compliance is third-trimester pregnancy. During the

TABLE 14-1. CAUSES OF DECREASED LUNG COMPLIANCE

Intrathoracic	Extrathoracic
Atelectasis	Flail chest
Pneumonia	Barrel chest
Pleural effusion	Pectus excavatum
Empyema	Pectus carinatum
Lung abscess	Kyphosis
Bronchospasm	Scoliosis
Pulmonary edema	Kyphoscoliosis
Bronchitis	Obesity
Asthma	Abdominal compartment syndrome
Emphysema	
ARDS	
Tension pneumothorax	

ARDS, acute respiratory distress syndrome.

third trimester, the abdominal contents are displaced upward, preventing the diaphragm from descending fully and decreasing the extent of chest wall expansion. Obesity and abdominal distention also prevent full movement of the diaphragm. The obese patient has decreased lung compliance as a result of the excess weight on the upper torso. The intercostal muscles cannot function efficiently as they attempt to lift the weight. Postoperative binders and chest splints decrease lung compliance over large segments of the thorax by limiting its expansion.

There are two types of compliance, static and dynamic. Static compliance (Cst) is the change in lung volume per unit airway pressure change when the lungs are motionless. Cst can be measured only when there is no flow of gases, at the end of inspiration or expiration. Measurements of Cst provide a reliable index of lung compliance when no airway disease is present, as the presence of airway disease alters the rate of gas flow from the mouth to the alveoli, resulting in inaccurate values. If airway disease is present, most of the resistance to airflow will be in the medium-sized bronchi.

Dynamic compliance (Cdyn) can easily be tested in the clinical area. To get an estimate of the Cdyn for the patient on mechanical ventilation, divide the tidal volume (VT) by the peak airway pressure (PAP). Normal dynamic compliance is about 35 to 55 mL/cm H_2O.

Airway resistance results from the impedance of gas flow by the walls of the airway or obstruction, changing the ratio of alveolar pressure against the rate of airflow. Airway resistance is increased by secretions, artificial airways, endotracheal tubes, bronchospasm, laryngeal or tracheal strictures, edema, emphysema, or space-occupying lesions. A measure of airway resistance can be made by comparing the Cst and Cdyn.

Elastic Recoil

Intra-alveolar septa are a major factor in the elastic recoil of the interstitial parenchyma. The thorax, pleura, and lung parenchyma have opposing elastic forces. The fluid lining the alveoli and the interstitial parenchymal tends to collapse the lungs, while the thoracic cage and pleura tend to expand them. As long as the thoracic cage and pleura are patent, these elastic forces balance each other. If the integrity of the pleura is compromised, the parenchymal forces become greater and the lung collapses.

Airflow

There are three basic types of airflow within the lung airways, turbulent, transitional, and laminar. Turbulent airflow occurs in large chambers such as the nose and oral pharynx (Fig. 14-13). Transitional airflow occurs in large to medium airways at points of bifurcation and/or narrowing. As air flows down the tracheo-bronchial tree, it branches into smaller and smaller tubes, creating transitional airflow (Fig. 14-14). Laminar airflow occurs in thin, flat, continuous sheets. The outermost layer of air has minimal contact with the walls of the air passage, providing slight filtering in the small peripheral airways (Fig. 14-15).

Lung Volumes

The total lung capacity (TLC) is the maximum amount of gas that the lungs can hold (Fig. 14-16). The normal amount is about 4000 to 7000 mL. The TLC is composed of four discrete lung volumes measured by spirometry: the inspiratory reserve volume (IRV), the tidal volume (V_T), the expiratory reserve volume (ERV), and the residual volume (RV). This relationship is expressed by the equation TLC = IRV + V_T + ERV + RV.

IRV is the amount of reserve or extra gas that can be inhaled at the end of a normal inspiration. Normal IRV may be as much as 3000 mL.

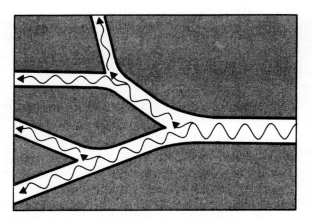

Figure 14-14. Transitional airflow.

V_T is the amount of gas that is exhaled or inhaled during normal breathing. Normal V_T is 5 to 10 mL/kg, or about 350 to 600 mL in a young adult.

ERV is the amount of gas that can be exhaled after a normal expiration. Normal ERV is about 1000 to 1500 mL.

RV is the amount of gas that always remains in the lungs and cannot be exhaled.

There are four lung capacities, which represent the combination of two or more lung volumes. The values listed for lung capacities are averages and will differ according to body size, weight, and age.

Vital capacity (VC) is the amount of gas that can be forcefully exhaled after a maximum inspiration (VC = V_T + IRV + ERV). Normal is about 4000 to 5000 mL.

The inspiratory capacity (IC) is the amount of gas that can be inhaled after a normal exhalation (IC = V_T + IRV). Normal is about 3500 mL.

The functional residual capacity (FRC) is the amount of air in the lungs after normal expiration (FRC = ERV + RV). Normal is about 2000 to 3000 mL.

These respiratory volumes and capacities can be used to establish a baseline and monitor the effectiveness of treatment modalities. Vital capacity, inspiratory force, and tidal volume are the most frequently measured parameters of respiratory muscle function.

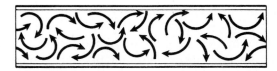

Figure 14-13. Turbulent airflow.

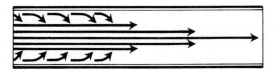

Figure 14-15. Laminar airflow.

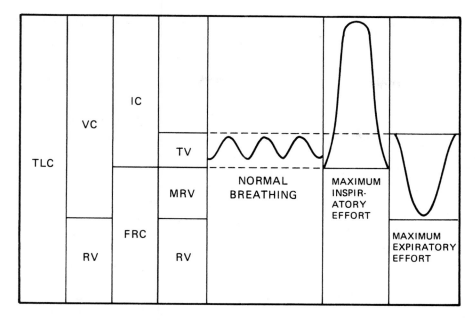

Figure 14-16. Lung volumes and capacities.

Dead Space

Dead space (VD) is the amount of inhaled gas that does not take part in gas exchange. Gas exchange occurs only in the terminal bronchioles and alveoli. There are two types of dead space, anatomic and physiologic. Physiologic dead space is the total amount of dead space in the lung. Anatomic dead space is estimated to be 150 mL or 1 mL/lb of ideal body weight (25% to 35% of VT). For a 500-mL tidal volume, approximately 350 mL reaches the alveoli.

The amount of inhaled air that reaches the alveoli and takes part in gas exchange is alveolar ventilation (VA). In a stable state, the arterial carbon dioxide is inversely related to alveolar ventilation and indicates adequacy of gas exchange. VA is equal to VE (minute ventilation) minus VD. VE is normally 5 to 10 L/min and is measured by multiplying VT × respiratory rate.

Phase II: Gas Diffusion

On inspiration, oxygen concentration or pressure is greater in the alveoli than in the erythrocytes, and the carbon dioxide concentration is greater in the erythrocytes than the alveoli. Therefore, the gas diffuses from the highest level of concentration toward the lower level of concentration.

The actual area of space the gases have to cross to diffuse is very thin; 0.2 to 0.5 μm. The alveoli and capillaries are so small and thin that, under the microscope, they look like a single sheet of blood. Instead, they are made up of six layers: the alveolus, alveolar membrane, interstitial space, capillary membrane, plasma, and erythrocyte membrane. The gases must diffuse through these layers, known as the respiratory membrane, for gas exchange to take place. If the membrane becomes thickened, as in pulmonary edema or interstitial pulmonary fibrosis, the diffusion of gases is slowed. Another factor affecting diffusion through the respiratory membrane is the available surface area. If an area of the lung is filled with fluid or pus, its presence will cause gas diffusion to be slowed or stopped completely. In emphysema, the alveolar septa collapse, destroying the alveolar structure and decreasing the surface area available for diffusion.

The specific composition of the alveolar, arterial, and venous compartments will directly affect the diffusibility of gases (Table 14-2).

TABLE 14-2. COMPOSITION OF PULMONARY GASES

Alveolar	Arterial	Venous	Atmospheric
$PH_2O = 47$	$PH_2O = 47$	$PH_2O = 47$	$PH_2O = 47$
$PACO_2 = 40$	$PaCO_2 = 40$	$PvCO_2 = 46$	$PICO_2 = 0$
$PAO_2 = 100-110$	$PaO_2 = 92$	$PvO_2 = 40$	$PIO_2 = 150$
$PAN_2 = 563$	$PaN_2 = 563$	$PvN_2 = 563$	$PIN_2 = 563$
			760 mm Hg

A, alveolar; a, arterial; CO_2, carbon dioxide; H_2O, water; I, inspired; N_2, nitrogen; O_2, oxygen; P, pressure or partial pressure; V, venous.

OXYGEN TRANSPORT

Once oxygen has penetrated the erythrocyte membrane, it is carried through the systemic circulatory system to all body tissues. Oxygen is transported in only two possible forms in the body, either dissolved in plasma or combined with hemoglobin. The amount of oxygen dissolved in the plasma is very small and amounts to 0.003 mL/100 mL of blood, or 3% of the total body oxygen. PaO_2 measures dissolved oxygen. The remaining 97% of oxygen is transported through the system's circulation in combination with hemoglobin (Hgb); this combination is called oxyhemoglobin. A gram of hemoglobin combines with approximately 1.34 mL of oxygen. The transport of oxygen to body tissues is influenced most by cardiac output, hemoglobin concentration, and oxygen-hemoglobin binding and releasing factors.

Cardiac output is usually 4 to 8 L/min. As the cardiac output varies, the quantity of blood oxygenated in the lungs also varies. In normal, healthy lungs, a slight decrease in cardiac output will not greatly alter oxygen content. A markedly decreased cardiac output will alter oxygen content, although the available blood will be maximally oxygenated. If hemoglobin is low, cardiac output will increase to help compensate and maintain an adequate oxygen content. The amount of oxygen transported per minute is determined by the cardiac output, even though there are other contributing factors.

Oxygen content (CaO_2) is the maximum potential amount of oxygen the blood can carry. It is expressed as milliliters of oxygen per 100 mL of blood. $CaO_2 \times Hgb \times 1.34$ (cubic centimeters of oxygen) $\times SaO_2 + (PO_2 \times 0.0031)$. In calculating the oxygen content, the dissolved oxygen in plasma (PaO_2) is usually not included because of its small contribution. Oxygen content is equal to the actual amount of oxygen in both the plasma and the erythrocytes.

Oxygen saturation (SaO_2) is the ratio comparing the actual amount of oxygen that could be carried with the amount actually carried, which is expressed as a percentage.

Oxygen Capacity

Hemoglobin has a natural affinity for oxygen. Once the oxygen diffuses through the erythrocyte membrane, it readily attaches to the hemoglobin molecule. With a hemoglobin level of 15 g/100 mL, 100 mL of blood will have enough hemoglobin to carry 20 mL of oxygen. Hemoglobin cannot be oversaturated; 100% is the maximum under human physiologic conditions.

Oxygen Transport

Oxygen transport/oxygen delivery (DO_2) is the amount of oxygen delivered to the cells expressed as milliliters of oxygen per minute. Oxygen transport (DO_2) = $CaO_2 \times$ cardiac output $\times$ 10, expressed in milliliters per minute. Normal oxygen transport is between 600 and 1000 mL/min, or 10 to 12 mL/kg.

The combination of oxygen content and oxygen transport is a more reliable index of oxygenation than the PaO_2 alone because the hemoglobin level and cardiac output are taken into consideration.

Oxygen Consumption

Oxygen consumption (VO_2) is the amount of oxygen used per minute. Normal VO_2 is approximately 3.5 mL/kg/min. A 70-kg person would use approximately 245 mL/min of oxygen at rest. Under normal circumstances, only 25% to 30% of the transported oxygen is used by the cells. If oxygen transport is 1000 mL/min and VO_2 is 250 mL/min, 25% of the oxygen transported is used. The oxygen extraction rate is the difference between the oxygen transported and the oxygen consumed. As the oxygen extraction rate increases, cellular oxygenation is threatened. Rates over 40% require assessment of oxygen transport and consumption components.

Oxyhemoglobin Dissociation

Factors affecting oxygen-hemoglobin binding and releasing include temperature, pH, PCO_2, acidosis or alkalosis, and 2,3-diphosphoglycerate (2,3-DPG). The oxyhemoglobin curve is an S-shaped curve representing the nonlinear relationship of the PaO_2 and the SaO_2 (Fig. 14-17).

The amount of oxygen dissolved in the plasma, the PaO_2, provides the driving pressure that forces oxygen to combine with hemoglobin. The driving pressure of dissolved oxygen exists until the alveolar (PAO_2) and arterial (PaO_2) pressures are almost equal. With the oxygen pressure gradient between the alveolus and the erythrocyte at equilibrium, the point of the normal curve is at the upper right. In the healthy person, the oxygen tension is 95 to 97 mm Hg with a hemoglobin saturation (SaO_2) of about 97%.

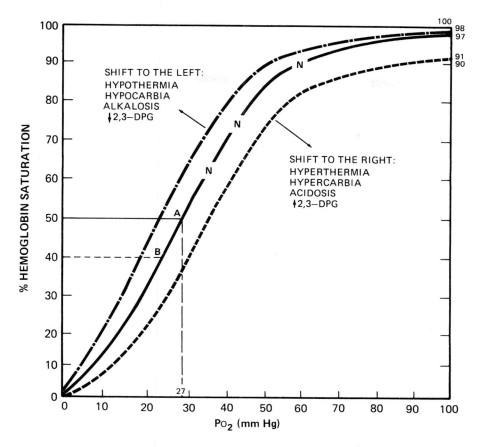

Figure 14-17. Oxyhemoglobin dissociation curve. (A) Hemoglobin 50% saturated with oxygen; (B), hemoglobin binds tightly with oxygen, preventing its release to the tissues, leading to hypoxia. N, normal curve.

There is a steep downslope portion to the curve, indicating a move from the lungs into the systemic circulation. The SaO_2 and the PaO_2 are dropping because the hemoglobin is readily giving up oxygen to the tissue capillaries. As the hemoglobin moves through the body, the PaO_2 drops and hemoglobin loses its affinity for oxygen, readily releasing it into the tissues. When SaO_2 drops to 50%, the P_{50}, the hemoglobin begins to give up to its oxygen much less readily. At the P_{50}, the partial pressure of arterial oxygen is about 27 mm Hg. The normal curve can be shifted to the right or to the left by many factors. A shift in either direction indicates a change from the normal SaO_2 and PaO_2 relationship.

A shift to the right occurs in acidosis, hypercarbia (increased carbon dioxide), and fever. A shift to the right means that there is less oxygen in the blood. It also means that oxygen is more readily given up to the tissues by the hemoglobin, preventing hypoxia. If shift persists, eventually the decreased oxygen content will not prevent tissue hypoxia.

A shift to the left occurs in alkalosis, hypocarbia, and hypothermia. In a shift to the left, hemoglobin binds oxygen much more tightly and releases less oxygen to the tissues. The arterial oxygen tension and hemoglobin saturation are only very slightly changed from the normal curve.

2,3-DPG is an important organic phosphate that will shift the normal curve to the right and left. It is a phosphate-type enzyme that is present in erythrocytes. An increase of 2,3-DPG in the hemoglobin of erythrocytes shifts the curve to the right and facilitates release of oxygen in the tissues. A decrease of 2,3-DPG in the hemoglobin of erythrocytes shifts the curve to the left and hinders the release of oxygen into the tissues.

Causes of Hypoxemia

Normal pulmonary anatomy accounts for the 2% to 5% of the blood flowing through the lungs that does not come in contact with inspired air for gas exchange. Anatomic shunt occurs when there is

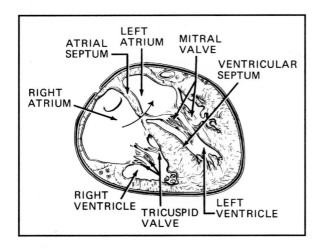

Figure 14-18. Anatomic shunt.

Decreased alveolar ventilation (VA) results in rising P_{ACO_2}, causing the displacement of oxygen and lowering of P_{aO_2}. Hypoventilation-induced hypoxemia is easily treated with oxygen therapy; however, the decreased VA must be improved or respiratory failure will occur.

Intrapulmonary, or physiologic, shunt is that portion of the pulmonary blood flow not exposed to functioning alveoli (Fig. 14-19). It provides a measure of efficiency of gas exchange in the lungs. Accumulated secretions, atelectasis, pulmonary edema, neoplasms, and foreign objects are only a few of many causes of obstruction.

Intrapulmonary shunts are also referred to as low ventilation/perfusion (V/Q) ratios. When alveolar ventilation is reduced without a subsequent reduction in perfusion, venous blood is not completely oxygenated. Normal venous oxygen levels are low (P_{vO_2} 35 to 45 mm Hg and S_{vO_2} 0.60 to 0.75), and more poorly oxygenated blood becomes mixed with oxygenated blood, resulting in hypoxemia (P_{aO_2} <60 mm Hg). Intrapulmonary shunt is measured by shunt equations or estimated from oxygen tension indices, such as the P_{aO_2}/F_{IO_2} ratio or a/A ratio. Normal P_{aO_2}/F_{IO_2} ratio is >286. The lower it becomes, the worse the intrapulmonary shunt. The hypoxemia of patients with intrapulmonary shunt will not respond dramatically to oxygen therapy, since the shunted blood will not come in contact with the increased alveolar P_{O_2}. Carbon dioxide elimination will usually not be affected and may

adequate ventilation to the alveoli but perfusion is absent or markedly decreased and blood does not have the chance to participate in gas exchange (Fig. 14-18). This can be due to an anatomic aberration of the circulatory system of the lungs, such as an anomaly in the pulmonary vasculature, which channels unoxygenated blood into the left atrium through the thebesian, pleural, and bronchial veins. The danger of this is that a low P_{aO_2} (<60 mm Hg) can produce pulmonary hypertension, increased breathing, and low S_{aO_2} levels.

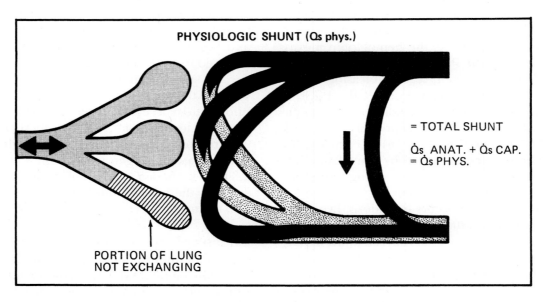

Figure 14-19. Physiologic shunt.

actually be low due to any increase in minute ventilation. Generally, if the PaO_2/FIO_2 ratio is below 200, the patient will not be able to maintain adequate oxygen levels in their blood without some form of supplemental oxygen therapy.

CARBON DIOXIDE TRANSPORT

Carbon dioxide is a by-product of metabolism. It is effectively eliminated only through respiration and is reflected in changes in $PaCO_2$ values. Carbon dioxide is transported in the blood in five different states: (1) dissolved in plasma, (2) as bicarbonate ion, (3) as carbonic acid, (4) in combination with hemoglobin, and (5) in an extremely small amount as the carbonate ion.

Much like oxygen, only a very small amount of carbon dioxide is transported in the dissolved state, making up about 7% of the total carbon dioxide. The presence of carbon dioxide in a dissolved state creates a pressure gradient or driving force measured as carbon dioxide tension, or $PaCO_2$. The pressure gradient of the dissolved carbon dioxide at the tissue level continues until the blood reaches the pulmonary capillaries. Since no carbon dioxide is normally inhaled, the pressure gradient is almost completely one-sided, pushing carbon dioxide from the capillary into the alveoli.

The dissolved carbon dioxide in the blood reacts with water to form carbonic acid. The amount of carbon dioxide that diffuses into the erythrocyte comes into contact with carbonic anhydrase, an enzyme and a strong catalyst, enabling dissolved carbon dioxide to convert to carbonic acid rapidly. About 70% of the body's carbon dioxide waste is handled by the lungs through exhalation. As soon as carbonic acid is formed, it is immediately broken down into hydrogen and bicarbonate ions through the process of dissociation. The hydrogen ions combine with hemoglobin, the bicarbonate ions diffuse into the plasma, and chloride ions diffuse into the erythrocytes to maintain homeostasis. Movement of the bicarbonate ion results in a chloride shift, allowing chloride to move into the erythrocytes. Since this is the body's most important way of transporting carbon dioxide, it is important to review the four steps of the chemical reactions.

1. Carbon dioxide enters the erythrocyte and does the following:
   a. Combines with hemoglobin

$$CO_2 + Hgb \rightarrow HgbCO_2$$

   b. Combines with water

$$CO_2 + H_2O$$
carbon dioxide + water
$$CA \leftrightarrow H_2CO_3$$

2. The carbonic acid of step B dissociates.

$$H_2CO_3 \leftrightarrow HCO_3^- + H+$$
carbonic acid $\leftrightarrow$ bicarbonate ion
+ hydrogen ion

3. Bicarbonate ion leaves the erythrocyte and enters the plasma, allowing the chloride ion to enter the erythrocyte (the chloride shift).

4. The hydrogen ion from step C binds with hemoglobin.

$$H^+ + Hgb \leftrightarrow HHgb$$

VENTILATION PHYSIOLOGY

The acid-base state in our bodies is kept within a very narrow range. An acid state that is not corrected will eventually result in coma and then death. A base or alkalotic state that is not corrected will eventually result in convulsion, tetany, and eventually death.

An acid is a chemical substance that dissociates into positive or negative electrically charged ions and gives up a hydrogen (H^+) proton to the solution. The positive ion is a cation and the negative ion is an anion. A base is a substance that can and will accept a hydrogen proton while in solution. Water is the most common and abundant base in the body. The pH represents the hydrogen ion concentration and is an expression of the hydrogen ion concentration as a negative logarithm.

Two types of acids are formed in the body: volatile acids and nonvolatile (fixed) acids. These acids are formed by the metabolism of food and by anaerobic glycolysis.

Volatile acids are those that can form a gas; because of an open system, they can be eliminated in their gaseous form. All volatile acids can, therefore, be eliminated by the lungs. The main source of volatile acids is the body's metabolism of glucose and fat. Carbonic acid is the major volatile acid in the body. It is made by the combination of carbon dioxide and water: $CO_2 + H_2O \leftrightarrow H_2CO_3$. The double-direction arrow indicates that the reaction readily moves in either direction.

Acids that cannot be converted into their gaseous form for elimination are termed non-volatile, or fixed, acids. Nonvolatile acids are excreted mainly by the kidneys via the urine and in the stool. Nonvolatile acid sources are anaerobic glycolysis, amino acid metabolism, and phosphoprotein/phospholipid metabolism. The kidneys excrete these fixed acids, totaling about 50 mEq/day. Disease can also produce nonvolatile acids.

ACID-BASE BALANCE

When there is any disruption in the acid-base balance of the arterial blood toward acidosis, the body has three main defense mechanisms: buffering, increasing alveolar ventilation, and/or increasing hydrogen ion elimination as well as increasing bicarbonate reabsorption.

Buffering

Buffering is an immediate response to an acid-base disturbance that prevents changes in hydrogen ion concentration. Increasing alveolar ventilation begins in 1 to 2 min. As the hydrogen ion concentration builds up, the lungs attempt to reduce their amount by increasing ventilation. The kidneys provide the strongest defense against acid-base disturbances by increasing hydrogen ion elimination and increasing bicarbonate ion reabsorption. Unfortunately, it takes from several hours to several days for the kidneys to rebalance the hydrogen ion concentration.

There are three major buffering systems: (1) the bicarbonate buffer system, (2) the phosphate buffer system, and (3) the protein buffer system. The bicarbonate buffer system is the most important system because the end products of the chemical buffer are regulated by both the kidneys and the lungs. The chemical reaction in this system is reversible and occurs extremely rapidly:

$$H^+ + HCO_3^- \leftrightarrow H_2CO_33 \leftrightarrow CO_2 + H^+$$

If the buffering moves toward the left, the bicarbonate ion is the end product, regulated by the kidneys. If the buffering moves toward the right, the end product is carbon dioxide, regulated by the lungs. The pH can be shifted up or down by either or both the renal system and/or the respiratory system.

The phosphate buffer system is similar to the bicarbonate system in function and buffers best at a slightly different pH than bicarbonate, mainly in the tubular fluids of the kidney. This system buffers strong acids (e.g., hydrochloric acid) and strong bases (e.g., sodium hydroxide) into weak acids and bases that have little effect on the blood pH.

The protein buffer system is the most inexhaustible buffering system in the body. All the plasma proteins and intracellular proteins, such as hemoglobin, buffer, and the supply of protein is infinite. Proteins buffer carbon dioxide quickly, and it buffers bicarbonate ions over a period of several hours. The importance of this system is that it helps buffer the extracellular fluids through diffusion of carbon dioxide and bicarbonate ion.

Increasing Alveolar Ventilation

If the buffering system has not rectified an acid-base disturbance within minutes, the respiratory system will become active. Alveolar hyperventilation increases the rate of carbon dioxide excretion, compensating for a metabolic acidosis. Alveolar hypoventilation does the opposite, compensating for a metabolic alkalosis. As alveolar ventilation increases, the $PaCO_2$ decreases. The decreased $PaCO_2$ results in a respiratory-induced alkalosis, forcing the hydrogen to combine with HCO_3^-. If alveolar ventilation decreases, the $PaCO_2$ level increases, resulting in a respiratory acidosis as a result of the increased availability of hydrogen.

Increasing Hydrogen Ion Elimination/ Bicarbonate Reabsorption

The final mechanism the body can utilize to alter acid-base disturbances is increasing hydrogen ion elimination and bicarbonate ion reabsorption. This defense mechanism involves both the lungs and the kidneys. The kidney function of acid-base disturbances reacts within a few hours of the disturbance; however, it is a slow-acting defense mechanism and may take several days to rebalance the acids and bases. The kidneys are able to excrete some hydrogen ions in relation to the excretion of nonvolatile acids. This is a very small amount of hydrogen ion elimination since the lungs excrete most of the hydrogen ions. At the same time, the kidneys reabsorb bicarbonate ions in the proximal tubule to equal the excessive number of hydrogen ions. As this reabsorption proceeds, carbon dioxide and water are formed:

$$H^+ + HCO_3^- \leftrightarrow H_2CO_3^- \leftrightarrow CO_2 + H_2O$$

If this reabsorption is not adequate to restore acid-base balance, sodium and hydrogen ions will trade places to maintain electrical neutrality and the sodium bicarbonate return from the kidney tubules to the plasma. If this does not reestablish acid-base balance, the kidneys will conserve still more bicarbonate by substituting ammonium ions (NH_4) for bicarbonate ions. Assuming that the acid-base disturbance continues and all of the possible bicarbonate ions have been retained, hydrogen ions will reach the distal tubules and combine with phosphates. These phosphates will be excreted in the urine. Alterations in potassium and extracellular fluid volume are final efforts of the kidney to restore acid-base balance.

ACID-BASE DISTURBANCES

The pH expresses the driving pressure of acid-base balance. The pH is a negative logarithm of the blood's hydrogen ion concentration. The smaller the value of the pH, the greater the concentration of hydrogen ions and the more acidic the solution. Conversely, the larger the value of the pH, the smaller the concentration of hydrogen ions and the less acidic the solution. The normal range of pH for arterial blood is 7.35 to 7.45.

Acidosis is an acid-base disturbance with a predominant quantity of acid. Acidemia is a state of increased hydrogen ions reflected in an arterial blood pH below 7.35. Alkalosis is an acid-base disturbance in which acids are insufficient in quantity or base is in excess. Acid insufficiency is more commonly a cause than is base excess. Alkalemia is a state of decreased hydrogen ions reflected in an arterial blood pH above 7.45.

There are only two ways by which the pH may be returned toward the normal 7.40 in acid-base disturbances: compensation or correction. Compensation occurs when the body attempts to respond to the acid-base abnormality. If the primary disturbance is respiratory, the kidneys will respond to shift the pH toward normal. If the primary disturbance is metabolic, the respiratory system will attempt to compensate for the alteration.

In respiratory acidosis, the lungs are responsible for the altered state. The kidneys will try to compensate by excreting more acid in the urine and increasing reabsorption of the bicarbonate ion. These two concurrent actions will move the pH nearly back to the normal value of 7.40. In respiratory alkalosis, the kidneys will try to compensate by increasing the amount of bicarbonate excreted.

In metabolic acidosis, the respiratory system is stimulated to increase alveolar ventilation. The hyperventilation increases the excretion of carbon dioxide as an acid waste product of metabolic processes. This is an effective and rapid way to decrease $PaCO_2$. The respiratory system can compensate in metabolic acidosis in just a few hours. In metabolic alkalosis, the respiratory system will hypoventilate, retaining carbon dioxide and shifting the pH toward normal. The body cannot fully compensate for metabolic alkalosis. The hypoventilation necessary for compensation causes a decrease in the PaO_2. When the oxygen level becomes too low, the respiratory system will respond to the decreased oxygen by increasing ventilation. Although this compensatory effort is rapid, it is not a complete compensation. The most significant fact about compensation as a defense mechanism in acid-base disturbance is that the body never overcompensates and will return the pH to near-normal (7.40), but it never "overshoots the mark."

RESPIRATORY IMBALANCES

Respiratory Acidosis

The normal $PaCO_2$ is 35 to 45 mm Hg. If the $PaCO_2$ is elevated above 45 mm Hg and the pH decreased below 7.35, respiratory acidosis is present, indicating acute or chronic hypoventilation. Respiratory acidosis indicates inadequate alveolar ventilation.

Any clinical condition that depresses the respiratory center in the medulla oblongata may precipitate hypoventilation and result in respiratory acidosis. These conditions include head trauma, oversedation, and general anesthesia. More rarely, neoplasms in the medulla oblongata or nearby areas with increasing intracranial mass, size, and pressure may cause a respiratory acidosis. Neuromuscular diseases—including myasthenia gravis, Guillain-Barré syndrome, multiple sclerosis, amyotrophic lateral sclerosis, and trauma to the cervical spinal cord—may cause hypoventilation and resultant respiratory acidosis. Inappropriate mechanical ventilation may cause respiratory acidosis. Too low a respiratory rate or tidal volume and too much dead space in the tubing may result in respiratory acidosis. Obstructive lung diseases may result in a degree of V/Q disturbance, increasing the risk for developing both acute and chronic carbon dioxide retention.

Respiratory acidosis can best be treated by improving ventilation. This includes nursing measures such as protecting the airway through positioning or the use of artificial airways. The key to treatment is to find the cause of the respiratory depression and correct it. A respiratory acidosis requires active treatment only if the increase in $PaCO_2$

results in a pH of about 7.25. The more alert the patient, the longer intubation and mechanical ventilation can be delayed. For the patient on mechanical ventilation, the respiratory rate is increased to decrease the $PaCO_2$ and maintain effective ventilation, or the tidal volume may be increased.

Respiratory Alkalosis

When the $PaCO_2$ is decreased below 35 mm Hg and the pH is increased above 7.45, respiratory alkalosis is present, indicating hyperventilation. Restrictive lung diseases are common pathologic causes of respiratory alkalosis. Other causes of respiratory alkalosis include anxiety, nervousness, agitation, hyperventilation via mechanical ventilation, and excessive Ambu bagging during a cardiopulmonary arrest.

A respiratory alkalosis is treated by finding the cause of the excessive breathing, such as anxiety, pain, fear, hypoxemic compensation for a metabolic acidosis, or central nervous system disturbance. Correcting the causative problem will correct the respiratory alkalosis. If the patient is on mechanical ventilation, decreasing the respiratory rate, decreasing the tidal volume, or adding additional tubing (dead space) may correct the imbalance. If the pH is greater than 7.55, more aggressive measures—such as administration of acetazolamide (Diamox), ammonium chloride, hydrochloric acid, or potassium chloride (KCl)—are used.

METABOLIC DISTURBANCES

Base Excess

The bicarbonate ion (HCO_3^-) and base excess are the parameters of the arterial blood gases used to identify nonrespiratory imbalances. Base excess is an easy guide to use in distinguishing metabolic acidosis from alkalosis. Base excess is the amount of base above the normal level after adjusting the level for hemoglobin. The normal midpoint value is zero. If the base excess is above +2, there is an excess of metabolic base in the body fluids and a metabolic alkalosis exists. If the base excess is below −2, there is not enough metabolic base in the body fluids and a metabolic acidosis exists.

Metabolic Alkalosis

Metabolic alkalosis is a condition with an excess base. The three most common causes are diuretic therapy, excessive vomiting, and excessive ingestion of alkaline drugs. Any condition that increases metabolic processes beyond the ability of the body to eliminate or neutralize the waste products results in an increase in bicarbonate ions. These conditions cause a loss of hydrogen ions (diuretics), chloride ions (vomiting), and potassium ions (hyperaldosteronism) through the kidneys. The effect is increased bicarbonate ion reabsorption in the kidneys, which forces excretion of the hydrogen, chloride, and potassium ions in the urine. Loss of gastric secretions from vomiting or through nasogastric suctioning results in metabolic alkalosis. Excessive ingestion of alkaline drugs, such as antacids and soda bicarbonate, may lead to metabolic alkalosis. Less commonly, treatment with corticosteroids, hyperaldosteronism, and Cushing's syndrome may result in a metabolic alkalosis.

A metabolic alkalosis is corrected by finding and treating the underlying cause. Most cases of metabolic alkalosis are due to electrolyte disturbances, such as hypokalemia (low potassium) or hyperchloremia (high chloride). In severe disturbances where the pH is greater than 7.60, hydrochloric acid or ammonium chloride may be administered.

Metabolic Acidosis

Metabolic acidosis occurs in the body when there is an increase in endogenous acid production (lactic acid, ketoacids), loss of bicarbonate (diarrhea, vomiting), or accumulation of endogenous acids (renal failure).

Metabolic acidoses are classified in two major groups: those with an increase in unmeasurable anions and those with no increase in unmeasurable anions. To calculate unmeasurable anions, add the serum chloride and the bicarbonate ion values and then subtract this sum from the serum sodium level. If the difference is greater than 15 mEq/L, there is an increase in unmeasurable anions known as the anion gap. No real anion gap exists since positive (cations) and negative (anions) ions must always be present in equal numbers. However, it appears as if the anion gap were present, since only the major ions (sodium, chloride, and bicarbonate) are measured.

Common causes of metabolic acidosis with an increase in unmeasurable anions (anion gap) include (the specific anion is in parentheses) diabetes mellitus (ketone bodies), uremia (phosphates and sulfates), lactic acidosis (lactate), aspirin poisoning (salicylate), methyl poisoning (formic acid), ethylene glycol poisoning (oxalic acid and formic acid), and paraldehyde poisoning.

There are several common causes of metabolic acidosis with no increase in unmeasurable anions (nonanion gap). Diarrhea is probably the most common cause. Large amounts of bicarbonate ion are in the intestines and are washed out in the diarrhea. The more severe the diarrhea, the greater the likelihood of metabolic acidosis. A general guide for the possible development of metabolic acidosis with no increase in unmeasurable anion is the presence below the umbilicus of a drainage tube (except a Foley catheter), such as that for drainage of the pancreas, or an ureterosigmoidostomy and other drainage tubes.

Another cause is uremia. In severe renal failure, the kidneys cannot excrete the acids normally formed daily by the body. As the acids build-up, uremia develops, resulting in an increase in unmeasurable anions.

Metabolic acidosis is the most difficult acid-base disturbance to correct. The high hydrogen ion concentration stimulates the body to attempt compensation by increasing both the depth and the rate of respiration (Kussmaul's breathing). Compensation is not usually enough by itself. The electrolytes are often quite abnormal and complicate the correction of the acid-base disturbance. A metabolic acidosis is treated by correcting the cause of the acidosis. Correction of the underlying cause will reverse the metabolic acidosis. Treatment with an alkali should be reserved for severe metabolic acidosis; pH less than 7.20. There is controversy over the benefit of using sodium bicarbonate ($NaHCO_3$) in a metabolic acidosis caused by the accumulation of a metabolized organic acid anion. Sodium bicarbonate may be ordered in a dose of 1 mEq/kg. If given judiciously, bicarbonate will begin to return the pH to normal while the underlying cause of the imbalance is identified and treated.

If tissue hypoxia is present, the lactate (normally <2 mmol) may increase. Lactate values greater than 4, when associated with a decreased pH, are warning signs of tissue hypoxia.

Diagnosis and Treatment of Pulmonary Disorders

EDITORS' NOTE

The PCCN exam will include questions that are related to ventilatory and oxygenation failure. You will be expected to perform a comprehensive pulmonary assessment and recognize changes related to therapy or decompensation. The PCCN exam will have questions related to interpretation of arterial blood gases (ABGs) and pulmonary medications. This chapter will familiarize you with the diagnostic techniques used to recognize these disorders and the pharmacologic interventions used to treat them.

INVASIVE AND NONINVASIVE DIAGNOSTIC STUDIES

Diagnostic studies used in identifying respiratory alterations include physical assessment, arterial blood gases, pulmonary function tests, and chest radiography.

Physical Assessment

Assessment of the respiratory system includes inspection, palpation, percussion, and auscultation of the lungs.

Inspection

Inspect the patient for respiratory pattern, chest symmetry, clubbing of the fingers, and color.

Five basic terms are used to describe breathing patterns: *eupnea, tachypnea, hyperpnea, bradypnea,* and *apnea.*

- Eupnea: regular rhythm and a respiratory rate of 12 to 20 breaths per minute (Fig. 15-1)
- Tachypnea: increased respiratory rate, above 24 breaths per minute, with normal depth of respiration
- Hyperpnea: increased depth of respiration at a normal respiratory rate
- Bradypnea: decreased respiratory rate, less than 10 breaths per minute, with normal depth of respiration
- Apnea: the absence of breathing (Fig. 15-2)

The four common patterns of respiration seen in critical care are (1) *central neurogenic hyperventilation* (Fig. 15-3)—regular, deep, rapid respirations without periods of apnea; (2) *Cheyne-Stokes respiration* (Fig. 15-4)—a pattern in which respirations start from apnea, reach a maximum in depth and rate, and then fade back to apnea; (3) *Kussmaul's breathing* (Fig. 15-5)—a tachypneic pattern of labored, deep breaths; and (4) *Biot's respirations* (Fig. 15-6)—regular, fast, shallow breaths with irregular, abrupt periods of apnea.

Central neurogenic hyperventilation is caused by neurogenic dysfunction. Cheyne-Stokes respirations are caused by alterations in acid-base status, an underlying metabolic problem, or neurocerebral insult. Kussmaul's breathing is associated with metabolic acidosis and renal failure. Biot's respiration is caused by central nervous system disorders; however, this pattern may be found in some healthy patients.

Pneumotaxic breathing occurs when the pneumotaxic center takes over control of ventilation. The pattern is irregular, deep, shallow breathing with random periods of apnea of varying lengths (Fig. 15-7).

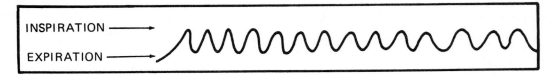

Figure 15-1. Spirometry pattern of normal ventilation.

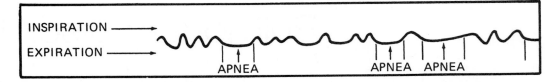

Figure 15-2. Spirometry pattern of apneustic breathing.

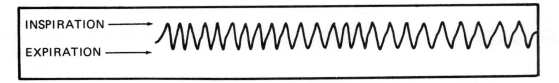

Figure 15-3. Spirometry pattern of central neurogenic hyperventilation.

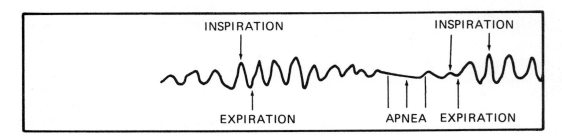

Figure 15-4. Spirometry pattern of Cheyne-Stokes breathing.

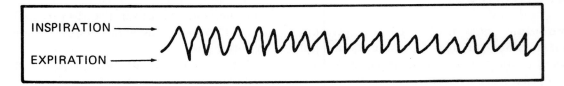

Figure 15-5. Spirometry pattern of Kussmaul's breathing.

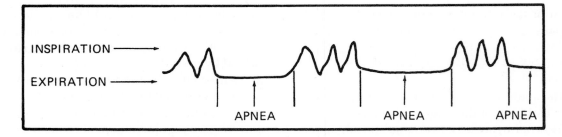

Figure 15-6. Spirometry pattern of Biot's (cluster) breathing.

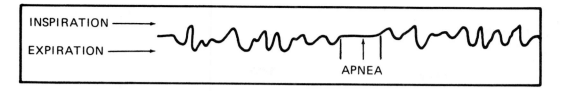

Figure 15-7. Spirometry pattern of pneumotaxic (ataxic) breathing.

Inspect the patient's color for signs of cyanosis. Peripheral cyanosis has little clinical value and often is the result of peripheral vasoconstriction. When you assess oxygenation from the physical examination, look at the mucosa of the oral cavity and mouth for signs of central cyanosis.

In diagnosing pneumothorax, it is important to inspect for chest wall symmetry and other processes that cause decreased or absent chest wall movement. Watch the patient breathe to determine whether the accessory muscles of ventilation—the scalene, trapezius, and sternocleidomastoid muscles—are being used. Their use suggests an increase in the work of breathing, which is often seen in patients with chronic obstructive pulmonary disease (COPD).

Clubbing of the digits indicates chronic oxygen deficit. The distal phalanges of the fingers become widened. This is most often seen in patients with cystic fibrosis, pulmonary hypertension, and end-stage COPD.

Palpation

Palpation of the chest wall can help further assess findings suggested by inspection. It is used to assess thoracic expansion, tactile and vocal fremitus, and subcutaneous emphysema.

Subcutaneous emphysema is assessed by the familiar crunching or popping that occurs on palpation. It is seen when a communication exists between the pleural space and subcutaneous tissue. By itself it is not dangerous and does not require treatment.

Percussion

Percussion is the assessment of the lung by striking or tapping on the thorax. It can help to identify areas of consolidation, hyperresonance, and diaphragmatic excursion. A flat or dull sound over the lung indicates that an air-filled space has been replaced with fluid or tissue.

Auscultation

Lung sounds are frequently described in general terms describing the quality of sound heard over each anatomic region. Tracheal and bronchial sounds reflect the airflow in the major airways. Bronchovesicular and vesicular sounds reflect the progression of airflow in more distal airways. The presence of bronchial sounds in the periphery or any place other than the bronchial area may reflect an abnormality. Any abnormal sound is referred to as an adventitious sound.

Crackles is the term used to describe the sounds heard during the reopening of airways secondary to changes in forces surrounding the airways. The airways collapse primarily on expiration and their sounds can be heard throughout the lungs. Crackles can have pulmonary or cardiac origins. Differentiation of pulmonary crackles from those of cardiovascular origin is based on the fact that cardiac crackles are position-dependent.

Wheezes are due to either partial or complete airway obstruction. They can be high or low pitched. The presence of a wheeze is assessed by identifying the location of the loudest wheeze and listening to the airflow distal to this point. The presence of airflow distal to the location of the loudest wheeze indicates airflow past the obstruction. If a wheeze disappears, the obstruction is either lessening or worsening. If airflow is more easily heard as the wheeze diminishes, the lung is improving. If airflow diminishes, the patient is worsening.

Lung sounds can be diminished by the presence of fluid or air between the lung and the stethoscope. For example, a pneumothorax or pleural effusion will diminish the intensity of lung sounds. On the other hand, consolidation of fluid in the lung itself will accentuate sound transmission. A pneumonia, for example, may accentuate the sound heard in the location of the pneumonia. A bronchial sound would be heard instead of the expected vesicular sound. Loss of airflow, as with bronchoconstriction or obstruction, differs from consolidation in that reduction in airflow generally diminishes breath sounds. For example, atelectasis or airway obstruction will reduce the intensity of breath sounds. It is up to the clinician to identify whether the source of the loss of breath sound is intrapulmonary (atelectasis, mucous plugs) or extrapulmonary (pneumothorax).

Interpreting Arterial Blood Gas Values

Basic acid-base disturbances can be identified by following a step-by-step procedure of analyzing arterial blood gas (ABG) values. The important values used to interpret ABGs are shown in Table 15-1.

When the pH and the arterial carbon dioxide pressure ($PaCO_2$) move in opposite directions, the primary cause of acid-base disturbance is respiratory. If the pH and the $PaCO_2$ move in the same direction, the primary cause is metabolic.

Step 1: Look at the pH to identify the presence of acidosis or alkalosis.

- If it is 7.35 to 7.45, the pH is normal.
- If the pH is less than 7.35, an acidosis exists.
- If the pH is greater than 7.45, an alkalosis exists.

Step 2: Look at the $PaCO_2$ to determine the primary disturbance.

- If the $PaCO_2$ is between 35 and 45, a normal level exists. If the value is below 35, a respiratory alkalosis exists. If the value is above 45, a respiratory acidosis exists.
- If the $PaCO_2$ moves in the same direction as the pH, the primary cause is metabolic.

Example 1:

$$pH = 7.25$$
$$PaCO_2 = 26$$

Since the $PaCO_2$ and pH moved in the same direction, the primary problem is a metabolic one. The pH is acidotic, therefore, a metabolic acidosis exists. A respiratory alkalosis exists as well, as evidenced by

the low $PaCO_2$. The respiratory alkalosis is an attempt to compensate for the metabolic acidosis but is unable to correct the acidosis.

Example 2:

$$pH = 7.24$$
$$PaCO_2 = 59$$

Since the $PaCO_2$ and pH moved in opposite directions, the primary problem is respiratory. As the $PaCO_2$ is elevated and the pH is depressed, a pure respiratory acidosis exists.

Step 3: Look at the bicarbonate ion (HCO_3^-) value.

- If it is 22 to 26, consider it normal.
- If it is less than 22, a metabolic acidosis exists.
- If it is greater than 26, a metabolic alkalosis exists.

Example 3:

$$pH = 7.25$$
$$PaCO_2 = 26$$
$$HCO_3^- = 17$$

A metabolic acidosis exists because the pH and $PaCO_2$ moved in the same direction. The low HCO_3^- level confirms a metabolic acidosis.

	Example 1	Example 2	Example 3
pH	7.19	7.35	7.52
$PaCO_2$	30	62	25
HCO_3^-	14	40	25

Practice ABG Interpretation

Example 1. Since the $PaCO_2$ and pH moved in the same direction, the primary problem is metabolic. The pH and HCO_3^- confirm a metabolic acidosis. The low $PaCO_2$, a respiratory alkalosis, is an attempt to correct for the metabolic acidosis. Since the pH is very low, this situation requires intervention to correct the metabolic acidosis.

Example 2. The $PaCO_2$ is elevated, indicating a respiratory acidosis, but the pH is normal. The only way this could occur would be if a compensation had occurred to offset the acidosis. The high HCO_3^- confirms that a metabolic alkalosis exists. The interpretation is respiratory acidosis compensated by a metabolic alkalosis. Since the pH is normal, no acute danger exists in this patient.

TABLE 15-1. NORMAL ARTERIAL BLOOD GAS VALUES AT SEA LEVEL

	Range	Midpoint	Mixed Venous
pH	7.35–7.45	7.40	7.36–7.41
PO_2	80–100 mm Hg	93	35–40 mm Hg
PCO_2	35–45 mm Hg	40	41–51 mm Hg
HCO_3^-	22–26 mEq/L	24	22–26 mEq/L
SaO_2	95%–100%	97%	70%–75%
Base excess	+2	0	+2

Example 3. Since the $PaCO_2$ and pH moved in opposite directions, the primary problem is respiratory. Because of the low $PaCO_2$ and high pH, a respiratory alkalosis exists. No compensation has occurred, as evidenced by the normal HCO_3^- level. In this case, a pure respiratory alkalosis exists.

The body's ability to compensate will not take the pH beyond midpoint. The direction the pH takes from midpoint can provide the clinician with a clue as to the primary problem. Intervention from clinicians can result in overcompensation.

The combination of an acidosis and an alkalosis is tolerated better by the body than two acidoses or alkaloses, as they tend to block compensation for each other, resulting in a severe acid-base and electrolyte disturbance.

Pulmonary Function Tests

Pulmonary function tests are used to evaluate the volumes and flow rate of the respiratory system with spirometry (Fig. 15-8).

Measurement of the flow of exhaled gas and the exhalation time helps distinguish between restrictive and obstructive lung diseases (Table 15-2). Forced vital capacity (FVC) measures the volume of air that the patient can forcibly exhale (i.e., his or her vital capacity) and suggests the maximum volume of air available for airway clearance.

FEV_1 is the forced expiratory volume in 1 s. The patient inhales as much as possible, holds his or her

TABLE 15-2. DIFFERENTIATING OBSTRUCTIVE FROM RESTRICTIVE DISEASE

Parameter	Obstructive	Restrictive
Vital capacity	Normal or ↓	↓
Functional residual capacity	↑	↓
Total lung capacity	↑	↓
Residual volume	↑	↓
FEV_1	↓	Normal or ↓

breath briefly, and then exhales as forcibly and quickly as possible. A decrease in the FEV_1 indicates obstruction to airflow.

Chest Radiography

The chest radiograph is used to evaluate the structures of the chest, the relationships between structures, and the presence of air and fluid in the thorax. It may be one of the early procedures performed when evaluating pulmonary symptoms. The thoracic cage is made up of 12 ribs, 7 attached (which are inserted in the sternum at a 45-degree angle) and 5 "floating" (not attached to the sternum). The trachea is at the midline and tubular. The cardiac silhouette appears anteriorly as a white solid structure in the left mediastinum. The width of the normal heart is less than half that of the thorax.

Review of the chest film begins with the bony structures. Look for the presence of the ribs and

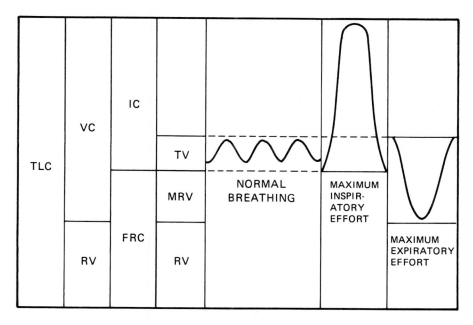

Figure 15-8. Lung volumes and capacities.

observe any notching or calcifications. Rib notching involves the third through the ninth ribs and is seldom seen in all the ribs of an individual patient. Rib notching has a number of causes, with the most common being coarctation of the aorta.

Determine that the major organs of the thorax are present and check their relationship to each other. Examine the cardiac silhouette for size and placement in the chest. The lungs are examined for expansion and any increased densities, such as those caused by fluid or masses.

Review the position of the hemidiaphragm. It is a rounded silhouette at the base of the thorax. The right side is slightly higher than the left. Flattening of the diaphragm is seen with chronic air trapping, COPD, and asthma. Proper placement of an artificial airway may be confirmed with a chest radiograph.

PULMONARY PHARMACOLOGY

Medications used in managing pulmonary disease include bronchodilators, orticosteroids, and anticholinergics.

Bronchodilators

Bronchodilators are divided into classes: methylxanthines and sympathomimetics.

Methylxanthines
Theophylline (anhydrous) is an example of a methylxanthine. It is usually given orally and metabolized in the liver; it has a half-life of 3 to 6 h. Its primary effect is bronchodilatation of the airways, although it also stabilizes mast cells and increases mucociliary clearance. The therapeutic range is 10 to 15 mcg/mL. Intravenous use is rare and reserved for the most extreme cases that are not responding to traditional therapy.

Side effects of theophylline include tachycardia, tremor, nervousness, palpitations, dizziness, sweating, dysrhythmias, increased blood pressure, irritability, vomiting, nausea, headache, and restlessness. Toxicity can be minimized by keeping the dose low. Clinicians need to be familiar with drug interactions and other factors that inhibit metabolism and/or decrease elimination of theophylline.

Overdose of theophylline is critical, as there is no antidote. Early indicators of theophylline overdose include central nervous system changes, headache, confusion, gastrointestinal upset, palpitations, tachycardia, and tachypnea.

Sympathomimetics
Sympathomimetic bronchodilators belong to the class of adrenergic receptor agonists that stimulate alpha, beta$_1$, and beta$_2$ receptors, controlling smooth muscle activity, cardiac muscles and glands, and metabolic processes. The lungs contain beta$_2$ receptors. Stimulation results in relaxation of bronchial smooth muscle, decreased mucus secretion, increased mucociliary clearance, and stabilization of the mast cell. Other beta$_2$ effects include dilatation of the major blood vessels, decreased blood pressure, and increased blood glucose levels.

Current therapy for acute bronchodilation is the use of short-acting selective beta$_2$ agonists such as albuterol, levalbuterol, terbutaline, and pirbuterol. Sympathomimetics are preferentially administered via metered-dose inhalers (MDIs) or by nebulized inhalation. Parenteral and oral administration should generally be avoided.

Long-term management of pulmonary disorders such as COPD and asthma is conducted through the use of long-acting beta agonists such as salmeterol or formoterol. Because these agents have a less rapid onset of action than the short-acting agents, their use in acute bronchodilation is limited. Recently, a nebulized form of arformoterol was approved; its role in controlling COPD is less well-defined.

Side effects of beta$_2$ agonists are dose-dependent, are higher for oral preparations than inhaled ones, and include stimulation of heart rate, contractility, and automaticity. They should be used with caution in patients with a history of tachycardia, dysrhythmias, ischemic heart disease, or uncontrolled hyperthyroidism. Tachycardia can be precipitated by vasodilation and a fall in blood pressure. Patients with diabetes may have increased hyperglycemia. Pregnant women in the third trimester may have delayed or prolonged labor with the use of beta$_2$ agonists. Central nervous system side effects include anxiety, irritability, insomnia, and fine tremor.

Overdose of sympathomimetics can result in excessive cardiac stimulation. Carefully administered beta blockers can be used to counteract the overdose; however, be prepared for the resulting beta blockade in the lung.

Epinephrine, isoproterenol, and ephedrine all have beta-adrenergic action. Epinephrine is the drug of choice for anaphylaxis because of its bronchodilating and cardiovascular effects. Subcutaneous epinephrine may be used to treat acute bronchospasm but should be reserved for patients who are refractory to inhaled sympathomimetics and steroids.

Corticosteroids

Corticosteroids are used to reduce inflammation and edema in the airway, stabilize mast cells, and restore bronchodilator response to sympathomimetics. Steroids can be given orally, parenterally, or nasally. Parenteral steroids, such as hydrocortisone, are used to treat severe bronchoconstriction. If prolonged therapy is needed, oral steroids such as prednisone may be used. Both parenteral and oral steroids have a systemic effect and can cause many side effects. These include edema, weight gain, hypernatremia, hypokalemia, hypertension, redistribution of body fat, osteoporosis, muscle weakness, and increased risk of peptic ulcer disease.

Dosage for hydrocortisone is 20 to 240 mg/day depending on the severity of the presenting symptoms. Prednisone dosage is 5 to 60 mg/day. The tapering of prolonged systemic steroids is done gradually to avoid withdrawal symptoms from adrenal insufficiency. Even 2 weeks of full-dose therapy can suppress the synthesis and release of cortisol into the bloodstream. Care must be taken when transitioning from systemic to inhaled corticosteroids.

Inhaled steroids provide the same reduction of inflammation and edema of the lung without the major systemic effects. They are supplied in MDIs or capsules for inhalation (budesonide respules). The most common ones include fluticasone, beclomethasone dipropionate, flunisolide, and triamcinolone acetonide. Inhaled steroids are used in conjunction with bronchodilator therapy. The effect of inhaled steroids takes weeks to achieve; therefore, they are not used to treat acute bronchospasm and bronchoconstriction. Inhaled steroids may reduce the need for oral maintenance of corticosteroids except in the most severe cases. Inhaled corticosteroids are usually graded based on low, medium, or high doses. Initial and maintenance doses are chosen based on underlying disease severity for either asthma or COPD.

The major side effect of inhaled steroids is topical infection with oral *Candida albicans* (thrush). Instructing the patient to rinse his or her mouth with water and expectorate after using the inhaler will prevent candidal development. Longer term studies among patients with COPD indicate an increased incidence of pneumonia among patients using inhaled corticosteroids. Other adverse events experienced with systemic corticosteroids are either absent or experienced less frequently with long-term use of inhaled agents.

Mast Cell Stabilizers

Cromolyn and nedocromil sodium are inhaled drugs used to stabilize the mast cells. They have no direct bronchodilator effect and are not used in acute situations. The drugs prevent the mast cells from releasing histamine and other mediators that lead to bronchoconstriction, edema, and inflammation of the airways. The availability of more effective agents has limited the use of both of these agents.

Anticholinergics

Anticholinergic drugs block the stimulation of cholinergic receptors by acetylcholine. Acetylcholine is a powerful bronchoconstrictor, stimulator of mucus production, and mast cell activator. The quicker acting ipratropium and the more sustained agent tiotropium are inhaled anticholinergics used as first-line therapy in chronic bronchitis and emphysema. These agents are used frequently in the treatment of COPD. Although these drugs have less cardiac-stimulating effects than beta agonists, ipratropium has been linked to some troubling increases in mortality among COPD-treated patients. Combination therapy, beta agonist and anticholinergic, may be beneficial in some patients. Recently, the use of tiotropium has been linked to improvement in quality of life, improved lung function, and fewer hospitalizations for exacerbations among patients with varying degrees of COPD.

ADJUNCTIVE RESPIRATORY MONITORING

Adjunctive respiratory monitoring includes pulse oximetry, venous oximetry, and capnography (Table 15-3).

Oximetry

Pulse Oximetry

Pulse oximetry (SpO_2 is oxygen saturation as measured by pulse oximetry) is a commonly used and excellent indicator of arterial oxygen saturation (SaO_2) values. It can decrease the need to obtain ABGs; however, it is recommended that an ABG be obtained initially to verify the accuracy of the pulse oximeter and to determine $PaCO_2$ levels. Pulse oximetry is most useful in trending saturation levels during weaning from oxygen therapy or positive end-expiratory pressure/continuous positive airway pressure levels. Spot checks or one-time pulse oximetry readings have little value and are not recommended. Pulse oximetry can be used to evaluate patients for the necessity of home oxygen. Typically, patients will be

TABLE 15-3. NORMAL VALUES FOR PULSE OXIMETRY, VENOUS OXIMETRY, AND CAPNOGRAPHY

Parameter	Value	Significance
Pulse oximetry		
(SpO$_2$)	>93%	**Normal**
	<93%	**Hypoxemia**
Venous oximetry		
(SvO$_2$)	60%–80%	**Normal**
	>80%	**Decreased oxygen consumption**
		Malposition of catheter
	<60%	**Increased oxygen consumption or decreased oxygen delivery**
(ScvO$_2$)	70%–80%	**Normal**
Capnography	1–5 mm Hg	**Normal**
(PETCO$_2$)	<PaCO$_2$	
	>5 mm Hg	**Widened gradient (Va/Q mismatch or increased dead space ventilation) can be due to pulmonary emboli, lung disease, or loss of cardiac output**

evaluated for desaturations during activity or with overnight oximetry looking for desaturations.

Oximetry measures functional, not fractional, SaO$_2$. Therefore, the pulse oximetry reading is expected to be 2% to 4% higher than SaO$_2$ measured by an ABG sample in the laboratory. Pulse oximetry must be used with caution when elevated values of abnormal hemoglobins are present. For example, the SpO$_2$ functional measurement will mistake carboxyhemoglobin for oxyhemoglobin and will display a value that reflects the total of the two versus just the oxyhemoglobin.

Complications associated with the use of pulse oximetry are skin breakdown at the probe site and inaccurate readings due to venous stasis, low blood pressure (below 90 mm Hg systolic), and low perfusion states. Forehead oximetry can be used in low perfusion states when traditional pulse oximetry is not able to pick up a reliable signal. Other potential sources of error with pulse oximetry may be excessive movement, dark (blue or black) nail polish, artificial nails, and ambient light effect on a loose-fitting probe.

Venous Oximetry

Mixed venous oximetry utilizes blood from the pulmonary artery to estimate overall oxygenation. The balance between oxygen transport and consumption is estimated by levels of mixed venous oxygen saturation (SvO$_2$). As long as blood flow to the capillaries is relatively normal, SvO$_2$ levels provide relatively accurate reflections of cellular oxygenation. Normal SvO$_2$ values, between 0.60 and 0.80, indicate an adequate balance between oxygen delivery and consumption. If the SvO$_2$ falls less than 0.60, either oxygen transport has decreased or oxygen consumption has increased indicating a risk for lack of oxygen at the tissue level. While limitations exist with SvO$_2$ use, it remains one of the more valuable tools in the assessment of global tissue oxygenation. The continuous SvO$_2$ levels will be higher, about 2%, than laboratory measured values, because it measures only oxyhemoglobin and reduced hemoglobin.

Complications associated with continuous SvO$_2$ monitoring include inadequate calibration of the monitor, infection from long-term catheter insertion, damage to the fiberoptics in the catheter, and possible malposition of the catheter.

True SvO$_2$ values can be obtained only from the pulmonary artery. Venous saturations obtained from large vessels near the right heart, core venous oxygen saturation (ScvO$_2$), can provide a similar assessment of global tissue oxygenation. A normal ScvO$_2$ is 0.70 to 0.80. Intermittent laboratory samples may be drawn from the distal lumen of a central venous cathether placed in or near the right atrium. Some catheters have continuous ScvO$_2$ capablilty.

Capnography

Arterial carbon dioxide levels are the key to determining the adequacy of alveolar ventilation. Capnography is a noninvasive method of assessing exhaled carbon dioxide. The peak exhaled carbon dioxide value, end-tidal carbon dioxide level (PETCO$_2$), is a close approximation of arterial carbon dioxide values (PaCO$_2$). It is usually slightly lower than arterial values (PaCO$_2$) by 1 to 5 mm Hg and can be used to approximate PaCO$_2$.

When an increase in physiologic dead space exists, the PETCO$_2$ may not equal the PaCO$_2$. The clinician can monitor the PaCO$_2$–PETCO$_2$ gradient as an indicator of the severity of the pulmonary dead space; the greater the gradient, the greater the dead space. Trends in the gradient are useful to the clinician in following changes in dead space. Some of the common clinical conditions that increase dead space are pulmonary embolism, low cardiac output states, and COPD. In patients with COPD, the gradient may rise to 10 to 20 mm Hg or higher as a result of the ventilation/perfusion mismatch.

A capnogram is a display of the PETCO$_2$ values or a recorded waveform of carbon dioxide concentration. Fast-speed capnograms are used for breath-to-breath analysis, while slow-speed capnograms are used for trending over time (Fig. 15-9).

Capnography has many valuable uses. It is excellent at detecting tracheal intubations since it will

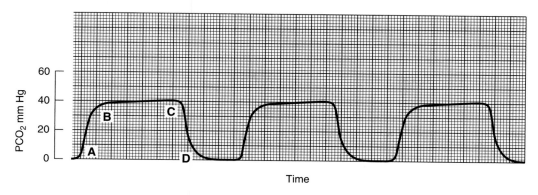

Figure 15-9. The normal capnogram. **(A)** Carbon dioxide concentration is zero, consists of gas from anatomic dead space. **(B)** Alveolar plateau; minimal rise in carbon dioxide near end of exhalation. **(C)** End-tidal carbon dioxide level (PETCO$_2$). **(D)** Inspiration, rapid fall in carbon dioxide.

reflect a CO$_2$ waveform. Capnography is a standard for intubation and ongoing monitoring of an artificial airway with mechanical ventilation. If an artificial airway becomes dislodged from the airway, the capnogram will reflect a loss of CO$_2$ waveform. Often the capnography alarm will alert the clinician before the ventilator alarm sounds. Capnography is also useful in assessing the effectiveness of cardiopulmonary resuscitation. Circulation is required to bring CO$_2$ from the cells to the lungs to be exhaled. When an arrest situation occurs, circulation will cease and the capnography waveform will reflect zero or a very low value. As circulation is reestablished, the capnogram and PETCO$_2$ values will increase, reflecting the return of circulation. During an arrest, lack of rise in capnography is indicative of a poor outcome since effective circulation has not been restored. Capnography—mainstream or real-time measurement—can be used to help identify end-exhalation on hemodynamic waveforms.

16

Alternative Methods of Ventilatory Support

EDITORS' NOTE

The PCCN exam will include questions related to ventilatory and oxygenation failure. This chapter reviews the treatment of these conditions. It is important to understand the concepts of mechanical ventilation, positive end-expiratory pressure/continuous positive airway pressure, noninvasive ventilation, and oxygen therapy.

OXYGEN THERAPY

Oxygen therapy is used to support oxygen transport while the underlying cause of oxygenation failure is being treated. There are two methods of delivering oxygen therapy, low- and high-flow systems (Table 16-1).

Low-Flow Oxygen Systems

Low-flow systems do not meet all inspiratory volume needs, requiring patients to entrain room air. The advantage of a low-flow oxygen system is its ease of use. In a low-flow oxygen system, the fraction of inspired oxygen level (FIO_2) fluctuates with varying depths of inspiration. A shallow breath has a higher FIO_2 than a deep one, even though the liter flow is the same, because less room air is entrained during inspiration. Low-flow systems provide FIO_2 levels between 24% and 44% with a nasal cannula or between 40% and 60% with a simple face mask (Table 16-2). Rebreathing masks can provide higher

levels of inspired oxygen; however, they are not as reliable as high-flow systems.

Low-flow oxygen systems are useful in the less acutely ill or mouth-breathing patient. The oral inspiration of air draws nasal gases simultaneously into the lungs, allowing for effective oxygen therapy.

High-Flow Oxygen Systems

High-flow oxygen systems meet all inspiratory volume and flow requirements independent of inspiratory changes. High-flow systems are more difficult to apply, requiring face masks or ventilator circuits. High-flow oxygen systems provide stable FIO_2 levels, with oxygen concentrations 24% to 100% (Table 16-3). Critically ill patients with oxygenation disturbances will almost always require high-flow oxygen systems. Oxygen therapy should not be removed until a stable SpO_2 or PaO_2/FIO_2 >286 is present.

Complications

As long as oxygen therapy generates an arterial oxygen pressure (PaO_2) level >60 mm Hg or an arterial oxygen saturation (SaO_2) level >0.90, no further increases in oxygen therapy should be instituted. Oxygen therapy is not without risk. An oxygen concentration in excess of 50% for more than 24 h increases the potential for the development of oxygen toxicity and lung damage. Alveolar type II cells, responsible for producing surfactant, are impaired by high oxygen levels.

One of the factors promoting alveolar expansion is the presence of nitrogen, the most plentiful gas, making up approximately 79% of the barometric

TABLE 16-1. LOW- AND HIGH-FLOW OXYGEN THERAPY

Low-Flow
Nasal cannula
Simple face masks
Rebreather masks
Nonrebreather masks

High-Flow
Venturi masks
Nebulizer-regulated FIO_2 systems
Ventilator circuits

TABLE 16-3. OXYGEN DELIVERY WITH THE VENTURI MASK SYSTEM

FIO_2 Desired	Liter Flow Required (L/min)	Air Entrainment Ratio	Liter Flow Delivered (L/min)
0.24	4	1:25	104
0.28	4	1:20	44
0.31	6	1:7	48
0.35	8	1:5	48
0.40	8	1:3	32
0.50	12	1:1.7	32

pressure. When 100% oxygen therapy is employed, nitrogen is completely displaced or washed out by the oxygen, resulting in a PaO_2 of 400 to 600 mm Hg. If perfusion exceeds ventilation, all oxygen can be absorbed from the alveoli, resulting in atelectasis.

Continuous Positive Airway Pressure

Continuous positive airway pressure (CPAP) is positive airway pressure above atmospheric levels applied throughout the respiratory cycle for spontaneous breaths. Continuous positive airway pressure stabilizes the airways during the expiratory phase. The PaO_2 values can be increased if the functional residual capacity (FRC) can be increased and the time for gas exchange to occur is increased. Continuous positive airway pressure increases FRC, improves distribution of ventilation, helps hold alveoli open, and opens smaller airways, improving oxygenation. It may help prevent microatelectasis and promote alveolar stability. Continuous positive airway pressure is most commonly used to treat obstructive sleep apnea, cardiogenic pulmonary edema, and obesity hypoventilation syndrome.

TABLE 16-2. APPROXIMATE FIO_2 WITH NASAL CANNULA AND FACE MASK

	Liter Flow (L/min)	Approximate FIO_2%
Nasal cannula	1	24
	2	28
	3	32
	4	36
	5	40
	6	44
Face mask	5–6	40
	6–7	50
	7–8	60

Positive End-Expiratory Pressure

Positive end-expiratory pressure (PEEP) is the application of a positive airway pressure at end-exhalation while the patient is on mechanical ventilation. It improves oxygenation by the same mechanisms as CPAP. Positive end-expiratory pressure is effective in raising PaO_2 and SaO_2 levels by maintaining alveolar airflow during expiration. Airways have a tendency to collapse during expiration as a result of increasing pressures outside the airway (Fig. 16-1).

Some clinicians believe in physiologic PEEP, a concept assuming that some PEEP is present in all people because of resistance of the airways. Low levels of PEEP, such as 3 to 5 cm H_2O, may be ordered even in patients without oxygenation problems so as to simulate physiologic PEEP.

PEEP is indicated to help reduce FIO_2 levels or to elevate PaO_2/SaO_2 values when high FIO_2 levels are unsuccessful, to drive lung water back into the vascular system, or to reduce mediastinal bleeding postoperatively.

Optimal PEEP levels are achieved by the lowest level of PEEP needed to raise the PaO_2/SaO_2 levels and do not result in cardiovascular compromise, such as decreased cardiac output, impeded right-heart filling, or tachycardia. The optimal PEEP level varies from patient to patient, although levels of PEEP higher than 20 cm H_2O are uncommon. Values between 5 and 15 cm H_2O are common in support of the patient with oxygenation problems.

Auto-PEEP

Auto-PEEP, also known as intrinsic PEEP, is the trapping of air in the alveoli, producing PEEP as the result of early airway closure or insufficient exhalation time. Patients at risk for the development of auto-PEEP include those with chronic obstructive pulmonary disease (COPD) or asthma or patients with increased minute ventilation (V_E) of 20 L/min

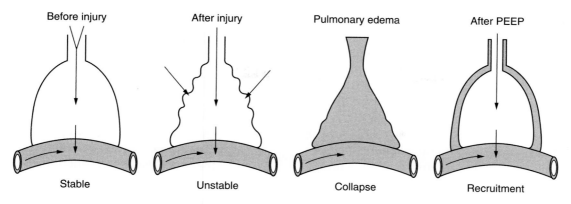

Figure 16-1. Effects of PEEP on airway stabilization, demonstrating recruitment of the alveoli.

or more; auto-PEEP may also develop with fast respiratory rates, including overly aggressive Ambu bagging. It can be measured by obstructing the exhalation port of a ventilator immediately prior to an inspiratory effort. Some mechanical ventilators will provide this assessment without manual occlusion of the exhalation port (Fig. 16-2).

Complications of auto-PEEP include increased work of breathing; barotrauma; hemodynamic compromise, such as decreased cardiac output and decreased venous return to the right heart; misinterpretation of filling pressure (PAOP/LAP [pulmonary artery occlusion pressure/left atrial pressure] or CVP/RAP [central venous pressure/ right atrial pressure]) readings; increased intracranial pressure; decreased renal function; passive hepatic congestion; and increased intrapulmonary shunt.

Complications of PEEP and CPAP

PEEP and CPAP have potential side effects related to the increased airway pressures. When PEEP or CPAP

is applied, the cardiac output must be carefully monitored. Cardiac output and stroke volume can fall as a result of the increased intrathoracic pressure, which impedes venous blood return to the right heart, producing a pseudohypovolemia. If cardiac outputs are not available, the heart rate and systolic blood pressure are monitored. Increases in the heart rate and falls in systolic blood pressure may signal a reduction in cardiac output and stroke volume.

Barotrauma and pneumothorax are also complications of PEEP and CPAP. Lung sounds should be monitored and the thorax percussed for potential development of pneumothorax. Sustained peak airway pressures greater than 40 cm H_2O increase the risk of barotrauma.

ARTIFICIAL AIRWAYS

In order to use a ventilator, the patient must have an artificial airway, such as an endotracheal or a tracheostomy tube.

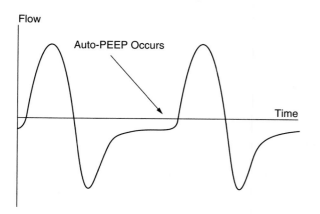

Figure 16-2. Airway flow showing incomplete exhalation and the presence of auto-PEEP.

Endotracheal Tubes

Endotracheal tubes may be inserted nasally or orally. Intubation should be attempted only by trained and experienced clinicians. Immediately after intubation, placement of the endotracheal tube in the airway can be confirmed by the presence of CO_2 through the use of capnography. All chest fields are auscultated to make sure that there are bilateral breath sounds. Physical examination should never substitute for CO_2 detection. Chest radiography is important to ensure whether the tip of the endotracheal tube is about 1 in.

(2 to 3 cm) above the carina. Reassessment of endo-tracheal tube placement is mandatory. Endotracheal tube position can change with coughing, patient movement, and suctioning. Continuous monitoring with end-tidal CO_2 can detect a loss of airway early. Daily chest radiography can help assess the tip position of the endotracheal tube.

Nasotracheal intubation is contraindicated in patients with increased intracranial pressure (ICP), head trauma, or chronic sinusitis. Disadvantages include the possibility of tissue necrosis, nosebleed, rupture of nasal polyps, and submucosal dissection. Increased mucus production as a result of the irritant properties of the tube increases the patient's susceptibility to infection, and stabilization of the tube is difficult if the patient is diaphoretic.

The advantages of orotracheal intubation are direct visualization and rapid intubation. Oral endotracheal tubes are repositioned to the opposite side of the mouth at least every 24 h to prevent necrosis of the lips. Disadvantages of oral intubation include increased dryness of oral mucosa, production of mucus, gagging, and susceptibility to infection.

Complications associated with intubation include laryngeal trauma, intubation of the right mainstem bronchus, and infection.

Tracheostomy

Tracheostomy, the formation of an opening into the trachea, may be performed if long-term ventilatory support is expected or in an emergency if a patient is unable to be endotracheally intubated. Tracheostomies bypass upper airway obstruction, decrease dead space, may help prevent aspiration, and may decrease the possibilities of necrosis and/or tracheoesophageal fistula formation. A sterile tracheostomy tube of the size used in the patient must be at the patient's bedside for emergency replacement. An endotracheal tube of the same or smaller size is also acceptable for maintaining the airway in an emergency. Care must be taken when replacing a displaced tracheostomy tube since tubes can be placed into false tracks and may not actually be in the airway. Tube placement should be confirmed with capnography.

Tracheostomy care consists of assessing the stoma for erythema, skin integrity, skin erosion, and purulent or bloody drainage. The stoma should be kept clean and dry. Avoid using cleansers that would be abrasive to the skin, such as hydrogen peroxide. Wound cleanser or a mild soap and water work best. If drainage is present, the use of a drain sponge will help absorb moisture and should be changed regularly.

The tracheostomy will be held in place with a special holder or surgical ties. Assess the neck for skin breakdown and change holder/ties if soiled. If a tracheostomy has a disposable inner cannula, it should be changed regularly to ensure patency. A resuable inner cannula should be removed and cleaned to keep the tracheostomy patent.

Patients who have long-term tracheostomies may become frustrated with the inability to vocalize. Vocalization may be accomplished through deflating the cuff of the trach, use of specialized "talking" trachs that allow air to pass by the vocal chords, or with one-way valves which allow the patient to inhale through the tracheostomy but exhale via normal anatomy.

Suctioning

Maintaining patency of the airway can be facilitated through suctioning. Suctioning can be accomplished with a closed-system multiple-use catheter or the traditional single-use catheter.

Hyperoxygenation of the patient prior to suctioning reduces hypoxemia associated with suctioning. Patients who benefit from hyperoxygenation include those receiving an FIO_2 of 0.40 or higher, those who have demonstrated decreased SaO_2 with suctioning, and those with cardiovascular compromise such as bradycardia or premature ventricular contractions (PVCs).

Suction pressures of less than 200 are generally adequate to remove secretions. The removal of viscous, thick secretions is difficult even with adequate suction. The lack of benefit of instillation of saline in the endotracheal or tracheostomy tube has been well documented, and such a maneuver increases the risk of ventilator-associated pneumonia (VAP). Thinning of pulmonary secretions is accomplished by adequate fluid intake. The stimulation of cough is a very effective aid to the clearance of secretions.

Cuff Management

Most endotracheal tubes and tracheostomy tubes for initiation of mechanical ventilation have inflatable cuffs. The cuff provides a closed system with a seal and reduces aspiration of fluids into the lungs. Soft, low-pressure cuffs are preferred because they minimize tracheal necrosis and fistula development. Pressure is distributed over a large area, and only sufficient pressure to provide a seal is necessary. High-volume, low-pressure cuffs negate the need to deflate the cuff for a specified period of time each hour. Cuffs can be inflated with a variety of materials, with the most common being air. Foam cuffs are usually self-inflating and require manual deflation on a scheduled basis. Sterile water may be used to inflate specific cuffs. It is important for the clinician to be familiar with the specifics of the cuff that is on the artificial airway being used.

Policies vary from hospital to hospital regarding the measurement of cuff pressures. Generally, a minimal occlusive pressure is maintained at 25 cm H_2O or less, or 20 mm Hg, to prevent tracheal damage. If more pressure is required, the patient may need to have a larger tube inserted. Cuff pressure can be checked by using a blood pressure manometer, syringe and stopcock, or pressure manometer specifically designed for measuring cuff pressures. This may be a shared responsibility with the respiratory care practitioner.

Deflation of the cuff is not recommended while mechanical ventilation is in place. During the weaning process, the patient may have periods of time off ventilation when the tracheostomy tube can be deflated. Before deflating the cuff, the patient should be suctioned carefully, especially orotracheally, to remove any secretions that may have accumulated on the top of the cuff. The patient must be monitored carefully for potential aspiration.

Complications

The major complication of a cuffed tube is obstruction from dried secretions (airway plugging). The increased production of mucus stimulated by the foreign body puts the patient at increased risk for airway plugging. The maintenance of adequate hydration and suctioning will help reduce the risk of plugging. Biofilm development on the artificial airway can lead to narrowing of the tube lumen. Additional potential complications include laryngeal edema, muscosal erosion, development of granulomas, vocal chord paralysis, and tracheal stenosis.

Endotracheal tubes can become displaced easily, leading to loss of airway, carinal rupture, unilateral lung ventilation, tension pneumothorax, and atelectasis. Signs of tube misplacement include loss of the end-tidal CO_2 waveform, diminished or absent lung sounds, loss of tidal volume, low pressure alarm on the ventilator, little, if any, chest excursion on the contralateral side, expiratory wheezing, and sometimes uncontrollable coughing. Tension pneumothorax may occur in the lung that has become intubated; this is one of the most serious complications of ventilatory support. The only treatment is insertion of a chest tube to relieve the pressure and remove air. Without adequate treatment, tension pneumothorax can be rapidly fatal.

If a tracheostomy tube's position fluctuates with the patient's pulse, it is possible that the tube is rubbing against the innominate artery; in such a case, the physician is notified immediately. Erosion of the artery usually results in exsanguination and death. A tracheostomy tube may become misplaced, causing subcutaneous and/or mediastinal emphysema or pneumothorax. Progressively deteriorating blood gases, loss of capnography waveform, poor air movement, and/or difficulty in suctioning should alert the clinician to a possible shift in the tracheostomy tube.

Tracheal dilatation, ischemia, and necrosis may occur because tracheostomy tubes and endotracheal tubes are round, whereas the trachea is oval. If ischemia and necrosis progress, a tracheoesophageal (TE) fistula may occur. This may be minimized by the use of low-pressure cuffs.

The longer an endotracheal tube or tracheostomy tube is in place, the greater the danger of infection. Frequent oral hygiene, including manual plaque removal with teeth brushing, use of chlorhexidine oral rinse, and tube care will make the patient more comfortable and help to reduce the risk of infection. Keeping the head of bed elevated higher than 30 degrees can help prevent aspiration and decrease the risk of ventilator-associated pneumonia.

The PCCN exam with have questions regarding ventilation through a tracheostomy. Most of these patients will have basic ventilatory modes. Focus on the understanding of the principles of mechanical ventilation and assessment so you can recognize changes that require intervention.

MECHANICAL VENTILATION

Mechanical ventilation is indicated for one of three reasons: to improve or support alveolar ventilation, to reduce the work of breathing, or to aid in supporting oxygenation. Improvement of alveolar ventilation (VA) is most obviously needed when $PaCO_2$ levels are increasing along with a falling pH. Reducing the work of breathing may be necessary when respiratory rates are in excess of 30 breaths per minute (Table 16-4). All modes of mechanical ventilation are designed to support one of these three functions. Mechanical ventilation should be considered early in the disease process in order to prevent the emergent need.

TABLE 16-4. SIGNS OF FAILURE OF SPONTANEOUS BREATHING

Respiratory rate	>35 breaths per minute
Tidal volume (V_T)	<2 mL/kg
Minute ventilation (V_E)	<5 or >12 L/min
$PaCO_2$	Increasing by more than 10 mm Hg from baseline
End tidal CO_2	Rising trend
pH	<7.30 with a rising $PaCO_2$
Blood pressure	Increase in systolic of 20 mm Hg
Heart rate	Increase of >20 beats per minute over resting heart rate

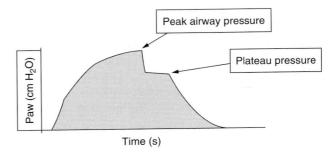

Figure 16-3. Peak and plateau airway pressure curves.

Mechanical ventilation is delivered by either negative or positive pressure. Negative-pressure ventilators include the iron lung or thoracic cuirass, which are usually not used in acute respiratory failure. Positive-pressure ventilators force air into the lungs, reversing normal breathing pressures and applying alveolar ventilation support.

The reversal of the normal negative inspiratory pressure to a positive pressure has a direct effect on the cardiovascular system. The increased intrathoracic pressure impedes venous return to the right heart, thus reducing stroke volume and cardiac output. The initial response may be a reflex increase in the heart rate to maintain output.

A complication of positive-pressure ventilation is pulmonary barotrauma/volutrauma. The peak airway pressure (PAP) on the ventilator should be monitored to assess excessive airway pressures. The PAP reflects the pressure required to deliver the tidal volume (V_T). It takes into account the resistance of the ventilator circuit, airway resistance, and compliance of the lungs. High PAPs can be monitored through dynamic compliance by dividing the PAP into the V_T. Normal dynamic compliance is 40 to 55 cm/mL. Values lower than 30 cm/mL place the patient at increased risk for barotrauma/volutrauma. Plateau pressures are more reflective of alveolar pressure. Plateau pressures are measured at the end of inspiration and require a brief inspiratory hold or pause to be assessed. Plateau pressures higher than 30 mm Hg place the patient at risk of barotrauma/volutrauma (Fig. 16-3).

Modes of Mechanical Ventilation

Ventilator breaths can be delivered by several modes and are subdivided into categories that determine the method by which the breath is terminated: volume, pressure, or time. Some of the newer modes will blend these functions. Respiratory rate and V_T are manipulated to achieve specific endpoints such as levels of oxygenation or V_E.

Volume-Limited Modes

The most common modes of mechanical ventilation are volume-limited modes. The ventilator breath will be delivered until the preset volume (V_T) is reached. The pressure required to deliver that breath will be variable. For safety, an upper pressure limit is set to prevent excessive pressures in the thoracic cavity. If the upper pressure limit is reached, the ventilator will cease delivering the breath. Continuous mandatory ventilation (CMV), assisted mandatory ventilation (AMV or assist/control), and synchronized intermittent mandatory ventilation (SIMV) are examples of volume-limited modes (Fig. 16-4). V_T on all modes is initially set at 6 to 8 mL/kg with a respiratory rate between 8 and 20 breaths per minute.

Continuous Mandatory Ventilation. This mode is used to support patients with little or no ventilatory drive or to gain control over excessive ventilatory drive. The ventilator delivers the preset V_T at the preset rate without sensitivity to patient inspiratory effort. The patient is unable to initiate breaths or to change the breathing pattern in any way. CMV is rarely used.

Assisted Mandatory Ventilation. This mode delivers constant preset V_T and a minimum number of breaths determined by the preset respiratory rate. The patient can initiate more breaths; however, they will be delivered at the preset V_T. The patient can alter the respiratory rate and pattern, not the V_T. The advantage of AMV is a reduction in the work of breathing. It can be used in weaning from mechanical ventilation by incorporating a spontaneous breathing trial (SBT) with T-piece or CPAP trials.

Synchronized Intermittent Mandatory Ventilation. This mode delivers a preset respiratory rate and V_T but allows the patient to breathe spontaneously between the preset V_T and rate. The ventilator

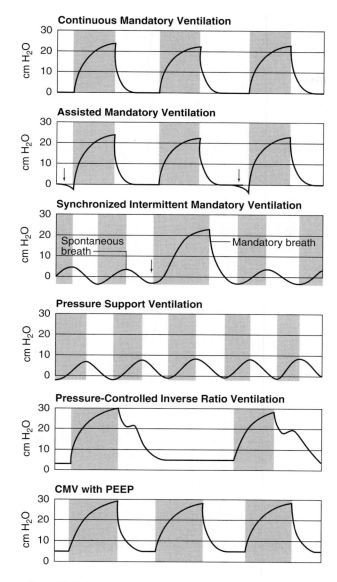

Figure 16-4. Pressure waveforms of differing modes of mechanical ventilation.

ventilation will augment the spontaneous breaths over the set ventilator rate and decrease the work of breathing. Weaning can be accomplished by a gradual decrease in the set rate, allowing the patient to assume more of the work of breathing. SIMV does not offer an advantage in weaning over SBT and may lead to respiratory muscle fatigue.

Pressure-Limited Modes

Pressure-limited modes of mechanical ventilation will deliver a breath until a preset pressure is reached. Pressure becomes constant but the VT achieved is variable. The VT obtained is dependent on the compliance of the lungs. The more compliant the lung, the larger the VT obtained, and the less compliant the lower the VT obtained. PSV and pressure-control ventilation (PCV) are the most common examples of this mode.

Pressure-Support Ventilation. In PSV, the ventilator delivers a preset positive pressure as the patient determines the inspiratory time, rate, and inspiratory flow rate. The patient is assisted during the inspiratory phase and must initiate a breath to receive the support. When inspiration ceases, the pressure support drops to ambient or PEEP. For safety, a back-up apnea mode can be set on the ventilator; then, in case the patient fails to initiate a breath, the ventilator will revert to the back-up mode after a predetermined time. The level of pressure support is set to achieve a VT of 6 to 8 mL/kg. Low levels of PSV, 3 to 6 cm H_2O, are valuable as an adjunct to overcoming endotracheal tube and ventilator circuit resistance. PSV can be used in weaning from mechanical ventilation by gradually decreasing its level. The combination of low levels of CPAP and PSV can be used for trials of spontaneous breathing. PSV can be added to spontaneous breaths in the SIMV mode.

Pressure-Control Ventilation. PCV can be used to limit excessive airway pressures. If excessive airway pressures are being obtained during volume-limited modes of mechanical ventilation, switching to PC may be an option. Pressures will be capped or controlled and not allowed to go higher than the combination of the preset drive pressure plus the set PEEP. The drive pressure is the pressure that delivers the breath. VT and VE will be variable so, must be closely monitored by the clinician. Lung compliance will affect the VT achieved. A respiratory rate can be set on PC.

is synchronized with the patient's ventilatory effort in an attempt to reduce competition between the ventilator and the patient.

There are many controversies about SIMV. It may increase the work of breathing at a low respiratory rate of 6 breaths per minute or less because the patient performs most of the work of breathing through the high-resistance ventilator circuit. High SIMV rates approximate AMV, as there is no time for the patient to initiate a spontaneous breath at his or her own VT. Many clinicians use a combination of SIMV and pressure-support ventilation (PSV). Pressure-support

Blended Modes of Ventilation

Blended modes or dual modes of mechanical ventilation use elements from both volume- and pressure-limited modes. The desire is to achieve the guaranteed VT and minimize the plateau pressure. Currently, there is no clinical evidence to suggest that one mode of mechanical ventilation is superior to another.

Volume Control Plus. In the volume control plus mode, breaths are pressure-controlled with a guaranteed minimum volume, based on feedback with patient ventilation to ventilator logic. This can occur within a breath or breath-to-breath adjustment. The ventilator delivers test breaths, then adjusts pressure and flow to deliver a minimum VT. Patients may experience less dysynchrony with this mode since the flow of gas is adjusted to meet their demand. This mode is named differently by various ventilator manufacturers such as pressure-regulated volume control (PRVC), volume-targeted pressure-controlled, or autoflow.

Airway Pressure Release Ventilation. Airway pressure release ventilation (APRV) cycles between a high continuous positive airway pressure (P high) and a low continuous positive airway pressure (P low). A high continuous positive airway pressure (P high) is delivered for a long duration (T high) and then falls to a lower pressure (P low) for a shorter duration (T low). The transition from P high to P low deflates the lungs and eliminates carbon dioxide. Conversely, the transition from P low to P high inflates the lungs. Alveolar recruitment is maximized by the high continuous positive airway pressure. The difference between P high and P low is the driving pressure which, along with the lung compliance, will determine the VT achieved. The time spent in T high and T low determines the rate or frequency of inflation and deflation. Spontaneous breathing can occur during the entire cycle of APRV. Further research is needed; however, APRV may decrease the PAP, improve alveolar recruitment, increase ventilation of the dependent lung zones, and improve oxygenation.

Noninvasive Ventilation

Noninvasive positive-pressure ventilation (NPPV) can be used to support a patient in hypercarbic or hypoxic respiratory failure. If successful, NPPV will allow the patient to avoid intubation and be supported until the acute event has been reversed. The earlier NPPV is applied, the greater its success. It can also offer a transition for patients who require support following weaning, allowing for earlier weaning from mechanical ventilation and avoiding reintubation. NPPV can be used for sleep-related breathing disorders and obesity hypoventilation syndrome. It is provided through a tight-fitting face mask or nasal mask. Patients who are not candidates for NPPV are those who have an immediate need for intubation, are hypotensive, are unable to clear secretions, or are unable to cooperate or tolerate the mask. NPPV is given with portable ventilators that provide pressure support. Standard mechanical ventilators can also be used to provide NPPV; however, the circuits and alarms make their use more difficult. The inspiratory (IPAP) and expiratory (EPAP) pressures are set to provide the necessary level of support for each patient's need. The respiratory rate and inspiratory time can also be adjusted according to the patient's need. Patients requiring support for hypercarbic respiratory failure will require a higher IPAP to ensure adequate VT and VE. Patients requiring support for hypoxemia will require higher EPAP levels. Initiation and titration of NPPV can be labor intensive, as a properly fitting mask must be ensured and the patient must be coached. Sleep studies will be required to find appropriate settings for patients with sleep-related disorders. Complications of NPPV include mask discomfort; skin breakdown; facial, oropharyngeal, and eye dryness; sinus congestion; gastric insufflation; and aspiration. Hemodynamic compromise of positive-pressure ventilation may also be seen with NPPV.

Complications of Ventilator Support

Hypotension may occur secondary to decreased cardiac output when a patient is put on a ventilator or when ventilator adjustments are increased. All positive-pressure ventilators exert a continuous positive pressure, which decreases venous return to the heart, thus decreasing cardiac output. This may result in a decreased urine output and cardiac dysrhythmias. Cardiac monitoring is essential. Hypotension may be caused by hypovolemia; and intravenous fluids may correct this problem. Vasopressors are indicated if preload is increased and the cardiac output is decreased.

Infection is among the most common complications of mechanical ventilation. The warm, moist environment of the ventilator equipment makes it an ideal place for organism growth. Strict adherence to sterile technique with good hand hygiene, changing ventilator circuits only when grossly soiled, keeping the head of bed elevated 30 degrees, aggressive oral hygiene, and weaning the patient as soon as possible are all important factors to decrease the risk of infection. As soon as a culture identifies an infecting organism and not colonization, specific antibiotic therapy is started. Aggressive pulmonary hygiene procedures are vital nursing interventions in preventing infection.

Atelectasis often occurs with mechanical ventilation. Bronchial hygiene is extremely important to prevent further complications once atelectasis has developed. Accidental disconnection from the ventilator may occur. Immediately reconnect it or use a manual resuscitator. Continuous monitoring of capnography will alert the clinician early when disconnection occurs.

Pneumothorax is not unusual when PEEP is used with mechanical ventilation. Treatment is insertion of a chest tube. Without adequate treatment, pneumothorax can be rapidly fatal.

Overventilation may occur, decreasing $PaCO_2$ more than desired. Reducing rate or V_T may be necessary to correct this problem.

WEANING FROM MECHANICAL VENTILATION

Weaning is the progressive removal of mechanical ventilatory support to spontaneous breathing. The first step in the weaning process is to determine whether the patient is ready for weaning. Assessment includes progress toward correction of the underlying reason for mechanical ventilation and respiratory mechanics; respiratory muscle endurance; and efficiency and work of breathing.

Lung-function tests used to assess readiness for weaning may include V_T, vital capacity, V_E, respiratory rate, negative inspiratory force (NIF) or peak inspiratory effort (PIP), the rapid-shallow-breathing index (respiratory frequency/V_T). The routine use of these indexes is limited as they will not have a positive prediction as to which patients will be successfully weaned. Low indices can indicate a negative prediction and identify which patients may not be ready to wean. The most useful of the indices is the rapid-shallow-breathing index. V_E is the amount of air exchanged in 1 min. Normal V_E is 5 to 10 L/min. NIF or PIP is the maximal inspiratory effort the patient can generate as measured by an inspiratory manometer. Normal PIP or NIF is −70 to −90 cm H_2O (Table 16-5). An NIF of at least −20 cm H_2O is the minimum for successful removal of ventilatory support. These assessments are limited by

TABLE 16-5. WEANING PARAMETERS

Muscle Efficiency	
Tidal volume (V_T)	2–5 mL/kg
Minute ventilation (V_E)	5–10 L/min
Vital capacity	>10 mL/kg
Respiratory rate	<30 breaths per minute
NIF/PIP	>−20 cm H_2O
Rapid shallow breathing index	>105 breaths per minute/L
Oxygenation	
PaO_2	>60 mm Hg on FIO_2 <0.40
Hemoglobin	>10 g/dL
Cardiac index	>2.5 L/min
Pao_2/FIO_2 ratio	>200
Carbon Dioxide Elimination	
$Paco_2$	35–45 mm Hg or at the patient's baseline level to maintain pH between 7.35 and 7.45
Dead space/tidal volume (V_D/V_T)	<60%

NIF, negative inspiratory force; PIP, peak inspiratory effort.

the effort the patient and therapist put into the assessment. It is important to correct as many of the patient's medical problems as possible before beginning the weaning process (Table 16-6).

There are a number of weaning techniques, including reduction of SIMV rates, reducing levels of PSV, alternating AMV with spontaneous breathing trials (SBT) via T-piece trials, or CPAP/PSV. Weaning through the SIMV circuit may increase the work of breathing, promote respiratory muscle fatigue, and increase oxygen consumption. This method is the least successful method of weaning. Spontaneous

TABLE 16-6. CONSIDERATIONS PRIOR TO INITIATING WEANING

Acid-base abnormalities
Airway secretion management
Cardiac abnormalities
   Arrhythmias
   Decreased cardiac output
   Anemia
Hyperglycemia
Infection
   Fever
Level of consciousness
Pain
Renal failure
   Electrolyte abnormalities
   Fluid imbalance
   Protein loss
Shock
Sleep deprivation

breathing trials are the most effective method of liberating patients from the mechanical ventilator. They should be brief, lasting from 30 to 120 min. Care should be taken not to fatigue a patient through a prolonged SBT before extubation. Patients who fail SBTs after having the underlying process reversed may require a longer, slower wean along with physical reconditioning. Tracheostomy placement may be required to facilitate patient comfort and physical reconditioning in patients who are failing weaning trials and require a longer, slower wean. Daily readiness-to-wean assessment, having clinician-driven weaning protocols, and using weaning teams have all been shown to decrease time spent on the ventilator. Monitoring throughout the weaning process includes assessment of mental status, vital signs, respiratory muscle fatigue (RR, V_T, use of accessory muscles, rapid shallow breathing index), oxygenation (SpO_2), $PaCO_2$ ($PETCO_2$), and electrocardiographic (ECG) changes (Table 16-7).

Extubation

Once the patient has been successfully weaned from mechanical ventilation, the decision to extubate must be addressed. A contraindication to extubation is lack of a gag reflex and inability to protect the airway. Extubation should be done when clinical support is available to replace the endotracheal tube if necessary. Baseline vital signs, pulse oximetry, and $PETCO_2$ are obtained. The head of the bed is elevated 45 to 90 degrees. The airway is carefully suctioned to remove any secretions that may have accumulated on top of the cuff. After the cuff is deflated, the endotracheal tube is

TABLE 16-7. CRITERIA FOR TERMINATION OF WEANING

Change in level of consciousness
Change in vital signs
    Diastolic blood pressure >100 mm Hg
    Fall in systolic blood pressure
    Heart rate >110 beats/min or >20 beats/min increase over baseline
    Respiratory rate >30 breaths/min or >10 breaths/min increase
        over baseline
Falling pulse oximetry saturation
Tidal volume <250 mL
Rising end-tidal CO_2 values
ECG changes
    PVCs >6/min
    Salvos of PVCs
    ST-segment elevation
    Ventricular conduction changes

ECG, electrocardiographic; PVCs, premature ventricular contractions.

removed at the end of inspiration so that the patient will be able to cough and exhale forcefully to prevent the aspiration of secretions during tube removal.

The caregiver must be prepared for reintubation if upper airway obstruction, such as glottic edema, occurs. Inspiratory stridor is treated with inhaled racemic epinephrine 0.5 mL in 1 to 3 mL of normal saline to reduce edema. The dose is repeated at 20- to 30-min intervals one or two times. If this does not relieve the stridor, immediate intubation is recommended.

The respiratory pattern will change following extubation for approximately 60 min. V_E increases by as much as 2 L/min, there is a slight increase in the V_T, an increase in the respiratory drive and rate, and a decrease in paradoxical abdominal movement. After about an hour, the respiratory pattern will return to preextubation patterns.

17

Acute Respiratory Dysfunction

EDITORS' NOTE

Several questions on the PCCN exam can be expected to address the concepts of acute and chronic respiratory failure. It is important to understand key physiologic events that produce the clinical symptoms of these conditions as well as the likely therapeutic events that might improve pulmonary function. This chapter provides a concise review of the major areas that the PCCN exam is likely to cover with respect to these topics.

CHRONIC OBSTRUCTIVE PULMONARY DISEASE

Chronic obstructive pulmonary disease (COPD) is a preventable and treatable disease characterized by airflow limitation that is not fully reversible. It manifests as chronic bronchitis or emphysema with some patients having features of both. Chronic bronchitis is defined as productive cough on most days of the week for at least 3 month's total duration in 2 successive years. Emphysema is characterized by permanent enlargement of the air spaces that are distal to the terminal bronchioles with destruction of lung parenchyma leading to loss of elastic recoil and loss of alveolar septa and lung hyperinflation. COPD is the fourth leading cause of death in the United States and this is expected to rise given the aging population. The prevalence of COPD increases with age and occurs more frequently in men. It is caused by inhalation exposure and/or genetic factors. The most common inhalation exposure is cigarette smoking. Other inhalation risk factors may include exposure to passive cigarette smoke, air pollution,

and occupational dust (e.g., mineral dust, cotton dust) or inhaled chemicals. The primary genetic disorder leading to COPD is alpha$_1$-antitrypsin deficiency. It is the most common cause of emphysema in nonsmokers and increases the risk of COPD in smokers. It may take years to develop symptoms of COPD.

Pathophysiology

Inhalation exposure leads to an inflammatory response in the airways leading to tissue destruction, bronchoconstriction, and increased mucus production. Airflow limitation is caused by airway obstruction, loss of elastic recoil, or both. Airway obstruction is caused by inflammation-mediated mucus hypersecretion, mucous plugging, mucosal edema, bronchospasm, peribronchial fibrosis, or a combination of these mechanisms. Enlarged alveolar spaces sometimes consolidate into bullae; defined as air spaces ≥ 1 cm in diameter. These changes lead to loss of elastic recoil and lung hyperinflation. Increased airway resistance and lung hyperinflation increase the work of breathing. Hypoxia from ventilation to perfusion mismatch occurs. Some patients with COPD will develop hypercarbia. Patients with COPD can develop pulmonary hypertension due to hypoxic pulmonary vasoconstriction and severe right heart failure (cor pulmonale). Patients are prone to respiratory infections.

Signs and Symptoms

Patients with COPD present with progressive dyspnea and productive cough that develop over several years. Some have learned to adapt their lifestyle and have become very sedentary to avoid activity that causes dyspnea. Usually, there is a >20-year pack smoking history before symptoms begin. Dyspnea can be exertional or persistent. Auscultation of the lungs will reveal decreased breath sounds, prolonged expiratory phase of respiration, and wheezing. An increase in the anterior/posterior diameter of the chest may occur that is often described as a "barrel chest." Use of accessory muscles may be observed, and some patients may breath through pursed lips. Weight loss is the result of decreased caloric intake related to dyspnea and increased caloric need because of the increased work of breathing. Signs of right heart failure will be apparent in advanced stages of the disease (distended neck veins, hepatic congestion, dependent edema).

Diagnosis

Diagnosis of COPD is based on history, physical examination, chest radiograph, and pulmonary function tests. The chest radiograph in emphysema will reveal flattened diaphragms and lung hyperinflation. Bullae may also be noted. An enlarged pulmonary vasculature will be seen in patients who have pulmonary hypertension and cor pulmonale. In patients with chronic obstructive bronchitis, chest radiographs may be normal or may demonstrate a bibasilar increase in bronchovascular markings as a result of bronchial wall thickening. A computed tomographic (CT) scan has greater sensitivity and specificity in the diagnosis of emphysema; however, it is not as clear with chronic bronchitis. Pulmonary function tests show reductions of FEV1, FVC, and the ratio of FEV1/FVC, which are the hallmark of airflow limitation. Alpha$_1$-antitrypsin level determination will be necessary to confirm alpha$_1$-antitrypsin deficiency. Other adjunctive testing could include arterial blood gases (ABGs) looking for hypoxia and elevated PaCO$_2$. An elevated hematocrit may be seen on a complete blood count (CBC) from chronic hypoxia. Echocardiography (ECG) may be done to assess the presence of right heart failure. An ECG will be nonspecific and demonstrate low-voltage QRS due to lung hyperinflation.

Treatment

Treatment of stable COPD consists of bronchodilators (beta agonist and anticholinergics) and inhaled corticosteroids. Supportive care may consist of supplemental oxygen, smoking cessation, nutrition, vaccinations (pneumococcal and influenza), and exercise therapy. The goal is to prevent exacerbations, improve exercise tolerance, improve health status, and prevent further deterioration. Some patients may qualify for lung transplantation or lung volume reduction surgery.

Treatment goals for COPD exacerbation are to ensure adequate oxygenation and near-normal blood pH, reverse airway obstruction, and treat any underlying cause. Oxygen therapy is given with the goal of increasing PaO$_2$ >60 mm Hg and SaO$_2$ >90% using care not to raise oxygen levels high enough to precipitate hypercapnia. Start with a nasal cannula and increase therapy as needed to achieve goals. Inhaled short-acting bronchodilators (beta agonists and anticholinergics) should be administered by metered-dose inhalers or nebulized treatments. Systemic bronchodilators do not show any benefit over inhaled bronchodilators and can lead to increased side effects. All patients should have a chest radiograph to rule out the possibility of pneumonia. The most common organisms found in patients with COPD exacerbations are *Streptococcus pneumonia, Haemophilus influenzae,* and *Moraxella catarrhalis. Pseudomonas aeruginosa* has been seen in severe cases of COPD exacerbation. Appropriate antibiotics to cover the most common organisms should be administered.

Exacerbation

Exacerbation of COPD can be mild to severe and present as worsening dyspnea, purulent sputum, and an increase in sputum volume. Acute exacerbations can be triggered by infections (viral or bacterial) or environmental exposure. It may not be possible always to identify the trigger of the exacerbation. Patients with mild exacerbations can be treated as outpatients; however, severe exacerbations may be life threatening and require hospitalization. Symptoms may show moderate to severe acute hypoxemia, acute respiratory acidosis, new arrhythmias, and/or deteriorating respiratory function. Systemic corticosteroid therapy is beneficial and may be necessary for a short while following the exacerbation. Antibiotic therapy has been shown to be beneficial, especially in moderate to severe exacerbations. Patients with worsening respiratory distress, worsening hypercapnia, worsening respiratory acidosis, worsening hypoxemia, and worsening dyspnea may require noninvasive positive pressure ventilation (NPPV) or mechanical ventilation. Early NPPV may prevent the need for intubation and mechanical ventilation while supporting the patient until symptoms resolve. Care should be taken to provide adequate exhalation time with ventilation. Lower respiratory rates should be set to avoid auto–positive end-expiratory pressure (auto-PEEP) which can result from inadequate exhalation.

ACUTE RESPIRATORY FAILURE

Acute respiratory failure (ARF) is the result of abnormalities in ventilation, perfusion, or compliance, leading to hypercapnia and/or hypoxemia. Respiratory failure is a medical emergency that can result from long-standing, progressively worsening lung disease or from severe lung disease that develops suddenly. The lungs are unable to maintain adequate oxygenation and carbon dioxide elimination to support metabolism, leading to respiratory acidosis. Acute respiratory failure develops rapidly over minutes to hours, whereas chronic respiratory failure develops more slowly. It is necessary to identify the underlying condition in order to initiate appropriate treatment.

Pathophysiology

ARF presents as an oxygenation or ventilation disturbance that may be life threatening. An alteration in oxygenation is the most common form of respiratory failure. Perfusion (Q) exceeds ventilation (V) (a low V/Q ratio or increased intrapulmonary shunt), causing decreased oxygenation of venous blood and a mixing of less oxygenated blood with arterial blood. The effect is a reduced arterial oxygen pressure (PaO_2) value or hypoxic respiratory failure.

In ARF, due to high V/Q ratios or increased dead space (V_D), there is a marked increase in the work of breathing. The patient increases minute ventilation (V_E) to compensate for an increased dead space in an effort to maintain adequate alveolar ventilation. Inadequate alveolar ventilation and failure to eliminate carbon dioxide cause acute increases in arterial carbon dioxide ($PaCO_2$) levels, resulting in respiratory acidosis, hypercapnic respiratory failure.

Etiology and Risk Factors

Respiratory failure can arise from an abnormality in any of the components of the respiratory system, including the airways, alveoli, central nervous system, peripheral nervous system, respiratory muscles, and chest wall. Patients at risk for developing ARF include those with COPD, restrictive lung disease, respiratory center depression, pulmonary edema, and pulmonary emboli, among many other conditions (Table 17-1).

Chronic lung disease complicated by a pneumonia, left ventricular (LV) failure resulting in pulmonary edema (cardiac), inhalation injuries, and acute respiratory distress syndrome (ARDS) are examples of ARF with alterations in oxygenation.

TABLE 17-1. CAUSES OF ARF

Oxygenation disturbances

ARDS
Pulmonary edema
Pneumonitis
Pneumonia

Alveolar ventilation disturbances

Central nervous system depression
Medication or anesthetic effect
Head or cervical cord trauma
Cerebrovascular accident
COPD
Interstitial pulmonary fibrosis
Pneumothorax

Ventilation/perfusion disturbances

Pulmonary emboli
Bronchiolitis
COPD
Lung trauma

Left-to-right shunt

Atelectasis
Oxygen toxicity
Pulmonary edema or emboli
Pneumonia

COPD, chronic obstructive pulmonary disease; ARDS, acute respiratory distress syndrome.

Acute respiratory failure caused by a depressed central nervous system (CNS) or a high V/Q ratio causes an increase in $PaCO_2$.

Signs and Symptoms

Ventilation failure due to CNS depression presents with a slowed rate of breathing. Few other obvious physical symptoms may exist. If the ventilation failure is due to increased dead space, the respiratory rate and depth increase; the respiratory rate may exceed 30 breaths per minute. The patient may also complain of shortness of breath and appear anxious.

Assessment findings include tachycardia, atrial cardiac dysrhythmias, pedal edema, tachypnea, dyspnea on exertion or at rest, labored breathing pattern, use of accessory muscles of respiration, crackles, wheezes, and a hyperresonant chest on percussion in patients with advanced COPD (Table 17-2).

Invasive and Noninvasive Diagnostic Studies

Arterial blood gas values can deteriorate suddenly, indicating acute pulmonary insufficiency. Findings

TABLE 17-2. SYMPTOMS OF OXYGENATION-INDUCED RESPIRATORY FAILURE

Shortness of breath
Orthopnea
Pao_2 <60 mm Hg
Sao_2 <0.90
Spo_2 <0.93
Anxiety
Increased respiratory rate (>30 breaths per min)
Possible labored breathing
Increased intrapulmonary shunt
   Pao_2/Fio_2 ratio <200
   Qs/Qt >20%
   a/A ratio <25%
   A–a gradient >350 on 100% oxygen

include a Pao_2 <60 mm Hg, requiring an increase in the fractional inspiratory oxygen pressure (Fio_2) and a $Paco_2$ >45 mm Hg. Other measures of oxygenation include a decreased a/A ratio (<0.25), a widened A–a gradient, and a decreased Pao_2/Fio_2 ratio (<200). The patient may present with an elevated hematocrit (above 52%) and an elevated hemoglobin (>18 g/dL) if this is a chronic problem and there is an underlying component of COPD. As the heart rate increases, cardiac output may fall.

Nursing and Collaborative Diagnosis

Potential diagnoses include but are not limited to:

- Impaired gas exchange
- Ineffective breathing patterns
- Intolerance of activity
- Inability to sustain spontaneous ventilation
- Potential for ineffective airway clearance
- Anxiety
- Potential for infection

Goals and Desired Patient Outcomes

Goals and desired patient outcomes include but are not limited to:

- Adequate oxygenation: Pao_2 60 to 100 mm Hg, Sao_2 >90%/Spo_2 93%
- Adequate ventilation: pH 7.35 to 7.45, $Paco_2$ at baseline or 35 to 45 mm Hg
- Ability to sustain spontaneous ventilation

Management of Patient Care

Management priorities include correction of hypoxia and acidosis, respiratory muscle rest, control

of shock, decreasing the risk of infection, and nutritional repletion.

Establishment or assurance of an adequate airway is needed to provide supportive treatment. Correction of hypoxia may require the use of oxygen therapy, continuous positive airway pressure (CPAP), noninvasive positive-pressure ventilation (NPPV) or endotracheal intubation with mechanical ventilation, and positive end-expiratory pressure (PEEP).

When medication is the cause of respiratory failure, discontinuation of the medication may reverse the respiratory depression and is the treatment of choice. When respiratory failure is due to trauma or increased intracranial pressure (ICP), treatment is focused on relieving the increased ICP.

When the problem is a high V/Q ratio (increased dead-space ventilation), reestablishing perfusion is the key. If a pulmonary embolism exists, thrombolytic therapy may be indicated. If low perfusion is due to a low cardiac output, the cardiac output must be improved.

Supportive treatment includes oxygen therapy, PEEP, and mechanical ventilation. Treatment of LV failure producing pulmonary edema focuses on resolving the cardiac dysfunction. If a pulmonary infection is the underlying cause, antibiotic therapy is indicated.

Complications

Complications associated with ARF include severe respiratory and metabolic acidosis, infection, failure to wean from mechanical ventilation, and lack of adequate nutritional support.

ACUTE RESPIRATORY INFECTIONS

Acute respiratory infection can lead to pneumonia, an acute inflammatory response of the lungs caused by a bacterial, fungal, or viral organism. The organisms can enter the lung directly by inhalation, by aspiration (microorganisms or macroorganisms), or via the blood. Pneumonia can be community-acquired, health care-associated (dialysis centers, nursing homes), or hospital-acquired (nosocomial). Pneumonia is a common and potentially serious illness.

Community-Acquired Pneumonia

Common clinical features of community-acquired pneumonia (CAP) include cough, fever, pleuritic chest pain, dyspnea, and sputum production. A leukocytosis is often present. The presence of an infiltrate on plain chest radiograph is considered the "gold standard" for diagnosing pneumonia when clinical and microbiologic features are supportive. The causative agent of community-acquired pneumonia remains unidentified in 30% to 50% of cases. *Streptococcus pneumoniae* is the most commonly identified pathogen in community-acquired pneumonia, although many other organisms have been identified (Table 17-3). Community-associated methicillin-resistant *Streptococcus aureus* (MRSA) typically produces a necrotizing pneumonia with high morbidity and mortality. Viral pneumonias, transmitted by airborne droplets, are usually community-acquired, although they can be nosocomial. Patients with a viral upper respiratory infection (URI) are at risk for the development of a secondary bacterial infection. Patients with comorbidities are at the highest risk of severe infection.

Hospital-Acquired (Nosocomial) Pneumonia

Patients who require mechanical ventilation are at risk for the most frequent nosocomial infection: ventilator-associated pneumonia (VAP). The presence of an artificial airway predisposes a patient to aspiration and colonization of the airway with organisms. VAP occurs in 10% to 20% of patients who are mechanically ventilated for more than 48 h. Development of VAP increases length of stay, hospital cost, and mortality. Risk factors for VAP include reintubation, self-extubation, prolonged mechanical ventilation, extremes of age (<6 years and >65 years), lying flat in bed, gastric distention, nasogastric tubes, inadequate endotracheal cuff pressure, routine changing of ventilator circuits, and stress ulcer prophylaxis. Care must be taken to determine whether a positive sputum culture represents colonization or an actual infection before beginning antimicrobial treatment. Colonization is the presence of an organism in the sputum without the signs and symptoms of an infection. VAP can be prevented by weaning as soon as possible, aggressive hand hygiene, maintaining the head of the bed at >30 degrees of elevation, draining ventilator circuits away from the patient, checking for gastric distention and preventing gastric residuals, careful oral suctioning to prevent pooling of secretions on top of the endotracheal tube cuff, and performing oral care.

Pathophysiology

When an organism enters the lung, macrophages and the lymph system work to remove them and prevent infection. When the lungs' normal defense mechanisms fail, the organisms multiply, filling the alveoli with exudate. This results in areas of low ventilation and normal perfusion and increased intrapulmonary shunt. Hypoxic vasoconstriction reduces blood flow to the affected area. The organisms cause edema of the airway and stimulate goblet cells to increase mucus production. The increase in secretions and airway edema increase airway resistance, leading to an increased work of breathing.

Etiology and Risk Factors

Patients at risk for the development of pneumonia include older adults; persons with dehydration, immobility, malnutrition, or COPD; those on mechanical ventilation; the immunosuppressed; and those taking drugs that impair airway clearance.

Signs and Symptoms

Signs and symptoms of bacterial pneumonia include fever, shaking chills, pleuritic chest pain that is worse on inspiration, increased sputum production, and cough. Sputum color ranges from reddish to green.

Viral pneumonia presents with a sudden onset of fever, dry cough, headache, myalgia, retrosternal

TABLE 17-3. ACUTE RESPIRATORY INFECTIONS: CAUSATIVE ORGANISMS

Community-acquired infections
  Streptococcus pneumoniae
  Klebsiella
  Haemophilus influenzae
  Staphylococcus aureus (MRSA or MSSA)
  Legionella species
  Mycoplasma pneumoniae
  Chlamydia pneumoniae
Viruses
  Pneumocystis carinii
Hospital-acquired (nosocomial) infections
  Staphylococcus aureus (MRSA or MSSA)
  Pseudomonas aeruginosa
  Streptococcus pneumoniae
  Klebsiella
  Haemophilus influenzae
  Escherichia coli
  Serratia
  Acinetobacter
  Enterobacter
  Stenotrophomonas maltophilia

MRSA, methicillin-resistant *Streptococcus aureus;* MSSA, methicillin-sensitive Streptococcus aureus.

chest pain unaffected by respiration, dyspnea, and cough.

Invasive and Noninvasive Diagnostic Studies

The chest film will reveal lobar infiltrates and may show pleural effusion. The ABGs may show a decreased PaO_2. Elevated leukocyte counts with a left shift and elevated bands may be seen. Sputum may be cultured to identify the organism; however, routine sputum cultures are not recommended for community-acquired pneumonia unless the patient does not respond to therapy or is immunocompromised. A positive sputum culture on a mechanically ventilated patient should be evaluated for colonization versus infection. Treatment is reserved for positive cultures when the patient has the additional signs of infection outlined above. A bronchial alveolar lavage (BAL) specimen examined for cell count can be useful in determining the presence of infection. A BAL specimen with high polymorphonuclear neutrophil (PMN) count indicates infection.

Nursing and Collaborative Diagnoses

Diagnoses include but are not limited to:

- Impaired gas exchange related to increased shunt
- Ineffective airway clearance related to retained secretions
- Activity intolerance related to breathlessness
- Dyspnea related to alveolar hypoventilation

Goals and Desired Patient Outcomes

Goals and desired patient outcomes include but are not limited to:

- Improved oxygenation; $PaO_2 \geq 60$ mm Hg, $SaO_2 \geq 90\%$
- Increased activity tolerance
- Reversal of dyspnea
- Decreased breathlessness on exertion
- Clearance of airway secretions

Management of Patient Care

Management of pneumonia includes administration of the appropriate antibiotic by intravenous, oral, or intramuscular routes. The current recommendation regarding antibiotic therapy is to begin with broad coverage and narrow coverage as soon as an organism is identified. The more specific the antibiotic therapy given for the shortest possible duration, the less likely the patient is to develop resistance. Hydration is important to keep secretions thin and prevent them from becoming thick and tenacious. Aggressive pulmonary hygiene—such as deep breathing, coughing, early ambulation, and aerosol treatments—is used to help remove secretions. Bronchodilators are used to increase airway size and relax airway muscles. Analgesics are recommended to treat muscle aches and fever.

Complications

Complications of pneumonia include hypotension, sepsis, ARDS, and death.

STATUS ASTHMATICUS

Status asthmaticus is a severe continuing attack of asthma that fails to respond to conventional drug therapy. It can last for days to weeks; even with optimal therapy, it may be fatal.

Pathophysiology

Status asthmaticus is characterized by airway hyperreactivity or hyperresponsiveness, airway obstruction, and airway inflammation. The increased airway responsiveness is manifest by narrowing of the airways secondary to bronchial constriction and excessive mucus obstruction, thus increasing the work of breathing, interfering with gas exchange, and producing hypoxemia (Fig. 17-1). Air trapping with resulting hyperinflation of the lungs is a common clinical feature.

When an inhaled substance elicits a hypersensitivity response, immunoglobulin E (IgE) antibodies stimulate mast cells in the lung to release histamine. Histamine causes inflammation, irritation, and edema in the smooth muscles by attaching to receptor sites in the bronchi. There is a release of inflammatory mediators from the epithelial cells as well as the epithelial mast cells and macrophages. Eosinophils and neutrophils alter the integrity of the epithelium, and changes occur in the autonomic neural control of the airway, mucociliary function, and airway responsiveness. Prostaglandin production is stimulated and further enhances the effects of

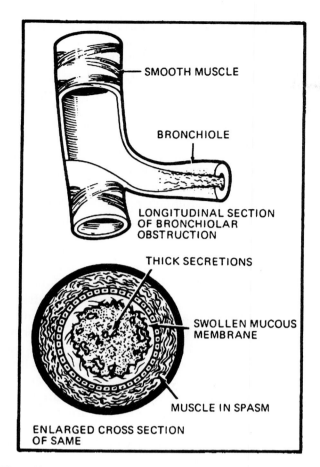

Figure 17-1. Appearance of respiratory bronchioles in asthma (bronchiolar obstruction on expiration by muscle spasm, swelling of mucosa, and thick secretions).

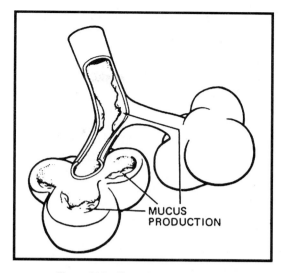

Figure 17-2. Airway lumen in bronchitis.

histamine, stimulating goblet cells to secrete excessive tenacious mucus and leading to airway narrowing (Fig. 17-2).

As the attack continues unabated, the bronchial walls hypertrophy and the clearance of secretions is diminished, causing bronchiolar obstruction, reducing alveolar ventilation, and causing hyperinflation of the lung.

Early airway closure causes increased intrathoracic pressure on exhalation, thus inhibiting alveolar ventilation. As alveoli fill with the excessive mucus, blood is shunted by nonfunctioning alveoli and intrapulmonary shunt increases. Diminished ventilation results in a respiratory acidosis.

Etiology and Risk Factors

Status asthmaticus is a complication of asthma. The three most common causes of status asthmaticus are:

(1) exposure to allergens, (2) noncompliance with the medication regimen, and (3) respiratory infections. It can result from a reaction to an allergen or nonallergen such as exercise and can be precipitated by irritants such as cold air, odors, chemicals, or changes in the weather. Environments that become unusually hot, cold, or dusty often trigger status asthmaticus because of the effect of inspired air on the lungs. Other triggers include psychological and emotional stimuli, aspirin, nonsteroidal anti-inflammatory drugs, beta-adrenergic agents, overuse of bronchodilators, and autonomic nervous system imbalance.

Signs and Symptoms

Patients with status asthmaticus are extremely dyspneic, with a hyperpneic respiratory pattern and a sensation of chest tightness. Inspiratory and expiratory wheezing is usually audible, with a prolonged expiratory phase as the patient tries to exhale the trapped air through narrow airways. Physical examination reveals tachypnea; tachycardia; a rapid, thready pulse; use of accessory respiratory muscles; distant heart sounds; hyperresonance on percussion; flaring nares; pallor, cyanosis; increased work of breathing; and fatigue. The disappearance of wheezing may be an ominous sign, as the airway may have become completely obstructed. The patient may have pulsus paradoxus, a drop in the systolic blood pressure of 12 mm Hg or more during inspiration.

Invasive and Noninvasive Diagnostic Studies

Arterial blood gases (ABGs) initially show a low $PaCO_2$ with a respiratory alkalosis. When the $PaCO_2$ normalizes or begins to rise that is an ominous sign since the patient is now tiring and generally requires intubation and mechanical support. The ABGs may reveal a normal or falling PaO_2. Chest radiography will probably not be helpful, showing a hyperinflated lung that is normal or translucent. Pulmonary function tests are not useful during the acute phase, as the patient is unable to move enough air to complete the test.

Nursing and Collaborative Diagnoses

Diagnoses include but are not limited to:

- Impaired gas exchange related to alveolar hypoventilation
- Ineffective airway clearance related to excessive mucus production
- Ineffective breathing pattern related to increased work of breathing
- Risk of inability to sustain spontaneous ventilation related to respiratory muscle fatigue

Goals and Desired Patient Outcomes

Goals and patient outcomes include but are not limited to:

- Maintenance of a patent airway
- Reversal of respiratory acidosis; pH 7.35 to 7.45
- Control of airway secretions
- Spontaneous ventilation
- Reversal of bronchospasm
- Adequate oxygenation; PaO_2 >60 mm Hg

Management of Patient Care

Management of status asthmaticus includes support of ventilation and respirations. Hypoxemia is the most common cause of death in asthma. Oxygen is the primary therapeutic modality. Supplemental oxygen must be provided for any patient who presents with status asthmaticus. Oxygen helps to correct V/Q mismatch.

Rapid-onset beta-agonist agents, typically albuterol or terbutaline, are the mainstays of acute therapy in asthma. The inhaled route of administration is generally the most effective one, although some patients with severe refractory status asthmaticus may benefit from intravenous administration. Inhaled beta agonists can be administered intermittently or as continuous nebulized aerosol in a monitored setting. Corticosteroids, such as methylprednisolone or prednisone, are critical in the therapy of status asthmaticus and are used to decrease the intense airway inflammation and swelling in asthma. Other treatments include anticholinergics, subcutaneous epinephrine, and magnesium. The use of theophylline in acute asthma has fallen into disfavor as the data suggest little or no benefit and significant additional toxicity, which includes tachycardia, arrhythmias (irregular heartbeat), nausea, and vomiting.

Helium and inhaled anesthetics may be used in severe cases. Helium is an inert gas that is less dense than nitrogen. The administration of a helium-oxygen mixture (Heliox) reduces turbulent airflow across narrowed airways, which can help to reduce and, thus, relieve the work of breathing and improve delivery of inhaled medication. Improved gas exchange with decreased respiratory acidosis will be seen. Heliox can be delivered via face mask or through a mechanical ventilator. Inhaled anesthetic agents, although potentially effective, are difficult to administer outside the operating room.

Mechanical ventilation may be necessary to support respiration while the above therapies take effect. There are no widely agreed upon guidelines for when asthmatic patients require intubation. Intubation and mechanical ventilation are difficult and dangerous for the asthmatic and hence are avoided if at all possible. Intubation should be approached cautiously in patients with status asthmaticus because manipulation of the airway can cause increased airflow obstruction due to exaggerated bronchial responsiveness. The narrowed airways, positive-pressure ventilation, and delayed emptying can lead to dynamic hyperinflation (DHI), placing the patient at risk for barotrauma and cardiac compromise. Interstitial emphysema, pneumothorax, pneumomediastinum, subcutaneous emphysema, and/or pneumoperitoneum can result from barotrauma. To minimize the development of DHI, a controlled hypoventilation should occur with settings that allow for a low minute ventilation, low respiratory rate (RR), long exhalation time, and low tidal volume (6 mL/kg). Care must be taken to assess for auto-PEEP, peak airway, and plateau pressures. Keeping plateau pressures less than 30 and auto-PEEP less than 10 cm H_2O is the goal. Sedation is usually required, with neuro muscular blockade (NMB) being necessary in extreme cases. Additional therapies include hydration, monitoring of oxygenation with ABGs or pulse oximetry, and antibiotics only if signs of infection are present.

Be aware of a decreasing level of consciousness, diminished wheezing, or a rising $PaCO_2$. These may signal a worsening of the asthmatic episode.

Complications

Complications include pneumothorax, hypoxemia, respiratory acidosis, and hypoxia. Status asthmaticus can cause respiratory failure and death.

PULMONARY HYPERTENSION

Pulmonary hypertension (PH) is a condition in which pressure in the pulmonary arteries is abnormally high often leading to right heart failure. Pulmonary hypertension is defined as a mean pulmonary artery pressure greater than 25 mm Hg at rest or 30 mm Hg with exercise, as measured by right heart catheterization.

Pathophysiology

PH can be idiopathic, familial, or associated with many other disease processes. Formerly, it was classified as primary or secondary, however, that has been revised by the World Health Organization (WHO). The WHO has classified PH into five groups that reflect the underlying etiology (Table 17-4). The primary cause of significant PH is almost always increased pulmonary vascular resistance (PVR). Increased flow alone does not usually cause significant pulmonary hypertension because the pulmonary vascular bed vasodilates and recruits vessels in response to increased flow, so that little, if any, increased pressure results. Similarly, increased pulmonary venous pressure alone does not usually cause PH. However, both increased flow and increased pulmonary venous pressure can increase pulmonary vascular resistance. The right ventricle hypertrophies in response to the pressure. If severe enough, the right ventricle dilates and cardiac output falls.

Etiology and Risk Factors

Pulmonary hypertension, WHO group 1 is a rare disease with an incidence of about two to three cases per million per year. Adult women are almost three times more likely to present with PH than adult men. The incidence of PH from other underlying causes is higher.

TABLE 17-4. CLASSIFICATIONS OF PH

Pulmonary arterial hypertension

Idiopathic
Familiar
Associated
    Collagen vascular diseases
    Congenital systemic-to-pulmonary shunts
Portal hypertension
HIV infection
Drugs and toxins
    Other (thyroid disorders, glycogen storage disease, Gaucher's disease, hereditary hemorrhagic telangiectasia, hemoglobinopathies, myeloproliferative disorders, splenectomy)
Associated with significant venous or capillary involvement
    PVOD
    PCH
    Persistent pulmonary hypertension of the newborn

Pulmonary hypertension with left heart disease

Left-sided atrial or ventricular heart disease
Left-sided valvular heart disease

Pulmonary hypertension associated with lung diseases and/or hypoxemia

Chronic obstructive pulmonary disease
Interstitial lung disease
Sleep-disordered breathing
Alveolar hypoventilation disorders
Chronic exposure to high altitude
Development abnormalities

Pulmonary hypertension due to chronic thrombotic and/or embolic disease

Thromboembolic obstruction of proximal pulmonary arteries
Thromboembolic obstruction of distal pulmonary arteries
Non-thrombotic pulmonary embolism (tumor, parasites, foreign material)

Miscellaneous

Sarcoidosis, pulmonary Langerhans' cell histiocytosis, lymphangiomatosis, compression of pulmonary vessels by adenopathy, tumor, fibrosing mediastinitis, or other process

PCH, pulmonary capillary hemangiomatosis; PVOD, pulmonary veno-occlusive disease.

Clinical Manifestations

Patients with PH may initially complain of dyspnea on exertion, lethargy, and fatigue. As the disease progresses and right ventricular failure develops, exertional angina, exertional syncope, and peripheral edema may develop. The initial physical finding of PH is usually increased intensity of the pulmonic component of the second heart sound, which may even become palpable. Evidence of right ventricular hypertrophy or failure may also exist. Patients may have signs of jugular venous distention, elevated central venous pressure (CVP), right upper quadrant pain, and anorexia from gastrointestinal congestion. Prognosis relates to how well the right ventricle functions under this increased workload. The prognosis is generally poor but varies according to the severity of the underlying cause, the functional abnormalities, and the hemodynamic abnormalities.

Invasive and Noninvasive Studies

Patients with pulmonary hypertension undergo a variety of tests with the goal of confirming the diagnosis and to attempt to identify an underlying cause. Chest radiography will show enlargement of central pulmonary arteries and, depending on the stage, may show enlarged right heart. The electrocardiogram may demonstrate signs of right ventricular hypertrophy or strain. Echocardiography is performed to estimate the pulmonary artery systolic pressure and to assess right ventricular size, thickness, and function as well as valvular function. The echocardiogram is not the most precise way to determine pulmonary artery pressures. Echocardiography can be performed during exercise to identify patients with exercise-induced PH. Pulmonary function tests can identify possible underlying lung conditions (obstructive pattern is suggestive of COPD, whereas restrictive disease suggests interstitial lung disease, neuromuscular weakness, or chest wall disease) that are contributing to PH. Overnight oximetry can determine underlying causes such as obstructive sleep apnea that cause hypoxemia and pulmonary vasoconstriction. Thrombolytic components may be assessed by V/Q scan or spiral CT scan. Right heart catheterization is necessary to confirm the diagnosis of PH and accurately determine the severity of the hemodynamic derangements as well as the presence of any congenital abnormalities.

Nursing and Collaborative Diagnoses

Potential diagnoses include but are not limited to:

- Intolerance of activity
- Anxiety
- Potential for infection
- Alteration in tissue perfusion related to decreased cardiac output

Goals and Desired Patient Outcomes

Goals and patient outcomes include but are not limited to:

- Increased activity tolerance
- Ability to maintain adequate tissue perfusion
- No evidence of infection
- Decreased anxiety

Management of Patient Care

There is no cure for pulmonary arterial hypertension. Treatment, however, has improved dramatically during the past decade, offering relief from symptoms and prolonged survival. Lung transplantation was the ultimate treatment option; however, with the improvement of vasodilator therapy, the need for transplantation has decreased. Treatment should be aimed at the causative underlying disease whenever possible. The mainstays of

TABLE 17-5. TREATMENT OPTIONS FOR PH

Pulmonary arterial hypertension
No primary therapy Advanced therapy options
Pulmonary hypertension with left heart disease

Treatment of underlying disease
    Avoid advanced therapy unless treatment of underlying disease
    (e.g., following mitral valve replacement)

Pulmonary hypertension associated with lung diseases and/or hypoxemia
Supplemental oxygen Advanced therapy for NYHA class III or IV only after correction of hypoxemia (inhaled nitric oxide, inhaled iloprost, and oral sildenafil)
Pulmonary hypertension due to chronic thrombotic and/or embolic disease
Anticolagulation Surgical thromboendarterectomy Advanced therapy to bridge to surgery or if NYHA class III or IV after intervention
Miscellaneous
Treatment of underlying cause Intravenous epoprostenal or oral bosentan
All Groups of PH
Diuretics Oxygen Anticoagulation Digoxin Exercise
Advanced Therapy Options for PH
Prostanoids (epoprostenol, treprostinil, iloprost) Endothelin receptor antagonists (bosentan, ambrisentan) Phosphodiesterase-5 (PDE5) inhibitors (sildenafil, tadalafil) Calcium channel blockers (nifedipine, diltiazem, or amlodopine;   verapamil should be avoided) if positive vasoreactive test

NYHA, New York Heart Association.

current medical therapy fall into several classes, including vasodilators, oxygen therapy, anticoagulants, antiplatelet agents, anti-inflammatory therapies, and vascular-remodeling therapies depending on the WHO classification of PH. Continuous intravenous administration of the prostanoids carries with it a risk of thromboembolism or line infection. The endothelin receptor antagonists require frequent monitoring of liver enzymes given their association with hepatic damage. Also, medication interactions are a predominant concern with this class of drugs. As such, provision of care with many of these agents in these advanced-stage patients takes highly specialized care.

Lung transplantation remains a treatment option for patients who do not respond to the other therapies. The earlier PH is diagnosed, the more responsive it will be to therapy. Patients should be referred to specialized treatment centers where clinicians have expertise in treating PH. Patients with PH should undergo an invasive hemodynamic assessment and an acute vasoreactivity test prior to the initiation of advanced therapy. Agents commonly used for vasoreactivity testing include epoprostenol, adenosine, and inhaled nitric oxide. An acute vasoreactivity test is considered positive if the mean pulmonary artery pressure decreases at least 10 mm Hg and to a value less than 40 mm Hg, with an increased or unchanged cardiac output and a minimally reduced or unchanged systemic blood pressure. Patients with a positive vasoreactivity test are candidates for a trial of calcium channel blocker therapy. In contrast, patients with a negative vasoreactivity test should be treated with an alternative agent because calcium channel blockers have not been shown to be beneficial in these patients and may be harmful. Table 17-5 outlines treatment options by the WHO classification. Creation of a right-to-left shunt by atrial septostomy has been performed in some patients with syncope or severe right heart failure in an attempt to increase systemic blood flow by bypassing the pulmonary vascular obstruction.

Complications

Severe right heart failure (cor pulmonale) with resultant low cardiac output is the ultimate progression of pulmonary hypertension. Chronic hepatic congestion from the severe right heart failure leads to hyperbilirubenemia and cirrhosis. Patients on intravenous medications are at risk for line infections. Patients with untreated PH have a median survival of 2 to 3 years from time of diagnosis.

18

Acute Pulmonary Embolism and Aspiration

EDITORS' NOTE

Pulmonary embolism is a likely content area for questions in the PCCN exam. Pulmonary emboli are best understood when applied to concepts in pulmonary physiology relative to disturbances of ventilation and perfusion (Chap. 14). However, it is important to remember the physical presentation and treatment discussed in this chapter for purposes of the test.

ACUTE PULMONARY EMBOLISM

An acute pulmonary embolus (PE) is a thrombus that occurs in the body, travels through the venous circulation to the pulmonary circulation, and partially or completely occludes a pulmonary artery. A massive PE is one that occludes more than 50% of the pulmonary artery bed.

Pathophysiology

The lung is capable of filtering small clots and other substances through fibrolytic mechanisms in the lung. The lung cannot dissolve large clots or multiple small clots. Most PEs occur when a lower extremity, deep venous thrombus breaks loose from its attachment and flows through the venous circulation, entering the right ventricle and then lodging in small pulmonary arteries (Fig. 18-1). The embolus will most often lodge in the right lower lobe because of increased regional blood flow. Once in the lung, the embolus may be dissolved, grow in size, or fragment

into many smaller pieces. An embolus can be composed of platelets, thrombin, erythrocytes, leukocytes, air, fat, fluid, tumors, or amniotic fluid (Table 18-1). Nonthrombotic emboli have a greater potential for entering the left heart because they can change shape easily and pass through the pulmonary capillary bed into the systemic circulation. Compromise will occur more readily if there is underlying chronic obstructive pulmonary disease (COPD), congestive heart failure (CHF), or other chronic conditions.

Obstruction of the pulmonary vasculature elicits neurohumoral stimuli, increasing pulmonary artery pressure and pulmonary vascular resistance. Because there is a disruption in the blood flow to alveoli, they become nonfunctioning units, not participating in the exchange of carbon dioxide and oxygen; there is, therefore, increased dead space. In an effort to maintain adequate gas exchange, ventilation is preferentially shifted to the uninvolved areas of the lung. This results in constriction of the distal airways, leading to alveolar collapse and atelectasis.

Etiology and Risk Factors

Patients at risk for the development of thrombus formation include those with three factors referred to as Virchow's triad: (1) damaged vascular endothelium, (2) venous stasis, and (3) hypercoagulability of the blood. Natural processes of clot dissolution may cause release of fragments; or external mechanisms such as direct trauma, muscle contraction, or changes in perfusion may contribute to the release of the thrombus.

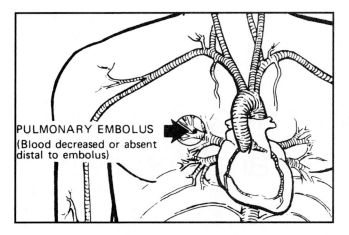

Figure 18-1. Pulmonary embolism.

Pulmonary emboli may develop in patients with no predisposing factors. Some acquired predisposing factors include stasis of venous blood resulting from immobilization, obesity, pregnancy, estrogen use, aging, major trauma or surgery within 4 weeks, malignancy, previous deep venous thrombosis (DVT) indwelling catheters or electrodes in the great veins or right heart, CHF, and acquired thrombotic disorders (heparin-induced thrombocytopenia, postsplenectomy, antiphospholipid antibodies). Hereditary factors that can cause thromboembolic disease include deficiency of antithrombin, protein C or S, resistance to activated protein C (factor V Leiden), prothrombin gene mutation, raised plasminogen-activator inhibitor, plasminogen disorders, and high plasma concentration of factor VIII. Rare occasions of thrombus formation include thrombus formation in the heart secondary to acute myocardial infarction, atrial fibrillation, subacute bacterial endocarditis, and cardioversion.

Signs and Symptoms

Increased respiratory rate, dyspnea, and tachycardia are the most common signs of PE. These may present with or without pleuritic chest pain and hemoptysis. The signs and symptoms of PE must be divided

TABLE 18-1. ETIOLOGY OF PEs

Deep venous thrombosis
Air embolus
Septic embolus
Fat embolus
Tumor embolus
Amniotic fluid embolus

PE: pulmonary embolus.

into the clinical pictures of a massive embolism and a submassive embolism. Massive embolism (<50% of pulmonary circulation obstructed) occurs suddenly and is associated with acute right heart failure (elevated pulmonary artery systolic pressure and pulmonary vascular resistance). Cardiac output falls as a result of the right heart's inability to fill the left heart. The patient may have crushing substernal chest pain and appear to be in shock, with hypotension, elevated right heart pressures, dyspnea, cyanosis, apprehension, or coma. Respirations are rapid, shallow, and gasping. The arterial pulse is rapid and the volume is diminished. If awake, the patient may express feelings of impending doom.

If capnography is available to the patient, the end-tidal CO_2 ($P_{ET}CO_2$) will suddenly decrease with a PE. The arterial CO_2 ($PaCO_2$) may decrease as well owing to hyperventilation. However, the $P_{ET}CO_2$ decreases more because of loss of blood flow in the lungs. This loss of blood flow causes an increased dead space, lowering the $P_{ET}CO_2$. PaO_2 levels may not change substantially. The difference between the $PaCO_2$ and the $P_{ET}CO_2$ will widen. However, in large PEs, hypoxemia is common.

Submassive PE may present only fleeting minimal symptoms or may be asymptomatic. If the submassive PE has occluded a medium-sized artery, tachypnea, dyspnea, tachycardia, generalized chest discomfort, and pleurisy-type chest pain may develop within a few hours. Fever, cough, and hemoptysis may occur over several hours or days. A pleural friction rub and a pleural effusion may develop. Usually, no hemodynamic compromise is seen in minor or submassive PE since no right heart failure occurs.

A subacute massive PE can develop as a result of multiple small emboli that accumulate over several weeks. Since the obstruction occurs gradually, the right heart has time to adapt and the degree of right heart failure is less than that which occurs with the sudden massive PE. Symptoms include dyspnea on exertion, exercise fatigue, elevated central venous pressure (CVP), and an S_3 gallop. Cardiac output is usually preserved unless the build-up of clot becomes unusually large; then the signs and symptoms will be similar to those of a sudden massive PE.

Invasive and Noninvasive Diagnostic Studies

No single noninvasive test is sufficient to diagnose PE in all patients. Diagnostic tests should be used, along with the degree of clinical suspicion, given the patient's presentation and risk factors. Identifying a proximal lower extremity DVT can be helpful since 70% of patients with PE are positive for DVT. If no DVT is identified, then the patient is unlikely to have a PE; however, additional workup based on clinical suspicion may be needed to completely rule out the presence of a PE. Routine chest films may be normal, but about 20% of such cases may show some consolidation. The chest film may be inconclusive within the first few hours after embolism. Things to look for on the chest film include pulmonary disease, atelectasis, pleural effusion, elevated diaphragm, and a prominent pulmonary artery.

The electrocardiogram (ECG) may be normal but most often shows sinus tachycardia or right ventricular (RV) strain. In an extensive PE, the ECG will show right axis deviation, transient right bundle branch block, ST-segment depression, T-wave inversion in leads V_1 and V_4, and tall peaked P waves in leads II, III, and aVF. If the embolus is massive, the ECG may show pulseless electrical activity (PEA).

Arterial blood gases (ABGs) are unreliable indicators of PE. If the arterial oxygen pressure (PaO_2) is >80 mm Hg on room air, a PE is less likely, although one may exist and not occlude major arteries. The ABGs may show a decrease in PaO_2 and $PaCO_2$. Patients on a mechanical ventilator with continuous end-tidal CO_2 monitoring will show a sudden decrease in the $PETCO_2$ value and a widened $PETCO_2$ gradient due to increase in dead-space ventilation.

An elevated brain natriuretic peptide (BNP) or N-terminal pro-brain natriuretic peptide (NT-proBNP) predicts RV dysfunction and strain. An elevated troponin I or troponin T level was shown to be associated with an increased risk of short-term mortality.

Echocardiography can be useful in identifying right heart failure or strain that is associated with a massive PE. On rare occasions a transesophageal echocardiography can see a massive PE in the central pulmonary artery. Usually, only the indirect signs of massive PE are noted; however, echocardiography can be useful in ruling out other causes of hemodynamic compromise (cardiac tamponade, aortic dissection, septal rupture) in an unstable patient.

A common test is a ventilation/perfusion (V/Q) scan. A V/Q lung scan that is normal usually rules out a PE. If a lung scan shows perfusion defects on segments that appear normal on chest radiography, PE is likely. A lung scan may be abnormal simply because of COPD. The V/Q scan is reported in terms of probability of the scan being positive for PE. A V/Q scan with a high probability means that the patient has multiple perfusion defects with normal ventilation. This type of patient has an 85% chance of having a PE. Patients with low or intermediate probability on a V/Q scan must be viewed in light of clinical suspicion. A normal or low-probability V/Q scan in a patient with low clinical suspicion may not receive treatment for PE, whereas a patient with high clinical suspicion may still receive treatment and/or undergo other diagnostic evaluation.

Spiral computed tomography (CT) with injection of contrast can be a valuable and reliable test for determining a PE. It is faster, less complex, and less operator-dependent than pulmonary angiography. The spiral CT also provides the clinician with other valuable information about the lungs, such as pneumonia, detection of masses, and pleural effusions. Right ventricular dilation may be detected on spiral CT, helping to identify the massive PE that is potentially fatal.

Pulmonary angiography should be considered when other tests are inconclusive. A positive angiogram will reveal filling deficits or sharp cutoffs in blood flow. A magnetic resonance imaging scan can also be used to detect changes in pulmonary blood flow or pinpoint an embolus.

Nursing and Collaborative Diagnoses

Diagnoses include but are not limited to:

- Impaired gas exchange related to increased dead-space ventilation
- Ineffective breathing pattern related to alveolar hypoventilation
- Anxiety related to difficulty breathing
- Decreased cardiac output related to RV failure
- Altered peripheral tissue perfusion related to thrombus formation
- Risk for inability to sustain spontaneous ventilation related to increased dead space and decreased alveolar ventilation

Goals and Desired Patient Outcomes

Goals and desired patient outcomes include but are not limited to:

- Adequate oxygenation
- Reversal of the clot
- Reduction in risk for additional clot formation
- Prevention of pulmonary infarction
- Improved V/Q ratio

Management of Patient Care

Intravenous anticoagulants are administered to prevent clot progression. Heparin or lowmolecular weight heparins (LMWHs) such as enoxaparin or dalteparin are the drugs of choice. The semisynthetic anti-Xa agent fondaparinux has also been approved for the treatment of venous thromboembolism, but lack of clinical experience limits its use in many centers.

Heparin and LMWHs impede clotting by preventing fibrin formation. Treatment with unfractionated heparin is based on body weight; the dosage is titrated based on the partial thromboplastin time (PTT). Each institution sets a range for therapeutic anticoagulation based on PTT based on their available testing methods. A continuous infusion of heparin maintains a steady therapeutic blood level; in contrast to a heparin bolus every 4 to 6 h. The bolus causes peak levels for short times and subtherapeutic levels for the remaining time before another bolus is due. Heparin or LMWHs are usually continued for around 5 days or until oral anticoagulation (warfarin) can become effective. Adverse reactions associated with heparin therapy include bleeding, hyperkalemia, osteoporosis, and thrombocytopenia.

Compared with unfractionated heparin, LMWHs offer distinct advantages: they have a longer biologic half-life, they can be administered subcutaneously once or twice daily, dosing is fixed, and laboratory monitoring is not required. One disadvantage of LMWHs is that their renal elimination precludes their use in individuals with severe renal dysfunction. Aside from bleeding risks that are equivalent to heparin, LMWHs offer fewer adverse events in comparison to heparin.

Oral anticoagulants such as warfarin are often started 3 or 4 days before the heparin or LMWHs are stopped in order to avoid a period without anticoagulant therapy. Heparin or LMWHs can be stopped after combined therapy with warfarin if the international normalized ratio (INR) of prothrombin clotting time exceeds 2 for 24 h. Oral anticoagulants are usually given for at least 3 months in both provoked and unprovoked venous thromboembolism. In provoked (idiopathic) thromboembolism, consideration for life-long anticoagulation must be made.

Streptokinase, urokinase, and tissue plasminogen activator (tPA) are thrombolytic enzymes used to dissolve or lyse the emboli. These agents are administered only by intravenous infusion. Therapeutic action begins immediately and ceases with the interruption of the intravenous administration. However, residual effects may last for as long as 12 to 24 h. Thrombolytics are used in the treatment of patients with massive acute PE who are in acute right heart failure.

Surgery is reserved for those patients who do not respond to anticoagulants, who have rebound effects to heparin, or who have recurrent emboli. Procedures may include ligation or clipping of the inferior vena cava, filter placement in the vena cava, and embolectomy. Embolectomy is a serious operation and is usually reserved for massive emboli or for the decompensating patient who cannot be stabilized. The vena caval filter (inserted in the inferior vena cava) may filter emboli. The inferior vena caval filter (IVCF) will prevent further emboli from reaching the lung, thus preventing further pulmonary and hemodynamic compromises. The utilization of IVCFs has historically been the treatment of choice for DVT in those individuals with contraindications to standard anticoagulation or those with ongoing embolism despite appropriate anticoagulation therapy. Systemic anticoagulation should be provided to individuals with IVCFs after resolution of their contraindications to therapy have been resolved. Prevention of thrombus formation is critical. Patients should ambulate as much as their clinical condition allows. Elevating the legs, use of pneumatic devices and antiembolic hose, and active and passive exercises including range of motion will help prevent stasis of venous blood in nonambulating patients. It is important to educate the patient and family about risk factors of embolism development and preventive measures.

Complications

A complication of PE is pulmonary hypertension from pulmonary arterial obstruction. If the obstruction is partial or develops slowly, the patient may survive to be treated. However, if the obstruction is rapid and total, the patient may suffer sudden death. Chronic pulmonary hypertension does not usually occur with a single embolus. It usually results from multiple emboli of middle-sized vessels.

Complications of PE may include pulmonary infarction due to the extension of emboli. Any embolus that is large enough to alter hemodynamics can cause complications. These include stroke, myocardial infarction, cardiac dysrhythmias that are not amenable to therapy, liver failure and necrosis secondary to congestion, pneumonia, pulmonary abscesses, acute respiratory distress syndrome, shock, and death.

PULMONARY ASPIRATION

Pulmonary aspiration is the inhalation of foreign fluid or particulate matter into the lower airways.

Pathophysiology

Aspiration of foreign substances into the lung results in a chemical pneumonitis. When an acidic fluid is aspirated, it immediately causes alveolar-capillary breakdown, resulting in interstitial edema, intra-alveolar hemorrhage, atelectasis, increased airway resistance, and, commonly, hypoxia. These changes usually start within minutes of the initiating event and may worsen over a period of hours. Nonacidic fluid aspiration destroys surfactant and thus causes alveolar collapse, atelectasis, and hypoxia. Aspiration of particulate food matter causes both physical obstruction of the airway and a later inflammatory response caused by the presence of a foreign body. It can progress to a necrotizing process, resulting in lung abscess and empyema.

Etiology and Risk Factors

Pulmonary aspiration can be the result of inhalation of gastric contents, fluids (as in a near drowning), or saliva. Patients at risk for aspiration include the elderly and patients with neurologic compromise (e.g., a cerebral vascular accident, seizures, or dementia). Head trauma, drug and alcohol overdose, vomiting, intestinal obstruction, and gastroesophageal reflux are all risk factors for aspiration.

Signs and Symptoms

Signs and symptoms include fever, breathlessness, tachycardia, tachypnea, wheezing, cough, and pleuritic pain.

Invasive and Noninvasive Diagnostic Studies

Chest radiography may reveal patchy infiltrates or large areas of fluid in the lung. The right middle and/or lower lobes are the most common sites of infiltration. The ABGs may be normal or show a falling Pao_2 depending on the amount of the lung involved. Gram's stain and sputum cultures may be used to identify any organism.

Nursing and Collaborative Diagnoses

Diagnoses include but are not limited to:

- Impaired gas exchange related to increased shunt
- High risk for infection related to aspiration of foreign material
- Ineffective breathing pattern related to breathlessness
- Ineffective airway clearance related to retained secretions

Goals and Desired Patient Outcomes

Goals and desired patient outcomes include but are not limited to:

- Improved oxygenation
- Elimination of infection
- Reversal of breathlessness
- Removal of secretions

Management of Patient Care

Treatment of aspiration pneumonitis is mainly supportive, consisting of oxygen and ventilatory support with positive end-expiratory pressure (PEEP). Patients with particulate aspirate may need bronchoscopy to remove large obstructing pieces. Management includes bronchodilators, intravenous fluids, and aggressive pulmonary hygiene. Routine use of antibiotics is not recommended. Steroids are not recommended because they have not been shown to be effective.

Complications

The consequences of pulmonary aspiration depend on the type of material aspirated and its volume and pH. Complications include pneumonia, necrotizing pneumonitis, lung abscess, acute respiratory distress syndrome (ARDS), and empyema.

Thoracic Trauma and Air-Leak Syndromes

EDITORS' NOTE

This chapter reviews chest trauma in order to give you the information you need about the assessment and treatment of chest injuries. Chest trauma, particularly from an assessment point of view, is also better understood if it is considered along with concepts in pulmonary physiology. The PCCN exam may have questions related to thoracentesis and chest tube insertion and management. The goal of this chapter is to provide enough information to help you understand how to assess and treat key pulmonary injuries but not overwhelm you with unnecessary information.

THORACIC TRAUMA

Thoracic injuries are common in multiple traumatic injuries. The more systems involved in the trauma, the more critical each injury becomes. Thoracic injuries are especially serious in the elderly, the obese, and patients with cardiac or pulmonary disease. The older the patient, the more likely he or she is to have underlying health problems and diminished physiologic reserve. Thoracic trauma accounts for 25% of all trauma-related deaths. The injury can be the result of blunt or penetrating injury. Blunt trauma can result from direct injury to the chest or from deceleration injury. Thoracic trauma occurs in 6 of 10 motor vehicle accidents.

Pulmonary Contusion

The most common visceral injury is pulmonary contusion. The next most common visceral injury is pulmonary laceration.

Pathophysiology

Pulmonary contusion is damage to the lung parenchyma, resulting in localized edema and hemorrhage. The thorax hits an object, such as the steering wheel, compressing the thoracic cage, diminishing its size, and compressing the lungs as a result of the increased intrathoracic pressure. As the thorax rebounds from the steering wheel or other blunt traumatic force, the thoracic cage increases in size, decreasing the intrathoracic pressure and the pressure on the lung parenchyma. The lung parenchyma, under pressure, expands, rupturing capillaries and resulting in hemorrhage (Fig. 19-1). Such blunt lung injury develops over the course of 24 h, leading to poor gas exchange, increased pulmonary vascular resistance, and decreased lung compliance.

If the force of the injury is sufficient to lacerate the lungs, there is commonly bleeding, which is potentially dangerous. Laceration may occur from tearing due to rib fractures or direct puncture.

Etiology and Risk Factors

Contusions may occur as the result of blunt thoracic trauma or penetrating lung trauma. Motor vehicle crashes are the most common cause of lung contusion.

Signs and Symptoms

Depending on the severity of the trauma, symptoms may include tachypnea, tachycardia, hypoxemia, and blood-tinged secretions. Crackles may be heard throughout all lung fields as a result of retained secretions. Obvious signs of chest wall damage may be present (bruising, abrasions, broken ribs, flail chest); however, these are often absent.

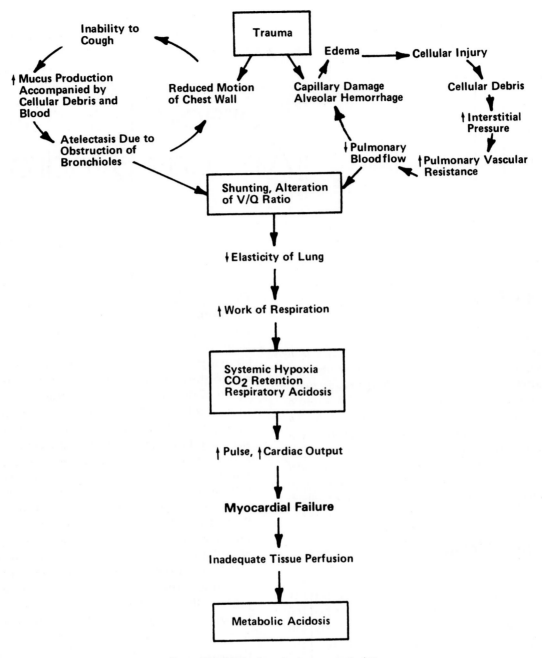

Figure 19-1. Mechanism of pulmonary contusion.

Invasive and Noninvasive Diagnostic Studies

The diagnosis of pulmonary contusion due to blunt trauma is difficult since symptoms may not occur from 24 to 72 h following trauma. Pulmonary contusion is rarely diagnosed by physical examination alone. The mechanism of injury should alert the clinician to the possibility of damage. Chest radiographs may be normal or may reveal localized opacification in the injured area. The affected area may be larger than revealed by the chest film, with the film lagging behind the development of clinical symptoms. Computed tomography (CT) is very sensitive for identification of pulmonary contusion and may allow differentiation from areas of atelectasis or aspiration. The CT scan will accurately reflect the area of damage; however, most contusions that are visible only on a CT scan are not clinically relevant in that they are not large enough to impair gas exchange and do not worsen outcome. Arterial blood gases (ABGs) will show decreased carbon dioxide ($PaCO_2$) and oxygen pressures (PaC_2) and worsening of the PaO_2/FIO_2 ratio, indicating increasing intrapulmonary shunt (Qs/Qt).

Nursing and Collaborative Diagnoses
Diagnoses include but are not limited to:

- Impaired gas exchange related to increased ventilation/perfusion (V/Q) mismatch
- Ineffective breathing pattern related to chest pain
- Pain related to thoracic injury
- Risk for fluid volume imbalance related to lung parenchymal injury
- Ineffective airway clearance related to retained secretions

Goals and Desired Patient Outcomes
Goals and desired patient outcomes include but are not limited to:

- Patent airway
- Improved oxygenation: PaO_2 above 60 mm Hg, oxygen saturation (SaO_2) at least 90% (SpO_2 >93%)
- Adequate pain control without respiratory depression
- Improved shunt fraction
- Restoration of normal lung function
- Effective airway clearance
- Fluid balance: central venous pressure (CVP) within normal levels

Management of Patient Care
Management of a pulmonary contusion is supportive, allowing for the injury to heal. If the contusion is mild, monitoring and supplemental oxygen by mask may be sufficient. Severe pulmonary contusions are treated like an acute respiratory distress syndrome (ARDS) because of the large amount of lung tissue damage, refractory hypoxemia, and decreased lung compliance. An estimated 40% of patients with pulmonary contusion will require mechanical ventilation.

Agitation and anxiety may indicate the presence of hypoxia and may be a first sign of impending deterioration. Pain from chest wall injury will affect the ability to ventilate and clear secretions. Management of a blunt chest injury, therefore, includes adequate analgesia.

Since moderate to severe pulmonary contusions are often accompanied by multisystem injuries, the fluid administration must be balanced against hemodynamic and pulmonary function. Fluid overload is associated with poor outcomes. Intake and output, CVP, and hemodynamics should be monitored. Steroids were formerly used to reduce lung edema but they are no longer recommended because they have been found to be ineffective.

Nasotracheal suctioning and humidification may help with removal of secretions.

Complications
Complications include pulmonary laceration, hemothorax, respiratory failure, atelectasis, pneumonia, and ARDS. A pulmonary contusion will usually resolve in 3 to 7 days provided that no secondary injury occurs. A pulmonary laceration occurs when the force of the injury is sufficient to lacerate the lung from a rib fracture or direct puncture, causing bleeding and hemothorax. Tracheal lacerations can occur; they are life threatening and require immediate surgery.

Fractured Ribs

Rib fractures are common injuries, which occur most often following blunt thoracic trauma but can also result from severe coughing, athletic activities (e.g., rowing, swinging golf club), or penetrating injury from gunshot wounds. Complications range from mild discomfort to life-threatening conditions such as pneumothorax, splenic laceration, and pneumonia.

Pathophysiology
It is not common to have a fracture of the first rib. Such a fracture is life threatening and indicates severe force and possible underlying thoracic and/or abdominal injuries. Fractures in ribs 1, 2, or 3 may be associated with mediastinal injury. When a very strong force is applied to the upper thoracic cage, the result is a "starburst" fracture—that is, pieces of bone going in all directions. Sternal fracture is suspected when there is paradoxical movement of the anterior chest wall.

Middle ribs (ribs 4 to 8) are the most commonly fractured. If a single rib is fractured, pain relief is usually the only treatment necessary. The intact rib on each side of the fractured rib stabilizes the fracture and keeps it in alignment for healing. Fractures of ribs 9 to 12 suggest possible laceration and/or rupture of the spleen and/or liver as well as diaphragmatic tears.

Etiology and Risk Factors
Rib fractures occur as the result of a blunt force that does not penetrate the chest wall. Motor vehicle collisions, falls, and violent assaults are the common causes of closed thoracic injury.

In an adult patient with blunt trauma, a hemothorax, pneumothorax, or pulmonary contusion seen on a chest radiograph will almost always be associated with a rib fracture, whether or not identified clinically or by radiography.

Signs and Symptoms

Symptoms include pain, dyspnea, ecchymosis, and splinting on movement. Often, point tenderness is noted over the site of the fracture. Bony crepitus may be present. The patient should be examined for neck injuries, brachial plexus injury, pneumothorax, aortic rupture or tear, and thoracic outlet syndrome.

Invasive and Noninvasive Diagnostic Studies

Rib fractures can be diagnosed by chest radiography. It may be difficult to see hairline fractures initially. Simple rib fractures are more easily seen as they begin to repair and lay down additional calcium at the injury site. Compound rib fractures and fractures with overlying bone are more easily detected by chest radiography.

Nursing and Collaborative Diagnoses

Diagnoses include but are not limited to:

- Pain related to thoracic cage injury
- Ineffective breathing pattern related to splinting of the injured area
- Impaired gas exchange related to alveolar hypoventilation

Goals and Desired Patient Outcomes

Goals and desired patient outcomes include but are not limited to:

- Pain control without ventilatory compromise
- Adequate oxygenation: PaO_2 <60 mm Hg, SaO_2 at least 90% (SpO_2 <93%)
- Stabilization of the rib fractures
- Prevention of atelectasis and pneumonia

Patient Management

Management of chest wall injury is directed toward protecting the underlying lung and allowing adequate oxygenation, ventilation, and pulmonary toilet. Management includes relief of pain so that pulmonary hygiene can be achieved. A continual epidural is one of the most efficient forms of analgesia and may be placed in the thoracic or high-lumbar position. Epidurals will provide excellent pain relief with local anesthetic and/or opioid agents and do not interfere with coughing, sighing, and deep breathing. Patient-controlled analgesia (PCA) and intercostal nerve block can also be used in relieving pain.

Bronchial hygiene and physical therapy are used to prevent the development of atelectasis and pneumonia. Binders are not recommended because they decrease excursion over a wide area of the thorax, predisposing the patient to hypoxemia and atelectasis. Sternal fractures may be stabilized internally with endotracheal intubation, mechanical ventilation, and positive end-expiratory pressure (PEEP).

Complications

Complications include atelectasis, fever, pneumonia, retained pulmonary secretions, and ARDS.

Flail Chest

The term *flail chest* refers to two or more adjacent ribs with two or more fractures, anteriorly or laterally. The flail thorax may be an especially severe injury if it is associated with a transverse fracture of the sternum. Sternal fracture is suspected when there is paradoxical movement of the anterior thoracic wall.

Pathophysiology

A section of the chest wall becomes detached from the thoracic cage. The involved portion of the thoracic wall may be so unstable that it will move paradoxically or opposite to the rest of the thoracic wall when the patient breathes (Fig. 19-2). During

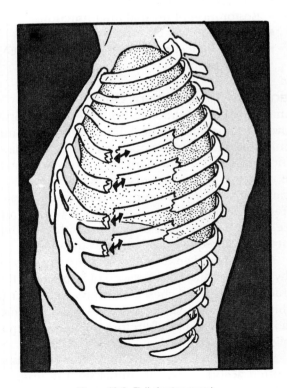

Figure 19-2. Flail chest segment.

inspiration, negative intrathoracic pressure increases and the chest wall moves outward. With a flail chest, the injured segment moves inward. On expiration, intrathoracic pressure decreases, the chest wall moves inward, and the flail section moves outward. This results in atelectasis and alveolar collapse because the alveoli cannot fill with air.

Etiology and Risk Factors

Causes include fight injuries, motor vehicle collisions, blast injuries, and athletic injuries.

Signs and Symptoms

Symptoms of flail injuries to the thorax include rapid, shallow respirations, cyanosis, severe thoracic wall pain, shock, bony crepitation at the site of fracture, and paradoxical thoracic movement. There may be signs of pulmonary contusion, bruised thorax, and tender chest on palpation. Hypotension, tachycardia, hypoxemia, and hemoptysis may also be present.

Invasive and Noninvasive Diagnostic Studies

Chest radiography confirms the diagnosis of flail chest. The ABGs may show a falling PaO_2, increasing $PaCO_2$, and a pH below 7.35, indicating respiratory acidosis.

Nursing and Collaborative Diagnoses

Diagnoses include but are not limited to:

- Impaired gas exchange related to alveolar hypoventilation
- Ineffective breathing pattern related to a flailing chest wall segment
- Pain related to chest wall injury

Goals and Desired Patient Outcomes

Goals and desired patient outcomes include but are not limited to:

- Adequate oxygenation: PaO_2 at least 60 mm Hg, SaO_2 at least 90% (SpO_2 >93%)
- Stabilization of flail segment
- Prevention of atelectasis and pneumonia
- Maintenance of fluid balance
- Avoidance or removal of retained secretions

Patient Management

Specific treatment of flail chest is stabilization of the flail segment and restoration of normal breathing. In an emergency, anything can be used to stabilize the thoracic wall and help immobilize the segment, (e.g., sandbags or hands). In the critical care unit,

intubation, positive-pressure ventilation, and PEEP may be used to stabilize the flailing segment. Neuromuscular blockade may be used to paralyze the patient and allow the ventilator to help stabilize the chest wall. Adequate sedation and analgesia must be provided when neuromuscular blockade is used.

Pain control is a top priority. Patients are medicated to achieve adequate pain control and reduce the work of breathing. The strategies for controlling pain with rib fractures can also be utilized with a flail chest.

Complications

Complications include pulmonary contusion, pneumothorax, hypoxia, pulmonary laceration, and cardiac contusion.

Hemothorax

Hemothorax is an accumulation of blood in the thorax. It is often accompanied by a pneumothorax.

Pathophysiology

The three major effects of a hemothorax are the accumulation of blood in the lungs, collapsing alveoli, and systemic hypovolemia. Shock can occur quickly with the development of a hemothorax. Trauma to the thorax may cause bleeding from the intercostal, pleural, lung parenchymal, or mediastinal vessels or from the internal mammary artery. As blood fills the pleural space, the underlying lung tissue is compressed, causing alveolar collapse. A hemothorax may be self-limiting, especially if its origin is venous. As the blood accumulates in the chest, the increasing pressure may reduce or stop the source of bleeding. Arterial injury, which is less common, will not be self-limiting.

Etiology

Hemothorax is caused by blunt or penetrating thoracic trauma, iatrogenic causes, lacerated liver, or perforated diaphragm. It may also result from thoracic surgery, anticoagulant therapy, or a dissecting thoracic aneurysm.

Signs and Symptoms

The symptoms of a hemothorax depend on the size of the blood accumulation. Small amounts of blood (i.e., 400 mL or less) will cause minimal symptoms. Larger amounts of blood (i.e., 400 mL or more) usually present with signs of shock: tachycardia, tachypnea, hypotension, and anxiety. Breath sounds may be diminished or absent, and the chest is dull on percussion.

Invasive and Noninvasive Diagnostic Studies

The chest film may show pleural fluid or a mediastinal shift. The ABGs will show a normal or decreased PaO_2, an increased $PaCO_2$, and a falling pH. If there has been a large amount of bleeding, the hematocrit and hemoglobin levels may be decreased. Central venous pressure or positive airway pressure (PAP) may be low if fluid volume depletion is evident. Ultrasound examination can detect smaller hemothoraces, although in the presence of a pneumothorax or subcutaneous air, ultrasound may be difficult or inaccurate. A CT scan will detect a hemothorax and is especially useful in identifying one in the presence of other multiple traumatic injuries.

Thoracentesis is used for both diagnosis and treatment. A large-bore needle is inserted into the chest and aspirated for blood or serosanguineous fluid.

Nursing and Collaborative Diagnoses

Diagnoses include but are not limited to:

- Impaired gas exchange related to alveolar hypoventilation
- Ineffective breathing pattern related to decreased lung volume
- Fluid volume deficit related to hemorrhage
- Pain related to thoracic injury
- High risk for infection related to traumatic injury
- Anxiety related to pain and traumatic injury

Goals and Desired Patient Outcomes

Goals and desired patient outcomes include but are not limited to:

- Stabilizing the patient's hemodynamic status
- Adequate oxygenation: PaO_2 at least 60 mm Hg, SaO_2 at least 90% (SpO_2 >93%)
- Restoring and maintaining fluid balance
- Reexpansion of the affected lung
- Control of pain
- Reduction of anxiety

Patient Management

Small hemothoraces may resolve spontaneously because of low pulmonary system pressure and the presence of thromboplastin in the lungs. Large hemothoraces are treated with the insertion of one or more thoracic tubes in the fifth or sixth intercostal space in the midaxillary line (Fig. 19-3). The thoracic tube is sutured in place and covered with a sterile dressing after being connected to an underwater seal with suction. Autotranfusion may be used

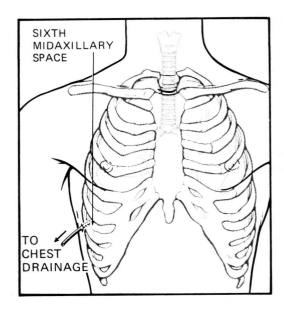

Figure 19-3. Chest tube insertion for hemothorax.

for patients with a blood loss of 1 L or more. Severe or uncontrollable hemothorax may require thoracotomy to remove the blood and fluid from the lung and correct the source of bleeding. Adequate venous access is critical so that fluid resuscitation and blood product administration can occur.

It is important to monitor the patient's ability to expel secretions and to suction when necessary so as to prevent hypoxia and atelectasis. Analgesics are recommended for relief of pain.

Complications

Complications of a hemothorax include atelectasis, lung collapse, hypoxemia, and mediastinal shift. Failure to adequately drain a hemothorax initially results in residual clotted hemothorax, which will not drain via a chest tube. If left untreated, these retained hemothoraces may become infected and lead to empyema formation.

Diaphragmatic Rupture

Pathophysiology

The immediate result of a significant tear in the diaphragm is herniation of the abdominal contents into the thoracic cavity. The rupture allows air to enter the thorax, causing increasing intrathoracic pressure. In the majority of cases, the left hemidiaphragm is injured, perhaps because of the protection by the liver on the right side.

Etiology and Risk Factors

Rupture of the diaphragm is associated with both blunt and penetrating trauma, especially gunshot wounds of the lower abdomen and chest. The incidence of diaphragmatic rupture is doubled in patients with a fractured pelvis. It is almost always accompanied by intraperitoneal and multisystem injuries.

Signs and Symptoms

Symptoms are related to the amount of herniated viscera in the thorax. Primary symptoms of a ruptured or herniated diaphragm include auscultation of bowel sounds in the chest, increasing shortness of breath, unequal diaphragmatic movement on palpation, elevated diaphragm and hyperresonance to percussion, marked or increasing respiratory distress, severe shoulder pain on the same side as the tear, and shock.

Invasive and Noninvasive Diagnostic Studies

The initial chest film may be normal in 50% of cases of rupture of the diaphragm. The chest film may reveal an elevated, arched shadow of a high left hemidiaphragm, a mediastinal shift to the right, shadows above the diaphragm, and abnormal air-fluid levels. The chest film may also reveal a nasogastric tube in the left thorax or air bubbles in the left chest, indicating visceral herniation. Ultrasound and CT can also be useful in making the diagnosis of diaphragmatic rupture. The CT scan is the best available test to confirm the diagnosis.

Nursing and Collaborative Diagnoses

Diagnoses include but are not limited to:

- Impaired gas exchange related to alveolar hypoventilation
- Ineffective breathing pattern related to increased intrathoracic pressure
- Fluid-volume deficit related to hemorrhage
- Pain related to thoracic injury
- High risk for infection related to traumatic injury
- Anxiety related to pain and traumatic injury

Goals and Desired Patient Outcomes

Goals and desired patient outcomes include but are not limited to:

- Stabilizing the patient's hemodynamic status
- Adequate oxygenation: PaO_2 at least 60 mm Hg, SaO_2 at least 90% (SpO_2 >93%)
- Control of pain
- Reduction of anxiety
- Surgical repair of the rupture

Management of Patient Care

Immediate treatment of rupture of the diaphragm is to establish adequate respiratory function. This is most frequently accomplished by endotracheal intubation and mechanical respiration. It may or may not be possible to stabilize a patient in shock prior to surgery depending on the severity of the rupture. Definitive therapy consists of surgical repair of the torn diaphragm and replacement of the abdominal organs in the abdominal cavity.

The patient's respiratory status should be monitored to ensure adequate oxygenation. Increased intrathoracic pressure and abdominal contents in the thoracic cavity will usually cause marked hemodynamic compromise.

Complications

Complications include strangulation of the bowel or bowel obstruction, cardiovascular collapse, and death.

AIR-LEAK SYNDROMES

A pneumothorax is accumulation of air in the pleural space. It may be the result of blunt or penetrating trauma or rupture of a bleb or emphysematous bulla, or it may have an iatrogenic cause, such as mechanical ventilation or high levels of PEEP (Table 19-1). There are three types of pneumothorax: closed, open, and tension.

TABLE 19-1. SIGNS AND SYMPTOMS OF PNEUMOTHORAX

Inspection
Asymmetrical chest wall movement
Hyperexpansion
Chest wall rigidity on the affected side
Palpation
Subcutaneous emphysema
Decreased vocal fremitus
Mediastinal shift
Tracheal deviation
Tympany on the affected side
Percussion
Hyperresonance on the affected side
Auscultation
Decreased or absent breath sounds on the affected side

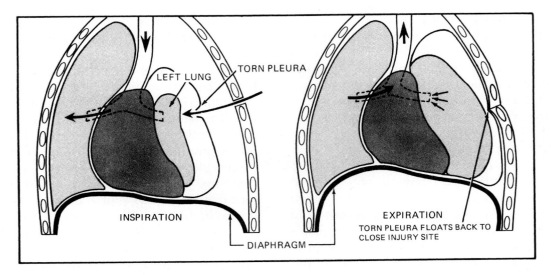

Figure 19-4. Open pneumothorax.

The closed pneumothorax occurs when air enters the pleural space through the airways. If the air cannot escape the chest, intrapleural pressure increases, pressure on the other lung and the heart will continue, and a tension pneumothorax is possible.

An open pneumothorax is caused by a penetrating injury that allows air to enter and exit the pleural space (Fig. 19-4). The open pneumothorax is less dangerous than a closed pneumothorax because of the reduced likelihood of developing a tension pneumothorax.

Tension pneumothorax is potentially life threatening. Air accumulates in the pleural space but cannot escape. During inhalation, air is sucked into the pleura through a tear; on exhalation, the torn pleura closes against the parenchyma, creating a one-way valve that prevents the air from being exhaled (Fig. 19-5).

Pathophysiology

The lungs are contained in the visceral pleura. The parietal pleura line the thorax. The potential area between these two pleura, the pleural space, is lined by a thin layer of lubrication. If air or fluid enters the space, the surfaces are separated. The pressure of the intrapleural space is -5 cm H_2O. When air or fluid

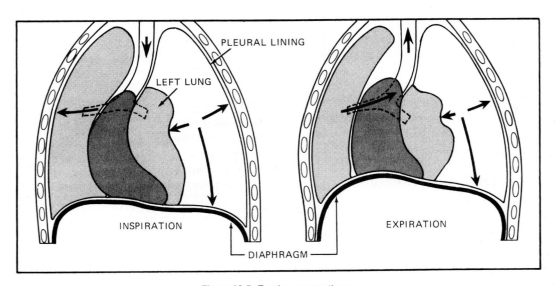

Figure 19-5. Tension pneumothorax.

enters the pleural space, the pressure becomes positive. This positive pressure leads to lung collapse, decreased lung compliance, decreased total lung capacity, and decreased vital capacity. Hypoxia is the result of the increasing V/Q mismatch. If the pressure cannot escape, as in tension pneumothorax, the intrathoracic pressure continues to build, leading to hemodynamic compromise and cardiovascular collapse.

The tension pneumothorax quickly produces hemodynamic and cardiopulmonary compromise. On inspiration, more air is drawn in through the tear; however, it has nowhere to escape. The accumulation of air in the thorax causes increasing intrathoracic pressure that leads to severe hemodynamic imbalances.

Signs and Symptoms

A simple pneumothorax may present with only mild respiratory distress, asymmetric chest wall expansion, vague complaints of difficulty in catching the breath, and chest pain (Table 19-1).

Tension pneumothorax produces symptoms that include dyspnea and restlessness, progressive cyanosis, diminished or absent breath sounds on the affected side, decreased chest wall movement, signs of increasing respiratory distress, chest pain and tracheal shift toward the *unaffected* side, asymmetric chest wall movement, and rigidity on the affected side. The mediastinum, trachea, and point of maximum intensity (PMI) all shift away from the affected side. If the patient is on volume-limited mechanical ventilation, the peak airway pressure will increase; and if the resistance is great enough, the high-pressure alarm will activate and the patient will not receive the full set tidal volume. Patients who are on pressure-limited mechanical ventilation will demonstrate a decreased tidal volume, but since the pressure is limited, it will remain unchanged. A tension pneumothorax is a medical emergency requiring immediate treatment.

Invasive and Noninvasive Diagnostic Studies

The chest film will show an accumulation of air in the pleural space. A mediastinal shift may be evident. The ABGs will show a decreased PaO_2 and an increased pH (respiratory alkalosis) due to the tachypnea. If respiratory compromise occurs, a rising $PaCO_2$ and a falling pH will be seen.

Nursing and Collaborative Diagnoses

Diagnoses include but are not limited to:

- Impaired gas exchange related to decreased lung tissue for ventilation
- Ineffective breathing pattern related to the collapsed lung
- Anxiety related to increasing difficulty in breathing
- Dyspnea related to decreased alveolar ventilation
- Risk for decreased cardiac output related to increased intrapulmonary pressures

Goals and Desired Patient Outcomes

Goals and desired patient outcomes include but are not limited to:

- Reexpansion of the collapsed lung
- Adequate oxygenation
- Maintenance of cardiac output
- Reduction and control of pain
- Maintenance of chest drainage system

Patient Management

A small pneumothorax may not require treatment. If no serious breathing problems occur, the air will be reabsorbed in a few days. Drainage of air and fluid from the pleural space requires an evacuation system that allows air and fluids to exit but not to reenter. If the pneumothorax is small enough, needle aspiration or thoracentesis may be sufficient treatment to reexpand the lung. Smaller catheters are being used to evacuate air from the thorax, resulting in less traumatic punctures and increased patient comfort. A catheter with a flutter valve may be used to allow the air to escape without reaccumulating. Because of the small diameter of the tubes, they are not recommended for draining fluid or blood.

If a tension pneumothorax is suspected and the patient is experiencing hemodynamic compromise, decompression with a needle is necessary before placement of a chest tube. Tension pneumothorax is a life-threatening condition that demands urgent management. If this diagnosis is suspected, do not delay treatment in the interest of confirming the diagnosis. Although a needle thoracostomy is not the definitive treatment for tension pneumothorax, emergent needle decompression does arrest its progression and serves to restore cardiopulmonary function. Insert a large-bore (i.e., 14- or 16-gauge) needle with a catheter into the second intercostal space, just superior to the third rib at the midclavicular line, 1 to 2 cm from the sternal edge. Listen for the hissing sound of air escaping, and remove the needle while leaving the catheter in place.

If a chest tube is used, it is inserted in the second or third intercostal space at the midclavicular line to remove the air (Fig. 19-6). Chest tubes are sutured in place and connected to a water-seal or suction drainage system. The insertion site of the tube is covered with a sterile dressing and connected to a water-seal drainage system.

The most common pleural units are single plastic units that can serve as one-, two-, or three-chamber units depending on the patient's needs. Some pleural units place a collection chamber before the water-seal chamber to avoid the effect of increasing resistance to air evacuation. As fluid accumulates in the water seal, the hydrostatic resistance to air leaving the pleural space increases. The collection chamber before the water-seal chamber reduces this problem. The water seal is situated at the end of the pleural tube to provide minimal resistance to pressure changes in the pleural space. Suction chambers have been developed to accelerate reexpansion of the pleural space. Although the value of suction is controversial, many physicians routinely order low-suction levels between 10 and 40 cm H_2O. Low levels are employed to avoid injury to pulmonary parenchymal tissue.

Air leaving the pleural space is readily seen by the bubbling in the water-seal chamber. When air has ceased leaking from the pleural space, this bubbling ceases. Evacuation of fluid is noted by measuring the amount of fluid in the collection chamber.

For the evacuation of air, chest tubes are placed superiorly and anteriorly in a patient lying flat, near the second intercostal space in the midclavicular line. Chest tubes are placed in gravity-dependent positions, near the fifth intercostal space in the midaxillary line, to facilitate fluid evacuation. Placement lower than the fifth intercostal space increases the risk of puncturing abdominal viscera.

Chest tubes should not be clamped if bubbling is present in the water-seal chamber. There is the potential for a tension pneumothorax in a situation where a tube is clamped while air is still exiting the pleural space. If no air is leaking from the pleural space, the clamping of a chest tube is generally not a problem, provided that there is no major accumulation of blood. In the event the pleural drainage system is accidentally broken or severely cracked, allowing atmospheric pressure into the system, insert the uncontaminated end of the connective tubing into a bottle of sterile water or saline to a depth of 2 cm until a new unit can be set up.

Milking and stripping of chest tubes is not recommended, as it has been shown to create suction pressures of up to −400 cm H_2O. This can cause damage to lung tissue and disruption of suture lines.

Chest films are used to verify the position of the chest tubes and monitor the reexpansion of the lung.

Complications

Complications of pneumothorax depend on the patient's size, rate of development, and underlying cardiopulmonary status. Cardiac and pulmonary failure can result from the sudden development of a large pneumothorax or a tension pneumothorax.

BIBLIOGRAPHY

The Acute Respiratory Distress Syndrome Network (2000). Ventilation with low tidal volumes as compared with traditional tidal volume for acute lung injury and acute respiratory distress syndrome. *New England Journal of Medicine, 342,* 1301–1307.

Ahrens, T. (2004). Monitoring carbon dioxide in critical care: The newest vital sign? *Critical Care Nursing Clinics of North America, 16*(3), 445–451.

Ahrens, T., Kollef, M., Stewart, J., & Shannon, W. (2004). Effect of kinetic therapy on pulmonary complications. *American Journal of Critical Care, 13*(5), 376–383.

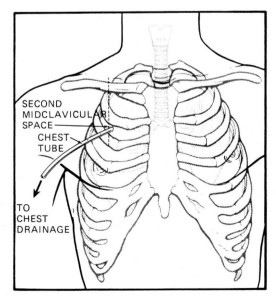

Figure 19-6. Chest tube insertion for removal of air.

Alsaghir, A. H., & Martin, C. M. (2008). Effect of prone positioning in patients with acute respiratory distress syndrome: A meta-analysis. *Critical Care Medicine, 36,* 603.

The ARDS Clinical Trial Network; National Heart, Lung and Blood Institute; National Institute of Health (2003). Effects of recruitment maneuvers in patients with acute lung injury and acute respiratory distress syndrome ventilated with high positive end expiratory pressure. *Critical Care Medicine, 31,* 2592–2597.

Barnes, PJ. (2000). Chronic obstructive pulmonary disease. *New England Journal of Medicine, 343,* 269–280.

Bokhari, F., Brakenridge, S., & Nagy, K. (2002). Prospective evaluation of the sensitivity of physical examination in chest trauma. *Journal of Trauma, 53*(6), 1135–1138.

Bonten,M. J., Kollef, M. H., & Hall, J. B. (2004). Risk factors for ventilator pneumonia: From epidemiology to patient management. *Clinical Infectious Diseases, 38,* 1141–1149.

Brochard, L., Ranes, A., Benito S., et al. (1994). Comparison of three methods of gradual withdrawal from ventilatory support during weaning from mechanical ventilation. *American Journal of Respiratory and Critical Care Medicine, 150,* 896–903.

Brook, A. D., Ahrens, T. S., Schraff, R., et al. (1999). Effect of a nursing-implemented sedation protocol on the duration of mechanical ventilation. *Critical Care Medicine, 27,* 2609–2615.

Buist, A. S. (2003). Similarities and differences between asthma and chronic obstructive pulmonary disease: Treatment and early outcome. *European Respiratory Journal, 21,* 30S–35S.

Burns, S. (2005). Mechanical ventilation of patients with acute respiratory distress syndrome and patients requiring weaning: The evidence to guide practice. *Critical Care Nurse, 25,* 14–23.

Busse, W. W., & Lemanske, R. F. (2001). Asthma. *New England Journal of Medicine, 344,* 350–362.

Chan, S. S. (2003). Emergency bedside ultrasound to detect pneumothorax. *Academy of Emergency Medicine, 10*(1), 91–94.

Chastre, J., & Fagon J. Y. (2002). Ventilator-associated pneumonia. *American Journal of Respiratory and Critical Care Medicine, 165,* 867–903.

Collins, J. (2000). Chest wall trauma. *Journal of Thoracic Imaging, 15*(2), 112–119.

Derdak, S., Mehta, A., Stewart, T. E., et al. (2002). High frequency oscillatory ventilation for acute respiratory distress syndrome in adults. *American Journal of Respiratory and Critical Care Medicine, 166,* 801-808.

Erickson, S. E., Martin, G. S., Davis, L. J., el al. (2009). Recent trends in acute lung injury mortality:1996–2005. *Critical Care Medicine, 37,* 1574.

Esteban, A., Frutos, F., Tobin, M. J., et al. (1995). A comparison of four methods of weaning patients from mechanical ventilation: Spanish Lung Failure Collaborative Group. *New England Journal of Medicine, 332,* 345–350.

Farber, H. W., & Loscalzo, J. (2004). Pulmonary hypertension. *New England Journal of Medicine, 351,* 1655.

Fedullo, P. F., & Tapson, V. F. (2003). The evaluation of suspected pulmonary embolism. *New England Journal of Medicine, 349,* 1247–1256.

Forsythe, S. M., & Schmidt, G. A. (2000). Sodium bicarbonate for the treatment of lactic acidosis. *Chest, 117,* 260–267.

Hagler, D. A., & Traver, G. A. (1994). Endotracheal saline and suction catheters: Sources of lower airway contamination. *American Journal Critical Care, 3,* 444–447.

Ho, M. L., & Gutierrez, F. R. (2009). Chest radiography in thoracic polytrauma. *American Journal of Roentgenology, 192,* 599.

Hull, R. D., Raskob, G. E., Rollin, F., et al. (2000). Low-molecular-weight heparin vs heparin in the treatment of patients with pulmonary embolism. *Archives of Internal Medicine, 160,* 229–235.

Johnson, J. L., & Hirsch, C. S. (2003). Aspiration pneumonia. *Postgraduate Medicine, 113*(3), 99–112.

Karmakar, M. K., & Ho, A.M. (2003). Acute pain management in patients with multiple rib fractures. *Journal of Trauma, 54,* 615.

Kollef, M. H. (1999). The prevention of ventilator-associated pneumonia. *New England Journal of Medicine, 340,* 627–634.

Kollef, M. H., Shapiro, S. D., Fraser V., et al. (1995). Mechanical ventilation with and without 7 day circuit changes. A randomized controlled trial. *Annals of Internal Medicine, 123,* 168–174.

Kollef, M. H., Prentice, D, Shapiro, S. D., et al. (1997a). Mechanical ventilation with and without daily changes of in-line suction catheter. *American Journal of Respiratory and Critical Care Medicine, 156,* 466–472.

Kollef, M. H., Shapiro, S. D., Silver, P., et al. (1997b). A randomized controlled trial of protocol-directed versus physician directed weaning from mechanical ventilation. *Critical Care Medicine, 25,* 567–574.

Kress, J. P., Pohlman, A. S., O'Connor, M. F., & Hall, J. B. (2000). Daily interruption of sedative infusions in critically ill patients undergoing mechanical ventilation. *New England Journal of Medicine, 342,* 1471–1477.

Mandell, L. A., Wunderink, R. G., Azueto, A., et al. (2007). Infectious Disease Society of America/American Thoracic Society consensus guidelines on the management guidelines of community-acquired pneumonia in adults. *Clinical Infectious Diseases, 44,* s2-s27.

McLaughlin, V. V., Archer, S. L., Badesch, D. B., et al. (2009). ACCF/AHA 2009 expert consensus document on pulmonary hypertension: A report of the American College of Cardiology Foundation Task Force on Expert Consensus Documents and the American Heart Association: Developed in collaboration with the American College of Chest Physicians, American Thoracic Society, and the Pulmonary Hypertension Association. *Circulation, 119,* 2250.

Meade, M. O., Cook, D. J., Guyatt, G. H., et al. (2008). Ventilation strategy using low tidal volumes, recruitment maneuvers, and high positive end expiratory pressures for acute lung injury and acute respiratory distress syndrome: A randomized control trial. *Journal of the American Medical Association, 299,* 637.

Nijkeuter, M., Sohne, M., Tick, L. W., et al. (2007). The natural course of hemodynamically stable pulmonary embolism: clinical outcomes and risk factors in a large prospective cohort study. *Chest, 131,* 517.

Papazian, L., Gainnier, M., Marin, V., Donati, S., et al. (2005). Comparison of prone positioning and high-frequency oscillatory ventilation in patients with acute respiratory distress syndrome. *Critical Care Medicine, 33,* 2162–2171.

Pierre, E. J., & Candiotti K. A. (2009). Basic concepts of trauma care. *Current Review of Nurse Anesthetists, 32*(7), 81.

Riedel, M. (2004). Diagnosis of pulmonary embolism. *Postgraduate Medicine Journal, 80,* 309–319.

Rose, L., & Hawkins, M. (2008). Airway pressure release ventilation and biphasic positive airway pressure: a systematic review of definitional criteria. *Intensive Care Medicine, 34,* 1766.

Safdar, N., Dezfulian, C., Collard, H. R., & Saint, S. (2005). Clinical and economic consequences of ventilator associated pneumonia: A systematic review. *Critical Care Medicine, 33,* 2184–2193.

Shang, X. L., Zhang, Y. Z., & Zhang, X. L. (2002). Diagnoses of bronchus and lung trauma by computed tomography and x-ray examination in 37 cases: A comparative study. *Di Yi Jun Yi Da Xue Xue Bao, 22*(4), 380–381.

Sutyak, J. P., Wholtmann, C. D., & Larson, J. (2007). Pulmonary contusions and critical care management in thoracic trauma. *Thoracic Surgery Clinics, 17,* 11.

Swanson, K. L., & Edell, E. S. (2001). Tracheobronchial foreign bodies. *Chest Surgery Clinics of North America, 11*(4), 861–872.

Tang, B. M. P., Craig, J. C., Eslick, G. D., et al. (2009). Use of corticosteroids in acute lung injury and acute respiratory distress syndrome: A systematic review and meta-analysis. *Critical Care Medicine, 37,* 1594.

Tapson, V. F. (2008). Acute pulmonary embolism. *New England Journal of Medicine, 358,* 1037.

Van der Molen, T., Ostrem A., Stallberg B., et al. (2006). International primary care respiratory group (IPCRG) guidelines: Management of asthma. *Primary Care Respiratory Journal, 15,* 35.

Ware, L. B., & Matthay, M. A. (2005). Clinical practice: acute pulmonary edema. *New England Journal of Medicine, 353,* 2788.

Weinert, C. R., Gross, C. R., & Marinelli, W. A. (2003). Impact of randomized results on acute lung injury ventilation therapy in teaching hospitals. *American Journal of Respiratory and Critical Care Medicine, 167,* 1304–1309.

West, J. B. (2004). *Pulmonary Physiology—The Essentials,* 7th ed. Baltimore, MD: Lippincott Williams & Wilkins.

Pulmonary Practice Exam

Question 1 refers to the following scenario:

A 51-year-old man is in the intensive care unit with the diagnosis of acute respiratory failure, possibly secondary to sepsis. His last vital signs and laboratory data were as follows:

Blood pressure	108/60 mm Hg
Pulse	70 (normal sinus rhythm)
Respiratory rate	12
Temperature	38.8
Pulse oximetry (SpO$_2$)	0.99
pH	7.52
PaCO$_2$	29
PaO$_2$	109
HCO$_3^-$	29

1. Based on the above ABGs, what is your interpretation of this patient's condition?
   (A) Uncompensated respiratory alkalosis
   (B) Respiratory acidosis with a compensating metabolic alkalosis
   (C) Compensated metabolic alkalosis
   (D) Uncompensated respiratory acidosis

2. The upper airway serves three of the key functions listed below. Select the one function that is NOT served by the upper airway.
   (A) Humidification of air
   (B) Removal of particles
   (C) Warming of inspired air
   (D) Participation in gas exchange

3. Which part of the trachea is relatively avascular, allowing for emergency placement of artificial airways in this area?
   (A) Thyroid cartilage
   (B) Cricothyroid cartilage
   (C) Laryngopharynx
   (D) Glottis

4. The left and right mainstem bronchi divide from the trachea at which of the following locations?
   (A) Carina
   (B) Sternoclavicular junction
   (C) Lingula
   (D) Larynx

5. Right mainstem bronchus intubations are more likely to be performed than left bronchus intubations for which of the following reasons?
   (A) The right mainstem bronchus has more ciliary clearance of mucus, facilitating passage of the endotracheal tube.
   (B) The left mainstem bronchus is located several inches lower than the right.
   (C) The left mainstem bronchus, although wider than the right, sits posterior to the right mainstem bronchus.
   (D) The right mainstem bronchus is wider and has less angulation than the left.

Questions 6 through 8 refer to the following scenario:

A 69-year-old woman is admitted at 0700 with persistent right-sided chest pain that is not affected by respiration or position. She had a V/Q scan at 0900 that showed intermediate probability for a pulmonary embolism. The pain fluctuates and is now not very severe. She has crackles in her right middle lobe. Her ECG shows no signs of ischemia. She is not intubated but is on a 35% high-humidity face mask. She has the following vital signs and ABGs:

Blood pressure	94/56 mm Hg
Pulse	108 (sinus tachycardia)
Respiratory rate	26
Temperature	36.7
SpO$_2$	0.98

pH	7.26
$Paco_2$	30
Pao_2	98
HCO_3^-	18
Lactate	4.8

The patient's physician has told you that he would call at about 1600 (4 P.M.). The current time is 1100. You are to call him only if her physical or laboratory values are SIGNIFICANTLY abnormal.

6. Based on the above information, interpret the ABGs.
   (A) Respiratory alkalosis with a compensating metabolic acidosis
   (B) Metabolic acidosis with a compensating respiratory alkalosis
   (C) Uncompensated respiratory alkalosis
   (D) Uncompensated metabolic acidosis

7. Based on the above information, what is your interpretation of her oxygenation status?
   (A) She shows signs of poor tissue oxygenation based on the elevated lactate, low HCO_3, and pH.
   (B) Her oxygenation is adequate at present based on the normal Spo_2 and Pao_2.
   (C) Her oxygenation is inadequate based on the Fio_2 of 0.35, generating a Pao_2 of only 98.
   (D) Her oxygenation is adequate at present based on the Fio_2 of 0.35, generating a Pao_2 of only 98 and an Spo_2 of 0.98.

8. What intervention should you make at this time?
   (A) Do not notify the physician but increase the Fio_2 per standing orders.
   (B) Notify the physician because of significantly abnormal values.
   (C) Wait until the physician calls at 1600 to report because while some values are abnormal, they are not significantly abnormal.
   (D) Continue to monitor the patient but make no changes in her current therapy.

9. What is the name of the lipoprotein secreted by alveolar type II cells that promotes alveolar expansion by increasing the surface tension of the alveoli?
   (A) Surfactant
   (B) Phagocytes
   (C) Alveolar epithelium
   (D) Pulmonary parenchyma

10. Cheyne-Stokes breathing is characterized by which of the following respiratory patterns?
    (A) Rapid shallow breathing
    (B) Short periods of apnea followed by respirations of increasing depth that then slow again to apnea
    (C) Regular deep breathing patterns that alternate with shallow breathing patterns over a period of several minutes
    (D) Slow deep breaths

11. Normal arterial Po_2 levels (at sea level) fall within which of the following ranges?
    (A) 20 to 35 mm Hg
    (B) 35 to 45 mm Hg
    (C) 60 to 80 mm Hg
    (D) 80 to 100 mm Hg

12. Normal arterial hemoglobin saturation (Sao_2) falls within which of the following range?
    (A) 0.40 to 0.60
    (B) 0.60 to 0.80
    (C) 0.80 to 0.90
    (D) Greater than 0.95

13. In comparison of finger oximetry values (Spo_2) with Sao_2 levels, which of the following statements is most accurate?
    (A) Spo_2 values underestimate Sao_2 values.
    (B) Spo_2 values overestimate Sao_2 values.
    (C) Spo_2 values should equal Sao_2 values.
    (D) Spo_2 values do not correlate with Sao_2 values.

Questions 14 and 15 refer to the following scenario:

A 75-year-old man is admitted to the unit with the diagnosis of pneumonia. He is short of breath and has circumoral cyanosis. He has crackles throughout both lungs. His initial ABGs and vital signs are:

Blood pressure	122/62	pH	7.25
Pulse	114	$Paco_2$	53
Respiratory rate	30	Pao_2	34
Temperature	37.4	HCO_3^-	25
Spo_2	0.77		

The physician requests the following:

I. Place him on 40% oxygen via a face mask.
II. Start gentamicin 80 mg IV tid.
III. Do not give sedatives.

The physician asks that you call when there are any changes that indicate the patient's condition is worsening. After you start the oxygen, the circumoral cyanosis goes away. The patient states he feels about the same. His repeat ABGs and vital signs reveal:

Blood pressure	116/58	pH	7.21
Pulse	115	$Paco_2$	59
Respiratory rate	30	Pao_2	61
Temperature	37.5	HCO_3^-	25
Spo_2	0.91		

14. Based on the above information, what do you think of the patient's condition?
    (A) He is getting better based on his improved Spo_2 and Pao_2.
    (B) He is about the same based on his blood pressure, pulse, respiratory rate, and HCO_3^-.
    (C) He is getting worse based on his pH and $Paco_2$.
    (D) You cannot tell from the data provided if the patient is better or worse.

15. What action is necessary, if any, for the above situation?
    (A) No action is necessary because he has improved.
    (B) Call the physician based on the abnormal data.
    (C) Repeat ABGs in 1 h but do not call the physician because the patient's condition has not markedly changed.
    (D) Continue to monitor the patient but make no changes in his current therapy.

16. Which of the following best describes vital capacity?
    (A) Maximal inspiration followed by maximal expiration
    (B) Normal inspiratory volumes
    (C) The amount of air vital to the person in 1 min
    (D) The amount of air in the lungs at rest

17. The amount of air that does NOT participate in gas exchange is referred to by which of the following terms?
    (A) Minute ventilation
    (B) Alveolar ventilation
    (C) Dead-space ventilation
    (D) Bronchial ventilation

18. Which of the following is the most common cause of hypoxemia?
    (A) Diffusion barriers
    (B) Hypoventilation
    (C) Changes in barometric pressure
    (D) Intrapulmonary shunts

19. Which of the following is an estimate of intrapulmonary shunting?
    (A) Pao_2/Fio_2 ratio
    (B) Diffusion capacity
    (C) Mixed venous oxygen tensions
    (D) FEV_1 (forced expiratory volume in 1 s)

20. Which of the following is the best description of Fio_2 (fraction of inspired oxygen)?
    (A) The molecular weight of oxygen
    (B) The percentage of oxygen during inspiration
    (C) The amount of oxygen (in milliliters) during inspiration
    (D) The fraction of oxygen versus carbon dioxide during inspiration

21. Which of the following would be a normal oxygen tension (Pao_2) on exposure to 100% oxygen?
    (A) 60 to 100 mm Hg
    (B) 100 to 250 mm Hg
    (C) 250 to 400 mm Hg
    (D) 400 to 600 mm Hg

22. The oxyhemoglobin dissociation curve is best described as illustrating which of the following?
    (A) The ability of oxygen to dissociate into different ions
    (B) The amount of oxygen carried in the blood per minute
    (C) The amount of oxygen carried in the dissolved state
    (D) The ability of hemoglobin to bind with oxygen

23. An acid is best described as which of the following?
    (A) A substance that gives up a hydrogen ion
    (B) A substance that accepts a hydrogen ion
    (C) An entity preventing oxygen from taking the electron split from hydrogen
    (D) A substance that depletes free-floating hydrogen from the blood

24. The pulmonary response to a change in hydrogen ion concentration occurs in which time frame?
    (A) Within 24 h
    (B) Within 48 h
    (C) Within 1 week
    (D) Within 5 min

25. The renal response to a change in hydrogen ion concentration occurs in which time frame?
(A) Within 24 h
(B) Within 48 h
(C) Within 1 week
(D) Within 5 min

26. Which of the following is the basis for the primary renal buffering mechanism for a change in hydrogen ion level?
(A) Bicarbonate
(B) Phosphate
(C) Protein
(D) Sulfate

Questions 27 through 33 require you to interpret a set of blood gas values:

27. What is the correct interpretation of the following blood gas values?

pH	7.35
$Paco_2$	72
HCO_3^-	41

(A) Respiratory acidosis alone
(B) Respiratory acidosis with compensating metabolic alkalosis
(C) Metabolic alkalosis alone
(D) Metabolic acidosis with compensating respiratory alkalosis

28. What is the correct interpretation of the following blood gas values?

pH	7.22
$Paco_2$	64
HCO_3^-	24

(A) Respiratory acidosis alone
(B) Respiratory acidosis with compensating metabolic alkalosis
(C) Metabolic acidosis alone
(D) Metabolic acidosis with compensating respiratory alkalosis

29. What is the correct interpretation of the following blood gas values?

pH	7.53
$Paco_2$	36
HCO_3^-	35

(A) Respiratory acidosis alone
(B) Respiratory alkalosis with compensating metabolic alkalosis
(C) Metabolic alkalosis alone
(D) Metabolic acidosis with compensating respiratory alkalosis

30. What is the correct interpretation of the following blood gas values?

pH	7.55
$Paco_2$	21
HCO_3^-	26

(A) Respiratory alkalosis alone
(B) Respiratory alkalosis with compensating metabolic acidosis
(C) Metabolic alkalosis alone
(D) Metabolic acidosis with compensating respiratory alkalosis

31. What is the correct interpretation of the following blood gas values?

pH	7.36
$Paco_2$	24
HCO_3^-	14

(A) Respiratory acidosis alone
(B) Respiratory acidosis with compensating metabolic alkalosis
(C) Metabolic alkalosis alone
(D) Metabolic acidosis with compensating respiratory alkalosis

32. What is the correct interpretation of the following blood gas values?

pH	7.15
$Paco_2$	37
HCO_3^-	11

(A) Respiratory alkalosis alone
(B) Respiratory acidosis with compensating metabolic alkalosis
(C) Metabolic acidosis alone
(D) Metabolic acidosis with compensating respiratory alkalosis

33. A patient with the diagnosis of asthma is admitted to your unit. He received initial bronchodilator therapy in the emergency room. His blood gas values at that time were as follows:

pH	7.39
$Paco_2$	25
Pao_2	62
HCO_3^-	25
Fio_2	0.30

Which of the following sets of blood gas values would indicate a *worsening* of the asthmatic episode due to diminished alveolar air flow?
(A) pH 7.30, $Paco_2$ 48, Pao_2 70, Fio_2 0.40
(B) pH 7.35, $Paco_2$ 29, Pao_2 69, Fio_2 0.40

(C) pH 7.48, $PaCO_2$ 18, PaO_2 60, FIO_2 0.40
(D) pH 7.39, $PaCO_2$ 24, PaO_2 58, FIO_2 0.40

34. At which pH is an acidosis generally treated?
(A) Less than 7.25
(B) 7.25 to 7.35
(C) 7.35 to 7.45
(D) Any pH greater than 7.45

35. Which of the following is NOT a cause of acute respiratory failure?
(A) Central nervous system injury
(B) Right ventricular failure
(C) Excessive use of narcotics
(D) Left ventricular failure

36. A 34-year-old woman is in the unit with acute respiratory distress secondary to sepsis following a motor vehicle collision. She currently has a chest tube in place set at 20 cm H_2O suction. There is no bubbling in the water seal, although there is bubbling in the suction control chamber.

One of the unit technicians tells you that while you were at lunch, they clamped the chest tube to determine whether the suction level was still at 20 cm H_2O. It is still clamped when you return to the room. The patient does not complain of any change in symptoms. About the same time, the patient's physician comes into the room and notices the clamped tube. He becomes very upset and orders an immediate chest radiograph to see whether a tension pneumothorax has occurred. What should you do?
(A) Unclamp the tube and get the chest film as soon as possible.
(B) Excuse yourself while you find the technician.
(C) Explain that there is no need for the chest film because the water seal chamber was not bubbling.
(D) Explain that there is no need for the chest film since the patient has no symptom change.

37. Which of the following exerts the primary chemical control over breathing?
(A) Oxygen tension
(B) Carbonic acid level
(C) Bicarbonate level
(D) Carbon dioxide level

38. Which system gives more stable FIO_2 therapy?
(A) Simple face mask
(B) Nasal cannula
(C) Rebreathing mask
(D) Venturi mask

39. At which level of FIO_2 support is oxygen toxicity thought to develop?
(A) 30% to 40% for longer than 48 h.
(B) 40% to 50% for longer than 2 h.
(C) Greater than 50% for longer than 24 h.
(D) FIO_2 does not cause oxygen toxicity; high PaO_2 values are the cause of toxicity.

40. During a code, the physician is attempting to intubate the patient but is concerned that the endotracheal tube may not be the lungs. Breath sounds are present but difficult to hear. What should you do to help the physician?
(A) Call for a stat chest film and keep bagging the patient.
(B) Attach a carbon dioxide monitor to confirm tube placement.
(C) Call for someone in anesthesia to come intubate.
(D) Suggest that the physician pull the tube and start over.

Questions 41 and 42 refer to the following scenario:

A 63-year-old man is admitted with acute respiratory distress. Symptoms include marked shortness of breath and circumoral cyanosis. He is awake but is beginning to be less responsive. He has a history of COPD. Blood gases reveal the following information:

pH	7.22
$PaCO_2$	62
PaO_2	54
SaO_2	0.81
HCO_3^-	25
FIO_2	30%

41. Based on the preceding information, which condition is likely to be developing?
(A) Congestive heart failure
(B) Acute respiratory distress syndrome
(C) Acute respiratory failure
(D) Pulmonary emboli

42. What would be the first treatment indicated at this time?
(A) Increase the FIO_2
(B) Intubate and place on mechanical ventilation
(C) Postural drainage treatment
(D) Aminophylline aerosol treatment

43. Which of the following conditions produces both ventilation and perfusion disturbances?
    (A) Emphysema
    (B) Asthma
    (C) Superior vena cava syndrome
    (D) Chronic bronchitis or COPD

44. Which of the following is an example of the bronchodilator category of methylxanthines?
    (A) Terbutaline
    (B) Albuterol
    (C) Metaproterenol
    (D) Theophylline

Questions 45 and 46 refer to the following scenario:

A 70-year-old woman is admitted to your unit with the diagnosis of exacerbation of COPD. She is currently short of breath, is using accessory muscles to breathe, and complains of difficulty in eating over the past several weeks because of her shortness of breath. Her blood pressure is 142/88 mm Hg, pulse rate is 108. She has the following laboratory information:

pH	7.39
$Paco_2$	32
Pao_2	59
Fio_2	Room air
Hemoglobin	10

45. Based on the preceding information, which condition is likely to be present?
    (A) Oat cell carcinoma
    (B) Emphysema
    (C) Asthma
    (D) Pulmonary emboli

46. Which of the following treatments would most improve her oxygen transport status?
    (A) Oxygen therapy
    (B) Blood transfusion
    (C) CPAP therapy
    (D) Intermittent positive-pressure breathing (IPPB) treatment

47. Which combination of treatments is most effective in treating status asthmaticus?
    (A) Corticosteroids and bronchodilators
    (B) Methylxanthines and antibiotics
    (C) Postural drainage and bronchodilators
    (D) Incentive spirometry and bronchodilators

Questions 48 through 50 refer to the following scenario:

A 24-year-old woman is admitted to your unit in acute respiratory distress with the diagnosis of asthma. Lung auscultation reveals generalized wheezing. She is compliant with her medications at home. She has received epinephrine, oxygen, and albuterol in the emergency department with no improvement in her symptoms. Her blood gases reveal the following:

pH	7.48
$Paco_2$	27
Pao_2	59
Fio_2	4 L/min via nasal cannula
HCO_3^-	23

48. Based on the preceding information, which condition is likely to be developing?
    (A) Pneumonia
    (B) Status asthmaticus
    (C) Pulmonary emboli
    (D) Acute respiratory distress syndrome

49. Assume that the Fio_2 is increased to 6 L/min. Which of the following blood gas values would be an indication of a *worsening* status?

	(A)	(B)	(C)	(D)
pH	7.36	7.52	7.44	7.44
$Paco_2$	40	24	27	29
Pao_2	70	64	72	59

50. Physical assessment by the nurse is one of the keys to the evaluation of therapy. During auscultation of the asthmatic patient's lungs, what should the nurse be aware of if a reduction in the degree of wheezing were to occur?
    (A) The patient's condition may be worsening or improving.
    (B) Reduction in wheezing always indicates improvement.
    (C) RV failure is developing.
    (D) Pulmonary hypertension is being alleviated.

51. What is the definition of status asthmaticus?
    (A) The first episode of a newly diagnosed asthmatic
    (B) The preterminal asthmatic episode
    (C) An asthma episode that has failed to improve with conventional treatment
    (D) An asthma episode that is complicated by CHF

52. Pulmonary emboli produce all of the following physiologic changes but one. Which of the following is NOT likely to occur with pulmonary emboli?
    (A) Pulmonary hypertension
    (B) Arterial hypoxemia
    (C) Hypocarbia (low $Paco_2$)
    (D) LV heart failure

53. Which of the following tests is most diagnostic for pulmonary emboli?
    (A) Blood gas analysis
    (B) V/Q scans
    (C) Pulmonary angiography
    (D) Pulmonary function tests

54. Effects from recurrent emboli due to deep venous thrombosis can be avoided by which one of the following therapies?
    (A) Use of an inferior vena cava filter such as a Greenfield filter
    (B) Heparin
    (C) Warfarin
    (D) Use of lower extremity alternating compression devices

55. Which of the following features of pleural drainage systems indicates an active pleural leak?
    (A) Bubbling in the water-seal chamber
    (B) Bubbling in the suction control chamber
    (C) Fluctuation of water level in the water-seal chamber with respiration
    (D) No fluctuation of water level in the water-seal chamber with respiration

56. Which type of condition can lead to a tension pneumothorax?
    (A) Closed pneumothorax
    (B) Open pneumothorax
    (C) Subcutaneous emphysema
    (D) Pneumomediastinum

57. Which of the following findings would be an indication of a ruptured diaphragm?
    (A) Diminished bowel sounds
    (B) Tracheal shift toward the affected diaphragm
    (C) Irregular breathing
    (D) Bowel sounds in the chest

Questions 58 and 59 refer to the following scenario:

A 26-year-old man is admitted to your unit from the emergency department with chest injuries following a motor vehicle collision. He complains of chest pain and shortness of breath. The right side of his chest (between the fourth and seventh intercostal spaces) moves in on inspiration and out on expiration. A chest film shows fractured ribs of the third through eighth intercostal spaces.

58. Based on the preceding information, which condition is likely to be developing?
    (A) Tension pneumothorax
    (B) Hemopneumothorax

    (C) Pericardial tamponade
    (D) Flail chest

59. Which treatment would be best advised for this patient?
    (A) Open thoracotomy
    (B) Negative-pressure ventilation
    (C) External rib fixation with sandbags
    (D) Supportive therapy, such as oxygen therapy and pain relief

Questions 60 and 61 refer to the following scenario:

A 41-year-old woman is admitted to your unit having landed on her left chest after a fall from the roof of her single-story house. She complains of left chest pain, which increases in intensity with deep inspiration. An admission chest radiograph is unremarkable. She is coughing up small amounts of blood-tinged sputum. Her trachea is midline. Her ECG and heart tones are normal. Blood pressure is 140/80 mm Hg, pulse 120, respiratory rate 28. SaO_2 is 92% on room air.

60. Based on the preceding information, which condition would need to be ruled out?
    (A) Cardiac rupture
    (B) Cardiac tamponade
    (C) Pulmonary contusion
    (D) Pneumomediastinum

Four hours after admission, the patient appears agitated and complains of increasing shortness of breath. Her pulse rate is now 140 and her respiratory rate is 38. The pulse oximeter displays a reading of 85% on room air.

61. What further treatment would be indicated based on this scenario?
    (A) Repeat chest film and supplemental oxygen
    (B) Insertion of a left chest tube
    (C) Pericardiocentesis
    (D) Emergent intubation

Questions 62 and 63 refer to the following scenario:

A 23-year-old woman is admitted to your unit from the emergency department following a motor vehicle collision. She has no apparent injuries, although a chest film indicated a fourth rib fracture on the left and a fifth rib fracture on the right. Shortly after arrival in the unit, she develops marked shortness of breath and manifests a rightward deviation of the trachea and diminished breath sounds on the left. Her blood pressure is 94/62 mm Hg, pulse is 120, respiratory rate is 32.

62. Based on the preceding information, what condition is likely to be developing?
    (A) Open pneumothorax
    (B) Tension pneumothorax
    (C) Cardiac tamponade
    (D) Flail chest

63. What would be the best treatment for this condition?
    (A) Insertion of pleural chest tubes
    (B) Insertion of mediastinal chest tubes
    (C) Open thoracotomy
    (D) Pericardiocentesis

Questions 64 and 65 are based on the following scenario

A 34-year-old woman is admitted to your unit 3 weeks after a cesarean delivery with acute shortness of breath and right chest pain. She has no prior cardiopulmonary medical history. Her vital signs are blood pressure 90/55 mm Hg, heart rate 140, respiratory rate 36. A stat transthoracic echocardiogram shows acute right heart failure and pulmonary hypertension. She has the following blood gas values:

pH	7.46
$PaCO_2$	30
PaO_2	62
FIO_2	3 L/min

64. Based on the preceding information, which condition is likely to be developing?
    (A) Pneumonia
    (B) dissecting thoracic aneurysm
    (C) pleuritis
    (D) pulmonary emboli

65. Which treatment would most likely improve her immediate symptoms?
    (A) heparin
    (B) oxygen therapy
    (C) tissue plasminogen activator (tPA) or streptokinase
    (D) aminophylline

Pulmonary Practice Exam

Practice Fill-Ins

1. _____
2. _____
3. _____
4. _____
5. _____
6. _____
7. _____
8. _____
9. _____
10. _____
11. _____
12. _____
13. _____
14. _____
15. _____
16. _____

17. _____
18. _____
19. _____
20. _____
21. _____
22. _____
23. _____
24. _____
25. _____
26. _____
27. _____
28. _____
29. _____
30. _____
31. _____
32. _____

33. _____
34. _____
35. _____
36. _____
37. _____
38. _____
39. _____
40. _____
41. _____
42. _____
43. _____
44. _____
45. _____
46. _____
47. _____
48. _____

49. _____
50. _____
51. _____
52. _____
53. _____
54. _____
55. _____
56. _____
57. _____
58. _____
59. _____
60. _____
61. _____
62. _____
63. _____

Answers

1. A	18. D	35. B	52. D
2. D	19. A	36. C	53. C
3. B	20. B	37. D	54. A
4. A	21. D	38. D	55. A
5. D	22. D	39. C	56. A
6. B	23. A	40. B	57. D
7. A	24. D	41. C	58. D
8. B	25. B	42. B	59. D
9. A	26. A	43. D	60. C
10. B	27. B	44. D	61. A
11. D	28. A	45. B	62. B
12. D	29. C	46. A	63. A
13. B	30. A	47. A	64. D
14. C	31. D	48. B	65. C
15. B	32. C	49. A	
16. A	33. A	50. A	
17. C	34. A	51. C	

III

ENDOCRINE

Donna Prentice

III

ENDOCRINE

20

Introduction to the Endocrine System

EDITORS' NOTE

Endocrine concepts make up about 4% (six to eight questions) of the PCCN exam. According to the PCCN guideline from the American Association of Critical Care Nurses (AACN) Certification Corporation, the key areas of endocrine dysfunction covered in the exam include (1) diabetic ketoacidosis and (2) acute hypoglycemia. It is possible to expect questions related to performing an endocrine assessment, monitoring normal and abnormal diagnostic tests, administering medications and monitoring patient responses, and managing insulin infusions.

Although recent PCCN exams have not specifically addressed items such as thyrotoxic crisis, myxedema coma, and acute adrenal insufficiency/ pheochromocytoma, we have retained the chapters on these topics for two reasons. First, a review of these chapters may help give you insight into endocrine disturbances in general. Second, although questions on the exam may not specifically address these disorders, an understanding of the content may help answer questions that are indirectly related to these concepts.

As you review the following chapters on the endocrine system, focus on key concepts rather than minor details. Endocrine dysfunction is a difficult area for many nurses taking the PCCN exam. Do your best to acquaint yourself with the information in these chapters while also noting patients in your unit with endocrine disturbances. Relating material in this text to patients in your unit will strengthen your ability to recall key concepts in endocrinology and increase your chances of answering most of the questions on endocrinology correctly.

HORMONAL PURPOSE AND FUNCTION OF THE ENDOCRINE SYSTEM

The primary function of the endocrine system is to regulate the metabolic functioning of the body. The term *endocrine* refers to the internal secretion of biologically active substances, such as hormones, that help to regulate the functions of cells and organs. Metabolic functioning includes chemical reactions and the rates of these reactions, growth, transportation of chemicals, secretions, and cellular metabolism.

There is a close interrelationship between the nervous system (responsible for integrating body processes) and the endocrine system (responsible for appropriate metabolic activity). Neuronal stimulation is required for some specific hormones to be secreted and/or to be secreted in adequate amounts.

The endocrine system is composed of specific glands (Fig. 20-1) that secrete their chemical substances directly into the bloodstream. The major single endocrine glands are the pituitary (also called the hypophysis) (Fig. 20-2) and the thyroid. The parathyroids are usually four glands, not two sets of paired glands. The adrenals form one pair of endocrine glands. Other glands that contain endocrine components and function in both the endocrine system and another system are the ovaries and testes (collectively termed the gonads), and the pancreas. The thymus gland has a major role in immunology but is sometimes included in discussions of the endocrine system.

All endocrine glands are very vascular. They function by extracting substances from the blood to synthesize into complex hormones. Hormones are released from the specific endocrine glands into the veins that drain the glands themselves. The circulatory

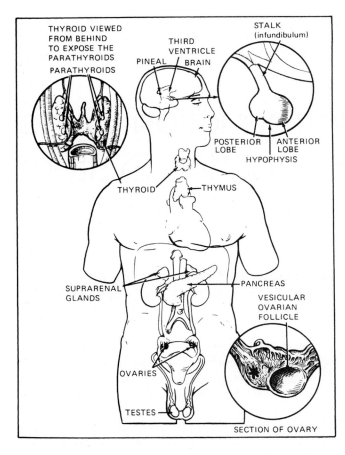

Figure 20-1. Overview of the endocrine system.

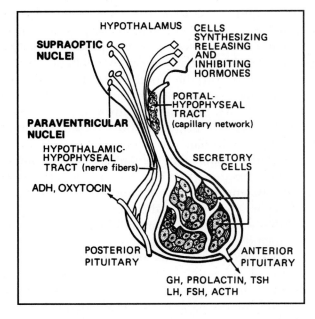

Figure 20-2. Paraventricular and supraoptic nuclei of the hypothalamus.

system transports endocrine substances to target glands and tissues throughout the body.

CLASSIFICATION OF HORMONES

The substances secreted by endocrine glands are chemicals called hormones. Hormones exert physiologic control over body cells. They bind specifically to hormone receptors expressed on the cell surface or within the cell. Local hormones are those released in specific areas (or tissues) and they exert a limited, local effect. Acetylcholine is an example of a local hormone having physiologic control at some synapses in the nervous system. General hormones are secreted by a specific endocrine gland and transported by the vascular system to a specific, predetermined site.

Important General Hormones

All of the general hormones play important roles in regulating various functions of the body. However, dysfunctional secretion of certain hormones would rarely, if ever, be a reason for admission to a critical care unit. General hormones include oxytocin, follicle-stimulating hormone (FSH), luteinizing hormone (LH), prolactin, melanocyte-stimulating hormone (MSH), corticosterone, deoxycorticosterone, and androgens (including estrogens, progesterone, and testosterone). These hormones are not discussed in detail in this text.

Those general hormones whose dysfunctional secretion may precipitate admission to a critical care area are listed in Table 20-1 and are covered in the following four chapters.

TABLE 20-1. ENDOCRINE GLANDS AND HORMONES OF SIGNIFICANT IMPORTANCE

Glands	Hormones
Adenohypophysis (anterior pituitary)	Adrenocorticotropin, somatotropin, or growth hormone, thyroid-stimulating hormone
Neurohypophysis (posterior pituitary)	Antidiuretic hormone, oxytocin
Thyroid	Thyroxine, triiodothyronine, calcitonin
Parathyroid	Parathyroid hormone (parathormone)
Adrenal medulla	Epinephrine, norepinephrine
Adrenal cortex	Glucocorticoids (cortisol), mineralocorticoids (aldosterone)
Pancreas	Insulin, glucagons

TYPES OF HORMONES

Hormones are classified on the basis of their class of action on a receptor (e.g., glucocorticoid, mineralocorticoid) and ligand or action type (e.g., agonist, partial agonist, antagonist). Hormones may be amines, peptides, proteins (or protein derivatives), or steroids. Prostaglandins are often considered tissue hormones. The first three types of hormones are water-soluble and do not require a carrier molecule for transportation throughout the body. Steroids and thyroxine are not water-soluble and must rely on a carrier substance to transport them to their site of action, the target cell.

Prostaglandins are unsaturated fatty acids, of which three types have been identified on the basis of their chemical structure. They are synthesized in the seminal vesicles, brain, liver, iris, kidneys, lungs, and other areas. Prostaglandins have a potent effect but are considered local hormones, not general hormones.

EDITORS' NOTE

Although the actions of hormones are important, remember that you should concentrate on general concepts rather than specific information. Terms such as amine hormone are introduced only for purposes of explanation. Do not expect to see this type of information on the PCCN exam.

ACTIONS OF HORMONES

Amine, Protein, and Peptide Hormones

Amine, protein, and peptide hormones include growth hormone (GH), adrenocorticotropic hormone (ACTH), thyroid-stimulating hormone (TSH), parathyroid hormone (PTH), calcitonin, insulin, the catecholamines, glucagon, antidiuretic hormone (ADH), FSH, LH, and prolactin. Since these hormones are water soluble and do not require a carrier substance, their concentrations may fluctuate rapidly and widely. These hormones are thought to react with specific surface receptors on the target-cell membrane. This alters the membrane's enzymes and leads to a change in the intracellular concentration of an enzyme. The hormone is called the first messenger and the intracellular enzyme is the second messenger. The second messengers are cyclic 3′,5′- adenosine monophosphate (cAMP), cyclic guanosine monophosphate (cGMP), calcium–calmodulin complex, and prostaglandins. Cyclic AMP (within the cell) activates enzymes, causes protein synthesis, alters cell permeability, causes muscle relaxation/contraction, and causes secretion. It is by the action of cAMP that many hormones exert control over the cells.

Steroids and Thyroxine

Steroids (sex hormones, aldosterone, and cortisol) and thyroxine are non–water-soluble hormones. These hormones are able to cross the cell membrane easily and then bind with an intracellular receptor. The hormone-receptor complex reacts with chromatin in the cell nucleus to synthesize specific proteins. Because these hormones are lipid chemicals, the reactions take longer to occur but are no less potent than the amine, protein, and peptide hormone reactions.

NEGATIVE-FEEDBACK SYSTEM

Some hormones are needed in very minute amounts in the body for variable amounts of time; some have prolonged action periods and some affect and interact with other hormones, producing a very complex, intricate system. A control system must exist to maintain this complex system.

Most control systems, including the endocrine system, act by a negative-feedback mechanism. When there is an increased hormone concentration, physiologic control is increased. The stimulus for hormone production received in the hypothalamus is decreased. This results in an inhibition of hormone-releasing factors that is negative in relation to the stimulus. In the same manner, when hormone concentrations are deficient or absent, a stimulus is received in the hypothalamus that results in an increased release of hormone-stimulating factors. This again is a negative (or opposite) response to the stimulus sent to the hypothalamus. The greater the need for the hormone, the greater the intensity of the stimulus; similarly, the greater the concentration of the hormone, the lower the intensity of the stimulus.

When a hormone concentration is deficient, the physiologic control of the body cells increases as more hormone is produced and/or secreted. With an increase in physiologic control, the feedback stimulus relayed to the endocrine gland decreases in intensity and release of the hormone decreases as

TABLE 20-2. RELEASING AND INHIBITING FACTORS PRODUCED BY THE HYPOTHALAMUS

Releasing Hormones	Inhibiting Hormones	Peripheral Hormones
Growth hormone–releasing hormone	Growth hormone–inhibiting hormone	Growth hormone
Prolactin-releasing hormone	Prolactin-inhibiting hormone	Prolactin
Corticotropin-releasing hormone	—	Adrenal steroids
Follicle-stimulating hormone–releasing hormone	—	Gonadal steroids
Luteinizing hormone–releasing hormone	—	Gonadal hormones
Thyrotropin-releasing hormone	—	Thyroid hormones

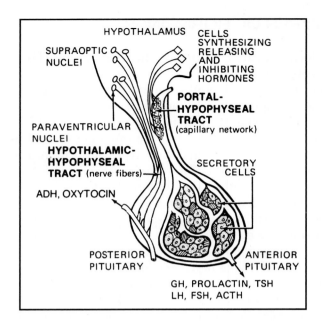

Figure 20-3. Portal-hypophyseal and hypothalamic-hypophyseal tracts of the hypothalamus.

homeostasis is achieved. The reverse process applies when the hormone concentration is excessive.

It is known that the hypothalamus produces releasing and inhibiting hormones (or factors) whose single target is the adenohypophysis, the so-called master gland. It is believed that all hormones have releasing and inhibiting factors produced by the hypothalamus, but only eight are known at this time (Table 20-2).

The principles of achieving regulatory control are similar with all the hormones listed in Table 20-1 with the exception of the hormones of the adrenal medulla.

The hormones of the adrenal medulla, epinephrine and norepinephrine, are under control of the autonomic nervous system. The hormones of the neurohypophysis (the posterior pituitary) are controlled by the concentration of the substance released from the target cell "feeding back" on the hypothalamus. The release of the hormone leads to a change in a plasma constituent that regulates hypothalamic activity rather than a change in the gland itself. Tropic hormones, secreted only by the adenohypophysis (the anterior pituitary), cause an increase in size and secretion rates of other endocrine glands and are controlled by the negative-feedback system as well as other factors.

All adenohypophyseal hormone–releasing and adenohypophyseal hormone–inhibiting factors (except the adrenal medulla) are carried by the hypothalamic-hypophyseal tract from the hypothalamus into the median eminence (Fig. 20-3) and then into the hypophyseal stalk.

EDITORS' NOTE

Remember, concepts of basic anatomy, such as the structure of the pituitary stalk, are usually not addressed on the PCCN exam. It may, in general, be helpful to understand such concepts, but do not spend too much time in trying to memorize this type of detail.

In the stalk, the hypophyseal portal system carries the releasing and inhibiting factors into the adenohypophysis for storage until needed.

The two neurohypophyseal hormone–releasing and neurohypophyseal hormone–inhibiting factors are formed in the paraventricular and supraoptic nuclei in the hypothalamus (see Fig. 20-3). They are then carried by nerve fibers into the neurohypophysis for storage.

Anatomy, Physiology, and Dysfunction of the Pituitary Gland

EDITORS' NOTE

As you review the functions of the pituitary gland, do not attempt to memorize basic anatomic features. Rarely would questions on anatomy, such as the type of tissue from which the pituitary arises, be on the PCCN exam. Skim these areas with the goal being to acquaint yourself with terms and concepts. Focus your attention on the key functions of the gland and how they may cause clinical disturbances.

The pituitary gland, or hypophysis, is a small gland about 1 cm in diameter and weighing about 0.5 g. It is located in the sella turcica, a depression in the sphenoid bone of the skull (Fig. 21-1), and is attached to the hypothalamus by the hypophyseal stalk.

ANATOMY OF THE HYPOPHYSIS

The hypophysis has two lobes, each of which derives from a different type of tissue. The anterior lobe, or adenohypophysis, is an outgrowth of pharyngeal tissue, which grows upward toward the brain in the embryo. The posterior lobe, or neurohypophysis, is an outgrowth of the hypothalamus, which grows downward in the embryo. A mnemonic may help you to keep these terms straight: anterior pituitary starts with the letter "a," as does adenohypophysis (*adeno* = anterior). The two lobes are separated by the pars intermedia, a small, almost avascular band of fibers whose function, other than keeping the two lobes separate, is unknown (Fig. 21-2).

The hypophysis is often referred to as the body's master gland because the hormones it secretes regulate many other endocrine glands.

Structure of the Adenohypophysis

The adenohypophysis is composed of epithelium-type cells (embryologic extensions of pharyngeal tissue). Many different types of epithelial cells have been identified for each hormone formed.

The hypothalamic-hypophyseal portal vessels in the adenohypophysis are made up of microscopic blood vessels (Fig. 21-3). These vessels connect the hypothalamus and the adenohypophysis (by passage through the pituitary stalk) and terminate in the anterior pituitary sinuses.

Substances carried in the hypothalamic-hypophyseal vessels are actually hormone factors and not hormones per se. These factors are releasing and inhibiting factors (see Table 20-2). For each adeno-hypophyseal hormone, there is an associated releasing factor. For some adenohypophyseal hormones, there are inhibitory factors.

Structure of the Neurohypophysis

Many cells of the neurohypophysis are called pituicytes, which are like the glial cells of the nervous system. The pituicytes provide supporting tissue for nerve tracts arising from the supraoptic and paraventricular nuclei of the hypothalamus. These nuclei form the neurohypophyseal hormones, which are carried by the nerve tracts through the hypophyseal stalk, a structure terminating in bulbous knobs in the neurohypophysis. The knobs lie on the surface of capillaries. As a hormone

229

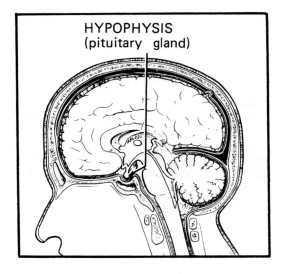

Figure 21-1. Location of the hypophysis (pituitary gland).

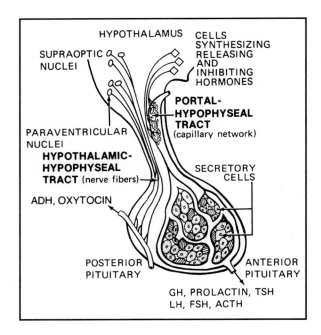

Figure 21-3. The hypothalamic-hypophyseal portal vessel.

formed in the hypothalamus and stored in the bulbous knobs is needed, exocytosis occurs. Exocytosis is the discharge of substances from a cell that are too large to diffuse through the cell membrane. The hormone is thus secreted from the bulbous knobs onto the capillaries and is absorbed into the vascular system. The adenohypophysis has a vascular relationship to the hypothalamus, whereas the neurohypophysis has a neural relationship.

PHYSIOLOGY

The various hormones control the activity of the target glands and target tissues. They exert an effect on target tissues by altering the rates at which cellular processes occur. There are two basic mechanisms of hormone action: cyclic 3′,5′-adenosine monophosphate (cAMP) and genetic activation. Cyclic AMP initiates actions characteristic of the target cell. For example, parathyroid hormone cells activated by cAMP form and secrete parathyroid hormone (parathormone); specific cells in the pancreas activated by cAMP form and secrete glucagon. Known hormones affected by cAMP include secretin, glucagon, parathormone, vasopressin, catecholamines, adrenocorticotropin, follicle-stimulating hormone, thyroid-stimulating hormone, and hypothalamic releasing factors.

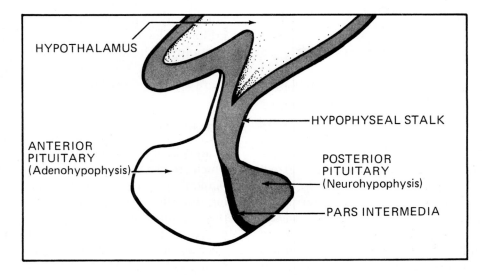

Figure 21-2. Lobes of the hypophysis.

Hormones of the Adenohypophysis

Hormone factors, all formed in the hypothalamus, are secreted by the adenohypophysis.

1. Thyrotropin-releasing hormone (TRH): causes the release of thyroid-stimulating hormone (TSH).
2. Growth hormone–releasing hormone (GRH): causes release of growth hormone (GH) or somatotropin (STH). Growth hormone–inhibiting hormone (GIH), or somatostatin, inhibits the release of growth hormone.
3. Corticotropin-releasing hormone (CRH): causes release of adrenocorticotropin (ACTH).
4. Gonadotropin-releasing hormone (GnRH): causes release of luteinizing hormone (LH) and follicle-stimulating hormone (FSH).
5. Prolactin-inhibiting hormone (PIH): causes inhibition of prolactin secretion.
6. Human chorionic gonadotropin (HCG).
7. Human placental lactogen (HPL).

All of the major adenohypophyseal hormones have an effect upon a target gland except growth hormone.

Growth Hormone and Metabolism

GH is also called somatotropin. Somatotropin has a general effect on bones, organs, and soft tissues; it is, therefore, considered a peripheral hormone. It influences the growth of body tissues.

GH has an important role in all aspects of metabolism. GH increases the rate of intracellular protein synthesis throughout the body. It is a factor in the mobilization of fatty acids from adipose tissue and in the conversion of these fats into energy. GH conserves carbohydrates by decreasing glucose utilization in the body.

Growth Hormone Factors

There are specific factors that stimulate or inhibit the release of GH.

The most common factors inhibiting the release of GH include hyperglycemia, sustained corticosteroid therapy at high levels, and the release of growth hormone–inhibiting factor (GIF) from the hypothalamus.

Common factors promoting release of GH include pituitary tumors, hypoglycemia, exercise, decreased amino acid levels, and the release of growth hormone–releasing hormone (GRH) from the hypothalamus.

Growth hormone secretion follows a diurnal pattern, with most release occurring in the first 2 h of deep sleep. This follows the pattern of the non–rapid eye movement (non-REM) stage of sleep.

Hormones of the Neurohypophysis

Two hormones are released by the neurohypophysis: antidiuretic hormone (ADH), also called vasopressin, and oxytocin. Oxytocin is not discussed in this text.

Antidiuretic hormone is formed mainly in the supraoptic nuclei of the hypothalamus. (The paraventricular nuclei mainly form oxytocin. The ratio of ADH to oxytocin formed in the supraoptic nuclei is 6:1, whereas the ratio is 1:6 in the paraventricular nuclei.) ADH is transported from the supraoptic nuclei by neurophysins. Neurophysins are protein carriers that bind very loosely with ADH and oxytocin to transport these hormones to the neurohypophysis for storage until needed.

Action of Antidiuretic Hormone

ADH works on the distal convoluted tubules and the collecting ducts of the kidney, altering the permeability of these tubules and ducts. Without ADH, the tubules and ducts are impermeable to water. In the presence of ADH, they become permeable to water, thus allowing large quantities of water to leave the tubules and collecting ducts and to reenter the hypertonic medullary interstitial fluid. This helps to conserve and balance the fluid content of the body.

Control of Antidiuretic Hormone

Serum sodium levels and extracellular fluid osmolality exert a major influence on ADH. Osmoreceptors shrink when hypertonicity of the extracellular fluid exists. The osmoreceptors emit impulses to the hypothalamus, and ADH is released from the neurohypophysis to reabsorb water from the kidneys and to reestablish homeostasis. When body fluids become diluted, stimulated osmoreceptors result in the inhibition of ADH, and water is *not* reabsorbed from the kidneys. Many factors control ADH in addition to the serum sodium and extracellular osmolality. Inadequate blood volume stimulates volume receptors in the periphery, the carotid sinus, the left atrium of the heart, and the aortic arch, leading to the release of ADH. The ADH response is much greater in hemorrhagic states than in altered-osmolality states. Trauma, stress, anxiety, exercise, pain, exposure to heat, nausea, hypoxia, nicotine, and phenytoin and other medications enhance ADH release. The release of ADH is inhibited by a decreased plasma osmolality, increased intravascular volume, alcohol ingestion, and pituitary surgery.

NEUROHYPOPHYSEAL DYSFUNCTION

There are two main neurohypophyseal disorders: diabetes insipidus and the syndrome of inappropriate ADH (SIADH).

Diabetes Insipidus

Diabetes insipidus is a disease of impaired renal conservation of water, resulting from either inadequate secretion of vasopressin from the neurohypophysis (central diabetes insipidus) or to an insufficient renal response to vasopressin (nephrogenic diabetes insipidus). When there are decreased levels of ADH, diuresis and dehydration occur. Decreased levels of ADH are found when there is damage to or destruction of the ADH neurons in the supraoptic and paraventricular neurons of the hypothalamus. Diabetes insipidus then results.

Symptoms
The symptoms of diabetes insipidus include dilute urine (until severe dehydration occurs) with a specific gravity between 1.001 and 1.005. Urinary output varies from 2 to 15 L/day regardless of fluid intake. Polyuria is often of sudden onset. Polyuria may not occur until 1 to 3 days postinjury owing to the utilization of stored ADH in the neurohypophysis. Polydipsia will occur unless the thirst center has been damaged. There is an increased serum osmolality and a decreased urine osmolality (100–200 mOsm/kg). A relative diabetes insipidus may occur in cases of high-dose, lengthy steroid therapy with a specific gravity of the urine ranging from 1.000 to 1.009, urine osmolality <500 mOsm/kg, and urinary volume about 6 to 9 L/day. Urine output >200 mL/h for 2 h should be reported to a physician.

Etiology
The two leading causes of diabetes insipidus are hypothalamic or pituitary tumor and closed head injuries with damage to the supraoptic nuclei and/or hypothalamus. Postoperative diabetes insipidus is usually transient. Other causes include inflammatory and degenerative systemic conditions, but these are not common. Central diabetes insipidus can be distinguished from nephrogenic diabetes insipidus by the administration of desmopressin (DDAVP), which will increase urine osmolality in patients with central diabetes insipidus but have little or no effect in patients with nephrogenic diabetes insipidus.

Treatment
The objective of therapy is first to prevent dehydration and electrolyte imbalances while determining and treating the underlying cause. A variety of replacement therapy modalities are available. Fluid support with hypotonic dextrose in water is essential. The goal is to return the urine volume milliliter for milliliter plus any insensible loss. The patient who is unable to manage his or her thirst may have a decreased level of consciousness or defective hypothalamic thirst center. It is essential to obtain the patient's weight daily in order to assess fluid loss. Exogenous vasopressin may be given as an intravenous bolus, as a continuous infusion, or subcutaneously. It is a short-acting ADH therapy with vasopressor activity. Desmopressin (1-deamino-8-D-arginine vasopressin [DDAVP]) is a synthetic ADH that can be used as an intravenous (central line only), subcutaneous, or nasal spray therapy. The advantage of DDAVP is a longer duration of action and negligible vasoactive properties. Following head trauma or neurosurgery, an aqueous vasopressin infusion of 5 to 10 units subcutaneously may be used to decrease the risk of dehydration and hypotension. If it is related to pituitary manipulation during surgery, diabetes insipidus may resolve in only a few days. In 50% of posttraumatic cases of diabetes insipidus, a three-phase cycle may occur. An initial diuretic phase is followed in 2 to 14 days by a period of antidiuresis. The oliguria is believed to be related to the release of stored vasopressin from the posterior pituitary with the resolution of the cerebral edema. The patient then demonstrates a permanent diabetes insipidus.

Nursing Interventions
Of prime importance is the accurate recording of the patient's intake and output. Monitoring body weight, electrolytes (especially potassium and sodium), urine specific gravity, osmolality, blood urea nitrogen, and being alert for signs of dehydration and hypovolemic shock will allow for early intervention in patients who are at risk for deterioration.

Syndrome of Inappropriate Secretion of ADH

The syndrome of inappropriate secretion of ADH (SIADH) is a condition of impaired water excretion with accompanying hyponatremia and hypoosmolality caused by the inappropriate secretion of ADH. In SIADH there is either increased secretion or increased production of ADH. This increase is unrelated to osmolality and causes a slight increase in total body water. Sodium (hyponatremia) and osmolar (hypoosmolality) concentration in extracellular fluid and serum are severely decreased.

Etiology

A number of disorders can cause SIADH. It is occasionally caused by a pituitary tumor but is much more commonly caused by a bronchogenic (small cell) or pancreatic carcinoma. Head injuries, other endocrine disorders (such as Addison's disease and hypopituitarism), pulmonary disease (such as pneumonia, lung abscesses, tuberculosis), central nervous system infections (and tumors), and drugs such as tricyclic antidepressants, oral hypoglycemic agents, diuretics, and cytotoxic agents are all possible causes.

Symptoms and Complications

Symptoms produced by SIADH reflect the interaction between the underlying condition and excessive water retention. Symptoms are mainly neurologic and nonspecific. The most common symptoms of SIADH are personality changes, headache, decreased mentation, lethargy, nausea, vomiting, diarrhea, anorexia, decreased tendon reflexes, seizures, and coma. Complications of SIADH include seizures, coma, and death.

Laboratory Recognition

The cardinal laboratory abnormality in SIADH consists of plasma hyponatremia (<130 mmol/L) and hypoosmolality (275 mOsm/kg) occurring simultaneously with inappropriate hyperosmolality of the low-volume urine. Urine will have an osmolality of >900 mOsm/kg with an increase in urine sodium. Another feature that separates SIADH from other conditions that produce hyponatremia is the high urinary sodium excretion. Other laboratory findings are nonspecific. Central nervous system symptoms are more evident as the serum sodium drops below 125 mmol/L. Seizures and coma are more likely to be present in the patient with a serum sodium <115 mmol/L.

Treatment

The first step in treating SIADH is to restrict fluid intake to prevent water intoxication. The objective of therapy is to correct electrolyte imbalances. Severity of symptoms will determine the rate of correction of the hyonatremia. In severe cases (severe hyponatremia with serum sodium levels <105 mEq/L), 3% hypertonic saline and/or intravenous furosemide are used. Rapid correction of sodium should be avoided in order to prevent osmotic demyelination. The initial rate of correction of 2 to 4 mEq/L in the first 2 to 4 h may be beneficial in patients with severe symptoms. Patients who are asymptomatic should receive a slower correction of the hyponatremia. Maximum rate of correction should be <10 mEq/L at 24 h and <18 mEq/L at 48 h. Supplemental potassium is usually necessary, with follow-up frequent monitoring of serum potassium and sodium levels every 2 to 4 h until the patient is stable. Daily weights are important measures of fluid gain. Vasopressin receptor antagonist may be given intravenously (conivaptan) or orally (tolvaptan) when other measures have proven to be ineffective. They produce a selective water diuresis without affecting sodium and potassium excretion. Demeclocycline (<2400 mg/day) and lithium carbonate (up to 900 mg/day) work by interfering with the normal ADH effect of increasing cAMP in the distal tubules and collecting ducts. These two agents are useful in the long-term management of SIADH.

Nursing Interventions

With SIADH it is necessary to maintain strict fluid restrictions and to monitor the patient for electrolyte imbalances, as indicated by confusion, weakness, lethargy, vomiting, and/or seizures. Fluid limitation may be set at 800 to 1000 mL/day. The oral intake should be equal to the urine output until the serum sodium is normalized. Fluids high in sodium should be selected. If hypertonic saline is given, it should be given slowly (1–2 mL/kg/h) and the patient monitored for congestive heart failure. All drips should be in a saline base. The nasogastric tube should be irrigated with normal saline instead of water, and enemas should be avoided. Accurate intake and output, daily weights, and laboratory monitoring of urine specific gravity and electrolyte levels are important.

Neurologic status should be assessed for subtle signs of decreasing level of consciousness, and precautions to prevent seizure should be taken. If the patient is comatose, turning, suctioning as needed, and standard nursing care procedures are required.

Frequent oral care, mouth rinsing without swallowing, and snacking on hard candy and chilled beverages will be helpful in coping with fluid restriction. Mouthwashes with an alcohol base and lemon and glycerin swabs should be avoided because of their drying effects. Cardiac monitoring will allow for early identification of impending hyperkalemia and its associated cardiac problems. The patient's nutritional needs must be met without increasing fluid intake. It is useful to provide emotional support to the alert patient, offering reassurance that his or her condition can be treated successfully. This will help to obtain the patient's cooperation unless he or she has an untreated psychologic problem.

22

Anatomy, Physiology, and Dysfunction of the Thyroid and Parathyroid Glands

EDITORS' NOTE

The PCCN guidelines do not discuss the care of patients with thyroid and parathyroid disturbances as part of the PCCN exam. However, understanding of thyroid and parathyroid function is useful for understanding other clinical conditions, particularly electrolyte and cardiovascular responses. You may be able to concentrate less heavily on this chapter.

ANATOMY OF THE THYROID GLAND

Location and Shape

The thyroid gland is in the anterior portion of the neck at the lower part of the larynx and the upper part of the trachea (Fig. 22-1). The thyroid has two lobes which, with a little imagination, resemble a butterfly's wings. The lobes lie on either side of the trachea and are connected by a narrow band of tissue called the isthmus, which lies anteriorly across the second and third tracheal rings.

Internal Structure

Each lobe of the thyroid is divided into lobules by dense connective tissue. Each lobule (Fig. 22-2) is composed of sac-like structures called follicles. The follicles are lined with cuboidal epithelium.

The follicular sacs are filled with a thick, viscous material called colloid. Colloid is actually thyroglobulin,

which is converted to thyroxine as needed. Storage, synthesis, and release of thyroxine are controlled by the hypothalamic-releasing hormone (factor) and the thyroid-stimulating hormone of the adenohypophysis.

PHYSIOLOGY OF THE THYROID GLAND

The thyroid gland secretes three important hormones: thyroxine, triiodothyronine, and thyrocalcitonin. Approximately 90% of the hormone is thyroxine (T_4) and 10% is triiodothyronine (T_3). In peripheral tissues, thyroxine is converted to triiodothyronine. The functions of these two hormones are essentially the same. Thyroid hormones stimulate metabolism of all body cells and produce effective function of multiple body systems. The intensity, speed of action, and formation of these hormones differ.

Iodide Trapping (The Iodide Pump)

To form thyroid hormones, iodides must be removed from blood and extracellular fluids and transported into the thyroid gland follicles. The basal membrane of the thyroid gland has the ability to transfer iodide into the thyroid cells. The iodide then diffuses throughout the thyroid cells and follicular sacs. This process is known as iodide trapping. The iodide is stored until thyroglobulin is needed. It then becomes ionized by the enzyme peroxidase and

235

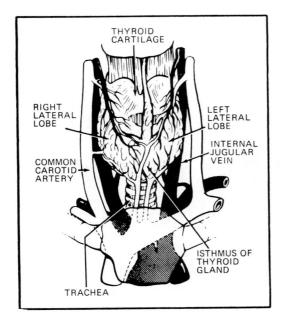

Figure 22-1. Location and shape of the thyroid gland.

hydrogen peroxide, converting the iodide into iodine at the point where thyroglobulin is released intracellularly. If the peroxidase system is blocked, production of thyroid hormone ceases.

Organification of Thyroglobulin

Thyroglobulin is the major component reacting with iodide to form thyroxine. Thyroid cells synthesize

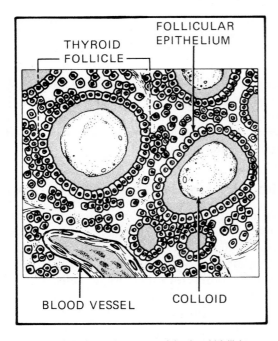

Figure 22-2. Internal structure of the thyroid follicles.

the glycoprotein thyroglobulin, which is the colloid filling the follicular sacs. The binding of iodide with the glycoprotein is termed the organification of thyroglobulin. The iodide is then an oxidized iodine. The oxidized iodine slowly bonds with tyrosine (an amino acid). In the presence of enzymes, this bonding is very rapid. Chemical reactions progress to yield thyroxine and triiodothyronine. The thyroid hormones are stored in an amount that is equal to the normal body requirements for 1 to 3 months.

Release of Thyroxine and Triiodothyronine

These two thyroid hormones separate from the thyroglobulin molecule. Separation is a multistep process involving several intermediate chemicals. The end result is that thyroxine and triiodothyronine are lysed from the glycoprotein. Once freed, these thyroid hormones enter the venous circulatory system of the thyroid gland itself and are carried into the systemic circulation. The strongest stimulation to release these hormones is cold temperature. Thyrotropin-releasing hormone (TRH) factors will stimulate release of thyroid-stimulating hormone (TSH), and thyroxine and triiodothyronine will be released from the thyroid gland (but not as rapidly as in response to cold).

The release of these hormones is inhibited by heat, insufficient hypothalamic-releasing factors (resulting in insufficient thyroid-stimulating hormones), and/or increases in plasma glucocorticoids.

Action of Thyroxine and Triiodothyronine

An interesting "rule of four" exists. Once these two hormones are in the peripheral tissues, triiodothyronine is four times as strong in initiating metabolic activities as thyroxine. Thyroxine's effect on the tissues will last four times as long as triiodothyronine's effect. So these two hormones balance each other very well.

Thyroxine Function

Approximately 1 mg of iodine per week is needed for normal thyroxine formation. Iodides are absorbed from the gastrointestinal tract. Two-thirds of ingested iodides are excreted in the urine and the remaining one-third is used by the thyroid gland to form the glycoprotein thyroglobulin.

The major effect of the thyroid hormones is to increase all metabolic activities of the body excluding those of the brain, spleen, lungs, retina, and testes. In children, the thyroid hormones also promote growth.

Production, Release, and Action of Calcitonin

Calcitonin is manufactured in special thyroid cells called parafollicular cells, or C cells. These cells are found in the interstitial tissue between the follicles of the thyroid gland.

An increase in the plasma concentration of calcium stimulates the release of calcitonin, as will the ingestion or administration of magnesium and/or glucagon.

Calcitonin functions in a relationship with parathyroid hormone more so than with the thyroid hormones. Calcitonin's major effect is on bones. Calcitonin reduces plasma calcium levels by immediate decrease in osteoclastic activity, a transient increase in osteoblastic activity, and a prolonged prevention of new osteoclast formation. Calcitonin also interacts with parathormone in the urinary excretion of calcium, magnesium, phosphates, and other electrolytes.

ANATOMY OF THE PARATHYROID GLANDS

Size and Location

The parathyroid glands are four small, flat, roundish glands located on the posterior surface of the lateral lobes of the thyroid (Fig. 22-3). Usually one parathyroid gland is located at the superior end of each thyroid lobe and another gland at the inferior end of each lateral lobe of the thyroid. This location may vary considerably. It is normal to have four glands; however, there may be fewer or more than four glands.

Internal Structure

Two types of cells have been identified in the adult parathyroid gland. Chief cells (Fig. 22-4) are the main cells in the adult. Oxyphil cells (see Fig. 22-4) are present in adults but are frequently absent in children. The function of oxyphil cells is unknown. There is a possibility that oxyphil cells are modified chief cells.

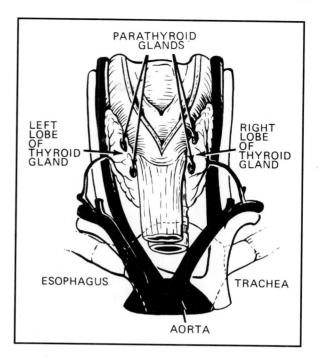

Figure 22-3. Location of the parathyroid glands (posterior view).

PHYSIOLOGY OF THE PARATHYROID GLANDS

Hormone Secretion

The parathyroid glands secrete a hormone termed parathormone (PTH). If two of the glands are inadvertently removed during a subtotal thyroidectomy,

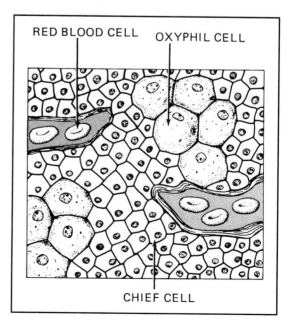

Figure 22-4. Chief cells and oxyphil cells of a parathyroid gland.

the remaining glands will produce sufficient PTH for the body's needs. Some parathyroid tissue should be preserved. This tissue will hypertrophy and continue to secrete PTH. Chief cells in the parathyroid gland are responsible for the secretion of PTH.

When hypothalamic releasing factors are stimulated by a decreased serum calcium level or an increased serum magnesium/phosphate concentration, a series of reactions occur, resulting in the secretion of PTH.

PTH release is also inhibited by hypothalamic factors when serum calcium is increased or when there is an excessive concentration of vitamin D.

Action of Parathyroid Hormone

The main action of PTH and calcitonin is conservation of normal blood calcium levels. PTH decreases renal tubular reabsorption of phosphates, sodium, potassium, and amino acids. It increases reabsorption of calcium, magnesium, and hydrogen ions.

Activated vitamin D is essential for PTH to function appropriately. The release of parathyroid hormone is controlled by a negative feedback mechanism between the blood calcium levels, the hypothalamus, and the parathyroid glands.

Target cells of the parathyroid glands include those of all bones (in a reciprocal relationship with calcium), the kidneys, and the gastrointestinal tract if there is sufficient ingestion of vitamin D.

THYROID DYSFUNCTION

Common disorders of the thyroid gland result primarily from autoimmune processes that either stimulate the overproduction of thyroid hormones (thyrotoxicosis) or cause glandular destruction and hormone deficiency (hypothyroidism). Hypothyroidism, also called myxedema, results from a lack of thyroid hormones. Myxedema coma is the result of severe deficiency or total absence of thyroid hormones. Hyperthyroidism is also called Graves' disease. The fulminant form of hyperthyroidism is called thyroid storm or thyrotoxic crisis. Thyroid storm, or crisis, may occur at any time.

Hypothyroidism (Myxedema)

Hypothyroidism is present when there is insufficient secretion of thyroid hormone. In hypothyroidism, the thyroid gland is usually small and consists of large amounts of fibrous tissue. Some 60% of all cases have autoantibodies present, caused by an autoimmune process.

Hypothyroidism is a chronic disease that is 10 times more common in women than in men and occurs in all age groups but is most commonly seen after 50 years of age. Physiologic signs and symptoms of hypothyroidism are the same regardless of the etiologic basis.

Etiology
The most common cause of hypothyroidism worldwide results from iodine deficiency. Autoimmune disease (Hashimoto's thyroiditis) and iatrogenic causes (treatment of hyperthyroidism) can also result in hypothyroidism. Hypothyroidism can result from a thyroidectomy. A more common cause is inadequate dosage of thyroid medications in known hypothyroid and postthyroidectomy patients. Lack of compliance with the prescribed medical regimen, cessation of medication, pituitary tumors, autoimmune processes, and idiopathic factors are other causes of hypothyroidism. Myxedema coma can develop from the decompensation of a preexisting hypothyroid state due to infection, trauma, exposure to cold, administration of sedatives, physical stress, or anesthesia.

Signs and Symptoms
A common symptom is edema of the face and puffiness of the eyelids (Fig. 22-5). Bloating of the face produces a broad, round shape. Lips become thickened and develop a cyanotic hue. Weakness, fatigability, exertional dyspnea, sensation of cold, paresthesia of the fingers, and loss of hearing are frequent symptoms. Lethargy, lack of concentration, failing memory, and alteration in mentation occur. Skin and hair changes are often early signs of hypothyroidism. The skin becomes dry and scaly and the hair, having become friable and dry, falls out. Total body hair may be involved. These signs increase as the condition progresses to myxedema coma.

Complications
The most serious complication of hypothyroidism is its progression to myxedema coma and death if untreated. Hypothyroidism is associated with an increased incidence of early severe arteriosclerosis. Anemia and increased sensitivity to hypnotic and sedative drugs may become serious problems. Resistance to infection is suppressed and response to treatment of infection is poor. Angina and

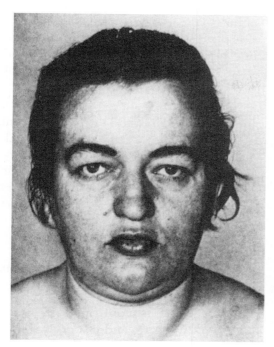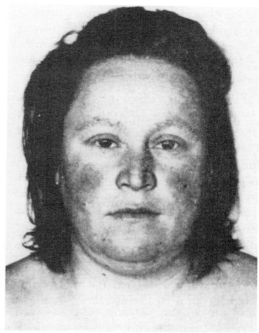

Figure 22-5. Facial appearance of two patients with myxedema.

myocardial infarction are especially common after starting replacement thyroid therapy. The therapy improves and increases myocardial action, but the arteriosclerosis prevents increased delivery of oxygen to the myocardium. Commonly, this results in ischemia and infarction.

Treatment

The optimal treatment for hypothyroidism is early intervention with the goal of restoring a euthyroid state. The only possibility for prevention of complications is the early recognition of hypothyroidism and close monitoring of medical therapy for the remainder of the patient's life. This, of course, necessitates the patient's compliance with the medical regimen.

The treatment of choice is synthetic thyroxin (T4). The advantage that T4 has over other thyroid preparations is that it allows a patient's own physiologic mechanisms to control the production of active hormone. T4 is a prohormone with very little activity. It is deiodinated in the peripheral tissues to make the active form of thyroid hormone T3. Most of the drug is absorbed and has a long plasma half-life. Once-a-day administration is sufficient to achieve a steady state. Levothyroxine (T4) preparations exist under several brand names. There may be slight variations between preparations, so if patients change from one form to another, they should have hormone levels checked as a follow-up to assess if dose adjustments are required. It should always be taken on an empty stomach. The mean daily dose is 150 mcg/day in men and 112 mcg/day in women but the dosage can range from 50 to 200 mcg/day. The elderly may need to start low and titrate up to the desired level. Other thyroid hormone therapies include T3 (liothyronine), desiccated thyroid, and/or mixtures of T4 and T3. These formulations have fallen out of favor for replacement because they can vary in their bioavailablity and, therefore, cause wide fluctuations in serum T3 levels.

EDITORS' NOTE

Do not attempt to remember all these dosages. For the PCCN exam, keep in mind basic concepts such as that hypothyroidism (if it is addressed at all) simply requires thyroid hormone replacement.

Myxedema Coma

Myxedema coma is a life-threatening emergency that is fatal without treatment. Myxedema coma results from untreated or inadequately treated hypothyroidism and can be precipitated by infections, acute illness such as cerebrovascular accident or myocardial infarction, acute trauma, excessive hydration, or administration of a sedative, narcotic, or potent diuretic drug. In addition, myxedema coma is most frequently associated with discontinuation of thyroid hormone therapy by the patient.

Clinical Presentation

Myxedema coma is characterized by hypothermia, hypoventilation, hyponatremia, hyporeflexia, hypotension, and bradycardia. The crisis is more common in winter than in summer because it occurs in response to exposure to cold. Myxedema crisis also occurs frequently following trauma, infection, and central nervous system depression.

The most frequent complication not already mentioned is seizures, which may be almost continuous as death becomes imminent.

Treatment

A multiple-systems approach must be used in treating this emergency. Mechanical ventilation is used to control hypoventilation, carbon dioxide narcosis, and respiratory arrest. Intravenous hypertonic normal saline and glucose will correct the dilutional hyponatremia and hypoglycemia. Warming techniques should be used to increase temperature gradually. These include warming blankets, warm inhaled ventilator gas, and intravascular devices. Hydrocortisone (100–300 mg daily) may be used to treat a possible adrenocortical insufficiency (a commonly associated problem). Thyroid therapy is started immediately without waiting for laboratory confirmation of the diagnosis. Levothyroxine sodium is the most commonly used drug in this emergency. Intravenous doses of 200 to 500 mcg are given during the first 24 h. Oral doses may then be tolerated. Vasoactive drugs may be used to support blood pressure. Bradycardia may require treatment with drugs or with a temporary pacemaker. Prior to the recognition of the need for intravenous levothyroxine sodium and for respiratory support, the mortality rate from myxedema coma was nearly 80%. Currently, the mortality rate is about 20% and is mostly due to the underlying or precipitating illness.

Hyperthyroidism

Toxic goiter and thyrotoxicosis are synonyms for hyperthyroidism. Hyperthyroidism due to Graves' disease is the most common cause of thyrotoxicosis and is thought to be an autoimmune process, although the terms are used interchangeably. Graves' disease results in the formation of autoantibodies that bind to the TSH receptor in thyroid cell membranes and stimulate the gland to hyperfunction.

Etiology

In hyperthyroidism, the thyroid gland enlarges, usually to two or more times the normal size. This releases excess thyroid hormones into the body, increasing the systemic adrenergic activity. Hyperthyroidism is thought to be caused by a failure of the negative-feedback system. Some cases are due to thyroid adenomas, goiters, or familial traits.

Clinical Presentation

Thyrotoxicosis of any cause produces many different clinical signs and symptoms. Patients may experience nervousness, restlessness, heat intolerance, increased sweating, fatigue, weakness, muscle cramps, tachycardia, palpitations, or weight change (usually loss). Exophthalmos (protruding eyeballs) is a clinical sign of hyperthyroidism or Graves' disease (Fig. 22-6). Additional common signs and symptoms are marked fatigue accompanied by insomnia, emotional lability, or irritability.

Diagnosis and Treatment

The diagnosis of hyperthyroidism is confirmed by the finding of increased thyroxine and triiodothyronine levels and an increased uptake of iodine 131 (^{131}I) by the thyroid. Some physicians maintain that the ^{131}I test is the only reliable index, along with the patient's symptoms, to establish a diagnosis of hypothyroidism or hyperthyroidism. Treatment may be medical or surgical. Beta blockers ameliorate the symptoms of hyperthyroidism that result from increased beta-adrenergic tone (palpitations, tachycardia, tremulousness, anxiety, and heat intolerance) and should be started as soon as the diagnosis has been made unless there is a contraindication for their use. Thionamides (propylthiouracil [PTU] or methimazole) are the primary drugs to treat Graves' hyperthyroidism, with the goal of achieving a euthyroid state in 3 to 8 weeks. Once the patient is euthyroid, ^{131}I, ablative therapy, or a subtotal thyroidectomy may be used as definitive therapy. After surgery, the patient usually requires daily thyroid medication for life.

Complications

Heart failure, malnutrition, and ventilatory failure (due to exhaustion) are common. A more life-threatening complication is thyroid storm.

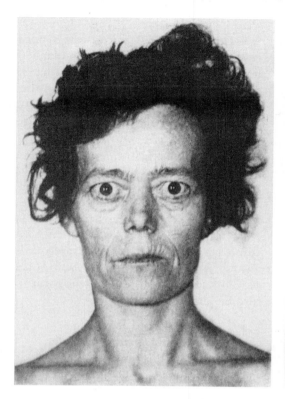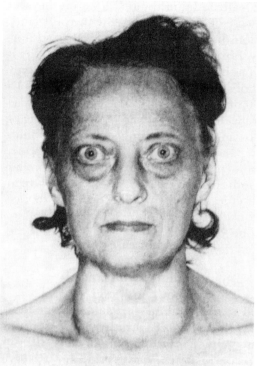

Figure 22-6. Facial appearance of two patients with hyperthyroidism.

Thyrotoxic Crisis (Thyroid Storm)

Thyrotoxic crisis, or thyroid storm, is a life-threatening hypermetabolic state due to hyperthyroidism. Thyrotoxic crisis is a metabolic emergency and has a >20% mortality rate.

Pathophysiology

This is the same as for hyperthyroidism.

Etiology

Any factor that increases the synthesis and secretion of thyroid hormones may cause a storm. Classically, thyroid storm occurs as a result of either previously unrecognized or poorly treated hyperthyroidism. Etiologic factors include subtotal thyroidectomy (due to release of thyroid hormones during the surgery), ketoacidotic states, abruptly stopping antithyroid drugs, or overdosing on thyroid medications (intentional or otherwise). Trauma, stress, infection, or an acute iodine load may precipitate a crisis.

Clinical Presentation

The thyroid storm syndrome characteristically includes hyperthermia (up to 106°F), hypertension with widened pulse pressure, and tachydysrhythmias (atrial fibrillation and paroxysmal atrial tachycardia).

An S_3 gallop may appear with pulmonary edema. Diarrhea, dehydration, diaphoresis, and altered neurologic status, including agitation, tremors, hyperkinesia, delirium, and stupor/coma, are common. Increased appetite, fatigue, proximal muscle weakness, atrophy, and amenorrhea are common. Nausea and vomiting with weight loss are common.

Treatment

Initial treatment of thyroid storm includes stabilization, airway protection, oxygenation, intravenous fluids, and monitoring. Treatment of thyroid storm is of an emergency nature. Treatment is started without waiting for laboratory confirmation of the diagnosis. The first objective is to support vital functions, which necessitates respiratory, cardiac, and renal monitoring and lowering body temperature. Nonaspirin antipyretics are used with a cooling blanket and ice packs to assist in reducing the fever. (The core temperature should be monitored.) Second, a reversal of peripheral effects of excessive thyroid hormone is achieved by intravenous beta blockers (propranolol, esmolol) to decrease the hypermetabolic activity. Third, a reduction in the available and circulating thyroid hormones must be achieved. Thionamides (methimazole, PTU) block new hormone synthesis within 1 to 2 h after administration; however, they will not block release of hormone from the thyroid gland. Iodine solutions may slow the release of thyroid hormones. They should be administered about 1 h after a thionamide has been given. The two most commonly used are Lugol's solution and sodium iodide. Lugol's solution is 30 drops of iodine mixed in milk or juice and given orally through a straw to prevent staining of the teeth. Slow intravenous administration of sodium iodide 1 to 2 g may block release of thyroid hormone. Iodinated radiocontrast agents may work in a similar manner to iodine solutions but there are no firm data on their efficacy. Fourth, glucocorticoids reduce T4 to T3 conversion and may improve outcome. Hydrocortisone 100 mg intravenously every 8 h is the recommended dose for a patient in thyroid storm.

Nursing Interventions

General symptomatic supportive care is appropriate. A quiet environment with limited visitors helps decrease external stress. Physiologic stress is often treated daily with hydrocortisone.

Cooling therapy is useful in hyperpyrexia. Cooling can be achieved with a variety of cooling blankets or intravascular catheters. Cooling to the extent of shivering and piloerection (hair on arms standing up—goose bumps) may have a rebound effect of raising the temperature even higher and increasing metabolic activity and should be avoided. Adjustment of room temperature is necessary; a cool room is desirable.

Fluids, electrolytes, and glucose are given to prevent dehydration and imbalances and to provide energy to meet metabolic needs. Sodium iodine may be given by nasogastric tube or intravenously to prevent release of thyroid hormones.

Complications

If untreated, thyroid storm results in heart failure, exhaustion, coma, and death. With treatment, the sequence is frequently the same. Thyroid storm is most often seen in the summer in undiagnosed or inadequately treated hyperthyroid persons. The presence of stress, infection, nonthyroid surgery, diabetic ketoacidosis, and trauma may result in thyroid storm so intense that it is not amenable to reversal.

PARATHYROID DYSFUNCTION

Hypoparathyroidism

A major parathyroid dysfunction is hypoparathyroidism. This state is a metabolic crisis. Hypoparathyroidism is often seen with hypocalcemia.

Pathophysiology

A deficiency of the PTH causes a hypocalcemic state, resulting in abnormal neuromuscular activity (calcium level <8.5 mg/dL). It is thought that this deficiency occurs secondary to a dysfunction in the calcium and phosphate concentration feedback loops' control systems.

Etiology

Acute hypocalcemia and hyperphosphatemia are usually secondary to ischemia or damage of the parathyroid gland during a thyroidectomy. Hypomagnesemia caused by malnutrition and malabsorption, increased renal secretion, and chemotherapeutic agents may also cause hypoparathyroidism. Very rarely, radiation therapy (with ^{131}I) of the thyroid may cause hypoparathyroidism, as can acute pancreatitis. Hypoparathyroidism may also be idiopathic.

Clinical Presentation

Nausea, vomiting, and abdominal cramps are common. Dyspnea may be accompanied by a laryngeal stridor and cyanosis. Neurologic signs and symptoms are prominent. There may be confusion, emotional lability, paresthesias of fingers and toes, and muscular twitching progressing to tetany and convulsions. (A decrease in the threshold for nerve and muscle excitation leads to muscle spasms, hyperreflexia, clonic-tonic convulsion, and laryngeal spasm.)

Diagnosis

Laboratory blood work will show hypocalcemia. Urine tests will reveal hypophosphaturia and perhaps hypocalciuria. Two signs are a positive Trousseau's and a positive Chvostek's sign, although these signs are not always present. Trousseau's sign is elicited by occluding circulation to the arm. This is done by inflating a blood pressure cuff to just above the systolic pressure level. If positive, the patient's hand will develop a carpopedal spasm within 3 min. A carpopedal spasm results in a hollow palm position and fingers rigid and flexed at the metacarpophalangeal joints. Chvostek's sign is elicited by lightly tapping the facial nerve in front of the ear. If positive, there is a unilateral contraction of the facial muscles.

Treatment

The objective of treatment is to raise serum calcium levels to normal. If seizures and tetany have not developed, oral calcium supplements are indicated, with additional vitamin D to promote calcium absorption. (Calcium may be given with food but not with milk because milk products will decrease calcium absorption.)

Some types of calcium chloride should be given only through a central line as infiltration in a peripheral line will result in tissue necrosis and sloughing. Calcium for infusion should be diluted in saline or dextrose solution to avoid vein irritation. The infusion should not contain bicarbonate or phosphate because this can form an insoluble calcium salt. If bicarbonate or phosphate administration is necessary, a separate IV line should be used.

Cardiac status must be monitored, especially if the patient is on digitalis. Digitalis and calcium have a synergistic action.

Complications

Complications include seizures, tetany, laryngeal spasm, shock, and death. A quiet environment with supportive equipment (ventilator, pacemaker) on standby may be useful in preventing potential complications.

Nursing Interventions

Preventive nursing care in hypoparathyroidism may avoid the complications of seizures and tetany. The environment should be modified to be as quiet as possible, including the limiting of visitors until the patient is well stabilized.

A respirator on standby will provide for immediate intervention in the advent of hypoventilation or deteriorating respiratory status as shown by serial arterial blood gas values. Emotional and physical stress often causes hyperventilation. In turn, hyperventilation causes alkalosis, which may precipitate tetany.

Cardiac monitoring is essential since calcium therapy may alter cardiac conduction times, with resultant dysrhythmias. Standard monitoring of intake/output, response to medication therapy, neurologic status, and such are applicable to these patients as the medication therapy will cause a change in their electrolytes and fluid balance.

Administration of calcium as ordered, with special attention to possible infiltration and precipitation if being given intravenously, and *avoiding* milk products if being given orally will help ensure maximum benefit with minimal side effects of the drugs.

23

Anatomy, Physiology, and Dysfunction of the Pancreas

EDITORS' NOTE

According to the PCCN exam blueprint, specific questions regarding pancreatic function are less likely to be addressed than questions regarding acute hyperglycemia and hypoglycemia and acute syndromes of glucose metabolism dysfunction. Focus your attention on disturbances in blood glucose and the clinical conditions associated with abnormal blood glucose levels. Bear in mind, however, that only a few (i.e., two to four) questions are likely in the content area covered by this chapter.

The pancreas has a dual classification. It is considered an accessory digestive gland because it produces many enzymes essential to digestion. These enzymes are released through exocrine glands (glands that release substances through ducts). The pancreas (Fig. 23-1) is also classified as an endocrine gland because it releases two hormones, insulin and glucagon, directly into the bloodstream.

ANATOMY

Two major types of tissues are found in the pancreas: the acini and the islets of Langerhans. The acini secrete digestive enzymes into the duodenum via exocrine glands. The islets of Langerhans are scattered throughout the pancreas; they may be called pancreatic islets in some texts.

Islets of Langerhans

Three structurally and functionally different cells make up the islets of Langerhans: alpha, beta, and delta cells (Fig. 23-2).

1. Alpha cells are located within the clusters of islet cells. They secrete the hormone glucagon, which is often called the hyperglycemic factor. Alpha cells secrete directly into the venous system of the pancreas.
2. Beta cells are located within the clusters of islet cells and are slightly smaller than alpha cells. They secrete insulin. The insulin molecules are very complex amino acid structures.
3. Delta cells are located within the clusters of the islet cells. They secrete a hormone called somatostatin. Somatostatin has an effect upon the secretion of glucagon and insulin.

PHYSIOLOGY

Glucagon

The alpha cells of the islets of Langerhans secrete the hormone glucagon, which affects many body cells, especially those of the liver. Glucagon is secreted when blood amino acid levels rise and in the presence of a decreased blood glucose level.

Glucagon acts primarily as an antagonist to insulin; its primary site of function is the liver. The most important aspect of this action is to increase

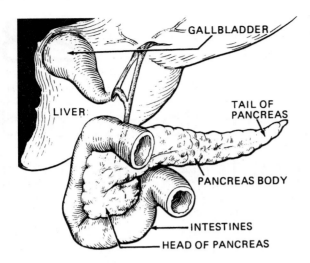

Figure 23–1. The pancreas.

blood glucose levels. Glucose metabolism is altered by two important actions of glucagon: glycogenolysis (the breakdown of liver glycogen stores) and the release of glucose. Gluconeogenesis (the formation of glucose from other substances) provides new glucose. There is also an increase in fatty acid oxidation and in urea formation as a natural response to glucagon.

Insulin

Insulin is a small protein comprising two amino acid chains. If the chains become separated, insulin loses its effectiveness. Once secreted into the circulatory system, insulin is removed by the liver and degraded. Most insulin circulates for only about 10 min before the degradation process occurs. This allows control and rapid initiation or cessation of insulin's action when it is being administered intravenously.

The target cells for insulin's action are skeletal muscle, adipose tissue, the heart, certain smooth muscle organs such as the uterus, and especially liver cells. The brain and erythrocytes do not require insulin. Factors that facilitate the secretion of insulin are an increase in blood glucose levels and growth hormone levels. A decreased insulin level results in hyperglycemia, ketosis, and acidosis.

Insulin's actions include transporting glucose across cell membranes, increasing fatty acid storage, enhancing protein synthesis, facilitating the transport of potassium, and decreasing the breakdown of triglycerides in cells.

DYSFUNCTION OF GLUCOSE METABOLISM

States of dysfunctional glucose metabolism that are treated in critical care areas include diabetic ketoacidosis, hyperglycemic hyperosmolar state, hyperglycemia of critical illness, and insulin shock.

Diabetic Ketoacidosis

Diabetic ketoacidosis (DKA) is an acute, life-threatening complication of diabetes occurring predominately in patients with type I (insulin-dependent) diabetes mellitus. It represents a state of relative insulin deficiency. The digestion of carbohydrates raises the blood glucose level, which stimulates the pancreas to secrete insulin. If insulin cannot be secreted or secreted in sufficient amounts, hyperglycemia develops.

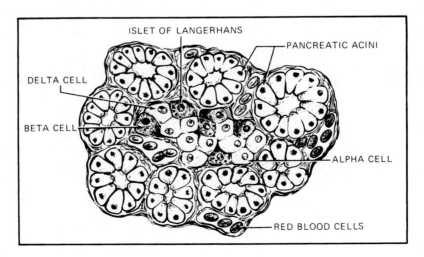

Figure 23–2. Cells of the pancreas.

Pathophysiology

A lack of insulin prevents peripheral cells from utilizing available blood glucose. The liver inhibits the production of glycogen, and such glycogen as is available is rapidly degraded. This releases free glucose into the blood, further raising the blood sugar level.

Since the cells cannot utilize the free glucose, protein stores release amino acids and adipose tissue releases fatty acids. The amino acids and free fatty acids are synthesized by the liver, which is producing excessive amounts of acetyl coenzyme A (acetyl-CoA). The acetyl-CoA is rapidly degraded into keto, acetoacetic, and beta hydroxybutyric acids. These acids are produced faster than the kidneys and lungs can dispose of them, causing a metabolic acidosis. Ketones (keto acids or ketoanions) are excreted by the kidneys, producing a positive urine acetone test. Acetoacetic acid and beta-hydroxybutyric acid are oxidized into acetone. The acetone is exhaled and is responsible for the sweet, fruity smell of the breath in these patients. (It is the acetone of the acetoacetic acid that has the odor; beta-hydroxybutyric acid is odorless.)

Etiology

The most common causes of DKA are failure to take insulin and/or increased stress due to illness, infection, trauma, surgery, cardiac conditions, and occasionally psychogenic trauma. Pregnancy and pancreatitis may also precipitate a diabetic ketoacidotic state. Previously undiagnosed type I diabetes mellitus can also present with DKA.

Clinical Presentation

The most common symptoms of DKA are polydipsia, polyuria, polyphagia (usually with weight loss), dyspnea, and a generalized malaise. Nausea, vomiting, anorexia, and abdominal pain may be present. Signs of dehydration, tachycardia, orthostatic hypotension, and weakness are usually present. Respirations are Kussmaul in character and may have an acetone smell. Mentation ranges from lethargy to coma.

Diagnosis

Three distinct clinical features are seen in DKA: hyperglycemia, ketonuria/ketonemia, and metabolic acidosis. Serum glucose levels are above 300 mg/dL. Serum ketones are present, as is an anion gap. Arterial pH <7.30 and serum bicarbonate <15 mEq/L are also seen. Metabolic acidosis can also result in potentially life-threatening electrolyte imbalances including hyperkalemia or hypokalemia. DKA should be ruled out in any patient who is comatose, dehydrated, and having deep, labored respirations.

Treatment

The objectives of treatment in DKA are to correct acidemia, hyperglycemia, hypovolemia, hyperosmolality, potassium deficit, and ketonemia. Underlying conditions responsible for DKA, such as infections, must be identified and treated concurrently.

Resolution of DKA is the most effective method of restoring normal acid-base balance.

Hypovolemia is corrected by rapid infusions of 0.9% or 0.45% normal saline. The average fluid loss is 3 to 6 L in DKA. Isotonic or hypotonic fluids are administered to counter the hyperosmolality that accompanies DKA. The goal is to correct the extracellular volume depletion without inducing cerebral edema due to too rapid reduction is serum osmolality. When the serum glucose level is decreased to 250 mg/dL, the fluids should be changed from saline to 5% glucose in 0.45% normal saline. This change will help avoid hypoglycemia, hypokalemia, and cerebral edema caused by the glucose diuresis. Correction of the hypovolemia usually corrects the hyperosmolality and, over a period of hours, the ketonemia. Successful progress is judged by frequent hemodynamic and laboratory monitoring. Patients may move from DKA coma to insulin shock without regaining consciousness if not closely monitored. The addition of glucose to intravenous fluids or, if the patient is alert and oriented, feeding the patient helps prevent this.

Hyperglycemia is corrected by insulin administration. Adequate fluid resuscitation will contribute to lowering serum glucose levels. Normally, an intravenous (IV) bolus of insulin is administered, followed by a slow continuous intravenous infusion. Insulin may be administered by subcutaneous (SQ) or intramuscular (IM) injections; however, this is not advocated in the crisis stage of DKA because of poor peripheral absorption. Rapid-acting subcutaneous insulin can be used to successfully treat mild to moderate DKA if the patient is not in a state of shock. The serum glucose level should fall approximately 100 mg/dL every 1 to 2 h. The brain does not require insulin and the blood-brain barrier prevents rapid movement of glucose out of the cerebrospinal fluid. To prevent cerebral edema, a slow decrease in the serum glucose is desired. The glucose is an osmotic particle and pulls fluid to the brain when the serum glucose is rapidly decreased. Regardless of the timing of when to switch over to the subcutaneous shorter acting and basal insulin, the intravenous infusion should be continued for an overlap of 1 to 2 h to prevent an acute fall in insulin levels and the return of hyperglycemia and/or ketoacidosis.

Both renal and gastrointestinal losses contribute to potassium depletion. Potassium deficits and other electrolyte imbalances may precipitate cardiac and/or neurologic disturbances. Potassium is usually added to intravenous fluids as the insulin forces potassium from the plasma back into the cells, producing hypokalemia. Initially, the serum potassium level may appear to be normal or high because of the shifting of potassium from the cells to the serum. Continuous monitoring and gradual changes to effect a correction over a 24-h period are safer than massive, rapid changes. The exception to this is the patient whose life is threatened by extremes of hypokalemia and hyperkalemia. The serum potassium should be maintained between 4 and 5 mEq/L.

Complications

Acidosis, electrolyte imbalances, acute renal failure, pulmonary edema, cerebral edema, seizures, cerebrospinal fluid acidosis, shock, and coma are the major complications of DKA.

Nursing Interventions

DKA requires frequent patient monitoring. It is essential to maintain a patent airway and suctioning as required to prevent aspiration. Monitoring respiratory status by observation and arterial blood gases will identify impending hypoxia.

Cardiac monitoring in response to electrolyte imbalances will reveal early dysrhythmias. With hypokalemia, U waves are normally present. In hyperkalemia, peaked or tented T waves are present. There may be tachycardia, which converts to bradycardia if the hyperkalemia increases.

Monitoring of urinary output and frequent auscultation of lung sounds to identify pulmonary edema, especially in the presence of underlying cardiac diseases, should be performed. Finger-stick glucose should be checked hourly. Once adequate urinary output is present, electrolytes are often added to the intravenous fluids to correct imbalances.

Blood sugar will initially be monitored hourly by bedside blood glucose monitoring to guide the administration of regular insulin. Long-acting insulin is not used in DKA crisis. Once the serum glucose reaches 250 mg/dL, the patient's intravenous fluids should be changed to 5% or 10% dextrose to prevent hypoglycemia. The American Diabetes Association (ADA) guidelines recommend a patient can be switched from IV to SQ insulin when the serum glucose is <200 mg/dL, serum anion gap is normal, serum bicarbonate is >18 mEq/L, and venous pH is >7.30. Patients may be restarted on their home insulin regimen once DKA has resolved. If the patient is able to eat, food may be given. The most common complication of treatment of DKA is hypoglycemia, and this can be significantly reduced with low-dose insulin and careful monitoring of blood glucose.

Potassium should be checked frequently since initially it moves from the cells into the blood and much is excreted in the urine. When insulin is given, potassium shifts back into the cells. In addition to the laboratory results, the cardiac monitor will show whether the patient's serum potassium is low, normal, or high.

Neurologic status is assessed hourly. Hyperglycemia does not have a deleterious effect on brain cells, but other electrolyte imbalances and cerebral edema do. Symptoms of cerebral edema usually appear 12 to 24 h after the initiation of treatment for DKA. Although more common in children, it can occur in adults. Headache is the earliest symptom, followed by behavior changes and lethargy. Deterioration can be rapid with seizures, papillary changes, bradycardia, incontinence, and respiratory arrest. Mortality can be high in patients who develop cerebral edema.

Controversy exists over the use of bicarbonate to correct the acidosis present in DKA. Typically, fluid and insulin administration will resolve any acidosis, making bicarbonate administration unnecessary. Bicarbonate given intravenously does not cross the blood-brain barrier. It causes a shift in the bicarbonate/carbonic acid ratio, releasing carbon dioxide. Carbon dioxide crosses the blood-brain barrier, dissolving in the spinal fluid. This raises the carbonic acid level and increases cerebral acidosis, which may prolong diabetic coma. Bicarbonate may be considered if the pH is <7 and if the patient shows signs of cardiac dysfunction or signs of life-threatening hyperkalemia. The venous or arterial pH may be used to monitor the effect and to adjust dosing.

Complications

Complications of DKA are related to treatment. Cerebral edema, hypoglycemia, hypokalemia, and hyperchloremic acidosis are the major concerns during the initial treatment of DKA.

Hyperglycemic Hyperosmolar State

Hyperglycemic hyperosmolar state ([HHS]; formerly known as hyperosmolar, hyperglycemic, nonketotic coma [HHNK]) is classified as hyperglycemia with profound dehydration without ketosis. In HHS coma, enough insulin is being released to prevent ketosis, but there is not enough of it to prevent hyperglycemia.

Pathophysiology

Hyperglycemia increases the solutes in the extracellular fluid, causing a hyperosmolality. Cellular dehydration occurs because of this, which is also the cause of diuresis. Without treatment, an osmotic gradient develops between the brain and the plasma, resulting in dehydration and central nervous system dysfunction. The end result of dehydration is a decreased glomerular filtration rate and the development of azotemia.

Typically, the HHS coma patient is older than 50 years, becomes ill, and experiences general malaise. Because of this, the patient is anorexic and eats and drinks poorly, which leads to dehydration. Since the patient is not eating, the body uses protein and fat for energy to maintain body processes. Almost the same pathophysiologic pattern of DKA appears in HHS coma. The difference is that in HHS coma, a sufficient amount of insulin is released to prevent the development of ketosis. The patient may be stuporous or comatose before being seen by a physician.

Etiology

One of the common causes of HHS coma is undiagnosed or untreated diabetes. Frequently, a mild diabetic state exists without any problems until the diabetic is under stress. Iatrogenic causes of some cases of HHS coma include hyperalimentation, the administration of hypertonic intravenous fluids, and the administration of steroids.

Clinical Presentation

Usually the patient, who is typically older than 50 years, is lethargic or comatose. Symptoms include polyuria, polydipsia, nausea, vomiting, and weight loss. Eventually, the urinary output begins to fall as fluid depletion becomes more severe. Dehydration is apparent, with dry skin and mucous membranes. Tachypnea as well as tachycardia, hypotension, and glycosuria are present.

Diagnosis

The three most outstanding signs may well be an elevated blood sugar level (commonly >1000 mg), plasma hyperosmolarity (>350 mOsm/kg), and an extremely elevated hematocrit. Urine and plasma are both negative for acetone. The blood urea nitrogen is usually elevated and there is marked leukocytosis.

Complications

Shock, coma, acute tubular necrosis, cerebral edema, and vascular thrombosis are common complications. Death can result with HHS coma if treatment is not quickly initiated.

Treatment

Correction of the fluid balance is one of the first objectives of treatment. It is essential that fluids be administered in order to correct the hyperosmolality and hypovolemia. If the patient has a cardiac history, slow administration of fluid (300 mL/h) may be performed. The hypoinsulinemia may be corrected by the use of insulin. Hyperglycemia is not known to have deleterious effects on the brain, but hyperosmolar dehydration may cause seizures. Return of the anion gap to normal levels may serve as an indication of success in the use of insulin therapy.

If metabolic acidosis is present, it is usually corrected by the administration of intravenous fluids. The use of sodium bicarbonate is controversial for the same reasons as it is in DKA. Any electrolyte imbalances, such as hypokalemia, should be corrected. Close and continuous monitoring is necessary to identify further changes or deterioration in the patient's electrolyte status. Cardiac monitoring and hourly neurologic checks will provide clues to changing status.

Nursing Interventions

The primary nursing responsibility is the administration of intravenous fluids to correct both dehydration and hyperosmolality without putting the patient into pulmonary edema. The average fluid loss in HHS is 8 to 10 L. The nurse must monitor breath sounds hourly to determine whether pulmonary edema is developing.

Cardiac monitoring is continuous to identify dysrhythmias due to electrolyte imbalances, especially hypokalemia/hyperkalemia. The patient must also be monitored to detect early signs of congestive heart failure.

Administration of insulin to correct hyperglycemia is usually accomplished by an insulin infusion as indicated by the blood glucose level. Continuous insulin infusion is used with caution to prevent hypoglycemia. The nurse should check the patient's blood glucose level hourly. Insulin therapy for HHS is the same as for DKA.

Neurologic status should be evaluated hourly to provide information on the efficacy of treatment. Skin and mouth care are important aspects of preventing infection and keeping the patient comfortable.

Hyperglycemia of Acute Illness

Stress-induced hyperglycemia in acutely ill nondiabetic patients is a common occurrence. The release of stress hormones—including glucagon, catecholamines, cortisol, and growth hormone, as well as their catabolic effects—causes increased gluconeogenesis and glycogenolysis and resultant hyperglycemia. In addition, these catabolic hormones induce tissue resistance to insulin. A number of additional factors including cytokines, epinephrine, and reactive oxygen species are also involved in initiating hepatic insulin resistance. The reported effects of hyperglycemia in critical illness include impaired immune function, increased inflammation, impaired wound healing, and endothelial cell dysfunction.

Formerly, hyperglycemia was not routinely controlled in an acute illness except in patients with known diabetes mellitus. Research on the benefits of moderate glycemic control has led to closer control of hyperglycemia in acutely ill patients. Intravenous insulin protocols to maintain moderate glycemic control, with serum glucose levels 140 to 180 mg/dL, have been shown to significantly reduce mortality rates and improve outcomes for critically ill patients. As a result, the management of hyperglycemia with the use of insulin protocols is becoming a new standard in critical and acute care. Nursing implications include oversight of intravenous administration of insulin, often with the use of protocols, and close monitoring of serum glucose levels. The risk of hypoglycemia from tight glucose control carries a significant mortality and should be avoided.

Hypoglycemic Reaction (Insulin Shock)

Pathophysiology

A decreased blood level of glucose is the criterion for the diagnosis of a hypoglycemic reaction, or insulin shock. The decrease may be due to a defect in the process of forming glucose, either glyconeogenesis or glycogenolysis, or by the removal of glucose by the use of adipose, muscle, or liver tissues.

Etiology

Hypoglycemia unrelated to exogenous insulin therapy is rare. Causes of hypoglycemia include an intolerance of fructose, galactose, or amino acids. Postgastrectomy patients may have hypoglycemia. A broad range of substances such as alcohol, insulin, and sulfonylurea drugs may be the origin. Endocrine dysfunctions, liver disease, severe congestive heart failure, and pregnancy may cause hypoglycemia. In diabetic patients, overdoses of exogeneous insulin or long-acting sulfonylureas and exercising without adjustment of insulin dosage are the common causes of insulin shock.

Clinical Presentation

The clinical presentation of hyperglycemia can vary between patients. The early signs and symptoms are restlessness, diaphoresis, tachycardia, and hunger. Beta blockers may hide these signs and symptoms. If the hypoglycemia progresses to <50 mg/dL, the central nervous system will be affected and the patient may exhibit bizarre behavior that can progress to a comatose state. Headache, dizziness, irritability, fatigue, poor judgment, confusion, visual changes, hunger, weakness, tremors, seizures, nausea, and personality changes are common signs and symptoms.

Diagnosis and Treatment

Treatment of hypoglycemia requires administration of glucose, either intravenously or orally. A glucose level <50 mg/dL with blood glucose monitoring is sufficient to require infusion of 50 mg of 50% dextrose intravenously. The patient will usually respond within 1 to 2 min. A sample of blood should be drawn prior to giving the glucose so that the diagnosis can be confirmed by laboratory tests. Glucagon 0.5 to 1.0 SQ or IM may be considered as another therapy for a patient who is unable to eat or drink. Glucagon will not be as effective in patients whose hepatic glycogen stores are low, in fasting patients, or in those patients who have been hypoglycemic for a prolonged time. Patients who are able to eat or drink may be given oral glucose solutions, juices, or food. Ingestion of 5 g of carbohydrate will raise the blood glucose by 15 mg/dL. Twenty-five grams of carbohydrate is usually necessary to correct hypoglycemia. Repeat administration of glucose may be necessary based on the action of the hypoglycemic agent. If hypoglycemia is present in a patient who does not have diabetes, additional tests must be performed to rule out endocrine disorders or tumors. If hypoglycemia is present in a known diabetic, the underlying cause of the insulin shock must be identified and corrected. Preventing hypoglycemic events can be possible by setting appropriate glucose goals, glucose monitoring, behavior modification, and patient/family education. The nurse must recognize factors that can lead to hypoglycemia during insulin administration. These include a delay in food after

Table 23-1. TYPES OF INSULIN AND THEIR ONSET, PEAK, AND DURATION

Type of Insulin	Onset (h)	Peak Effect (h)	Duration (h)
Long-acting			
Insulin glargine	3–4	None	≥24
Intermediate– to Long–acting			
Insulin detemir	3–4	3–9	6–23
Intermediate–acting			
Insulin NPH (isophane suspension)	1–2	4–12	14–24
Short–acting			
Insulin regular	0.5	2.5–5	4–12
Rapid–acting			
Insulin lispro	0.25–0.5	0.5–2.5	≤5
Insulin aspart	0.2–0.3	1–3	3–5
Insulin glulisine	0.2–0.5	1.6–2.8	3–4
Combinations			
Insulin aspart protamine suspension and insulin aspart	0.17–0.33	1–4	18–24
Insulin lispro protamine and insulin lispro	0.25–0.5	1–6.5	14–24
Insulin NPH suspension and insulin regular solution	0.5	2–12	18–24

premeal insulin administration, a decrease in food intake (oral, parenteral, or enteral) or stopping IV dextrose administration, heart failure, renal disease, liver disease, insulin dosage error, reduction in steroids, and failure to recognize a downward trend in blood glucose levels. Being alert to these contributing factors will decrease the incidence of hypoglycemic events. The nurse's understanding of time of onset, peak effect, and duration of action of the type of insulin administered is imperative to prevent hypoglycemia (Table 23-1).

Complications

The brain obtains almost all of its energy from glucose metabolism. If the glucose level is maintained below 45 to 50 mg/dL, cerebral ischemia, edema, and neuronal hyperexcitability occur. If the blood glucose level drops to 20 to 40 mg/dL, seizures may occur. If the blood glucose level drops below 20 mg/dL, coma develops. If it is not promptly reversed, the low blood glucose levels may cause irreversible brain damage, myocardial ischemia, infarction, and death.

Somogyi Effect

When too much insulin is administered, hypoglycemia occurs. This alerts the body's defense systems, which overreact. With hypoglycemia, certain anti–insulin hormones are secreted. These include epinephrine, glucagon, glucocorticoids, and growth hormones. The secretion of these hormones causes hyperglycemia. A cyclical pattern develops: hypoglycemia one day may be followed by one or more days of hyperglycemia. In some patients, the cycle is so short that periods alternate within the same day. Symptoms of hypoglycemia in a hyperglycemic patient may indicate a Somogyi effect. Blood sugar levels may reach dangerously high levels because of this rebound effect.

Dawn Phenomenon

Early-morning increases in blood glucose concentration can occur with no corresponding hypoglycemia during the night. This phenomenon is thought to be secondary to the nocturnal elevations of growth hormone.

24

Anatomy, Physiology, and Dysfunction of the Adrenal Glands

EDITORS' NOTE

Like thyroid disturbances, adrenal dysfunction is less likely to be specifically addressed on the PCCN exam; questions pertaining to adrenal dysfunction will usually appear in the context of another system. Consequently, read this chapter to introduce yourself to key concepts and to familiarize yourself with major functions of the adrenal glands.

ANATOMY

The adrenal glands are a pair of glands located on the top of each kidney (Fig. 24-1). Each of the two glands is identical to the other.

The adrenal gland is composed of two separate parts (Fig. 24-2): the adrenal cortex, the outer two-thirds of the gland, and the adrenal medulla, the inner one-third of the gland. A mnemonic for remembering where each part lies is the letter "M," standing for "medulla" and "middle."

Adrenal Cortex

The adrenal cortex is composed of three distinct regions, or zones (Fig. 24-3). The outermost zone is the zona glomerulosa. The middle zone is the zona fasciculata. The innermost zone is the zona reticularis. The zona glomerulosa functions by itself. The zona fasciculata and zona reticularis function together as a unit.

The zona glomerulosa is a thin zone located on the outer part of the cortex, directly under the capsular covering. The cells in this zone are arranged in clumps. The regulation of the hormone (aldosterone) secreted in the zona glomerulosa is completely independent of the regulatory controls over the zona fasciculata and the zona reticularis. The regulatory control of the zona glomerulosa is the release of adrenocorticotropic hormone (ACTH), releasing factors from the hypothalamus, and ACTH-stimulating factors from the adenohypophysis.

The zona fasciculata is the largest of the three zones. Its cells are arranged in straight rows. The zona reticularis is composed of an anastomosing network of cells. These two zones function together to regulate cortisol and androgenic hormones and are controlled by the same regulatory mechanisms of the adenohypophysis.

Adrenal Medulla

Cells of the adrenal medulla (Fig. 24-2) develop from the same embryologic source as the sympathetic neurons. These cells are also called chromaffin cells because of their histologic staining characteristics. Because of their origin, the cells of the adrenal medulla are related functionally to the sympathetic nervous system.

PHYSIOLOGY

Functionally, the adrenal cortex and the adrenal medulla are totally different. Without adrenocortical hormones or replacement therapy, death occurs in 3 to 14 days.

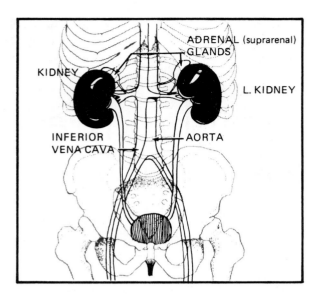

Figure 24-1. Location of the adrenal glands.

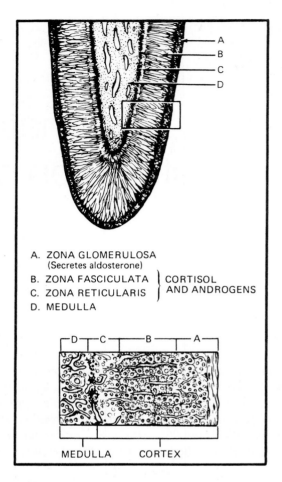

A. ZONA GLOMERULOSA
   (Secretes aldosterone)
B. ZONA FASCICULATA } CORTISOL
C. ZONA RETICULARIS } AND ANDROGENS
D. MEDULLA

Figure 24-3. Zones and medulla of the adrenal gland.

Adrenocortical Hormones

The hormones secreted by the adrenal cortex are classified as corticosteroids since they are synthesized from the steroid cholesterol. As a group, more than 30 corticosteroids may be referred to as corticoids.

The adrenal cortex secretes three classes of hormones: the glucocorticoids, the mineralocorticoids, and the androgenic hormones.

Glucocorticoids

Originally, the glucocorticoids were thought to control the body's blood glucose level. It has since been

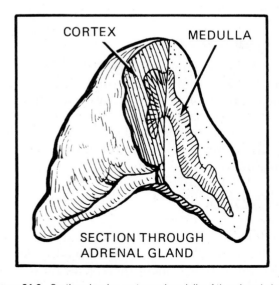

Figure 24-2. Section showing cortex and medulla of the adrenal gland.

discovered that glucocorticoids play a major role in utilization of carbohydrates, proteins, and fats.

Cortisol. This glucocorticoid is responsible for 95% of the adrenocortical secretory actions. Cortisol is the most important hormone of this class of steroid hormones, affecting all body cells (especially the liver). It is secreted by the zona fasciculata and the zona reticularis in response to stress (both physical and psychogenic), trauma, and infection.

Cortisol is active in all metabolic processes. These include the ability of the body to stimulate gluconeogenesis by the liver up to 10 times its normal rate. (It does this by increasing the migration of amino acids from the extracellular fluids to the liver, the migration of amino acids from muscles into the liver, and all of the enzymes needed to convert the amino acids into glucose in the liver.) Cortisol causes a moderate decrease in the rate of glucose utilization by the cells. Both the increased rate of gluconeogenesis and the moderate reduction in rate of glucose utilization by the cells cause the blood glucose concentration to rise. Cortisol decreases protein storage in all body cells except the liver, resulting in muscle weakness and decreased functions of immunity in the lymphoid tissues. The proteins stored in tissues are shifted to the liver (called mobilization of amino acids), which results in decreased protein synthesis.

Cortisol promotes fatty acid mobilization weakly, but that mobilization is sufficient to provide some fat for body energy in the absence of the normal glucose.

Cortisol has a strong anti-inflammatory effect and, in sufficient amounts, may block and/or reverse the inflammatory process.

Secretion of the glucocorticoids is controlled almost entirely by ACTH secreted by the anterior pituitary gland. The hypothalamus provides the negative-feedback mechanism responsible for cortisol-releasing factors (CRFs) and cortisol-inhibitory factors (such as exogenous intake of corticosteroids).

Mineralocorticoids

Mineralocorticoids are named as such since their action is chiefly with the extracellular fluid electrolytes (minerals) sodium and potassium. The most important mineralocorticoid is aldosterone, which is secreted in the zona glomerulosa.

Aldosterone. This mineralocorticoid's most important function is regulating the movement of sodium and potassium through the renal tubular walls. It also plays a minor role in hydrogen ion transport.

Aldosterone exerts its action on the distal convoluted tubules and the collecting ducts. There is a slight effect on sweat glands (to conserve salt in hot conditions). The primary action of aldosterone is to cause an increase in sodium reabsorption and potassium and hydrogen ion excretion by the kidney. Since water follows sodium, aldosterone secretion tends to change the extracellular fluid volume in proportion to its secretion.

Aldosterone excess may rapidly cause severe hypokalemia and alkalosis, including muscle weakness, and muscle paralysis if the potassium level is reduced to half its normal value. Hypertension may occur as a result of the increase in extracellular fluid volume.

The release of aldosterone is stimulated by an increased serum potassium level, the renin-angiotensin cascade, decreased serum sodium levels, and ACTH.

Decreased levels of aldosterone allow the extracellular level of potassium to rise to double the normal potassium level, resulting in severe hyperkalemia and cardiac toxicity, as evidenced by weakness of contractions. A concurrent decrease in serum sodium and increase in water loss occurs. A potassium level only slightly higher will cause cardiac death.

Androgens

Several androgens are secreted by the adrenal cortex, but their alterations are not usually a primary cause for treatment in a critical care area and are not covered in this text except to mention that they are secreted by the zona fasciculata and the zona reticularis.

Adrenal Medullary Hormones

The hormones secreted by the adrenal medulla are classified as catecholamines and have very far-reaching effects. Catecholamines are synthesized in the adrenal medulla as well as by the endings of sympathetic adrenergic nerve fibers, the brain, and some peripheral tissues. Both of the catecholamines secreted by the adrenal medulla have an effect on the adrenergic (sympathetic) receptor sites. There are three sites, termed alpha, beta$_1$ (β_1), and beta$_2$ (β_2). Table 24-1 lists the adrenergic receptors and their functions.

Ordinarily, the norepinephrine secreted directly in a tissue by adrenergic nerve endings remains active for only a few seconds, illustrating that its reuptake

TABLE 24-1. ADRENERGIC RECEPTORS AND THEIR FUNCTIONS

Alpha Receptor	Beta Receptor
Vasoconstriction (α_1, α_2)	Vasodilatation (β_2)
Iris dilatation (α_1)	Cardioacceleration (β_1)
Intestinal relaxation (α_1, α_2)	Increased myocardial strength (β_1)
Intestinal sphincter contraction (α_2)	Intestinal relaxation (β_2)
Pilomotor contraction (α_1)	Uterine relaxation (β_2)
Bladder sphincter contraction (α_1)	Bronchodilatation (β_2)
Ureter contraction (α_1)	
Vas deferens contraction (α_1)	
Uterus contraction (α_1)	
Uretheral contraction (α_1)	
Bronchioles constriction (α_1)	
Inhibit insulin release (α_2)	
Glucagon release from pancreas (α_2)	
Platelet aggregation (α_2)	
	Colorigenesis (β_2)
	Glycogenolysis (β_2)
	Lipolysis (β_1)
	Bladder relaxation (β_2)

and diffusion away from the tissue is rapid. However, the norepinephrine and epinephrine secreted into the blood by the adrenal medulla remain active until they diffuse into some tissue, where they are destroyed by enzymes. This occurs mainly in the liver. Therefore, the effects last about 10 times as long as compared to direct sympathetic stimulation.

Epinephrine (Adrenaline)

Epinephrine (adrenaline) accounts for 80% of the total catecholamine secreted by the adrenal medulla; it excites both alpha and beta adrenergic receptor sites equally.

A major action of epinephrine is the "fear, fight, flight" body response to stress. These actions would include positive effects on the cardiac muscle, shifting of blood to certain muscles, decreasing gastrointestinal function, bronchiolar dilatation accompanied by hyperpnea and tachypnea, and an increase in serum glucose level.

Epinephrine is released by sympathetic nervous system stimulation and other hormones, such as insulin and histamine.

Norepinephrine

Norepinephrine accounts for 20% of catecholamines secreted by the adrenal medulla. Norepinephrine excites mainly alpha receptors and to a slight degree beta receptors. The action of norepinephrine is similar to that of epinephrine with two notable exceptions. The effect of norepinephrine on cardiac and metabolic functions is not as intense as that of epinephrine. Also, norepinephrine has a more intense action than epinephrine on skeletal muscle vasculature. This increases peripheral vascular resistance as a result of the increased vasoconstriction.

The sites of action for norepinephrine are body cells and vascular beds, and releasing factors for norepinephrine are the same as for epinephrine.

DYSFUNCTION OF THE ADRENAL CORTEX

Adrenal insufficiency is a major life-threatening dysfunction of the adrenal cortex. It is also known as hypoadrenalism and/or hypocorticism.

Addison's Disease

Addison's disease is a chronic dysfunction of the adrenal glands, resulting in an inadequate adrenal secretion of cortisol and aldosterone (adrenal insufficiency). Addison's disease results from progressive destruction of the adrenals, with up to 90% or more of the glands being affected before adrenal insufficiency appears. Acquired forms of primary insufficiency are relatively rare, may occur at any age, and affect both sexes.

Pathophysiology

Adrenal cortex dysfunction results in a deficiency of mineralocorticoids and glucocorticoids. The major clinical feature is volume depletion and hypotension.

Mineralocorticoid decrease results in an aldosterone deficiency. Without aldosterone, there is an increased excretion of sodium chloride and water in the urine. The depletion of sodium leads to dehydration and hypotension. At the same time, there is a retention of potassium. If the potassium concentration increases sufficiently, first there is a flaccidity of the cardiac myocardium followed by cardiac cell paralysis as the potassium level rises. Hemoconcentration, acidosis, decreased cardiac output, shock, and death due to cardiac paralysis occur.

A decrease in glucocorticoids results in a cortisol deficiency with normal blood glucose concentration between meals. Anorexia, nausea, vomiting, and abdominal pain result in weight loss. The neurologic effects of cortisol deficiency include fatigue, lethargy, apathy, confusion, and psychosis. Cardiovascular effects include an impaired response to the vasoactive catecholamines. Energy-producing mechanisms—for example, decreased glucogenesis (resulting in hypoglycemia) and fat mobilization—are altered. The decreased cortisol level stimulates the hypophysis to secrete ACTH unrestrained. Resistance to both physical and psychogenic stress is decreased.

Melanin pigmentation (Fig. 24-4) is increased in most cases of Addison's disease. This pigmentation is unevenly distributed and is probably due to increased secretion of melanocyte-stimulating hormone (MSH) and ACTH from the adenohypophysis. Additional symptoms may include weakness and fatigability, weight loss, myalgias, arthralgias, fever, anorexia, nausea and vomiting, anxiety, and mental irritability.

Etiology

The most common cause of Addison's disease is related to autoimmune destruction of the adrenals. Primary atrophy, tubercular destruction of the cortex, or a cancerous tumor can also cause Addison's disease. Autoimmune Addison's disease can be associated with primary ovarian failure, testicular failure, and pernicious anemia.

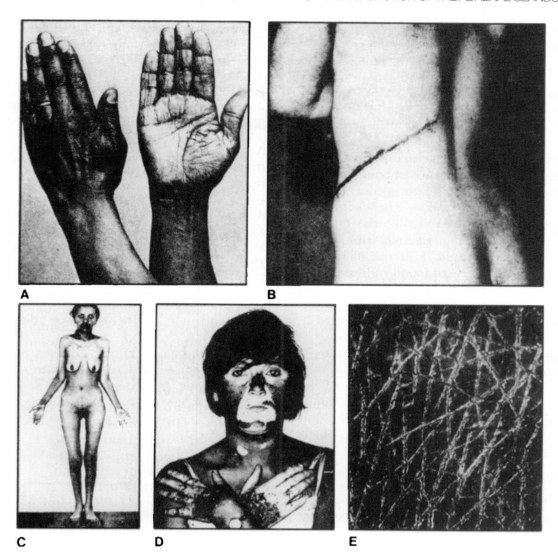

Figure 24-4. Melanin oversecretion in Addison's disease.

Treatment

If untreated, the patient dies within a few days to a few weeks. Replacement therapy of small amounts of mineralocorticoids and glucocorticoids may prolong life for years.

Strict adherence to a diet low in potassium and high in sodium will help prevent complications. If a tumor is the etiologic factor, surgery is performed.

Complications

Addisonian crisis may be fatal. Such a crisis may occur anytime there is an increase in stress, since the adrenal cortex cannot increase its production of cortisol. Steroids should be increased in patients with Addison's disease who are under stress. Even a slight cold necessitates increased steroid hormone levels. The only successful treatment of addisonian crisis is massive doses of glucocorticoids; often as much as 10 or more times the normal dose must be used to prevent death.

Acute Adrenal Insufficiency

Acute adrenal insufficiency is an emergency medical condition caused by insufficient cortisol. "Adrenal crisis" and "addisonian crisis" are synonyms for acute adrenal insufficiency and may be used interchangeably.

Etiology

Usually an underlying chronic condition (Addison's disease) is present before a crisis. In addition to this chronic disease, an infection, trauma, surgical procedure, or some other extra stress occurs and the patient develops acute adrenal insufficiency. Less common causes of acute adrenal insufficiency are adrenalectomy, Waterhouse-Friderichsen syndrome, abrupt cessation of steroid therapy, chemotherapy, and hypothalamic diseases. An autoimmune response may be a factor.

Clinical Presentation

Anorexia, nausea, vomiting, diarrhea, and abdominal pain lead to increased fluid and electrolyte disturbances. Fever may lead to alterations in consciousness. Hypotension precedes shock and coma.

Diagnosis

Patient history, physical examination, and presenting symptoms are usually sufficient to provide a tentative diagnosis and indicate the need for immediate treatment. Definitive laboratory studies are those evaluating endocrine function and identifying resultant system dysfunction or imbalances in the electrolytes.

Complications

Death is the common complication, although it is usually preceded by dysrhythmias, hypovolemia, shock, and coma.

Treatment

Adequate circulatory volume is vital. Continuous monitoring of vital signs to identify developing dysfunction provides for early intervention. Glucocorticoids must be replaced. An intravenous glucocorticoid such as hydrocortisone should be given. Physical and psychologic stress should be avoided.

Nursing Interventions

Continuous monitoring of the respiratory system with a ventilator on standby is indicated. If serial arterial blood gases show deteriorating respiratory status, the patient may be intubated and placed on a respirator. Standard nursing procedures for all artificially ventilated patients should be instituted.

Cardiac and hemodynamic monitoring will reveal early signs of impending dysrhythmias and shock, providing an opportunity for early intervention. Intake and output records will indicate renal function. Emotional support of the patient and family is of utmost importance in an attempt to decrease exogenous stress as much as possible.

Adrenal Insufficiency in Critical Illness

As a part of the normal stress response, the hypothalamic-pituitary-adrenal axis is activated, causing the release of cortisol. During critical illness states, adrenal insufficiency can develop due to dysfunction at the hypothalamic, pituitary, and/or adrenal level (HPA axis). The integrity of the HPA axis can be assessed with a random cortisol level. Dysfunction at the HPA axis will result in low circulating cortisol levels (<25 mcg/dL). A random cortisol level of <15 mcg/dL in a moderately stressed (vasopressor-independent) critically ill patient is suggestive of HPA dysfunction. Recent research indicates that adrenal failure is common in critically ill patients and that treatment with stress-level doses of glucocorticoids may be beneficial. Such treatment has been demonstrated to improve the survival of critically ill patients, especially those with septic shock.

A corticotropin-stimulation test is used to diagnose adrenal insufficiency in critically ill patients. A serum cortisol level of <20 mcg/dL 30 min after a low-dose corticotropin test is suggestive of primary adrenal failure. Failure of the corticotropin level to increase after the administration of human corticotropin-releasing hormone is suggestive of secondary adrenal failure.

Hypercortisolism (Cushing's Syndrome)

Hypercortisolism is a marked increase in the production of mineralocorticoids, glucocorticoids, and androgen steroids, resulting in the condition known as Cushing's syndrome (not to be confused with Cushing's triad).

Etiology

Cushing's syndrome is usually due to adrenal tumors or a pituitary tumor, which is typically very small (<5 mm). It occurs more frequently in women than in men. A pituitary tumor causes increased release of ACTH, which results in hyperplasia of the adrenal cortex. An ectopic ACTH-secreting adenoma of the lungs (most common), pancreas, thyroid, or thymus

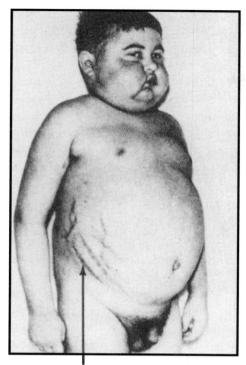
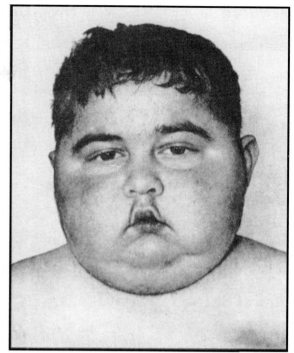

PURPLE STRIAE

Figure 24-5. Cushing's syndrome, showing "moon face," trunk fat, and purple striae.

and carcinoma of the gallbladder, cervix, or prostate may also cause hypercortisolism.

Clinical Presentation

An increase in glucocorticoids (cortisol) causes increased glucogenesis, resulting in hyperglycemia as well as increased wasting of protein tissue. It also causes increased fat, resulting in the typical "moon face," and increased trunk fat, or "buffalo hump" (Fig. 24-5).

The increased cortisol causes mood swings ranging from euphoria to depression. Changes in mental status—from depression, mood swings, and insomnia to severe psychotic paranoia—are seen, as are short-term memory deficits and decreased attention span.

Increased mineralocorticoids (aldosterone) results in increased potassium excretion, causing dysrhythmias, renal disorders, and muscle weakness. The increased aldosterone causes a decrease in sodium secretion. The increased sodium causes an increase in fluid retention, resulting in edema and usually an increase in blood pressure and weight. (Eighty percent of patients with Cushing's syndrome have hypertension.) Increased sex hormones (androgens) cause increased facial hair and acne.

The skin thins and becomes fragile and prone to injury secondary to protein wasting. Pink and purplish striae of the abdomen, underarms, and buttocks may be seen. There is easy bruising and hematoma formation.

Diagnosis

Patient history, physical examination, and presenting symptoms are usually sufficient to provide a tentative diagnosis. Definitive laboratory studies are those evaluating endocrine function and identifying resultant system dysfunction or imbalance. Hyperglycemia, acidosis, and increased cortisol levels are present.

Treatment

Treatment consists of removing the tumor, if possible, which will necessitate steroid replacement. A diet low in sodium and high in potassium is required.

Nursing Interventions

Routine postsurgical nursing care is required. In addition, the patient must be assessed for endocrine imbalance, indicating a need for replacement therapy. The patient's immune system will have been depressed because of the increased steroid levels prior to surgery, so signs of infection must be closely monitored. Education relating to diet therapy and medication regimens is essential to prevent recurrent endocrine crises.

Note: The increase in mineralocorticoids may also cause Conn's syndrome (increased sodium and blood pressure and decreased potassium levels due to a benign aldosterone-secreting tumor).

Hypofunction of the Adrenal Medulla

Hypofunction of the adrenal medulla does not cause systemic problems because the sympathetic nervous system will compensate for decreases in epinephrine and norepinephrine.

Hyperfunction of the Adrenal Medulla

Hyperfunction of the adrenal medulla can be life threatening, primarily because of the severe persistent or paroxysmal hypertension that leads to cerebrovascular accident and congestive heart failure. In hyperfunction, epinephrine increases blood pressure, cardiac output, pulse, and metabolism. Norepinephrine increases the blood pressure more than epinephrine does. Hyperfunction may be precipitated by stress and/or exertion, ingestion of tyrosine-containing foods, increased caffeine intake, external pressure on the tumor, and anesthesia.

Pheochromocytoma

Pheochromocytomas produce, store, and secrete catecholamines. Hyperfunction of the adrenal medulla is the most common cause of pheochromocytoma. Pheochromocytoma is an encapsulated, vascular tumor of chromaffin tissue of the adrenal medulla.

Diagnosis. Signs and symptoms are the major diagnostic clues associated with pheochromocytoma. However, hyperfunction of the adrenal medulla often resembles other disorders that must be ruled out. These include diabetes mellitus, essential hypertension, and psychoneurosis. Although pheochromocytoma occurs in less than 0.3% of hypertensive individuals, it is an important correctable cause of hypertension. Diagnosis is rarely confirmed and there is no consensus on the best test. The diagnosis is typically made by measurements of urinary and plasma fractionated metanephrine and catecholamines.

Clinical Presentation. The outstanding symptom in pheochromocytoma is the extremely high blood pressure (diastolic blood pressure <115 mm Hg) secondary to the excessive medullary hormones. Other signs and symptoms include increased sympathetic nervous activity, sweating, headache, palpitations and dysrhythmias, postural hypotension, apprehension, nausea/vomiting, tremor, pallor or flushing of the face, abdominal and/or chest pain, and hyperglycemia.

Treatment. Treatment of pheochromocytoma is its surgical removal, performed either laparoscopically or via an open laparotomy for very large, invasive tumors. Alpha-adrenergic–blocking agents are commonly administered preoperatively to control hypertension. After alpha-adrenergic therapy has been initiated, a beta blocker may be added to help control tachycardia. The prognosis is dependent on the timing of diagnosis and the presence of malignancy. The malignancy of a pheochromocytoma cannot be determined by histologic examination, and a tumor is considered malignant if metastases are present. Lifetime surveillance is usually required, as metastases may occur years afterward.

Nursing Interventions. Preoperatively, the nurse should promote rest and reassure the patient. Blood pressure should be monitored closely. Routine postoperative procedures are instituted; in addition, the patient must be closely monitored for shock, hypotension (due to decreased levels of epinephrine and norepinephrine), hypoglycemia, and hemorrhage (the adrenal glands being very vascular).

BIBLIOGRAPHY

AACE Diabetes Mellitus Clinical Practice Guidelines Taskforce (2007). AACE Diabetes Mellitus Guidelines. Diabetes management in a hospital setting. *Endocrine Practice, 13*(Suppl 1), 59–63.

Annane, D. (2003). Time for a consensus definition of corticosteroid insufficiency in critically ill patients. *Critical Care Medicine, 31*(6), 1868–1869.

Annane, D., Sebille, V., Charpentier, C., et al. (2002). Effect of treatment with low doses of hydrocortisone and fludrocortisone on mortality in patients with septic shock. *Journal of the American Medical Association, 288*(7), 862–871.

Beishuizen, A., & Thijs L. G. (2004). The immunoneuroendocrine axis in critical illness: Beneficial adaptation or neuroendocrine exhaustion? *Current Opinion in Critical Care, 10*(6), 461–467.

Biller, B. M., Grossman, A. B., Stewart, P. M., et al. (2008). Treatment of adrenocorticotropin-dependent Cushing's syndrome: A review of the Mayo Clinic experience. *Clinical Endocrinology (Oxf), 68,* 513.

Cefalu, W., & Weir, G. (2003). New technologies in diabetes care. *Patient Care, 37,* 66–78.

Chiasson, J. L., Aris-Jilwan, N., Belanger, R., et al. (2003). Diagnosis and treatment of diabetic ketoacidosis and the hyperglycemic hyperosmolar states. *Canadian Medical Association Journal, 168,* 859–866.

Cooper, M. S., & Stewart, P. M. (2003). Corticosteroid insufficiency in acutely ill patients. *New England Journal of Medicine, 348*(8), 727–734.

Cryer, P. E., Davis, S. N., & Shamoon, H. (2003). Hypoglycemia in diabetes. *Diabetes Care, 26,* 1902–1912.

Fahy, B. G., Sheehy, A. M., & Coursen, D. B. (2003). Glucose control in the intensive care unit. *Crit Care Medicine, 37*(5), 1769–1776.

Freeland, B. (2003). Diabetic ketoacidosis. *Today's Educator, 29,* 385–395.

Holcomb, S. S. (2002). Diabetes insipidus. *Dimensions in Critical Care Nursing, 21,* 94–97.

Kitabchi, A. E., Umpierrez, G. E., Miles, J. M., & Fisher, J. N. (2009). Hyperglycemic crises in adult patients with diabetes. *Diabetes Care, 32,* 1335.

Krumberger, J. Endocrine system. In M. Chulay & S. Burns (Eds.). (2005). *AACN Essentials of Critical Care Nursing* (pp. 357–399). New York, NY: McGraw-Hill.

Marik, P. E., Zaloga, G. P. (2003). Adrenal insufficiency during septic shock. *Critical Care Medicine, 31,* 141–145.

McGraw-Hill's Access Medicine (2005). Diabetic ketoacidosis. Accessed 12/26/05.

McGraw-Hill's Access Medicine (2005). Diabetes insipidus. Accessed 12/26/05.

McGraw-Hill's Access Medicine (2005). The endocrine system. Accessed 12/26/05.

McGraw-Hill's Access Medicine (2005). Acute adrenocortical insufficiency (adrenal crisis). Accessed 12/26/05.

Nayak, B., & Burman, K. (2006). Thyrotoxicosis and thyroid storm. *Endocrinology and Metabolism Clinics of North America, 35,* 663.

Nice Sugar Study Investigations (2009). Intensive versus conventional glucose control in critically ill patients. *New England Journal of Medicine, 360*(13), 1283–1297.

Nylen, E. S., & Muller, B. (2004). Endocrine changes in critical illness. *Journal of Intensive Care Medicine, 19*(2), 67–82.

Robinson, L. E., & van Soeren, M. H. (2004). Insulin resistance and hyperglycemia in critical illness: Role of insulin in glycemic control. *AACN Clinical Issues, 15*(1), 45–62.

Selig, P., Popek, V., & Pebbles, K. M. (2010). Minimizing hypoglycemia in the wake of tight glycemic control protocol in hospitalized patients. *Journal of Nursing Care Quarterly, 25*(3), 255–260.

Sprung, C. L., Annane, D, Keh, D., et al. (2008). Hydrocortisone therapy for patients with septic shock. *New England Journal of Medicine, 358*(2), 111–124.

Taylor, J. H., & Beilman, G. J. (2005). Hyperglycemia in the intensive care unit: No longer just a marker of illness severity. *Surgical Infections, 6*(2), 233–245.

Van den Berghe, G. (2004). How does blood glucose control with insulin save lives in intensive care? *Journal of Clinical Investigations, 114*(9), 1187–1195.

Van den Berghe, G., Wouters, P., Weekers, F., et al. (2001). Intensive insulin therapy in critically ill patients. *New England Journal of Medicine, 345,* 1359–1367.

Verbalis J. G., Goldsmith SR, Greenberg A, et al. (2007). Hyponatremia treatment guidelines 2007: Expert panel recommendations. *American Journal of Medicine.* 2007, *120,* S1.

Young, W. F, Jr. (2007). Adrenal causes of hypertension: pheochromocytoma and primary aldosteronism. *Review of Endocrinological and Metabolic Disorders, 8,* 309.

PART III

Endocrine Practice Exam

1. Which of the following stimulates insulin secretion?
   (A) Thyroid hormone
   (B) Growth hormone
   (C) Glucocorticoids
   (D) Prolactin

2. Which phrase best describes gluconeogenesis?
   (A) Utilization of oxygen stores due to deficits of serum glucose
   (B) Breakdown of protein
   (C) Formation of glucose from other substances
   (D) Breakdown of glycogen stores in the liver

Questions 3 and 4 refer to the following scenario:

A 67-year-old man is admitted to your unit with a decreased level of consciousness. He was brought to the hospital by the police after being found at a shopping mall "acting strange." He complains of fatigue and is disoriented as to time and place. His respiratory rate is deep and rapid. Vital signs and laboratory data are as follows:

Blood pressure	96/58
Pulse	114
Respiratory rate	34
Glucose	760
Osmolality	307
pH	7.28
$PaCO_2$	20
PaO_2	91
Na^+	156
K^+	5.0
HCO_3^-	14

The blood pressure also decreases when the patient changes from a lying to a sitting position.

3. Based on the preceding information, which condition is likely to be developing?
   (A) Adrenal crisis
   (B) Thyroid storm

   (C) Hyperosmolar, hyperglycemic, nonketotic (HHNK) coma
   (D) Diabetic ketoacidosis (DKA)

4. Which of the following would most likely be administered to this patient?
   (A) Glucocorticoids
   (B) Thyroxine
   (C) Sodium bicarbonate
   (D) Insulin and normal saline

5. Which blood gas change is usually present in DKA?
   (A) Respiratory acidosis alone
   (B) Metabolic acidosis alone
   (C) Respiratory alkalosis and metabolic acidosis
   (D) Respiratory acidosis and metabolic alkalosis

6. Initial insulin therapy for DKA is usually administered by which route?
   (A) Intravenous bolus
   (B) Intravenous bolus followed by a continuous infusion
   (C) Subcutaneously
   (D) Intramuscularly

7. Presenting signs and symptoms of DKA could include which of the following?
   (A) Shallow slow respirations
   (B) Decreased urine output
   (C) Tachycardia and orthostatic hypotension
   (D) Peripheral edema and dependent pulmonary crackles

8. Insulin therapy brings about which electrolyte change?
   (A) Increased serum potassium
   (B) Decreased serum sodium
   (C) Increased intracellular potassium
   (D) Decreased intracellular calcium

9. Hyperosmolar hyperglycemic syndrome (HHS) coma is differentiated from DKA by which of the following?
   (A) Hyperglycemia
   (B) Absence of ketosis
   (C) Serum osmolality
   (D) Serum potassium levels

10. Dehydration in HHS coma is primarily due to which event?
    (A) Lack of ADH
    (B) Inability of the kidney to concentrate urine
    (C) Nausea and vomiting
    (D) Osmotic diuresis from the high glucose level

Questions 11 and 12 refer to the following scenario:

A 69-year-old overweight man is in your unit following resection of a perforated bowel. He has a history of adult-onset diabetes and mild hypertension. The patient is alert and oriented with stable vital signs at the beginning of your shift. During your shift he becomes disoriented. His skin is cool and clammy; he has muscle tremors, and complains of nausea. Serum electrolytes are drawn; the laboratory results are as follows:

Na^+	133
K^+	3.7
Cl^-	100
HCO_3^-	25
Glucose	43
Osmolality	282

11. Based on the preceding information, which condition is likely to be developing?

    (A) Hyperosmolar hyperglycemic nonketotic acidosis
    (B) Hypoglycemia
    (C) Diabetic ketoacidosis
    (D) Diabetes insipidus

12. Which treatment would most likely be given to this patient?
    (A) Insulin bolus followed by infusion
    (B) Glucose (dextrose) bolus (D50)
    (C) Normal saline bolus with potassium
    (D) Glucocorticoids

13. Which of the following physical signs is more indicative of hypoglycemia than hyperglycemia?
    (A) Cool skin
    (B) Rapid breathing
    (C) Warm skin
    (D) Tachycardia

14. At which blood glucose level does change in mentation begin?
    (A) 10 to 20 mg/dL
    (B) 20 to 30 mg/dL
    (C) 30 to 40 mg/dL
    (D) Any level below 50 mg/dL

15. High serum glucose levels can directly cause which physical symptom?
    (A) Increased urine output
    (B) Decreased urine output
    (C) Hypotension
    (D) Decreased respiratory rate

Endocrine Practice Exam

Practice Fill-Ins

1. _____
2. _____
3. _____
4. _____

5. _____
6. _____
7. _____
8. _____

9. _____
10. _____
11. _____
12. _____

13. _____
14. _____
15. _____

PART III

Answers

1	B	5.	C	9.	B	13.	A
2.	C	6.	B	10.	D	14.	D
3.	D	7.	C	11.	B	15.	A
4.	D	8.	C	12.	B		

IV

IMMUNOLOGY AND HEMATOLOGY

Ruth M. Kleinpell
Sharon Manson

Physiology of the Immunologic and Hematologic Systems

EDITORS' NOTE

Immunologic and hematologic concepts account for 2% (approximately three to four questions) of the PCCN exam. The major content areas covered under immunology and hematology include anemia and life-threatening coagulopathies such as disseminated intravascular coagulation (DIC) and sickle cell crisis. The PCCN exam testable nursing actions for hematology/immunology include performing a comprehensive hematology/immunology assessment, monitoring normal and abnormal diagnostic test results and administering medications, treatment or interventions, and monitoring patient response. This chapter presents key information normally encountered on the PCCN exam regarding both major concepts and the principles necessary to achieve the understanding required for the PCCN exam.

As with most other chapters, concentrate on key principles rather than on details or points of pure anatomy and physiology. Nurses often find immunology and hematology to be a difficult area of the PCCN exam because of their lack of clinical familiarity with the concepts. Study this chapter and then try to apply the information during your work. The more you can integrate the information after reading it, the more likely you will be to retain the information for the test.

IMMUNE SYSTEM

Alterations in hemostasis and coagulation are common problems during acute illness. Therefore, having an understanding of the immune system and hematologic and immunologic disorders is important for the early detection and treatment of disorders. The immune system is a dynamic system, consisting of many cell types and structures. In fact, approximately 1 in every 100 of the body's cells is an immune cell. It is dynamic not only in the sense that it does not necessarily remain in one place—as does, say, the heart—but also in the sense that its many components are in a constant state of dynamic interaction.

The mature immune system is capable of performing three general types of functions: defense, homeostasis, and surveillance. In providing defense, resistance to infection is facilitated by both nonspecific innate mechanisms and more specific acquired immune responses that bring about the destruction of foreign antigens (anything recognized by the body as nonself; for example, microorganisms, proteins, and cells of transplanted organs). The maintenance of immunologic homeostasis involves keeping a balance between immune protective and destructive responses and the removal of senescent immune cells from the body. Although the function of the immune system is inherently protective, there are conditions in which natural immune responses become destructive to the host. Examples of such conditions are the numerous autoimmune diseases as well as allergic and anaphylactic reactions. Surveillance involves the recognition of microorganisms or cells bearing foreign antigens on their membranes. Some of the immune cells, lymphocytes in particular, are highly mobile and travel throughout the vascular and lymphatic systems in search of potentially harmful antigens. Some types of cancer cells, in particular, are sought out and destroyed by immune cells in this way.

Immune responses can be classified into two major types: natural, or innate, responses and acquired responses. Both types of responses play critical roles in host defense.

Innate Immune System

The innate immune system consists of natural or nonspecific mechanisms for the protection of an individual against foreign antigens. These natural defenses are present from birth and do not necessarily require exposure to specific antigens to develop. Natural defenses, the body's first line of defense, consist of anatomic, chemical, and cellular defenses against microbial invasion. Anatomic defenses include the skin, mucous membranes, and ciliated epithelia. Chemical defenses include gastric acid, lysozymes, natural immunoglobulins, and the interferons. Cellular defenses include leukocytes.

Anatomic and Chemical Defenses

The skin provides the initial physical barrier to external environmental antigens. The outermost skin layer, the stratum corneum, is the main barrier to microbial invasion. Certain conditions (pH, humidity, and temperature) influence the growth of potentially pathogenic organisms on the skin. Alterations in normal conditions related to these factors favor the development of infection. The normally acid pH of the skin inhibits the growth of microorganisms. When the acid-base balance of the skin is altered in favor of a higher pH, this protective mechanism is lost. When water loss from epidermal cells exceeds intake, the stratum corneum can dry and crack, predisposing the host to microbial invasion. On the other hand, excessive moisture decreases barrier efficiency.

Skin cells are constantly exfoliating, and in this process organisms are sloughed along with dead skin cells. In addition, the skin is colonized with normal flora (mainly aerobic cocci and diphtheroids), which, through various mechanisms, prevents the colonization of potentially pathogenic organisms. The resident flora maintains the skin's pH in the acidic range and competes effectively for nutrients and binding sites on epidermal cells, making it difficult for nonresident flora to survive. It is when the normal flora is altered, as occurs with long-term or broad-spectrum antibiotic therapy and with the use of disinfectants or occlusive dressings, that potentially pathogenic organisms become opportunistic. Opportunistic organisms take advantage of the lack of competition for nutrients and epidermal binding sites and then multiply to cause infection.

The sebaceous glands, mammary glands, respiratory epithelium, gastrointestinal mucosa, genitourinary mucosa, and conjunctivae all secrete a protective immunoglobulin (another term for antibody) called secretory IgA. Ciliated respiratory epithelial cells also facilitate the removal of bacteria and other foreign antigens from the respiratory tract; the low pH of the gastric mucosa prevents bacterial growth in the stomach.

Leukocytes

All leukocytes (white blood cells [WBCs]) develop as stem cells in the bone marrow. Leukocytes develop along two major lineages: the myeloid lineage and the lymphoid lineage. The myeloid lineage includes all leukocytes except the lymphocytes. The lymphoid lineage consists of T and B lymphocytes. Myeloid cells make up the backbone of the natural, or innate, defense system. Myeloid leukocytes can be further classified into two major groups: granulocytes and monocytes. The major function of both of these types of cells is phagocytosis.

Granulocytes. Granulocytes, commonly referred to as polymorphonuclear granulocytes (PMNs), or polymorphs, are produced in the bone marrow at the rate of approximately 80 million per day, and their average life span is about 2 to 3 days. Some 60% to 70% of all leukocytes are PMNs. These cells are sometimes called polymorphs because their nuclei are multilobed; they are called granulocytes because they contain intracellular granules. These intracellular granules contain hydrolytic enzymes that are cytotoxic to foreign organisms. Furthermore, granulocytes are classified, according to the histologic staining reactions of the granules, into three more distinct types: neutrophils, eosinophils, and basophils. Granulocytes may leave the circulation to become tissue phagocytes (Fig. 25-1).

Neutrophils are the most abundant cells in the bone marrow and blood, comprising about 90% of all granulocytes. Three forms of neutrophils can be identified in the peripheral blood: segmented neutrophils, bands, and metamyelocytes. Segmented neutrophils are fully mature, bands are slightly immature, and metamyelocytes are completely immature neutrophils. Neutrophils are strongly phagocytic: that is, they ingest microorganisms or other cells and foreign particles, and they digest the ingested material within their phagocytic vacuoles.

In conditions such as infection, there is an increased demand for neutrophils. The bone marrow responds by releasing more neutrophils into the

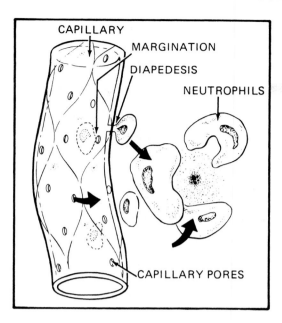

Figure 25-1. Diapedesis of WBCs.

circulation, and in this process immature cells, or band cells, are released along with the mature cells. As a result, the percentage of bands in the peripheral blood is increased. This condition is referred to as a "shift to the left" and indicates acute inflammation or infection. In more serious conditions, metamyelocytes will also appear in increased numbers in the peripheral blood. The normal neutrophil count in the adult is between 1000 and 6000/mm³ blood, or approximately 60% of the differential WBC count. Bands normally number about 600/mm³ blood, or approximately 0% to 5% of the differential WBC count. Metamyelocytes should not be present in the peripheral blood.

Eosinophils are weakly phagocytic cells that are seen in increased numbers in the circulation specifically during parasitic infections and allergic reactions. Eosinophils degranulate (release their cytotoxic granules) upon antigenic stimulation and kill organisms extracellularly. The normal eosinophil count is about 200/mm³ blood, or between 2 and 5% of the differential WBC count.

Basophils are responsible for anaphylactoid reactions to allergens. Like eosinophils, basophils are capable of releasing their cytotoxic granules when stimulated by certain antigens to effect extracellular killing. Basophils are morphologically identical to mast cells but can be differentiated from mast cells in that basophils are bloodborne and mast cells reside in tissues outside of the circulation. In other words, when a basophil migrates out of the circulation to reside in tissue, it becomes a mast cell. The

normal basophil count is about 100/mm³ blood, or about 0.2% of the differential WBC count.

Monocytes. The PMNs can be differentiated from monocytes by their multilobed nuclei and many intracellular granules. Monocytes are mononuclear cells and do not contain cytotoxic intracellular granules. They do, however, release the prostaglandin PGE_2, which is a mediator of the inflammatory response. The normal monocyte count is about 200 to 1000/mm³ blood, or about 5% of the differential WBC count.

A specific type of monocyte is the antigen-presenting cell (APC). APCs are formed in the epidermis, where they are called Langerhans' cells, and in the lymphoid system. The APCs play an important role in linking the innate immune system with the acquired immune system. They carry foreign antigens that enter the host via the respiratory or gastrointestinal tract, through the skin, or through the lymphatic system and present them to lymphocytes in the lymph nodes and spleen, thereby triggering cellular and humoral immune responses.

Phagocytosis. Monocytes, like granulocytes, may leave the circulation to become tissue macrophages. Together, blood and tissue macrophages comprise a highly mobile network of cells for first-line defense called the reticuloendothelial system. These cells are strategically and conveniently located in the liver, spleen, lymph nodes, kidney, lung, peritoneum, brain, and synovia.

Phagocytosis, which means "cell eating," is the first step in host defense. Phagocytes (or macrophages) have surface receptors that allow them to seek out and attack nonspecific foreign organisms, engulf them, and ultimately destroy them (Fig. 25-2). Phagocytosis is the process by which excess antigen and dead cells are removed from the body. Phagocytosis is also essential in the initiation of cellular and humoral immune responses by T and B lymphocytes.

Inflammation. Inflammation is an attempt to restore homeostasis. It is the body's initial reaction to injury and the first step in the healing process. Wound healing cannot occur if the inflammatory response is fully inhibited. During the inflammatory response, a series of cellular and systemic reactions is triggered; these responses serve to localize and destroy the offending antigen, maintain vascular integrity, and limit tissue damage.

Tissue injury provides the initial stimulus for activation of inflammatory mechanisms and results in the cellular release of vasoactive substances, such as

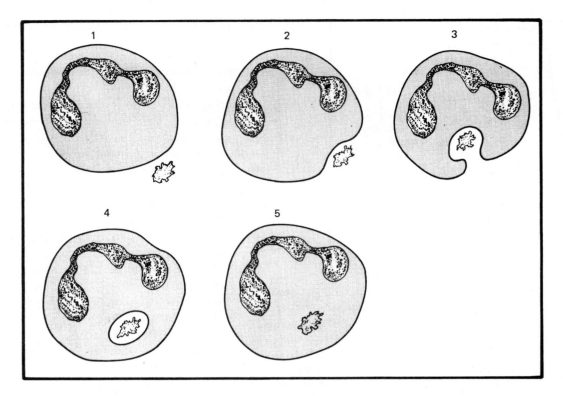

Figure 25-2. Phagocytosis of WBCs.

histamine, bradykinin, and serotonin. The circulatory effects are vasodilatation and increased blood flow to the affected site; increased vascular permeability, facilitating diapedesis of immune cells from the circulation to the tissues; and pain. The clotting system is activated in an attempt to "plug up" the injury. Increased blood flow and capillary permeability lead to local interstitial edema and swelling. Leukocyte migration occurs as phagocytes are attached to the affected site (chemotaxis), and dying leukocytes release pyrogens, which stimulate the hypothalamus to produce a state of fever. Pyrogens also stimulate the bone marrow to release more leukocytes, thus perpetuating the process.

Finally, the complement system is activated. The complement system consists of a complex set of approximately 20 interacting proteolytic enzymes and regulatory proteins found in the plasma and body fluids that attack antigens. The complement system is conceptually similar to the coagulation system in that complement proteins react sequentially in a series of enzymatic reactions in a cascading manner. Several factors are responsible for activation of the complement system: the formation of insoluble antigen-antibody complexes, aggregated immunoglobulin, platelet aggregation, release of endotoxins by gram-negative bacteria, the presence of viruses or bacteria in the circulation, and the release of plasmin and proteases from injured tissues. Complement proteins can mediate the lytic destruction of cells, including erythrocytes (red blood cells [RBCs]), WBCs, platelets, bacteria, and viruses.

The inflammatory response can be altered or suppressed in many situations: the administration of corticosteroids or other immunosuppressive drugs, malnutrition, advanced age, chronic illness, and prolonged stress. Conversely, the inflammatory response can become exaggerated in conditions such as anaphylaxis and septic shock.

The innate immune mechanisms just discussed will be called upon as the first line of defense in ridding the host of foreign antigens. However, if these mechanisms are not entirely successful, a second set of defenses, the acquired immune system, is activated to work in concert with the innate immune system. The acquired immune system is composed of lymphocytes and other lymphoid structures necessary for specific immune responses.

Acquired Immune System

The lymphoid system matures during the fetal and neonatal periods, when lymphoid stem cells differentiate into T and B lymphocytes. At this time, the mechanisms for conferring genetic specificity to lymphocytes develop. This property of specificity is what differentiates the lymphoid cell from the myeloid cell, which can react with any antigen. The process of lymphopoiesis (lymphocyte origination and differentiation into functional effector cells) begins in the yolk sac and then continues later in life in the thymus gland, the liver, the spleen, and finally the bone marrow, which is the primary site of lymphopoiesis in the full-term neonate.

Primary Lymphoid Tissue

Primary lymphoid tissue consists of central organs that serve as major sites of lymphopoiesis. Lymphoid stem cells originate in the bone marrow. These cells give rise to the various components of the acquired immune system.

Secondary Lymphoid Tissue

Secondary lymphoid tissue is peripheral tissue that provides an environment for lymphocytes to encounter antigens and proliferate if necessary. Secondary lymphoid tissue consists of the bone marrow, spleen, lymph nodes, thymus, liver, and mucosa-associated lymphoid tissue in the tonsils, respiratory tract, gut, and urogenital tract. Localization of secondary lymphoid tissue is not coincidental, as all of these structures provide major portals for the entry of foreign microorganisms into the body. Once in secondary lymphoid tissue, lymphocytes may migrate from one lymphoid structure to another by vascular and lymphatic channels.

Lymphatics. The lymphatic system consists of (1) a capillary network, which collects lymph (a clear, watery fluid in the interstitial spaces); (2) collecting vessels, which carry lymph from the lymphatic vessels back to the vascular system; (3) lymph nodes; and (4) lymphatic organs, such as the tonsils. Lymphatic channels provide a major transit system for lymphocytes while they carry out specific functions related to immunologic surveillance. Both superficial and deep lymphatics empty into the large thoracic duct, which drains into the left subclavian vein (Fig. 25-3).

Lymph Nodes. Lymph nodes are small oval bodies of lymphatic tissue encapsulated by fibrous tissue that are situated in the course of lymphatic vessels. The interior of the lymph nodes resembles a matrix of connective tissue that forms compartments densely populated with lymphocytes. Afferent lymphatics carry lymph to the lymph nodes, and efferent lymphatics serve as exit routes for lymphocytes from lymph nodes (Fig. 25-4). Lymph nodes are located at

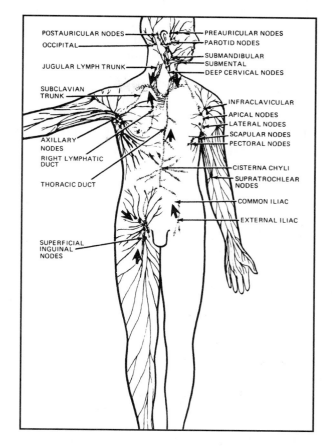

Figure 25-3. Location of lymph nodes in the body.

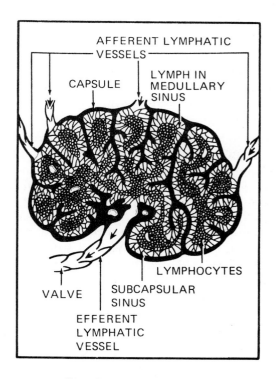

Figure 25-4. Typical lymph node.

the junctions of lymphatic vessels and form a complete network for the draining and filtering of extravasated lymph from interstitial fluid spaces.

Spleen. The spleen is a soft, purplish, highly vascular, coffee bean–shaped organ in the left upper quadrant. It lies between the fundus of the stomach and the diaphragm. It is covered by a fibroelastic membrane that invests the organ at the hilum to form fibrous bands (trabeculae) that constitute the internal framework of the spleen and contain the splenic pulp.

During fetal and neonatal life, the spleen gives rise to RBCs. The physiologic function of the spleen in adult life is not completely understood. However, a major function of the spleen seems to be the removal of particulate matter from the circulation. It is known that it has reticuloendothelial, immunologic, and storage functions. The spleen produces monocytes, lymphocytes, opsonins, and immunoglobulin M (IgM) antibody–producing plasma cells.

Blood flow within the spleen is sluggish, which allows phagocytosis to occur. The spleen clears the blood of encapsulated organisms (*Neisseria meningitidis, Haemophilus influenzae, Streptococcus pneumoniae*), and antigens in the rest of the body are phagocytosed and carried to the spleen to be eradicated by antibodies.

Postsplenectomy sepsis syndrome is seen predominantly in young immunosuppressed individuals who have been splenectomized, but this syndrome can occur in the healthy adult after splenectomy. The etiology of this often fatal syndrome is the loss of particulate filtering, coupled with IgM and opsonin production by the spleen.

Normally about 30% of the total platelet population is sequestered in the spleen, but this can increase to 80% with splenomegaly. Increased numbers of RBCs and WBCs will also be sequestered and destroyed in splenomegaly. Therefore, pancytopenia (anemia, leukopenia, and thrombocytopenia) occurs during splenomegaly.

Thymus. The thymus is a prominent organ in the infant, occupying the ventral superior mediastinum. In the older adult, it may be scarcely visible because of atrophy. The thymus is composed mostly of lymphocytes. Its only known function is the production of lymphocytes.

Lymphocytes

Lymphocytes are the primary defenders of the acquired immune system. Lymphocytes have surface receptors that are specific for surface molecules (antigens) located on the surfaces of foreign proteins and are, therefore, the only cells that have the intrinsic ability to recognize specific antigens.

There are two major types of lymphocytes: T lymphocytes (T cells) and B lymphocytes (B cells). T cells are involved in immunologic regulation and mediate what is called the cellular immune response. B cells produce antibodies and mediate what is called the humoral immune response.

T Lymphocytes (T Cells). Immature T cells develop under the influence of thymic hormones. As mediators of the cellular immune response, T cells defend against viruses, fungi, and some neoplastic conditions, and they destroy transplanted organs by mediating accelerated and acute rejection responses. T-cell function is inhibited by viral and parasitic infections, malnutrition, prolonged general anesthesia, radiation therapy, uremia, Hodgkin's disease, and advanced age.

T cells are divided into four functionally distinct but interactive cell populations, or subsets: cytotoxic, helper (T4), suppressor (T8), and memory T cells.

Cytotoxic and memory T cells are referred to as *effector cells* because they have a specific cytotoxic effect on antigen-bearing cells. Cytotoxic T cells bind to target cells and facilitate their destruction via substances known as lymphokines, which stimulate inflammatory cells, and via the production of cytolytic proteins.

Lymphokines are one of the two soluble products of lymphocytes, the other being antibodies. Lymphokines are inflammatory and regulatory hormones of the immune system that serve a variety of functions, such as the recruitment of macrophages to antigen sites (chemotaxis), augmentation of T-cell function in general, and inhibition of viral replication.

Lymphokines carry molecular signals between immunocompetent cells in order to amplify the immune response. Their role in amplification of the T-cell response is crucial to cellular immunity. Two of the most important lymphokines are interleukin-1 (IL-1) and interleukin-2 (IL-2). IL-1 stimulates T-cell proliferation, induces fever, stimulates the liver to produce acute-phase proteins, and stimulates the release of prostaglandin. IL-2 (T-cell growth factor) also stimulates T-cell proliferation. The reaction of T cells with IL-1 is necessary for the production of IL-2.

Memory T cells are T cells that have been sensitized to a specific antigen and then cloned to remember the antigen. Memory cells remain present in the body for many years and are, therefore, available for defense upon repeated exposure to an antigen. Repeated exposure to an antigen that the host has been previously sensitized to will result in a more rapid and accelerated immune response than on the first exposure.

Helper and suppressor T cells are *regulatory* in nature. Helper T cells are active in lymphokine-mediated events. They produce multiple lymphokines that promote the proliferation and activation of other lymphocytes and macrophages. Although the B cells can produce antibody by direct interaction with surface antigen on a macrophage, the assistance of helper T cells is required for most antibody production. They recruit cytotoxic T cells to antigen sites and interact with macrophages in the spleen and lymph nodes to facilitate antibody production by B cells. Helper and suppressor T-cell activity is normally balanced to maintain immunologic homeostasis. Too much suppressor T-cell function, for instance, will inhibit helper T-cell function.

B Lymphocytes (B Cells). B cells are effector cells that mediate the humoral immune response through the production of antibodies, which is their major function. B cells are important in defense against pyrogenic bacterial infections and can destroy transplanted organs by mediating hyperacute graft rejection. When a B cell is stimulated by a particular antigen, it differentiates into a lymphoblast. The lymphoblast differentiates into a plasmablast, which further differentiates into a plasma cell. Plasma cells, which are capable of producing and releasing antibody, do so until the antigen is destroyed. Memory of the offending antigen is retained for at least several months.

Antibodies are also referred to as immunoglobulins (Table 25-1). Immunoglobulins are specifically modified proteins present in serum and tissue fluids that are capable of selectively reacting with inciting antigens. The body produces several million antibodies capable of reacting with just as many antigens. However, each is specific and can usually recognize only one antigen. When viruses or bacteria, for instance, enter the body, their structural surface features are recognized by the body as not belonging to it. Antibodies are then formed and attracted to these foreign structures, for which they have identical matching receptors. In this way, antibodies are able to bind with antigens in a process called antigen-antibody complex formation. Mechanisms of antigen interaction by antibody include agglutination, precipitation, neutralization, and lysis.

Antibodies can be divided into five major classifications: IgM, IgG, IgA, IgD, and IgE. IgM is the principal mediator of the primary immune response. IgM is a natural antibody; that is, there is no known contact with the antigen that stimulated its production. About 10% of all antibodies are of the IgM type. IgG is the principal mediator of the secondary immune response, which requires repeated exposure to the same antigen. IgG is the major antibody against bacteria and viruses. About 75% of all antibodies are of the IgG type. IgA is the secretory immunoglobulin present in bodily secretions and offers natural protection against nonspecific foreign antigens. About 15% of all antibodies are of the IgA type. The function of IgD is not known, but about 1% of antibodies are of this type. Although only about 0.002% of antibodies are of the IgE type. IgE antibodies present on basophils and mast cells play a significant role in inflammatory and immune reactions.

Lymphocyte Responses

All cells express foreign antigens. Foreign cells, of course, express antigens that are genetically different from those of the host. It is through specific receptors on the surfaces of lymphocytes that B and T cells can be differentiated, and it is also through these receptors that B and T cells are able to recognize foreign antigens. During lymphocyte maturation, each B and T cell acquires specific cell membrane surface receptors that allow the cell to "match up" with certain foreign antigens. This matching between host lymphocytes and foreign antigens is the recognition phase of the acquired immune response. When this occurs, lymphocytes are activated to differentiate, proliferate, and then quickly mount an effective immune response against the offending antigen.

Cellular Immune Response. The cellular immune response is the immune response mediated by T cells. T cells recognize foreign antigens only after they are

TABLE 25-1. TYPES AND FUNCTIONS OF IMMUNOGLOBULINS

Type	Function
IgM	First antibody in fetal life
	First antibody after exposure to a new antigen
IgG	Major antibody of adult life
	Produced after repeated exposure to the same antigen
IgA	Found in secretions: tears, saliva, mucous secretions in gastrointestinal and respiratory tracts
	Meets antigen at port of entry
IgE	Mediates allergic reactions
IgD	Function unclear; may be regulatory in nature

displayed on the surfaces of macrophages or APCs. The cellular immune response can be summarized as follows:

1. Naturally, the presence of a foreign antigen is necessary to initiate the response.
2. Initially, macrophages encounter the antigen and begin to phagocytize it. Antigenic fragments are released and then carried to T cells in the lymph nodes by APCs.
3. Resting virgin or memory T cells are activated when the antigen-APC complex binds with the T-cell surface receptor.
4. The APCs are stimulated to produce IL-1, which summons helper T cells.
5. Helper T cells are then responsible for a number of actions, including the release of IL-2, which causes the differentiation and proliferation of T cells. The helper T cells also stimulate antibody production by B cells.
6. Clonal expansion greatly increases the sensitized T-cell population.
7. Ultimately, the antigen-bearing cells are destroyed by the direct cytotoxic effect of effector T cells. Some sensitized T cells are returned to the lymphoid system with the memory of the antigen for future challenge.

Examples of cellular immune responses include tumor cell surveillance, defense against viral and fungal infections, acute organ rejection, graft-versus-host disease, and autoimmune diseases.

Humoral Immune Response. The humoral immune response is mediated by B cells. Antigens trigger B cells by stimulating immunoglobulins on their surfaces. The humoral immune response can be summarized as follows:

1. Naturally, as with the cellular immune response, the presence of a foreign antigen is necessary to initiate the process. Unlike T cells, B cells can recognize an antigen in its native configuration.
2. Initially, macrophages encounter the antigen and begin to phagocytize it. Antigenic fragments are released and then carried to B cells in the lymph nodes and spleen by APCs. Resting virgin or memory B cells are activated when antigen binds to surface immunoglobulin.
3. IL-1 is released by APCs, and helper T cells stimulate the sensitization and clonal proliferation of effector B cells. B cells are activated to differentiate and produce

antibody when antigen binds to their receptors.
4. Antigen-antibody complexes form, and ultimately the antigen-bearing cells are destroyed.
5. As in the cellular immune response, some of the plasma cells with specific memory of the antigen are cloned and returned to the lymphoid system.

In addition, B cells can process and present antigen to T cells. Examples of humoral immune responses include resistance to encapsulated pyrogenic bacteria such as pneumococci, streptococci, meningococci, and *H. influenzae*, hemolytic transfusion reactions, and hyperacute organ rejection.

The first exposure of an antigen to an activated lymphocyte evokes a primary immune response. Repeated exposure of the identical antigen to activated lymphocytes evokes an accelerated secondary response. In the secondary immune response, the latent period is shorter and the amount of antigen required to initiate the response is less.

The differences between cell and humoral responses are listed in Table 25-2.

Hypersensitivity Reactions

When an adaptive immune response occurs in an exaggerated or inappropriate form, causing tissue damage, a hypersensitivity reaction is said to occur. Hypersensitivity reactions occur on second exposure to the causative antigen. Four types of hypersensitivity reactions are described: Types I to IV.

Type I

Type I hypersensitivity reactions (allergic or anaphylactic) are immediate in nature. This antibody (IgE)–mediated response results in the release of histamine by mast cells, which produces an acute inflammatory reaction. The distinguishing clinical feature of a type I hypersensitivity reaction is an immediate wheal-and-flare reaction.

Type II

Type II hypersensitivity reactions are caused by the presence of preformed circulating cytotoxic antibodies. These antibodies destroy the target cells on contact.

Examples of type II hypersensitivity reactions are transfusion reactions, autoimmune hemolytic anemia, and hemolytic disease of the newborn (HDNB). In a transfusion reaction, antibodies (IgM) to ABO anti-A and anti-B antibodies to blood group antigens present on red blood cells cause agglutination,

TABLE 25-2. COMPARISON OF B- AND T-CELL IMMUNITY

Characteristic	B Lymphocyte	T Lymphocyte
Type of immunity	Humoral	Cell-mediated
Immune functions	Antibody formation	Direct cytotoxicity
	Immediate hypersensitivity	Delayed hypersensitivity
		Immune surveillance
		(destruction of cancer cells)
		Graft rejection
		Immune regulation
Organisms protective against	Pyogenic bacteria	Intracellular bacteria
	Staphylococcus	*Pseudomonas*
	Haemophilus	*Listeria*
	Neisseria	Mycobacteria
	Viruses	Viruses
	Hepatitis B virus	Herpes simplex virus
	Adenovirus	Herpes zoster and varicella
	Enterovirus	zoster viruses
	Echovirus	Cytomegalovirus
		Epstein-Barr virus
		Retrovirus (excluding HIV)
		Fungi
		Candida
		Cryptococcus
		Aspergillus
		Pneumocystis carinii
		Protozoa
		Toxoplasma gondii

complement fixation, and intravascular hemolysis. A direct Coombs' test will confirm the presence of antibody on the RBCs. An indirect Coombs' test measures the degree of hemolytic activity. In autoimmune hemolytic anemia, antibodies against the body's own RBCs are produced. This reaction is provoked by allergic reactions to drugs, when a drug and antibody to the drug form a complex that attacks the RBCs. The HDNB occurs during the pregnancy of a mother who has been sensitized to blood group antigens on a previous infant's RBCs and makes IgE antibodies to them. The antibodies cross the placenta and react with the fetal RBCs, causing destruction. Rhesus D (Rh factor) is the most commonly involved antigen.

Type III

Type III hypersensitivity reactions are immune complex–mediated reactions. In this condition, large quantities of antigen-antibody complexes are deposited in the tissues and cannot be cleared from the body by the reticuloendothelial system. This leads to a condition known as serum sickness. Causes are persistent infection, autoimmune disease, and environmental antigens.

Type IV

In type IV (delayed-type) hypersensitivity reactions, when the host comes into contact with a foreign antigen, antigen-sensitized T cells release lymphokines that destroy the antigen. Allergic contact dermatitis, acute allograft rejection, and delayed hypersensitivity skin testing are examples of type IV hypersensitivity reactions.

Anaphylaxis

Anaphylaxis is an acute, generalized, and violent antigen-antibody reaction that may be rapidly fatal even with prompt emergency treatment.

Pathophysiology

Anaphylaxis results from a reaction to an allergen that causes the release of IgE, an antibody formed as part of the immune response. Upon first exposure to an antigen, IgE antibodies are formed and attach to mast cells in tissues and basophils in the vascular system. Once antibodies have been formed, a second exposure to the antigen results in an immune reaction (releasing histamine) that may vary from mild to fatal. In its severe form, the reaction is called anaphylactic shock.

The reaction of anaphylactic shock is primarily a histamine reaction, setting off a chain of multiple chemical reactions that cause further reactions. The more reactions that occur, the more severe the anaphylaxis and the greater the mortality.

The release of histamine results in vasodilatation of the capillaries (causing hypotension) and a markedly increased cellular permeability. The increase in intracellular fluid alters the cell shape, leaving spaces between the previously compact cells. This promotes movement from the vascular system, thus increasing the colloid osmotic pressure. As more colloids move into interstitial spaces, edema and a decreased circulating volume of blood occur. This has the effect of decreasing cardiac output.

Histamine occurs in two forms, H_1 and H_2. H_1 causes vasoconstriction of the bronchi and intestines. H_2 increases gastric acid secretion and minor cardiac stimulation. Both H_1 and H_2 are responsible for vasodilatation.

The release and action of histamines result in the release of other amines into the bloodstream. Bradykinin, serotonin, slow-reacting substances, a chemotactic factor attracting eosinophils, prostaglandins, and acetylcholine all play a role in the physiologic development of anaphylaxis. These chemicals may also activate the complement system. These amines increase arteriolar and venous dilatation, capillary permeability, and abnormal shift of fluid from the vascular tree into the interstitial compartment. This shift decreases circulating blood volume but does not decrease total blood in the body. With blood remaining in the microcirculation, decreased systolic and diastolic pressure occurs. These substances and H_1 and H_2 cause an intense bronchiolar constriction that leads to a general hypoxemia.

Etiology

Many substances known as allergens can cause anaphylaxis. Allergens can range from foods and food additives to drugs and insect-sting venom, including bee, wasp, and hornet (Table 25-3). Routes of entry for an allergen can include injection, ingestion, inhalation, and skin absorption. Drugs, especially antibiotics, are the major allergens in anaphylaxis. Other drugs, iodine-based contrast dye, and blood transfusions are also involved in anaphylaxis. More recently, food preservatives and additives have been attributed to an increasing number of cases of anaphylaxis.

Clinical Presentation

Clinical signs of anaphylaxis include generalized pruritus, respiratory distress, syncope, and apprehension, and can appear within several minutes of exposure to the antigen (Table 25-4). The severity of the reaction is directly related to the onset of symptoms, with early signs appearing with a severe reaction. Occasionally, biphasic reactions occur in which symptoms recur several hours after the initial reaction.

Angioedema is edema in membranous tissues and is most easily seen in the eyes and mouth. It also occurs in the tongue, hands, feet, and genitalia. There is a diffuse erythema occurring more in the upper body parts than in the lower. Occasionally, abdominal cramps, vomiting, and/or diarrhea may occur. Unconsciousness occurs early in severe anaphylaxis.

As fluid shifts from the capillaries into the interstitial tissue, edema of the uvula and larynx occurs. This edema may produce an acute respiratory obstruction. Laryngeal edema is accompanied by impaired phonation and a barking or high-pitched cough. If the patient is alert, he or she will show signs of increased anxiety and complain of air hunger.

Cardiovascular effects of anaphylaxis are the same as those associated with other types of shock—mainly hypotension, tachycardia, and changes in the

TABLE 25-3. COMMON ANAPHYLAXIS ALLERGENS

Foods	Food Additives	Medications	Others
Eggs	Monosodium glutamate	Antibiotics	Latex
Peanut butter	Autolyzed yeast	Aspirin	Exercise
Fish	Natural flavorings	Contrast dye	Insect venom
Shellfish	Yeast extract	Blood products	Animal hair/dander
Milk	Food coloring	Vaccines	Dust
Cheese		Narcotics	Pollen
Tomatoes		Local anesthetics	
Chocolate			
Nuts and seeds			

TABLE 25-4. CLINICAL SIGNS AND SYMPTOMS OF ANAPHYLAXIS

General
 Pruritus (generalized itching)
 Flushing
 Altered respiratory status/coughing
 Wheezing
 Urticaria (hives)
 Angioedema (edema of the lips/tongue)
 Restlessness
 Nausea/vomiting/diarrhea
Life-threatening
 Respiratory distress
 Stridor
 Bronchospasm
 Laryngeal edema

Source: Adapted from Kleinpell RM: Shock states, Gannett Healthcare Group, www.nurse.com. http://www.nurse.com. Used with permission.

electrocardiogram similar to those that occur in myocardial injury. Temporary changes in the ST segment and the T wave suggest coronary ischemia. However, the serum enzymes are normal.

Life-threatening signs and symptoms include respiratory distress, stridor, bronchospasm, and laryngeal edema. The changes in ventilation (causing hypoxia) and decreased circulating blood may result in convulsions and unconsciousness. Circulatory failure and respiratory distress are the usual causes of death in anaphylaxis.

Complications

Myocardial infarction (MI) secondary to venous dilatation and a decreased blood pressure may occur. With decreased blood pressure, increased tissue hypoxia occurs. This results in increased tissue anoxia and destruction. Hypoventilation occurs as a result of the decreased venous return of blood to the heart and increased tissue hypoxia.

Pulmonary status, already compromised by bronchiolar constriction, may be further damaged as a result of overadministration of the intravenous fluids used to compensate for the decreased vascular volume. Chemical reactions causing further imbalances may lead to central nervous system convulsions and coma. If the pulmonary, cardiac, or vascular system is refractory to treatment, anaphylaxis results in a shock state and can lead to cardiac, renal, pulmonary, and multisystem organ failure. Death in anaphylaxis can result from cardiovascular or respiratory distress.

Treatment

The treatment goals for anaphylactic shock include the "ABCs" of emergency care (airway, breathing,

and circulation) along with volume expansion. Hypotension can be managed with intravenous fluids to promote intravascular volume expansion. Vasoconstrictor agents may be required to reverse the effects of severe vasodilation and depressed myocardial function. Epinephrine is a first-line drug given to patients with anaphylaxis because it promotes bronchodilation and vasoconstriction and inhibits further mediator release. The primary objective of treatment is to dilate the bronchioles, which is accomplished by the administration of epinephrine either subcutaneously or intramuscularly. Antihistamines are used simultaneously to help control local edema and itching, but they cannot alter the circulatory failure and bronchoconstriction to a significant degree. After administration of epinephrine, the respiratory system may need to be supported by oxygen via face mask. The patient may need to be transferred to the intensive care unit if intubation and mechanical ventilation are required.

The second goal of therapy is to improve the patient's circulatory status. Promoting the movement of fluid from the interstitial compartment back into the vascular compartment is usually achieved through the use of intravenous fluids. The third-space loss of fluid is believed to be caused by leakage through the injured capillary walls. Glucocorticoids help to decrease cellular damage, reduce the severity of anaphylaxis, and prevent inflammation of the damaged tissues. Hydrocortisone given intravenously is the drug usually used. Steroids stabilize the membrane of the basophils, reducing the chemical reactions in anaphylaxis.

In addition to maintaining respiratory status, using epinephrine and antihistamines, and administering glucocorticoids (both those formed by the body in response to stress and synthetic forms), intravenous fluid will increase the circulating blood volume. Electrolytes may be added to intravenous fluids so as to control acid-base imbalances.

Nursing Intervention

Assessment of the signs and symptoms of anaphylaxis, especially respiratory distress and life-threatening hemodynamic instability is extremely important. Research has shown that laryngeal edema and hypotension are major factors causing death.

Anaphylaxis may occur in susceptible patients immediately or as much as an hour after injection of an antigen (drug, blood). Respiratory assessment includes identifying signs of stridor, the use of auxiliary muscles for breathing, and/or cyanosis; auscultating lung fields for crackles, rhonchi, or wheezes; pulse oximetry; and measuring arterial blood gases. Mechanical ventilation should be on standby if not already in use. Normal nursing interventions for patients on ventilators are applicable for these patients.

The patient's cardiac and circulatory status should also be monitored closely, as hypotension can precede the onset of anaphylactic shock. Death can occur within minutes if there is circulatory failure or pulmonary edema. Vital signs—including heart rate, blood pressure, respiratory rate, and pulse oximetry—should be observed continuously until the patient is stable and then at very frequent intervals (at least every 15 min for four times, then every 30 min for four times, and then every 1 to 2 h).

Antihistamines are not usually helpful in altering circulatory failure and bronchoconstriction. The use of antihistamines does not affect the release of histamine, but antihistamines do occupy receptor sites, thus preventing the attachment of histamine. Administration of these drugs requires close observation because of their depressive effects on the central nervous system. If epinephrine is used intravenously, it is essential to monitor for hypertension and cardiac dysrhythmias.

Renal status is monitored by Foley catheter to prevent fluid overload as the extracellular fluid moves back into the vascular system with appropriate drugs. In severe anaphylaxis, the patient is frequently comatose, and establishing the monitoring and support systems may leave little if any time for psychosocial support. As the patient's condition stabilizes and his or her level of consciousness returns to normal, emotional support is essential. Explaining to the patient what has happened, what all the monitoring equipment is being used for, and that these monitors will be removed as his or her condition improves will help to alleviate the patient's fear. In addition, prevention of anaphylactic shock through identification of patients at risk and careful monitoring of patient response to potential allergens including drugs, blood products, and blood are important components of nursing care.

HEMATOLOGIC SYSTEM

Red Blood Cell Formation and Anemias

Hematopoiesis

The bone marrow is a spongy substance within the bone where maturation of blood cells occurs. In the adult, bone marrow is primarily located in the long, flat bones (skull, ribs, sternum, pelvis, shoulder girdles, vertebrae, innominates). The mature erythrocyte, leukocyte, and thrombocyte all begin as primitive cells called stem cells. In response to specific stimuli, called colony-stimulating factors, a stem cell becomes "committed" to a particular cell line and matures to perform the functions of either an RBC, WBC, or platelet. Once the stem cell is committed, it is no longer capable of mitosis. It matures within the bone marrow and is released into the peripheral blood. Stem cells increase in number during times of increased demand (hypoxia, infection) in order to increase production of the needed blood cell type.

RBC production is stimulated by the hormone erythropoietin. Erythropoietin is released by the kidney in response to tissue hypoxia. This hormone results in increased erythrocyte production by (1) increasing the number of stem cells placed into the maturational process, (2) decreasing maturational time, (3) increasing hemoglobin synthesis, and (4) causing a premature release of reticulocytes from the bone marrow. Reticulocytes may appear in the peripheral blood within 2 days of increased demand, but an increase in mature erythrocytes is not apparent until 6 to 8 days. An increase in the peripheral reticulocyte count is an indication of increased RBC production.

The primary function of the RBC is the transportation of oxygen and carbon dioxide. Hemoglobin is the molecule responsible for this function. It is produced throughout most of the maturation of the RBC. Normal hemoglobin production depends on a sufficient iron supply, protoporphyrin, and globin.

The life span of the mature RBC in the circulation is approximately 120 days. As the cell becomes older, it is no longer able to traverse the microvasculature, and then it is phagocytized by the reticuloendothelial tissue.

Platelet Production

Platelet production is thought to be regulated by the hormone thrombopoietin. Platelets mature in the bone marrow and migrate to the spleen. They travel between the spleen and circulatory system in order to maintain a steady state of circulating platelets. Platelets contribute to hemostasis by forming a plug over an area of damaged endothelium. Plug formation requires an adequate number of functioning platelets as well as vascular integrity. Platelets are a source of phospholipids, which are necessary in the coagulation process.

Normal Coagulation and Pathologic Hematologic Conditions

Several sequential events occur to aid in preventing bleeding. Vasoconstriction and platelet aggregation are the first two events in hemostasis. Primary hemostasis is the process of platelet plug formation at the site of injury. This occurs within seconds of injury. Secondary hemostasis involves the reactions of the plasma coagulation system resulting in fibrin formation. This occurs within several minutes of injury.

Normal Coagulation

Blood clotting is a complex process that controls bleeding when tissues are injured. Normal coagulation depends on the presence of all clotting factors and the appropriate functioning of other separate but interrelated components. These components are the extrinsic cascade, the intrinsic cascade, and the common final pathway.

A cascade is similar to a row of dominoes standing on their ends. When the first domino falls, it strikes the next domino, starting a chain reaction that continues until all the dominoes have been toppled. This means that each domino must be positioned so that it will connect with the next. Within the circulating blood, there is a plethora of clotting factors to continue a cascade once initiated. It is interesting to note that there is at least one specific spot in each of the three cascades (extrinsic, intrinsic, and final common pathway) that requires calcium ions (Ca^{2+}, factor IV) to continue activation of these cascades. These sites are identified in Fig. 25-5, which shows the normal coagulation process.

Extrinsic Cascade. The extrinsic cascade (Fig. 25-6) is activated by injury to vessels and tissue. The end result of this cascade is the release of thromboplastin into the circulatory system.

A second mechanism for activating clotting factors is the release of phospholipids from platelets and damaged tissue. This is thought to increase the rate of blood coagulation through both the extrinsic and intrinsic cascades.

Intrinsic Cascade. The intrinsic cascade (Fig. 25-7) is initiated when factor XII (the Hageman factor, or the surface substance) comes into contact with collagen or the basement membrane of the blood vessel's damaged endothelium.

Common Final Pathway Cascade. Both the extrinsic and intrinsic cascades react to completion and, in the presence of calcium ions, join to form the common final pathway cascade shown in Fig. 25-8.

Syneresis is the final step in coagulation and the first step in clot stability. Syneresis is the process of particle suspension in a gel that begins to aggregate and form a compact mass—the clot. Clot retraction occurs soon after syneresis is complete. Platelets contain an enzyme called thromboplastin that causes the fibrin strands and cells in the clot to be drawn together, expressing a clear, serous fluid. Clot retraction is responsible for drawing the edges of damaged vessels together, which fosters healing.

Anticoagulation

When the vascular damage has been repaired, dissolution of the clot begins. This is termed fibrinolysis. Up to this point, the various cascades have clotted the injured vessels but have not caused massive intravascular clotting. Massive clotting is avoided because excess thrombin is carried away from the clot site by the circulating blood and antithrombin III is released from mast cells.

There are actually two mechanisms to prevent excessive clotting: the antithrombin system and the fibrinolytic system.

Antithrombin System. This system protects our bodies from excessive intravascular clotting by neutralizing the clotting capability of thrombin. Antithrombin III is the neutralizing agent. Heparin functions as an antithrombin III and inhibits all serine proteases in all cascades. These include Xa, Ha, Vt12, and thrombin. Heparin interrupts the action of thrombin on fibrinogen.

When clot retraction is complete, profibrinolysis is activated by factor XII. This activation results in fibrinolysin (plasmin), which phagocytizes the clot and other clotting factors present in excess of the normal amount. In this way, both intravascular clotting and bleeding are controlled.

Fibrinolytic System. Fibrinolysis, or clot lysis, begins immediately after the formation of a hemostatis plug. Three potential activators of the fibrinolytic system are the Hageman factor (factor XII), or plasma protein fragments; urinary plasminogen activator, or urokinase; and tissue plasminogen activator. These activators convert plasminogen, adsorbed to the fibrin clot, to plasmin, which lyses the clot. Clot lysis (fibrinolysis) is accomplished by two mechanisms: clearance of activated clotting factors by the reticuloendothelial system and the actual lysis

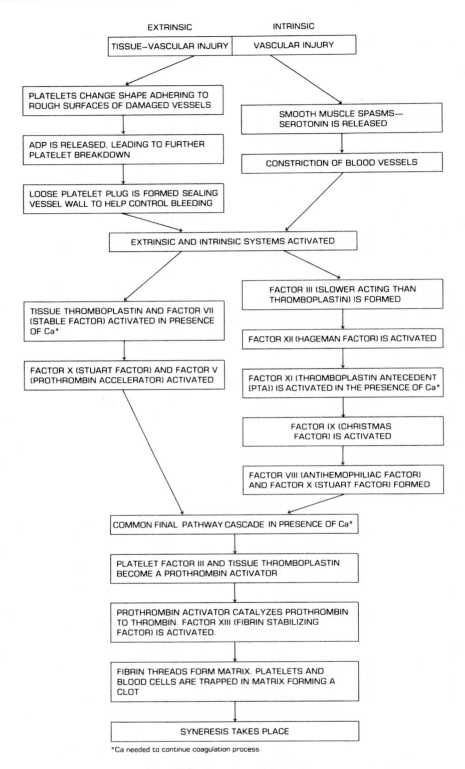

Figure 25-5. Normal coagulation process.

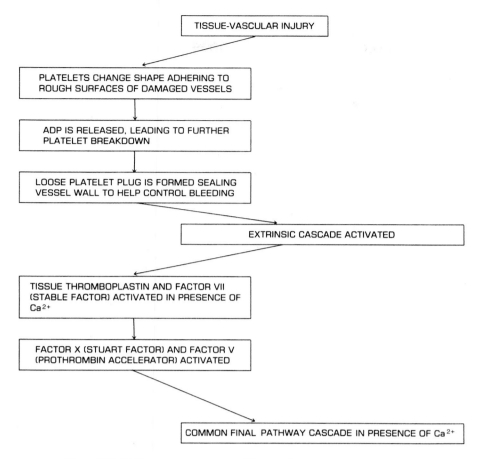

Figure 25-6. Extrinsic cascade segment of the overall normal coagulation process.

of the fibrin structure in the clot. Lysis of the clot is initiated by either the internal or external pathway. In the internal pathway, factor XII is activated to XIIa upon contact with an abnormal or irregular vascular lining. At the same time, XIIa catalyzes prekallikrein to kallikrein (a blood plasminogen activator). The extrinsic system provides tissue plasminogen activators from damaged vascular areas. Both types of plasminogen activators convert plasminogen to plasmin. Plasmin breaks the fibrin structure, causing the mesh holding blood components, such as platelets, to weaken and dissociate as a stable unit. The breakdown of the fibrin structure causes an increase in fibrin degradation products (or fibrin split products). An increase in fibrin degradation products may signal the onset of a coagulopathy such as DIC.

Antiplatelet, Anticoagulant, and Fibrinolytic Therapy. Antithrombotic agents—including antiplatelet drugs, anticoagulants, and fibrinolytic agents—are used to prevent thrombotic events, prevent or minimize complications of thrombotic events, and restore vascular patency. Table 25-5 outlines anticoagulant agents commonly used in progressive care. Fibrinolytic therapy in the treatment of acute MI and pulmonary emboli employs the principles of normal clot lysis. Normally, the fibrinolytic system converts plasminogen to plasmin, which degrades fibrin into soluble fragments. In the presence of large thrombi, this system cannot dissolve the fibrin mass. However, the introduction of exogenous plasminogen activators produces more plasmin, which depletes circulating fibrinogen and promotes lysis. Exogenous plasminogen activator also destroys coagulation factors V and VIII, causing a systemic lytic state that increases the potential risk of bleeding.

The fibrinolytic agents used most frequently include reteplase (rPA), alteplase (tPA), and streptokinase (SK). Streptokinase is derived from beta-hemolytic streptococci and activates the fibrinolytic

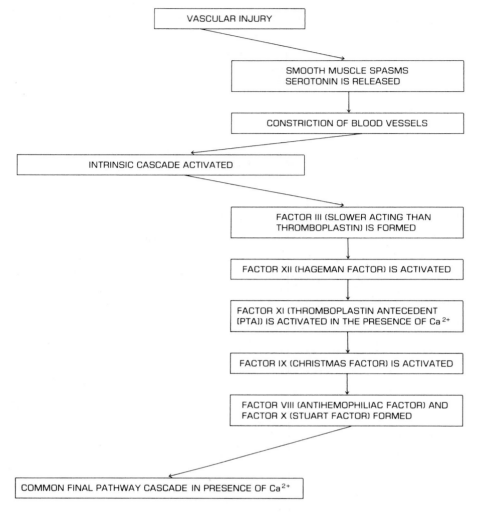

Figure 25-7. Intrinsic cascade segment of the overall normal coagulation process.

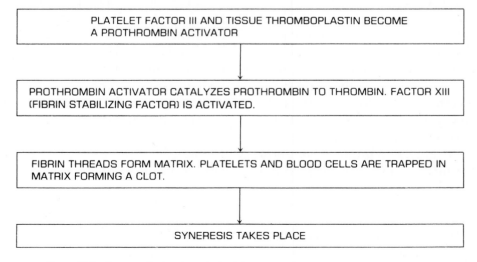

Figure 25-8. Common final pathway (cascade) segment of the normal coagulation process.

TABLE 25-5. ANTICOAGULANT AGENTS COMMONLY USED IN PROGRESSIVE AND ACUTE CARE

Antiplatelet agents	Aspirin
	Clopidogrel
	Dipyridamole
	Ticlopidine
	Prasugrel
Glycoprotein IIb/IIIA inhibitors	Abcixmab
	Eptifibatide
	Tirofiban
Unfractionated heparin	Heparin
Low molecular weight heparins	Enoxaparin
	Dalteparin sodium
Synthetic anti-X agent	Fondaparinux
Direct thrombin inhibitors	Bivalirudin
	Desirudin
	Argatroban
	Lepirudin
Fibrinolytic agents	Streptokinase
	Recombinant plasminogen activator
	Alteplase

Source: Adapted from "Hematology and Immunology Systems," by D. Dressler. In M. Chulay, & S. Burns (Eds.). *AACN Essentials of Progressive Care Nursing.* New York, NY: McGraw-Hill, 2010, pp. 283-294. With Permission.

process by forming an activator complex with plasminogen. It depletes fibrinogen and other coagulant factors, predisposing the patient to systemic bleeding. Allergic anaphylactic reactions can be induced upon a second exposure to the drug due to its nature as a bacterial protein. Alteplase was the first recombinant tissue–type plasminogen activator and is identical to a native tissue plasminogen activator. It is the fibrinolytic agent most often used for the treatment of coronary artery thrombosis, pulmonary embolism, and acute stroke. Reteplase is a synthetic second-generation recombinant tissue–type plasminogen activator that works more quickly and has a lower bleeding risk than the first-generation agent tPA.

Fibrinolysis is indicated for acute MI (if the patient presents within 12 h of symptom onset), coronary artery thrombosis, pulmonary embolism, acute stroke, and acute peripheral arterial occlusions. Bleeding complications can occur with fibrinolysis. For serious bleeding complications, the fibrinolytic agent should be stopped and supportive therapy instituted. Volume and/or transfusion may be indicated of blood or blood factors such as fresh frozen plasma and/or cryoprecipitate to replenish fibrin and clotting factors. If the patient has also been receiving heparin, protamine sulfate may be used to reverse the heparin effect. Aminocaproic acid, a specific antidote to fibrinolytic agents, may also be indicated.

26

Diagnosis and Treatment of Immunologic and Hematologic Problems

COMPLETE BLOOD COUNT

The red blood cell (RBC) count consists of the total number of circulating RBCs, the part of the blood that transports oxygen. Table 26-1 lists normal values. The hemoglobin (Hb) measures the oxygen-carrying capacity of the RBC, while the hematocrit (Hct) compares the RBC volume to the plasma volume. Other valuable indices include mean corpuscular volume (MCV), which is the average size of the RBC, and the mean corpuscular hemoglobin (MCH), which measures the average weight of the Hb per RBC. Finally, the MCH concentration (MCHC) measures the average percentage of Hb in an RBC. A peripheral smear allows the practitioner to examine the RBC and obtain data on composition, size, and shape.

Another useful test in evaluating the hematologic system is the reticulocyte count. This test identifies the bone marrow's ability to produce young erythrocytes. Reticulocytes are matured into RBCs in just under 24 h by reticulin. The life span of an RBC is approximately 120 days, after which it dies and releases Hb into the circulation; this is transported to the liver and spleen and ultimately broken down. Iron is then stored in the liver and spleen for future use and the remaining heme molecule is converted into bilirubin and excreted in the urine or stool.

The white blood cell (WBC) count measures the total number of white cells, or leukocytes. Further breakdown of the WBC count is called the differential. Components of the differential include neutrophils, monocytes, lymphocytes, basophils, and eosinophils. Absolute counts in the differential are more important because they are in direct relation to the WBC count. Abnormal components and causative agents of the differential are listed in Table 26-2.

The erythrocyte sedimentation rate (ESR) is often used in evaluating infectious diseases. It is a nonspecific test that examines the volume of RBCs that settle in 1 h. Elevation is usually seen with inflammation, infection, or malignancy.

Other helpful tests include radiographs, scans, and biopsies.

HEMOSTATIC SCREENING TESTS

Normal clotting has three stages: (1) vascular injury activates thromboplastin activity in both the extrinsic and intrinsic pathways, (2) thromboplastin converts prothrombin to thrombin, and (3) thrombin converts fibrinogen in the plasma at the site of injury to form a fibrin plug.

Specific tests can be performed to evaluate blood-clotting activity, identify abnormalities, and ascertain patient response to therapy.

Prothrombin Time

The prothrombin time (PT) measures the activity level and patency of the extrinsic clotting cascade and the common final pathway. The PT measures

TABLE 26-1. NORMAL LABORATORY VALUES FOR THE COMPLETE BLOOD COUNT

Red cell count (RBC)	
Women	$3.8–5.2 \times 10$/mL
Men	$4.4–5.9 \times 10$/mL
Hemoglobin (Hb)	
Women	11.7–15.7 g/dL
Men	13.3–17.7 g/dL
Hematocrit (Hct)	
Women	34.9%–46.9%
Men	39.8%–52.2%
Platelets	150,000–400,000
White cell count	3500–11,000/mL
Neutrophils	39%–79%
Lymphocytes	10%–40%
Monocytes	3%–8%
Basophils	0%–2%
Eosinophils	0%–5%
Reticulocyte count	0.5%–1.5%
Erythrocyte sedimentation rate	
Women	1–20 mm/h
Men	1–13 mm/h
Prothrombin time	11–16 s
Activated partial thromboplastin time	20–35 s
Bleeding time	<4 min
INR	1.0–2.0
Fibrinogen	200–400 mg/dL
Fibrin split products	2–10 mcg/mL
D-Dimer	<200 mg/mL

Normal values may vary between laboratories. Refer to local laboratory standard values in interpreting test results.
INR, international ratio.

factors I, II, V, VII, and X. Normal values are the same as control values (should be 11 to 16 s). The effectiveness of warfarin is assessed with the PT.

Activated Partial Thromboplastin Time

The activated partial thromboplastin time (aPTT) measures the activity level and patency of the intrinsic clotting cascade and common final pathway. Normal values of 20 to 35 s are used to assess all clotting factors except VII and XIII. The effectiveness of heparin is assessed with the aPTT.

Bleeding Time

Platelet plug formation time is measured with the bleeding time. Normal values are less than 4 min (Ivy), 1 to 4 min (Duke), and 1 to 9 min (Mielke). Bleeding times predominantly reflect platelet function, and conditions causing poor platelet function produce abnormal results.

Platelet Count

This is a specific count of platelets seen in a blood smear. Normal values are 150,000 to 450,000 platelets per microliter (mcL). Values below 100,000 are pathognomonic for thrombocytopenia, the cause of which must be determined. A lower platelet count results in excessive bleeding, since there is an insufficient number of platelets to clot. Counts <20,000 are associated with spontaneous bleeding.

HUMAN IMMUNODEFICIENCY VIRUS SCREENING TESTS

The enzyme-linked immunosorbent assay (ELISA), also referred to as an enzyme immunoassay (EIA), is the initial diagnostic test for human immunodeficiency virus (HIV). Although the EIA is an extremely sensitive test, it lacks full specificity, and a person with suspected HIV infection with an inconclusive EIA must have additional specific assay testing. The most commonly used confirmatory test is the Western blot, which captures the separation of HIV antigens based on their different molecular weights, which are detected as discrete bands. A positive Western blot is considered positive if antibodies exist to two of the three HIV proteins. If the result of the Western blot is indeterminate, the test should be repeated in 4 to 6 weeks. Other tests that may be performed include a p24 antigen capture assay, polymerase chain reaction, and nucleic acid sequence–based assay. Other diagnostic studies that have proven useful in tracking the progression of HIV and response to therapy are CD4 counts and HIV viral load. The CD4 cell is the primary target and binding site of HIV. As the virus progresses, the CD4 count drops, although with the new antiretroviral therapy available today, it is not uncommon to see the CD4 count rise significantly. A new diagnostic marker called HIV viral load is now available. It measures the free virus in the plasma. This test can also show response to new therapy or indicate the need for a treatment change.

TESTS FOR OTHER INFECTIOUS DISEASES

Diagnostic tests often ordered for patients with a suspected infectious disease include cultures, susceptibility, and Gram's stain. Samples for these procedures will be collected by the nurse or physician and sent to the microbiology lab. Sources include blood, sputum, urine, and drainage from wounds. In addition, the nurse should review subjective and objective assessments and be aware of the various signs of hematologic and immunologic diseases (Table 26-3).

BLOOD AND COMPONENT THERAPY

The primary reason for transfusing blood is to increase the oxygen available for preventing tissue hypoxia. Blood is administered primarily when the

TABLE 26-2. INFLUENCE OF DISEASE ON BLOOD CELL COUNT

Cell Type	How Affected
Neutrophils	**Increased by:** • Infections: osteomyelitis, otitis media, salpingitis, septicemia, gonorrhea, endocarditis, smallpox, chickenpox, herpes, Rocky Mountain spotted fever • Ischemic necrosis due to myocardial infarction, burns, carcinoma • Metabolic disorders: diabetic acidosis, eclampsia, uremia, thyrotoxicosis • Stress response due to acute hemorrhage, surgery, excessive exercise, emotional distress, third trimester of pregnancy, childbirth • Inflammatory disease: rheumatic fever, rheumatoid arthritis, acute gout, vasculitis and myositis **Decreased by:** • Bone marrow depression due to radiation or cytotoxic drugs • Infections: typhoid, tularemia, brucellosis, hepatitis, influenza, measles, mumps, rubella, infectious mononucleosis • Hypersplenism: hepatic disease and storage diseases • Collagen vascular disease, such as systemic lupus erythematosus • Deficiency of folic acid or vitamin B_{12}
Eosinophils	**Increased by:** • Allergic disorders: asthma, hay fever, food or drug sensitivity, serum sickness, angioneurotic edema • Parasitic infections: trichinosis, hookworm, roundworm, amebiasis • Skin diseases: eczema, pemphigus, psoriasis, dermatitis, herpes • Neoplastic diseases: chronic myelocytic leukemia, Hodgkin's disease, metastases and necrosis of solid tumors • Miscellaneous: collagen vascular disease, adrenocortical hypofunction, ulcerative colitis, polyarteritis nodosa, postsplenectomy, pernicious anemia, scarlet fever, excessive exercise **Decreased by:** • Stress response due to trauma, shock, burns, surgery, mental distress • Cushing's syndrome
Basophils	**Increased by:** • Chronic myelocytic leukemia, polycythemia vera, some chronic hemolytic anemias, Hodgkin's disease, systemic mastocytosis, myxedema, ulcerative colitis, chronic hypersensitivity states, nephrosis **Decreased by:** • Hyperthyroidism, ovulation, pregnancy, stress
Lymphocytes	**Increased by:** • Infections: pertussis, brucellosis, syphilis, tuberculosis, hepatitis, infectious mononucleosis, mumps, German measles, cytomegalovirus • Other: thyrotoxicosis, adrenal insufficiency, ulcerative colitis, immune diseases, lymphocytic leukemia **Decreased by:** • Severe debilitating illness, such as congestive heart failure, renal failure, advanced tuberculosis • Defective lymphatic circulation, high levels of adrenal corticosteroids, immunodeficiency due to immunosuppressives
Monocytes	**Increased by:** • Infections: subacute bacterial endocarditis, tuberculosis, hepatitis, malaria, Rocky Mountain spotted fever • Collagen vascular disease: systemic lupus erythematosus, rheumatoid arthritis, polyarteritis nodosa • Carcinomas, monocytic leukemia, lymphomas

TABLE 26-3. SIGNS AND SYMPTOMS OF HEMATOLOGIC AND IMMUNOLOGIC DISEASES

Subjective
Fatigue
Dyspnea
Inability to perform activities of daily living

Objective
Altered mental status
Fever
Tachycardia
Hypotension
Tachypnea
Cough
Dysrhythmia
Abnormal lab values
Positive cultures
Skin lesions
Poor urine output
Lymphadenopathy

Hb/Hct levels are low (generally when Hb levels are <7 g/dL), when intravascular volume is low, and to replace deficient or utilized substances such as protein, platelets, and clotting factors.

Whole Blood

One unit of whole blood is approximately 500 mL of blood cells, serum, platelets, proteins, and other intravascular nutrients and substances. Whole blood is the best substance to transfuse in hemorrhage since it replaces both volume and elements. Owing to shortages, the transfusion of whole blood is actually rare. Whole blood can be divided into packed RBCs (PRBCs), fresh frozen plasma (FFP), and cryoprecipitate, making it possible for more than one patient to benefit from the donation of 1 unit of whole blood. Whole blood can be stored for 5 weeks; however, factors V and VIII are labile and are significantly decreased after 7 days.

Normally, during the administration of a blood transfusion, the cold (due to storage) donor blood is rapidly warmed as it mixes with circulating blood at normal infusion rates. Rapid replacement with cold blood predisposes the patient to cardiac arrest, hypothermia, and coagulopathies. When massive, rapid transfusions are necessary, the blood can be passed through a warmer to reach body temperature, thus reducing these dangers.

Red Blood Cells

PRBCs provide the advantage of less blood volume (200 to 300 mL) to infuse, thereby decreasing the chance of fluid overload. PRBCs are used in severe anemias without blood loss and hemorrhage. One unit of PRBCs raises hemoglobin concentration by about 2 g/dL. PRBCs are given cautiously in patients with congestive heart failure, cardiac disease, or with renal failure related to the increased risk of fluid overload. In the average adult, 1 unit of RBCs raises the hemoglobin by 1 g.

Fresh Frozen Plasma

Fresh frozen plasma is the fluid portion of blood after centrifugation to remove the RBCs. When the plasma is frozen, all clotting factors (especially V and VII) except the platelets are preserved.

Administration of plasma is indicated when there is a coagulopathy or hypovolemia with little or no actual blood loss; for example, in burns and crush injuries. One unit of FFP raises most coagulation factor levels by about 20%. In an emergency, FFP may be used as a volume expander in hypovolemic bleeds until fresh whole blood is available. One unit of FFP can raise coagulation factors by 5% to 8% and fibrinogen by 13 mg/dL in the average patient.

Cryoprecipitates

Cryoimmunoglobulins are serum proteins that precipitate at temperatures <20°C. Cryoimmunoglobulins must be obtained and processed at temperatures >20°C and ideally before refrigeration, which may cause cryoproteins to be caught in the blood clots. Many authorities believe that cryoprecipitates are antigen-antibody protein compounds.

Cryoprecipitates usually compose 20 to 30 mL/unit of blood and must be infused immediately after thawing. Cryoprecipitates contain factors VIII and XIII and fibrinogen. One unit (20 to 50 mL) raises fibrinogen by about 75 mg/dL. It is not uncommon to infuse as many as 30 bags of cryoprecipitates at one time, using a special transfusion administration set.

Cryoprecipitate is useful to quickly raise the fibrinogen level in patients with disseminated intravascular coagulation (DIC). The administration of cryoprecipitates is also indicated in hemophilia A and von Willebrand's disease.

Platelets

Less than 40,000 to 50,000 platelets per cubic microliter (mcL) are considered inadequate for hemostasis. Prolonged bleeding time is a better index of the need for platelet transfusion than an actual platelet count. There is an approximate increase of $10,000/unit$ (platelets)$/mm^3$. A postplatelet transfusion bleeding time is the most accurate index of response to therapy.

In thrombocytopenia, splenomegaly, and DIC, platelet transfusions are useful until more definitive therapy can be instituted. Alloimmunity may require cross matching to have any value for platelet transfusion. One unit of single donor (pheresis) platelets is equivalent to 5 to 6 platelet concentrates. One concentrate of platelet can raise the platelet count by 5000 to 7000 Units/L. Platelets can be safely kept at room temperatures for up to 3 days and are inactivated if refrigerated.

Volume Expanders

Albumin, hetastarch, and in some institutions, dextran 40 and dextran 70 are used as volume expanders.

Salt-Poor Albumin

Albumin as 25% (25 g in 100 mL) is commercially available as a volume expander. It does not supply any clotting factors. Its sole value lies in expanding blood volume since it increases the colloid osmotic pressure for up to 24 h (although the time may be as low as 4 h).

Hetastarch

Hetastarch is a large glucose-based colloidal volume expander. It has approximately the same molecular weight as albumin and similar volume-expansion properties. Only about 20% of the volume of crystalloid solutions (lactated Ringer's or normal saline) is necessary with hetastarch to achieve similar hemodynamic responses. Normally, hetastarch is administered in a 6% solution. Hetastarch is cleared by renal excretion in about 24 to 36 h. Although hetastarch is similar to albumin in volume expansion, it has the advantage of costing only about one-third as much.

Dextran

Dextran is commercially available in two forms: dextran 70 or dextran 40 (low molecular weight dextran [LMWD]).

Dextran 70 is a 6% solution in 0.9 normal saline or D_5W composed of both small and large molecules. It has colloid effects similar to those of plasma.

Dextran's greatest value lies in its expansion properties in addition to its action in lowering of blood viscosity. The lower blood viscosity is due to a lower Hct and reduction of platelet and RBC aggregations, which improve tissue perfusion. The LMWD may help prevent a vascular thrombus occlusion of a vessel or graft.

Major complications of dextran use are allergic reactions, impaired coagulation (due to interference with platelet aggregation), and difficulty in future type-matching and cross-matching attempts for whole blood infusions. The allergic reactions may range from urticaria to anaphylaxis, which may occur immediately or after more than 30 min. Nausea, vomiting, and hypotension may occur.

Dextran therapy is not indicated in oliguric patients, patients with congestive heart failure (CHF), and patients with blood-clotting dyscrasias. Its use has markedly decreased over the past years.

Blood Substitutes

Several synthetic blood products have been proposed for use in transfusion therapy to increase oxygen-carrying capacity. Three products are undergoing continued clinical testing: two human (PolyHeme and HemoLink) and one bovine-based hemoglobin solution (Hemopure). Human polymerized hemoglobin (PolyHeme) is an oxygen-carrying resuscitative fluid that has been used in the treatment of acute blood loss. A whole blood substitute, Fluosol-DA, has also been proposed as a solution with increased oxygen-handling capability. These early-generation red cell substitutes are limited in their use, and testing of these agents in clinical trials continues.

Granulocytes

Centers performing leukapheresis have the ability to filter out granulocytes. Each unit is about 200 to 300 mL, and the recipient must be compatible with the donor. An infusion of granulocytes improves phagocytosis from the marginal cells without increasing the already circulating pool of WBCs. The marginal cells are those being released from the bone marrow.

It is common for the patient to have fever and chills during granulocyte infusion. Steroids and antihistamines given before the infusion will help control the fever, whereas meperidine hydrochloride (Demerol) will control the chills.

Reactions to Blood and Component Therapy

In spite of meticulous procedures for blood and component therapy, reactions do occur. There are four major reactions.

1. Circulatory overload occurs when too much fluid or too rapid an infusion is administered to patients with underlying cardiac, renal, liver, pulmonary, or hematologic disease. With proper monitoring and assessment, circulatory overload should not occur. If it does occur, prompt and appropriate intervention will remove sufficient fluid to restore the normal fluid status.
2. A bacterial reaction to transfusion therapy is the most common reaction and is characterized by the development of a fever in a previously afebrile patient. If the patient is febrile, a rising temperature may indicate a reaction.
3. Allergic reactions may occur with almost any product transfused. A slight reaction may be manifested by a mild urticaria. A severe allergic reaction is indicated by anaphylaxis that may or may not be reversible.
4. A hemolytic reaction usually occurs within the first 30 min of the transfusion. It results in actual hemolysis of the RBCs, and the transfusion must be stopped. A Coombs' test will diagnose this problem.

Clinical Presentation

The signs and symptoms will differ with the type of reaction, length of transfusion, substance being infused, and intensity of the reaction. Common signs and symptoms may include chills, fever, hives, hypotension, cardiac palpitations, tachycardia, flushing of the skin, headache, loss of consciousness, nausea and vomiting, shortness of breath, back pain, and hemoglobinuria. In some instances, warmth along the vein carrying the infusion may be detected.

Nursing Intervention

The nurse must immediately stop the infusion (saving the substance being transfused) and keep the vein open with 0.9 normal saline. Accurate assessment of patient status must be completed quickly and efficiently for comparison with pretransfusion baseline data. The physician and the blood bank are notified of the reaction, and the physician's orders are carried out. If the reaction is anaphylactic, emergency resuscitative measures are instituted while personnel contact the physician and laboratory and save the substance being transfused.

Nursing support of the patient and family is best achieved by rapid but efficient and professional conduct in instituting all necessary interventions. Education as to the cause of the reaction may prevent a recurrence.

Clotting Factors

Confusion often occurs with the nomenclature assigned to the specific clotting factors. Consequently, an international committee agreed that all clotting factors would be designated by roman numerals for the inactive clotting factors. It was further agreed that once activated, the clotting factors would be identified by a roman numeral and a lower case "a." Table 26-4 lists the clotting factors and their synonyms. There is no designated factor VI.

Most of the clotting factors are found in circulating blood, the blood elements, and tissues surrounding and within the microcirculatory system. Clotting factors I (fibrinogen), II (prothrombin), V, VII, IX, and X are synthesized in the liver. Factors XI and XIII may also be synthesized in the liver. Factor VIII is most likely synthesized by macrophages in the spleen. Lymphocytes and the bone marrow may work in conjunction with the macrophages to form factor VIII.

Four clotting factors—factors II, VII, IX, and X— are dependent on vitamin K for synthesis by the liver. Research indicates that factor XI may also be vitamin K dependent. It is known that at least 30 substances may be connected with the clotting process; however, the 17 listed in Table 26-4 are the most significant.

TREATMENTS FOR HEMATOLOGIC AND IMMUNOLOGIC DISORDERS

Neutropenia

Treatment for neutropenia involves administering colony-stimulating factors such as filgrastim or pegfilgrastrim. These medications stimulate granulocyte precursors and must be given intravenously or subcutaneously. The dosage is 5.0 to 7.5 mcg/kg three to seven times per week.

TABLE 26-4. CLOTTING FACTORS AND THEIR SYNONYMS

Factor	Synonym
I	Fibrinogen
Ia	Fibrin
II	Prothrombin
IIa	Thrombin
III	Thromboplastin
IV	Calcium
V	Ac-globulin (labile factor, proaccelerin)
VII	Proconvertin (autoprothrombin I)
VIIa	Convertin
VIII	Antihemophiliac globulin
IX	Christmas factor (autoprothrombin II), plasma thromboplastin component
IXa	Activated plasma thromboplastin component
X	Stuart-Prower factor (autoprothrombin III)
XI	Plasma thromboplastin antecedent
XII	Hageman factor
XIIa	Activated Hageman factor
XIII	Fibrin-stabilizing factor

TABLE 26-5. RISK FACTORS FOR IMMUNOCOMPROMISE

Age extremes: neonates and elderly

Malnutrition

Known diseases involving the immune system, such as HIV infection

Chronic disease, such as diabetes, renal or hepatic failure

Immunosuppressive agents: steroids, cancer chemotherapeutic agents, and transplant immunosuppressive agents

Radiation therapy

Invasive catheters, such as intravascular catheters, indwelling urinary catheters, wound drains, ventricular shunts

Prosthetic devices such as synthetic vascular grafts

Cardiovascular devices such as pacemakers, implantable defibrillators

Orthopedic hardware such as pins, plates, screws, artificial joints

Loss of skin integrity as a result of wounds, burns, presence of decubitus ulcers

Loss of protective epithelial barriers as a result of oral or nasogastric intubation

Source: Adapted from "Hematology and Immunology Systems," by D. Dressler. In M. Chulay, & S. Burns (Eds.). *AACN Essentials of Progressive Care Nursing.* New York, NY: McGrawHill, 2010. With permission.

Anemia

Certain anemias can be treated with epoetin injections. This is the erythropoietin hormone produced by recombinant DNA technology. Darbepoetin is a longer acting synthetic agent. The route must be intravenous or subcutaneous because of poor bioavailability by the oral route.

Infection

At the first indication of infection, the patient is pancultured, meaning cultures are obtained from all possible sources of infection such as the blood, urine, wound, and sputum. On an empiric basis, antimicrobial coverage is generally aimed at bacterial infection. Of course, once culture results are obtained, the antimicrobial regimen can be individualized. Antimicrobials have potentially serious side effects and require careful monitoring by the nurse. Some of the undesirable side effects possible with these agents include bone marrow suppression; a change in the normal body flora, allowing colonization by more pathogenic hospital-acquired organisms; development of resistance by the organism; and liver and kidney toxicity.

Often acutely ill patients in progressive care require a combination of antimicrobial therapies, thus making benefits versus adverse effects a delicate balance.

In using antibiotic therapy, careful attention must be given to the administration schedule as well as culture results. Organism resistance is becoming more evident. Vancomycin-resistant *Staphylococcus* has been reported in several cases, and vancomycin-resistant *Enterococcus* is evident in many hospitals in the United States. These examples are the main reason hospitals have antibiotic restriction policies.

Included in treatment should be appropriate infection control. Isolation should be used according to disease specifications. The goal is to decrease nosocomial infections (Table 26-5).

Immunodeficiency

Finally, the treatment for HIV/AIDS is ever changing. Combination antiretroviral therapy, or highly active antiretroviral therapy (HAART), is the cornerstone of management of patients with HIV infection. Currently, agents used for the treatment of HIV infection fall into five categories: (1) reverse transcriptase inhibitors, or those that inhibit the viral reverse transcriptase enzyme; (2) protease inhibitors, those that inhibit the viral protease; (3) fusion inhibitors; (4) entry inhibitors; and (5) integrase inhibitors. The reverse transcriptase inhibitors were the first class of drugs licensed for the treatment of HIV infection and are indicated for this use as part of combination regimens. Reverse transcriptase inhibitors include the *nucleoside analogues* zidovudine, didanosine, zalcitabine, stavudine, lamivudine, abacavir, and emtricitabine; the *nucleotide analogue* tenofovir; and the *nonnucleoside reverse transcriptase inhibitors* nevirapine, delavirdine, efavirenz, and etravirine. Protease inhibitors (saquinavir, indinavir, ritonavir, nelfinavir, amprenavir, lopinavir/ritonavir, atazanavir, tipranavir, darunavir) are used as part of initial regimens in combination with reverse transcriptase inhibitors and are effective in suppressing HIV replication. Enfuvirtide, the only Food and Drug Administration (FDA)–approved fusion inhibitor, is administered as a subcutaneous injection. It works by inhibiting fusion of the HIV envelope to the target cell membrane. Several additional fusion inhibitors are currently in clinical trials. Entry inhibitors (maraviroc) inhibit the binding of HIV to the chemokine receptor CCR5, which is the coreceptor used by monotropic strains of HIV. Its use is restricted to persons who are infected with monotropic, rather than T-cell tropic, strains of HIV. Integrase inhibitors (raltegravir) inhibit the viral integrase enzyme which mediates integration of the viral genome into the target cell DNA. Often, three-drug regimens are used in the treatment of HIV, and all require close monitoring because of their potential for causing numerous side effects, including bone marrow suppression, peripheral neuropathy, hepatomegaly, renal toxicity, and gastrointestinal upset.

27

Hematologic and Immunologic Failure and Its Effects on Other Organ Systems

EDITORS' NOTE

The PCCN exam may contain approximately two to four questions on disorders of the hematologic and immune systems. Although specifics of different types of diseases, such as cancers, are not likely to be addressed on the exam, it is important to understand the general concepts presented in this chapter. Immunologic concepts are sometimes difficult to apply clinically, but the major concepts are important to the assessment and therapeutic interventions associated with progressive-care immunology.

DISORDERS OF THE HEMATOLOGIC SYSTEM

Anemia

Definition and Etiology

Anemia is the most common problem of the erythrocyte (red blood cell [RBC]). It is a clinical condition defined as (1) a reduction in the number of RBCs, (2) a reduction in the quantity of hemoglobin, and/or (3) a reduction in the volume of RBCs. As RBC mass measurement is impractical, anemia is measured with an RBC count, hemoglobin (Hb) concentration, and hematocrit (Hct) concentration. The etiology of anemia is dependent on the underlying condition or disease that produced the anemia. There are numerous causes of anemia, which can be divided into those resulting from heredity, nutritional deficiencies, blood loss, immunologic and idiopathic causes, exogenous (medications) causes, chronic diseases, infections, and neoplasms. Table 27-1 outlines the classification of anemias.

Clinical Presentation

The signs and symptoms of anemia are the result of tissue hypoxia or the compensatory mechanisms activated to prevent damage resulting from hypoxia. Persons are symptomatic at varying levels. Someone with mild anemia may be asymptomatic. Anemia may be the first indication of a serious underlying disease such as cancer or renal failure. If it occurs gradually, adaptation allows for minimal signs and symptoms. A person with a rapid onset of anemia may be very symptomatic. The signs and symptoms associated with anemia are as follows: increased pulse, respiration, and pulse pressure; decreased blood pressure; palpitations; chest pain; dyspnea on exertion; fatigue; weakness; vertigo; bone tenderness; and delayed wound healing.

Diagnosis

Laboratory findings indicative of anemia are (1) decreased Hb and Hct, (2) decreased RBC indices, (3) increased reticulocyte count (may or may not be present dependent on cause of anemia), and (4) decreased erythrocyte count.

TABLE 27-1. CLASSIFICATION OF ANEMIA

I. Blood loss
   A. Acute
   B. Chronic
II. Deficient RBC production
   A. Iron deficiency
   B. Vitamin B$_{12}$ deficiency
   C. Folic acid deficiency
   D. Bone marrow failure or suppression
      1. Myelofibrosis
      2. Aplastic anemia
      3. Malignant infiltration of marrow by tumor
      4. Marrow toxin (drugs, radiation)
      5. Infectious agents
III. Excessive RBC destruction
   A. Hemolytic anemia
   B. Defective glycolysis (G6PD deficiency)
   C. Membrane abnormalities
   D. Physical causes (prosthetic heart valves)
IV. Defective hemoglobin synthesis
   A. Thalassemias
   B. Sickle cell anemia
V. Anemias of chronic disease
   A. Renal disease
   B. Inflammatory disease
   C. Liver disease
   D. Endocrine disorders
   E. Cancers

G6PD, glucose-6-phosphate dehydrogenase; RBC, red blood cell.

Nursing Intervention

Nursing interventions for the patient with anemia are based on the principles of minimizing complications, conserving energy, and instituting medical therapies. The key interventions include the following:

1. History
   a. Signs of blood loss
   b. Bleeding tendencies
   c. Exposure to marrow toxins (drugs, radiation, chemicals)
   d. Previous history of anemia
   e. Surgical history (e.g., gastric resection)
   f. Comorbid conditions
   g. Changes in nutritional status
2. Physical assessment
   a. Oxygenation: vital signs, lung sounds, tolerance of activity
   b. Skin, mucous membranes: pallor, jaundice, purpura, petechiae, IV-line sites, wounds, indwelling catheters, stomatitis
   c. Gastrointestinal: ascites, splenomegaly
   d. Mobility: paresthesias, impaired sensation, bone pain (sternum, ribs, vertebrae)

3. Administer therapy to correct anemia
   a. Packed RBC (PRBC) infusion
   b. Iron replacement
   c. Hematopoietic hormone (erythropoietin alfa, EPO [Epogen, Procrit], darbepoetin alfa [Aranesp]).
4. Minimize energy expenditure by:
   a. Organizing activities according to patient tolerance
   b. Planning rest periods
   c. Limiting external stimulation
   d. Preventing chills
5. Maintain skin integrity
6. Promote a diet adequate in protein, iron, vitamins, and minerals
7. Maintain physical safety (e.g., assist with ambulation if the patient is dizzy)
8. Institute an appropriate oral hygiene program

Thrombocytopenia

Thrombocytopenia, a quantitative decrease in the number of circulating platelets, is caused by one of three mechanisms: decreased bone marrow production, increased sequestration of platelets in the spleen, or accelerated destruction of platelets. Drug-induced thrombocytopenia can also result from many common drugs including antibiotics (sulfonamides, penicillins, cephalosporins), heparins (highest incidence is with unfractionated products), cardiovascular drugs (thiazide diuretics), and chemotherapeutic agents (carboplatin, alkylating agents, anthracyclines, antimetabolites). Normal platelet count is 150,000 to 300,000/mm^3. The risk of bleeding increases as the platelet count decreases. Usually persons are placed on bleeding precautions when the platelet count falls below 50,000/mm^3. The risk of spontaneous bleeding increases at a platelet count of less than 20,000/mm^3. Table 27-2 outlines common causes of thrombocytopenia.

Clinical Presentation

Signs and symptoms associated with thrombocytopenia include petechiae, ecchymosis, hematemesis, hemoptysis, hematuria, vaginal bleeding, rectal bleeding, blood in stool, anemia, and active bleeding from mucous membranes, wounds, indwelling catheters, and sites of invasive procedures.

Treatment

Platelet transfusions are administered to thrombocytopenic patients who are actively bleeding, undergoing invasive procedures, or at increased risk of

TABLE 27-2. COMMON CAUSES OF THROMBOCYTOPENIA

Symptom	Cause
Decreased production	Leukemia
	Lymphoma
	Multiple myeloma
	Metastatic cancer
	Chemotherapy
	Radiation therapy
	Drugs (thiazides, estrogen)
	Alcohol
Increased destruction of platelets	Autoimmune disorders
	Idiopathic thrombocytopenic as in purpura
	Malignant disorders
	Disseminated intravascular coagulation Infectious agents
Abnormal platelet function	Aspirin or ibuprofen qualitative dysfunction but not really thrombocytopenia
Decreased availability	Sequestration in spleen

spontaneous bleeding. Platelet transfusions can be from a random donor pooling or a single-donor human including those from a leukocyte antigen (HLA)–matched product. Upon exposure to an increasing number of platelet transfusions, the patient may become refractory to the benefits of the transfusion as a result of antibody formation to platelets. A person with fever usually has increased destruction of platelets. A 1- to 2-h posttransfusion platelet count is performed to document the effectiveness of the platelet transfusion. Reactions or complications of platelet transfusions are similar to those of whole-blood transfusions but also include a higher risk of reaction than transfusion of PRBCs secondary to the coadministration of plasma.

Nursing Intervention

Nursing interventions are based upon (1) protection of the patient from bleeding and associated complications and (2) early detection of bleeding. Most institutions have policies (bleeding precautions, platelet precautions) that are instituted when the platelet count is less than 50,000/mm³. A sign is placed near the patient to alert all health team members that the patient is at risk for bleeding. Key interventions include:

1. Bleeding precautions for a platelet count of less than 50,000/mm³
2. Assessment of sites of potential bleeding
   a. Skin
   b. Mucous membranes
   c. Indwelling catheter sites
3. Assessment of bodily excrement for occult and frank bleeding
   a. Urine
   b. Stool
   c. Sputum
   d. Pad count in menstruating women
4. Routine neurologic assessment
5. Prevention of trauma
   a. Use soft toothbrushes or toothettes for oral hygiene
   b. Use electric razors
   c. Coordinate blood sampling to avoid multiple venipunctures
   d. Institute bowel routine to prevent constipation
   e. Avoid intramuscular injections
   f. Avoid prolonged use of tourniquets
   g. Avoid use of urinary catheters, rectal tubes
   h. Use soft restraints only when absolutely necessary
   i. Use padded side rails when the patient is in bed
   j. Assist the patient with ambulation if indicated
   k. Institute measures to minimize vomiting
6. Avoid use of aspirin, aspirin-containing compounds, and ibuprofen
7. Control of temperature elevations
8. Monitor pertinent laboratory data
   a. Hemoglobin
   b. Hematocrit
   c. Platelet count
   d. Preplatelet and postplatelet transfusion counts

EDITORS' NOTE

It is unlikely that hemophilia and von Willebrand's disease will be on the PCCN exam. This section is included simply to provide a more complete description of abnormal coagulation concepts.

HEMOPHILIA AND VON WILLEBRAND'S DISEASE

Hemophilia is the name given to three inherited disorders that have bleeding in common. The bleeding is due to a lack of or deficiency in a plasma clotting factor. Von Willebrand's disease is included in this section since it also involves a deficient clotting factor.

Etiology

Hemophilias A and B are sex-linked recessive disorders. They affect men mainly but do occur rarely in women. It is more common that the woman is a "carrier" and genetically transmits these diseases to male offspring. Hemophilia C is an autosomal trait. Von Willebrand's disease has an autosomal dominant mode of inheritance, so it should occur equally among men and women. Von Willebrand's disease is an actual lack of factor VIII. A complete absence of this factor may occur, or there may be a reduced amount of structurally normal factor. Hemorrhaging may occur in a muscle mass, forming an extremely painful hematoma. These hematomas (masses) press against nerves, resulting in transient motor and/or sensory loss. Gastrointestinal bleeding is the next most common symptom, in which there is often no evidence of ulceration to account for the bleed. Epistaxis is also common.

Joint deformity with eventual crippling may occur. Hematuria is often present in hemophiliacs and may continue for weeks without a known cause.

Hemorrhage into the central nervous system (CNS) is rare in hemophiliacs but is extremely severe when it does occur. It is not uncommon for these patients to die secondary to hemorrhage into the CNS. This bleeding is often caused by trauma.

Hemophiliacs seem to fluctuate in the frequency and severity of the bleed during the year. They tend to bleed less with age. The reasons for these two variables are unknown at this time. All of these symptoms except hemarthrosis also occur in von Willebrand's disease.

Diagnosis

A familial tendency to excessive bleeding is usually known, and the family frequently reports the diagnosis as "the bleeding disease." The clinical condition can be verified by laboratory tests. The partial thromboplastin time (PTT) is prolonged. Factor assays reveal decreased factor VIII in hemophilia A and normal to decreased factor VII in von Willebrand's disease. Factor IX is decreased in hemophilia B. Platelet aggregation is normal in hemophilia but decreased in von Willebrand's disease.

Treatment

The goal of therapy is to prevent crippling deformities and prolong life expectancy. A cure is not available at this time. Stopping the bleed and increasing the plasma levels of the deficient factors will help prevent the degenerative stages of joint destruction.

In hemophilia A, cryoprecipitated antihemolytic factor (AHF) is administered to raise the factor to 25% of normal to allow coagulation. Surgery requires increasing the AHF to 50% of normal. If the AHF is not available, fresh frozen plasma or plasma fraction, rich in AHF, may be administered.

In hemophilia B, administration of fresh frozen plasma or of factor IX itself will increase the blood level of factor IX. In von Willebrand's disease, the infusion of cryoprecipitates or blood fractions rich in factor VIII and von Willebrand's factor (VWF) will shorten the bleeding time. Prior to surgery or in bleeding states, an intravenous infusion of cryoprecipitate or fresh frozen plasma is needed to raise the factor VIII level to 50% of normal.

A patient with hemophilia or von Willebrand's disease needs the care of a hematologist for surgical procedures and dental extraction.

Nursing Intervention

During hemophiliac bleeds, administration of the deficient clotting factor or plasma is ordered. AHF is effective for 48 to 72 h. This means that repeat transfusions may be required to stop the bleed.

Apply cold compresses to the injured area, raise the injured area if possible, and cleanse any wounds. Thrombin-soaked fibrin or sponge may be utilized for wound care in some institutions. Restrict activity for 48 h after the bleeding is controlled to prevent recurrence. Control pain with analgesics such as acetaminophen, propoxyphene hydrochloride, codeine, or meperidine. Avoid intramuscular injections to prevent a hematoma at the injection site. Aspirin and ibuprofen are contraindicated because they affect platelet aggregation. If the patient bleeds into a joint, immediately elevate the joint and immobilize it in a slightly flexed position. Watch for signs of further bleeding such as increased pain and swelling, fever, or possible shock-like symptoms. Monitor the patient's PTT.

In von Willebrand's disease, monitor the patient's bleeding time for 24 to 48 h after surgery and observe for signs of new bleeding. During a new bleed, elevate the injured part and apply cold compresses and gentle pressure to the bleeding site. Education as to the causative factors and treatment of minor injuries is indicated, as well as discussion of conditions for which the patient should seek medical attention.

Educate the patient and parents (if the patient is a child) in how to control minor trauma and warn against using aspirin or aspirin-containing drugs. Refer the parents to a genetic counseling service.

The National Hemophilia Society, local hemophilia groups, genetic evaluation, or psychotherapy may be useful for fostering better acceptance of the disease and forming an association with other patients who are managing successfully.

SICKLE CELL DISEASE

Sickle cell disease is an autosomal recessive disorder and life-long disease in which an abnormal Hb leads to chronic hemolytic anemia. Sickle cell disease is also referred to as sickle cell anemia because of the pathophysiology.

Pathophysiology

With an abnormal hemoglobin molecule known as hemoglobin S, the RBCs become insoluble when hypoxic. Because of this, RBCs become rigid, rough, and elongated. The hemoglobin becomes crescent or sickle shaped. Sickling decreases the cells' flexibility and results in a risk of various complications. The sickling occurs because of a mutation in the hemoglobin gene.

Sickling has a hemolyzing effect, and altered cells collect in the capillaries and small vessels. This impairs normal circulation and results in pain, swelling, tissue infarctions, and anoxia. Blood viscosity is, therefore, increased, causing further impairment of circulating blood. Blockages extend in the capillaries and small vessels, leading to further sickling obstruction. A vicious cycle is thus begun.

Etiology

Congenital hemolytic anemia occurs most often in African Americans and is due to genetic inheritance. The causative factor is a defect in the hemoglobin S molecule.

There is a homozygous and a heterozygous inheritance. Homozygous inheritance involves the substitution of the amino acid valine for glutamic acid in the beta-hemoglobin chain, resulting in the disease itself. In heterozygous inheritance, the patient carries the sickle cell trait but may be asymptomatic.

Clinical Presentation

Several types of crises occur, but common to all are the symptoms and physical findings of tachycardia, cardiomegaly, murmurs, pulmonary infarctions, chronic fatigue, dyspnea (with or without exertion), hematomegaly, jaundice or pallor, aching bones, chest pain, ischemic leg ulcers, and increased susceptibility to infection. Infection, stress, dehydration, and hypoxic states (e.g., strenuous exercise) may induce a crisis.

Sickle cell disease may lead to various acute and chronic complications, including vaso-occlusive crises which are caused by sickle-shaped RBCs that obstruct capillaries and restrict blood flow to an organ, resulting in ischemia, pain, and often organ damage.

The frequency, severity, and duration of these crises vary considerably. They do not usually develop for the first 5 years but then appear sporadically. They are due to the obstruction of blood vessels by rigid, tangled sickle cells. Tissue anoxia and possibly also necrosis occur, causing severe thoracic, abdominal, muscular, and bone pain. Jaundice may occur along with dark urine and a low-grade fever. After a crisis resolves, infection may occur within 4 days to several weeks secondary to occlusion and necrosis of the blood vessels.

Autosplenectomy occurs with long-standing disease. It is the process of splenic damage and scarring, inducing shrinkage of the spleen such that it is no longer palpable. After autosplenectomy, the patient is very susceptible to diplococcal pneumonia, which is rapidly fatal without immediate aggressive treatment. Lethargy, sleepiness, fever, and/or apathy occur as signs and symptoms of infection.

Aplastic (megaloblastic) crisis is a result of bone marrow suppression and is often associated with a viral infection. Signs and symptoms include fever, markedly decreased bone marrow activity, pallor, lethargy, dyspnea, possible coma, and RBC hemolysis.

Acute sequestration develops in some children aged 8 months to 2 years. There is a sudden, massive entrapment of RBCs in the liver and spleen. Symptoms of this rare crisis are lethargy and pallor. If not treated, it progresses to hypovolemic shock and death. This is the leading cause of death in sickle cell children younger than 1 year. (Following the first episode, splenectomy is usually performed.

Sequestration is often associated with aplastic crisis and parvovirus B19 infection.)

A hemolytic crisis is rare and is usually confined to those who have a glucose-6-phosphate dehydrogenase (G6PD) deficiency. This crisis usually occurs as an infectious response to complications of sickle cell disease rather than to the disease itself.

Diagnosis

A family history and the clinical picture point toward sickle cell disease. A blood smear shows sickle-celled RBCs rather than normal RBCs. Hemoglobin electrophoresis showing hemoglobin S is pathognomonic.

Treatment

There is no specific treatment for the primary disease; palliative measures are used to manage care. Painful crises are treated with hydration and analgesics; pain management requires opioid administration at regular intervals until the crisis has been resolved. For milder crises, a subgroup of patients may need nonsteroidal anti-inflammatory drugs (NSAIDs). For more severe crises, most patients require inpatient management for intravenous opioids. Oral hydroxyurea increases hemoglobin F concentration, thus preventing the formation of hemoglobin S polymers, and has been found to be an effective pharmacologic treatment to reduce pain events and the need for transfusions; it decreases thrombotic events/crisis and is often used for patients with a history of severe vaso-occlusive events and acute chest syndrome. Treatment of aplastic crisis includes transfusion of PRBCs, oxygen, and supportive therapies. In sequestration crisis, treatment includes whole-blood transfusion, oxygen, and large amounts of oral or intravenous fluids. Folic acid supplementation and transfusions may be used for aplastic or hemolytic crises. The use of pneumococcal vaccination can reduce the incidence of infections with pneumococci.

Nursing Intervention

Supportive care during exacerbations will help avoid such crises and provide a more normal life. Pain management is a key area of focus. During the crisis, apply warm compresses to painful areas and cover the child with a blanket. Avoid cold compresses since their use may result in vasoconstriction and prolong the crisis. Encourage bed rest and administer analgesics, antipyretics, and antibiotics as ordered.

Education of the patient and family will help avoid some crises. Such education would include avoidance of drinking large amounts of cold fluids, swimming in cold water, clothing that restricts circulation, and any activity that would produce hypoxia, such as flying in small (unpressurized) aircraft. A large fluid intake will prevent dehydration and decrease blood viscosity, reducing the chance of another crisis. Stress the importance of childhood immunizations and prompt treatment for infections.

IMMUNE SYSTEM

Cells of the Immune System

The ultimate effect of immunodeficiency is an impaired ability of the body to defend against foreign antigens. This leads to an increased susceptibility to infection and certain other diseases believed sometimes to be linked to an impaired immune status, such as cancer and autoimmune disorders. The incidence of infection, the most common complication of immunosuppression, increases with both the duration and the severity of the immunodeficiency. In fact, the highest risk of infection occurs when the leukocyte (white blood cell [WBC]) count is $<1000/mm^3$ and the neutrophils number $<500/mm^3$. The infections that develop are related to the underlying immune defect and the organisms to which the individual is now most susceptible. Most infections associated with immunosuppression are opportunistic or secondary to endogenous organisms that do not cause infection in the presence of a normally functioning immune system. However, many of the organisms colonizing a hospitalized patient are actually acquired during the hospitalization. Also, the infections that develop in immunosuppressed patients tend to be more severe, to be of longer duration, and to have a greater potential for dissemination than those seen in the general population. The lung is the most common site of serious infectious complications. Table 27-3 reviews common infections in the immunocompromised host.

IMMUNOSUPPRESSION

The immune system serves many functions, such as surveillance, homeostasis, and defense. Immunosuppression is an alteration in normal immune protective responses, a state of decreased responsiveness of the immune system. Immunosuppression can also occur as a result of injury, including surgery, shock, infection, and sepsis.

TABLE 27-3. COMMON INFECTIONS IN THE IMMUNOCOMPROMISED HOST

Site of Infection	Bacteria	Viruses	Fungi	Protozoa
Skin	Staphylococcus aureus Staphylococcus epidermidis	Herpes simplex virus Herpes zoster and varicella zoster viruses	Candida	
Oropharynx		Herpes simplex virus	Candida	
Gastrointestinal tract	Gram-negative rods	Herpes simplex virus (esophagitis)	Candida	Giardia lamblia
	Mycobacterium avium intracellulare	Cytomegalovirus		Cryptosporidium Entamoeba histolytica
Urinary tract	Gram-negative rods		Candida	
Lungs	Gram-negative rods Mycobacterium tuberculosis Mycobacterium avium-intracellulare	Cytomegalovirus	Candida Aspergillus, Mucor Histoplasma capsulatum	Pneumocystis carinii Toxoplasma gondii
CNS	Listeria monocytogenes	Herpes zoster and varicella zoster viruses	Cryptococcus neoformans	Toxoplasma gondii
	Streptococcus pneumoniae Pseudomonas aeruginosa Haemophilus influenzae	Herpes simplex virus	Aspergillus	
Blood	Gram-negative rods		Candida	

The individual who cannot mount an effective immune response is said to be anergic. Anergy can occur as a natural phenomenon in the life cycle, as in the very young and the elderly, or it can occur as a result of intentional and unintentional immunosuppression, as in organ transplantation and human immunodeficiency virus/acquired immunodeficiency syndrome (HIV/AIDS). Alterations in cell-mediated immunity can result from underlying disease (e.g., congenital defects in cell-mediated immunity, Hodgkin's disease, AIDS), or they may occur as a result of malignancies (such as acute leukemias) or antineoplastic or immunosuppressive treatment (e.g., treatment of lymphoma or transplant rejection).

Opportunistic Infections

Immunosuppressed individuals are vulnerable to opportunistic infections. Such infections are caused by organisms that are ubiquitous in the environment (internal and external) but rarely cause disease in the immunocompetent host. Patients with alterations in cell-mediated immunity are especially susceptible to infections caused by intracellular pathogens such as *Listeria monocytogenes, Mycobacterium* spp., *Cryptococcus neoformans,* and other fungi (such as *Aspergillus* and *Candida*), and herpesviruses (herpes simplex virus [HSV], cytomegalovirus [CMV]), as well as *Pneumocystis carinii.* Patients with humoral immune dysfunction (e.g., untreated multiple myeloma, patients who have undergone splenectomy) are susceptible to

infections caused by encapsulated organisms, particularly *Streptococcus pneumoniae* and *Haemophilus influenzae.* Natural protection from opportunistic infection depends on the presence of normal and intact innate and acquired immune mechanisms.

The three major determinants of nosocomial infection are the hospital environment, microorganisms, and host defense. Hospitalization and the acute care environment alone predispose an individual to an increased risk of infection. Hospitalization initiates the conversion of normal cutaneous flora to colonization of a new microbial population that is prevalent in the hospital. Colonization by itself is not harmful to the individual. However, when the first lines of defense are broken or bypassed, colonization opens the way to infection.

Some 50% of patients admitted to ICUs become colonized with Gram-negative bacteria within 72 h. The major vector of these bacteria is the human hand. Infection is more prevalent in teaching hospitals and on surgical services. The most frequent types of nosocomial infection are urinary tract infections, wound infections, respiratory infections, and septicemia, in that order.

Other factors that predispose acutely ill patients to infection include surgery, trauma, malnutrition, renal failure, liver failure, splenectomy, broad-spectrum antibiotic or corticosteroid therapy, and obesity.

Immunosuppressed individuals are usually neutropenic (see Chap. 25 for a discussion of the anatomy and physiology of neutrophils; see Chap. 26

TABLE 27-4. CAUSES OF DEATH IN NEUTROPENIC PATIENTS

Complication	Percentage (%) of Patients
Infection	35
Hemorrhage	27
Progression of disease	18
Other	20
Renal insufficiency	
Myocardial infarction	
Pulmonary edema	

for treatment). The longer the patient is neutropenic, the greater the chance for mortality (Table 27-4). In part, this is due to the fact that signs and symptoms of infection—redness, tenderness, swelling, and erythema—are often absent as a result of the lack of granulocytes. Patients with circulating granulocyte counts below 500 are especially susceptible to infections caused by Gram-negative bacilli (including *Pseudomonas aeruginosa*) and staphylococci. Sometimes, the only sign is fever. The immunosuppressed patient can be infected with bacteria, fungi, viruses, or a combination of these. Patients treated with corticosteroids are at significantly increased risk for bacterial, fungal, and *P. carinii* infections.

Nursing Care

Nursing care of the patient who is immunosuppressed is based on the nursing diagnosis of potential for infection related to specific and often multiple immunodeficiencies or a disruption in the natural protective barriers to microorganisms (Table 27-5). The patient requires frequent and thorough physical assessments because the signs and symptoms of infection are often subtle in the immunocompromised host. Important points regarding assessment and interventions are outlined below.

Assessment

1. History
    a. Age
    b. Past infections
    c. Medications, noting those that are immunosuppressive
    d. Treatment that can be immunosuppressive (e.g., radiation therapy)
    e. Presenting signs and symptoms
    f. Coexisting systemic symptoms (e.g., weight loss, malaise)
2. Physical examination
    a. Inspect skin carefully, particularly noting conditions of skin folds, pressure points, and perirectal area (frequent site of infection in the immunocompromised host). Observe for:
        i. Localized redness or swelling (may not be present with neutropenia or lymphopenia)
        ii. Excoriation
        iii. Rash suggestive of herpes simplex virus or herpes zoster
        iv. Lesions, infections, or Kaposi's sarcoma
        v. Lymphadenopathy
    b. Closely inspect the mouth and throat, a frequent site of infection in the immunocompromised host. Note:
        i. Condition of teeth and gums (if infected, can cause sepsis)
        ii. Lesions (candidiasis, herpes simplex, Kaposi's sarcoma)
    c. Monitor temperature and note pattern of elevation.
        i. An elevated temperature is the best indication of infection in the immunosuppressed.
        ii. A temperature over 38°C for 12 h or more is probably indicative of infection.
        iii. Fever is also part of the disease process of some disorders associated with immunosuppression (leukemia, lymphona, HIV infection).
    d. Assess central line and peripheral intravenous lines for signs of infection.
    e. Assess breath sounds.
        i. Adventitious sounds are frequently absent or minimal at the onset of infection in the immunosuppressed patient.
        ii. Note respiratory rate, presence of cough, and character of sputum.
        iii. Be prepared with oxygen support, as alterations in respiratory status can occur.
    f. Note complaints of tenderness and localized pain, as they may be indicators of infection.
        i. Back pain
        ii. Burning on urination
        iii. Rectal discomfort with bowel movements
3. Laboratory data
    a. WBC (leukopenia or leukocytosis)
        i. WBC differential
        ii. Absolute granulocyte count, especially if <500/mm^3
        iii. Lymphocyte count

TABLE 27-5. ETIOLOGY OF ACQUIRED IMMUNODEFICIENCY

Etiologic Condition	Immune Defect
Injury/Disease	
Burns	Disruption of natural barrier Impaired phagocytosis Deficient/delayed hypersensitivity
Uremia	Abnormal neutrophil function Impaired cell-mediated immunity
Diabetes mellitus Cancer	Impaired neutrophil function
Solid tumors	Deficiency in cell-mediated immunity Impaired neutrophil function
Leukemias	Deficiency in humoral and cell-mediated immunity
Hodgkin's disease	Impaired cellular immunity
Non-Hodgkin's lymphoma	Impaired humoral or cellular immunity (depends on type of lymphocyte involved)
Multiple myeloma	Impaired humoral immunity
AIDS	Impaired cell-mediated immunity with subsequent deficiency in humoral immunity
Certain infections (influenza, cytomegalovirus, Epstein-Barr virus, mononucleosis, tuberculosis, candidiasis)	Depression of lymphocyte and monocyte function
Treatment/Medication	
Surgery	Disruption of natural barriers Lymphopenia
Splenectomy	Impaired humoral immunity
Radiation therapy	Neutropenia Lymphopenia
Anesthetic agents	Inhibition of phagocytosis Impaired humoral and cell-mediated immunity
Cytotoxic drugs (cancer chemotherapy)	Disruption of natural barriers (mucositis) Neutropenia/lymphopenia Deficiencies in humoral and cell-mediated immunity
Steroids	Anti-inflammatory Suppressed functioning of neutrophils Deficiencies in humoral and cell-mediated immunity
Immunosuppressive agents (azathioprine, cyclosporine, tacrolimis, antilymphocyte globulin)	Impaired cell-mediated immunity
Certain antibiotics (pentamidine gentamicin, Septra)	Leukopenia Neutropenia
Miscellaneous	
Extremes of age	Deficiencies in humoral and cell-mediated immunity
Protein-calorie malnutrition	Impaired phagocytosis Deficiencies in humoral and cell-mediated immunity
Stress	Exact mechanism of immunodeficiency unknown

AIDS, acquired immunodeficiency syndrome.

b. T_4 count; T_4:T_8 ratio (indicators of immune status in patients with AIDS)

Interventions

1. Meticulous personal hygiene
   a. Prevent skin breakdown by turning the patient and using pressure-relieving devices.
   b. Avoid injury (will provide a port of entry for microorganisms), keep nails trim, use electric razor.
   c. Provide meticulous perirectal care.
      i. Avoid taking rectal temperatures and using rectal suppositories and enemas because of fragile rectal mucosa and

the possibility of causing a break in the mucosa.

ii. Initiate a bowel regimen to avoid constipation and/or control diarrhea.

2. Good oral hygiene
   a. Brush oral cavity, using a soft toothbrush or toothettes.
   b. Moisturize lips and mucosa with water-soluble lubricant.
   c. If stomatitis is present, rinse mouth with normal saline every 2 to 4 h.
   d. Avoid commercial mouthwashes.
   e. Advise patient to avoid smoking and use of alcohol.
   f. Encourage a soft bland diet and cool foods or provide nutritional support.
   g. Control pain.
      i. Viscous lidocaine.
      ii. Chlorhexidine gluconate mouth rinse to decrease colonization.
      iii. Mixture of sodium bicarbonate (5 mL), Maalox (5 mL), 2% viscous lidocaine (5 mL), and diphenhydramine (5 mL). Every 4 h, swish in mouth for 3 min and then swallow.
   h. Obtain order for appropriate antimicrobials if secondary infection is present.

3. Aseptic technique
   a. Minimize invasive procedures.
   b. Use smallest gauge lumens possible on all invasive devices.
   c. Provide meticulous care of vascular access.
   d. Coordinate blood studies.
   e. Keep all systems closed as much as possible.
   f. Avoid transparent, occlusive dressings over drainage wounds (the presence of WBCs collecting under the dressing is required to clean out the wound).

4. Manipulation of the environment to minimize exposure to organisms
   a. Eliminate sources of stagnant water (sources of Gram-negative bacteria).
      i. Change disposable tubing on ventilators daily.
      ii. Avoid cold-mist humidifiers.
   b. Remove live plants and flowers from the room (sources of *Aspergillus*).
   c. Institute protective isolation when the WBC count is less than 1000/mm^3 or the absolute granulocyte count is less than 500/mm^3.
   d. Restrict exposure to persons with infection.

   e. Evaluate the appropriateness of a low bacterial diet.
      i. Eliminate raw, unpeeled fruits and vegetables and uncooked eggs and meat from the diet.
      ii. Effectiveness in decreasing the incidence of infection is controversial.

5. Adequate nutrition
   a. Nutritional intake may be compromised by anorexia, fatigue, stomatitis, dysphagia, nausea and vomiting, and taste changes caused by some medications, including chemotherapy.
   b. Encourage a high-calorie, high-protein diet.
   c. Enteral feedings are preferable to parenteral nutrition because of decreased risk of infection.

6. Alleviation of stress
   a. Allow rest periods.
   b. Maintain day/night schedule as much as possible.
   c. Minimize environmental noise.
   d. Maximize comfort.
   e. Attend psychosocial needs.

DISORDERS OF THE IMMUNE SYSTEM

Acquired Immunodeficiency Syndrome

The acquired immunodeficiency syndrome is the endpoint of infection by HIV, a retrovirus found in the body fluids of infected individuals. The disease caused by HIV is a spectrum ranging from primary infection, with or without the acute syndrome, to the asymptomatic stage, to advanced disease. It is transmitted by sexual contact (either heterosexual or homosexual), exchange of bloods and body fluids, and perinatally. The profile of the high-risk groups affected by the disease to date include male homosexuals and bisexuals, intravenous drug users, hemophiliacs, blood transfusion recipients prior to 1985, and sexual partners of any of these individuals. In most developed countries, including the United States, there has been a gradual shift in that there is a greater total percentage of heterosexuals and intravenous drug users among new cases of AIDS than of homosexual individuals. HIV infection/AIDS is a global pandemic, with cases reported from almost every country.

Since recognition of the disease in 1981, much has been learned about the spectrum of HIV infection. Individuals who are infected may range from being asymptomatic to having systemic symptoms such as generalized persistent lymphadenopathy, fever, night sweats, diarrhea, and weight loss. AIDS itself is diagnosed when specific "indicator" diseases (i.e., diseases that indicate an underlying immunodeficiency) are present. Under most circumstances, the diagnosis also requires the person to be HIV seropositive. This is determined by enzyme-linked immunosorbent assay (ELISA) and Western blot laboratory tests, which screen for the antibody to HIV. The antibody develops an average of 6 to 12 weeks after exposure to the virus. The pattern of disease will vary from person to person. Some people experience rapid progression of the disease, whereas others are considered long-term survivors.

Clinical Presentation

The immunodeficiency of AIDS is multifaceted. HIV primarily infects the T_4 cell, and because of the rule of the T cell as the main coordinator of the immune response, devastating deficiencies occur in both the cell-mediated and humoral immune responses. The viral effects on the immune system include a profound lymphopenia and a reverse T_4:T_8 ratio (<1). As a result, the person with AIDS develops opportunistic infections. These infections tend to be severe and become disseminated, but they also tend to recur upon discontinuation of antimicrobial therapy. Most patients with AIDS die as a result of infection due to an organism normally protected against by T cells.

The establishment of a chronic, persistent infection is the hallmark of HIV disease. Some of the infections frequently seen with AIDS include cytomegalovirus retinitis, cryptococcal meningitis, toxoplasmosis, mycobacterial infections and, most commonly, *Pneumoncystis jiroveci* pneumonia (PCP). The onset of PCP is usually insidious, characterized by a gradually increasing shortness of breath, dry cough, fever, and—on chest radiography—pulmonary infiltrates. The respiratory status of a patient with PCP can deteriorate rapidly, necessitating admission to a critical care unit. Hypoxemia and dyspnea may require ventilatory support. Drug therapy usually includes administration of a 21-day course of intravenous pentamidine or trimethoprim/sulfamethoxazole. Occasionally, high-dose steroids are given. In many patients, it may take 7 to 10 days for a clinical response

to be seen. It is not unusual for a relapse of PCP to occur; when it does, it is often fulminant in nature and associated with a mortality rate of approximately 40%. For this reason, patients are commonly started on prophylactic therapy, which may consist of maintenance doses of oral trimethoprim/sulfamethoxazole or aerosolized pentamidine.

Secondary cancers, namely Kaposi's sarcoma and non-Hodgkin's lymphoma (NHL), can also occur in association with AIDS. Kaposi's sarcoma, which arises from the endothelium of either lymphatic or blood vessels, is characterized by skin and mucosal lesions ranging in color from dark red or purple to nearly black. The lesions also tend to develop in the oropharynx, lymph nodes, gastrointestinal (GI) tract, lungs, and skin. NHL is typically high grade, of B-cell origin, and present in extranodal sites. In approximately 20% of those with NHL, the cancer presents as a primary lymphoma of the brain—a very rare occurrence in the general population. Generally, the AIDS-related malignancies are much more aggressive and respond more poorly to therapy than the same cancers in the general population.

Neuropsychiatric manifestations accompany AIDS in over 60% of patients, and in some cases are diagnostic of the disease. The most common disorder of this type is AIDS dementia complex, a subcortical dementia manifested by changes in cognition, behavior, and motor functioning. Symptoms initially include memory loss, difficulty in concentrating, and lethargy; these may progress to withdrawal, aphasia, ataxia, paresis, and seizures. The condition is secondary to HIV infiltration of the brain. The virus is known to infect macrophages, which themselves are not destroyed by the virus but serve to transport HIV across the blood-brain barrier.

Also identified as part of the clinical picture associated with AIDS is the HIV wasting syndrome. This is defined as loss of over 10% of the usual body weight, accompanied by diarrhea, weakness, or fever of a chronic nature. Multiple factors may contribute to development of the syndrome, including difficulty in maintaining adequate nutrition. However, like the cachexia seen with cancer, muscle wasting seems to exceed what would be expected.

Treatment

Treatment is aimed at the secondary diseases that develop with AIDS. Systemic NHL, usually widely disseminated at the time of diagnosis, necessitates treatment with an intensive chemotherapy regimen that is fairly toxic and usually poorly tolerated by the patient with AIDS. Primary lymphoma of the brain usually has a good initial response to cranial radiation, but relapse soon occurs, generally within the CNS. Therapy for Kaposi's sarcoma, commonly initiated when the patient develops pain or lymphatic obstruction or when the lesions are cosmetically disturbing, is palliative and consists of chemotherapy and/or radiation. These cancer therapies, particularly chemotherapy, induce myelosuppression and compound the already existing immunodeficiencies of AIDS, making the patient even more susceptible to the development of infection (see Chap. 26 for specific medication treatment).

Nursing Intervention

In addition to requiring nursing care relevant to immunosuppression, patients with AIDS, especially those with PCP, require aggressive pulmonary care and close monitoring of arterial blood gases. Decisions regarding intubation and ventilation should be made prior to severe respiratory dysfunction. As cognitive impairment can occur secondary to hypoxemia, AIDS dementia, opportunistic infection, or CNS malignancy, a close assessment of mental status is required in order to detect any changes from baseline. If impaired concentration and memory are noted, it is necessary to give the patient simple explanations and directions and to provide a safe environment. Nutritional support must also be addressed. If diarrhea is present—a common problem due to either HIV enteropathy or opportunistic infection—enteral feedings may not be possible. As is evident, the patient with AIDS presents an array of problems with complex etiologies requiring advanced nursing skills in assessment and symptom management.

Leukemias

Leukemias are a group of malignancies that occur when immature WBCs proliferate uncontrollably and accumulate in the bone marrow and peripheral blood. Leukemias are classified according to the type of cell that is predominant and whether the disease is acute or chronic. The four general categories of leukemia are acute lymphocytic or lymphoblastic (ALL), acute nonlymphocytic or myelogenous (ANLL or AML), chronic lymphocytic (CLL), and chronic myelogenous (CML).

The accumulation of leukemic cells, which do not function normally, impedes the adequate production of normal RBCs, WBCs, and platelets. This, along with infiltration of other organs by the

TABLE 27-6. MANIFESTATIONS OF LEUKEMIA

Rationale	Signs and Symptoms
Bone marrow failure	Anemia
	Thrombocytopenia
	Leukocytosis (primarily blast cells)
	Granulocytopenia (if ALL, CLL)
	Lymphopenia (if ALL, CML)
Organ infiltration	Bone pain
	Lymphadenopathy
	Splenomegaly
	Hepatomegaly
	Testicular mass or swelling
	Headache, nausea, vomiting (CNS involvement)
Hyperleukocytosis	Stroke
	Adult respiratory distress syndrome
	Splenic infarction
Hypercatabolism and rapid cell turnover (tumor lysis syndrome)	Disseminated intravascular coagulation
	Hyperuricemia
	Hyperkalemia
	Hypocalcemia
	Weight loss

ALL, acute lymphocytic or lymphoblastic leukemia; CLL, chronic lymphocytic leukemia; CNS, central nervous system.

leukemic cells, underlies the clinical presentation of leukemia. Table 27-6 presents a summary of the signs and symptoms.

Complications

The patient with leukemia requires an acute care setting when complications, due to either the disease or its treatment, arise. Both the disease itself and the intensive chemotherapy used to treat it are associated with severe and often prolonged myelosuppression. The total WBC count may be less than $100/mm^3$ for a period of a week or more after high-dose chemotherapy. As a result, infection is the major cause of morbidity and mortality in the patient with leukemia. Common pathogens causing infection in immunocompromised patients are Gram-negative bacteria (*Escherichia coli, Klebsiella, Pseudomonas*) and fungi (*Candida, Aspergillus*). Frequent presentations include cellulitis, pneumonia, and perirectal infections. Sepsis is common and must be treated immediately and aggressively.

Also contributing to the likelihood of infection is the disruption that can occur in the natural barriers of the skin and mucous membranes, allowing easy entry to microorganisms. The chemotherapy, depending on the drugs and the doses, can cause severe stomatitis and mucositis. In patients who have received bone marrow from a donor, graft-versus-host disease

(GVHD) can occur as the transplanted marrow recognizes the host tissue as foreign. One of the tissues that the engrafted T cells attempt to reject is the skin. In acute GVHD, this usually starts as a rash and may progress to desquamation. The treatment for GVHD includes immunosuppressive drugs; thus, compounding the already existing immunodeficiencies. Target tissues for acute GVHD are skin, liver, GI tract, and immune system.

Another reason for admission of a leukemia patient to the progressive care unit is bleeding. This phenomenon occurs secondary to thrombocytopenia induced by the disease process and/or the chemotherapy. It is not unusual for the platelet count to be <20,000/mm^3, which puts the patient at risk for spontaneous bleeding. Of particular concern is the possibility of a pulmonary or intracranial hemorrhage. Because of the multiple platelet transfusions required, single-donor leukocyte-poor products are administered

Bleeding may also be seen in association with disseminated intravascular coagulation (DIC), a complication of leukemia, especially progranulocytic leukemia, a subtype of AML. It is caused by the release of tissue thromboplastin from tumor cells. The clotting cascade is triggered, leading to accelerated coagulation and the formation of excessive thrombin. With the ongoing coagulation, the fibrinolytic system is activated. Thus, clotting and bleeding continue until the cycle is interrupted by treatment of the cause. Besides hemorrhage, organ dysfunction can occur as a result of thromboemboli. Chemotherapy should be initiated immediately; however, initiation of chemotherapy can potentially exacerbate DIC owing to the destruction of promyelocytes. Heparin, although its use is controversial with other etiologies of DIC, has been found to be an effective supportive therapy in acute progranulocytic leukemia. Newer therapies for acute promyelocytic leukemia (APL), a subtype of AML, include the use of *all*-transretinoic acid (ATRA). This is a form of "differentiation therapy" as ATRA activates a retinoid receptor and causes promyelocytes to differentiate (to mature), which deters them from proliferating. There is a differentiation syndrome associated with ATRA (and arsenic used for relapsed APL) which consists of leukocytosis fever, weight gain, edema, pulmonary infiltrates, pleural and pericardial effusions, hypotension, and renal dysfunction. Treatment should be initiated with dexamethasone 10 mg q 12 h.

Leukostasis can also be life threatening. Leukostasis can occur with a WBC count of >100,000/mm^3, consisting mostly of blasts. Leukemia blasts plug capillaries, causing rupture, bleeding, and organ dysfunction. Intracerebral hemorrhage is the most common and most lethal complication. Management includes the administration of fluids and allopurinol or rasburicase to counteract the hyperuricemia associated with cell lysis. Appropriate chemotherapy must be initiated. As an emergency measure, leukapheresis may be necessary.

Treatment

A first step in treatment of the acute leukemias is to obtain complete remission, which is defined as normal peripheral blood with resolution of cytopenias, normal bone marrow with no excess blasts, and normal clinical status. The acute leukemias require immediate treatment with chemotherapy, and the type of initial chemotherapy depends on the subtype of leukemia. Treatment is approached in three phases. The initial phase, called induction therapy, consists of a combination of chemotherapeutic drugs given in high doses in order to achieve remission. Complete remission occurs when the number of leukemic cells is below detection, hematopoiesis is restored, and signs and symptoms of the disease are no longer present. However, because leukemic cells remain, even though they are microscopically undetectable, a consolidation phase of therapy is necessary to further decrease or eliminate these cells. This cycle of chemotherapy, also very intensive, is usually administered 6 to 8 weeks after induction. The third phase, maintenance therapy, involves the administration of moderate doses of chemotherapy over a prolonged time. It is given with the intent of maintaining remission, but its effectiveness is controversial (not indicated with AML but is used with ALL).

By comparison, chronic leukemia is treated with oral chemotherapeutic agents, which are associated with much less toxicity. More aggressive therapy may be initiated as the disease progresses, particularly in patients with CML who undergo an end-stage blast crisis, which resembles an acute leukemia. Patients with CLL are often treated with intravenous chemotherapy, which can increase the risk of infection.

The rate of relapse—that is, the recurrence of detectable leukemic cells either in the bone marrow, peripheral blood, or extramedullary sites—varies with the type of leukemia. However, once relapse occurs, it is more difficult to induce a second remission. One treatment alternative that is available to patients with ALL, ANLL, and CML who meet specific criteria is bone marrow transplantation. This involves the administration of dosages of chemotherapy and radiation therapy that, although ablative to the bone marrow, are also more cytotoxic to cancer cells. Prior to the cytotoxic therapy, bone marrow cells are harvested from the patient or a matched donor. If the patient is to receive his or her own marrow, special techniques are used in an attempt to completely eliminate all leukemic cells before infusion. The bone marrow is reinfused at the time the blood counts reach their lowest point. Engraftment of the bone marrow and functional immune recovery takes approximately 4 weeks, but patients often remain immunosuppressed for a period of 1 year or more.

Nursing Intervention

In the patient with leukemia, nursing care centers on monitoring for potential infection and injury (bleeding). In addition to the assessments previously reviewed, assessment of neurologic status is important because of the possibility of CNS complications, including intracranial bleeding or stroke. Fluid and electrolyte balance must also be carefully monitored because of the large volume of fluids given and the possibility of tumor lysis syndrome or septic shock. Multisystem failure can occur secondary to leukemic infiltration, leukostasis, DIC, sepsis, or the toxicity of cancer chemotherapy. In addition to the continual assessments, the nurse will administer the extensive supportive therapy required, including multiple antibiotics, blood and blood product transfusions, and usually total parenteral nutrition. Nursing care of the patient with leukemia is a challenge, particularly in terms of protecting the patient from infection amid all of the acute care interventions.

Other Malignancies Associated with Immunodeficiency

Lymphomas

The term *lymphoma* encompasses a group of cancers that affect the cells that play a role in the immune system, and primarily represents cells involved in the lymphatic system of the body. Lymphomas, in which the malignant cell is either a lymphocytes B or T cell or their subtypes, are broadly classified in one of two major categories: Hodgkin's lymphoma ([HL], previously called Hodgkin's disease) and all other lymphomas (non-Hodgkin's lymphomas [NHLs]). These two types occur in the same places,

may be associated with the same symptoms, and often have similar gross physical characteristics. However, they are readily discriminated via microscopic examination.

Hodgkin's lymphoma develops from a specific abnormal B lymphocyte lineage. NHLs may derive from either abnormal B or T cells and are distinguished by unique genetic markers.

There are five subtypes of HL and about 30 subtypes of NHL. Although similar in many respects, the distinguishing feature of HL is the presence of Reed-Sternberg cells, whose origin and nature are uncertain. The incidence of HL peaks during the second and third decades and again after 60 years of age. NHL occurs primarily in older individuals and is four times more common than HL. The World Health Organization's Classification of Lymphoid Malignancies further divides lymphoid malignancies into B- and T-cell neoplasms based on morphologic, clinical, immunologic, and genetic information.

Lymphoma is the most common type of blood cancer in the United States. It is the sixth most common cancer in adults and the third most common in children. NHL is far more common than HL. Lymphoma can occur at any age, including childhood. HL is most common in two age groups: young adults aged 16 to 34 years and in older adults aged 55 years and older. NHL is more likely to occur in older persons.

The pathology of lymphomas is the transformation of the lymphocyte into a malignant cell at some stage of its development, which accounts for the different histologic subtypes of both HL and NHL. What triggers this transformation is unknown, although there is evidence linking HL to a viral etiology (Epstein-Barr virus [EBV]), particularly when it occurs in the young. In the case of NHL, there is a strong association with a preexisting immunodeficiency. Regardless of the histology, the lymphocytes proliferate uncontrollably and invade body organs, although the degree of aggressiveness varies.

The disease usually presents as one or more enlarged lymph nodes, usually in the cervical region (cervical region predisposition is normally seen in HL). Occasionally, the initial site of disease is the gastrointestinal tract. Approximately one-third of patients also exhibit systemic symptoms consisting of fever, night sweats, and loss of over 10% of the usual body weight. Staging procedures are done to determine the extent of disease, as this has implications for treatment. Hodgkin's lymphoma tends to spread from one lymph node group to an adjacent group, whereas NHL tends to skip to non-contiguous groups. The workup must determine the involvement, if any, of lymph node groups, the bone marrow, liver, and spleen. Sometimes an exploratory laparotomy may be necessary, especially with HL.

The "staging," or evaluation of extent of disease, for both HL and NHL, are similar.

- Stage I (early disease)—Lymphoma located in a single lymph node region or in one area or organ outside the lymph node
- Stage II (locally advanced disease)—Lymphoma located in two or more lymph node regions all located on the same side of the diaphragm or in one lymph node region and a nearby tissue or organ. (The diaphragm is a flat muscle that separates the chest from the abdomen.)
- Stage III (advanced disease)—Lymphoma affecting two or more lymph node regions, or one lymph node region and one organ, on opposite sides of the diaphragm
- Stage IV (widespread or disseminated disease)—Lymphoma outside the lymph nodes and spleen that has spread to another area or organ such as the bone marrow, bone, or central nervous system

Both HL and NHL are further classified with letters.

- An "A" or "B" designation indicates whether the person with lymphoma had symptoms such as fevers, night sweats, and/or weight loss at the time of diagnosis. "A" indicates no such symptoms, and "B" indicates symptoms.
- An "E" designation indicates that the tumor spread directly from a lymph node into an organ or that a single organ outside the lymphatic system is affected with no apparent lymphatic involvement.

Treatment for lymphoma depends on the type and stage. If the lymphoma is localized, radiation therapy is initiated and is usually given with or after chemotherapy to disease sites. In HL, this consists of total nodal irradiation and radiation to the spleen (if not removed at laparotomy). For early-stage disease, radiation is given with curative intent, although it is generally more effective in HL than in NHL. Chemotherapy is given for more widespread systemic disease, and sometimes, in the case of NHL, is recommended as the treatment of choice for localized disease. Both chemotherapy and radiation therapy, if given to areas of major bone marrow activity, are myelosuppressive. Another side effect that is sometimes associated with the chemotherapeutic treatment of NHL is tumor lysis syndrome.

Cure is expected in over 50% of patients with lymphoma. However, if the disease recurs, therapy is more poorly tolerated because of the depressed bone marrow reserve as a result of the initial therapy. Potential complications representing oncologic emergencies that can occur with progressive disease are superior vena cava syndrome, tumor lysis syndrome, and spinal cord compression. In superior vena cava syndrome, the vena cava is obstructed by tumor or enlarged nodes. The impaired venous drainage causes cough, dyspnea, neck vein distention, and facial, trunk, and arm edema. Immediate treatment with radiation is required to relieve pressure on the superior vena cava. The other complication treated on an emergency basis is spinal cord compression, usually due to lymph node extension into the epidural space. Paraplegia can result if treatment is not initiated with radiation therapy or, if the neurologic deterioration is rapid, a decompression laminectomy.

Multiple Myeloma

Multiple myeloma is a relatively uncommon malignancy of the plasma cell, the antibody-producing form of the B cell. A disease of older adults (median age at presentation is 65 years), multiple myeloma is

TABLE 27-7. CLINICAL MANIFESTATIONS OF MULTIPLE MYELOMA

Rationale	Signs and Symptoms
Bone marrow involvement by plasmacytomas (plasma leukopenia cell tumors)	Anemia (common) Thrombocytopenia
Skeletal involvement by plasmacytomas and tumor activation of osteoclasts	Bone pain Osteolytic lesions
Pathologic fractures	Hypercalcemia
Production of light chains called Bence-Jones protein (part of immunoglobulin)	Proteinuria Renal insufficiency due to tubular damage
Hyperviscosity	Occlusion of small vessels Headache Mental status changes Visual disturbances Retinal hemorrhage Intermittent claudication
Hypervolemia	Congestive heart failure

a malignancy of plasma cells characterized by replacement of the bone marrow, bone destruction, and paraprotein formation. In this disease, excessive amounts of a single type of immunoglobulin are produced. Table 27-7 lists the clinical manifestations of myeloma. The disease, commonly advanced at the time of diagnosis, is treated palliatively. Most commonly patients require treatment because of bone pain or other symptoms related to the disease. Renal dysfunction and failure is common. The treatment of myeloma is rapidly changing. Although combination chemotherapy has frequently been used, nonchemotherapeutic options with new and investigative agents are being tested. Autologous stem cell transplantation can be used for management after the initial disease has been controlled. Clinical trials employing combination therapy of new biologic agents are also under way. Although the disease is not curable, most patients survive for many years.

28

Organ Transplantation

EDITORS' NOTE

Organ transplantation is not included in the PCCN exam, but the content is provided here for supplemental information to provide a comprehensive overview of acute care conditions.

Organ transplantation is the established treatment for the failure of vital organs such as the kidneys, pancreas, liver, heart, or lung. Kidneys are the most common type of organ transplant. Organ transplantations can be divided into three categories based on the similarity between the donor and the recipient: autotransplants, which involve the transfer of tissue or organs from one part of an individual to another part of the same individual; allotransplants, which involve the transfer from one individual to another individual; and xenotransplants, which involve transfers across species. Autotransplants are the most common type of transplants and include skin grafts, vein grafts for bypasses, bone and cartilage transplants, and nerve transplants. No immunosuppression is required for autotransplants, as the donor and the recipient are the same. Allotransplants are performed for most solid-organ transplantations. Immunosuppression is required for allograft recipients in order to prevent rejection. The most common organ transplants in the United States are heart, lung, liver, kidney, and pancreas. Table 28-1 presents a historical overview of transplantation. Because the posttransplant course is difficult, only those candidates who meet strict requirements are offered transplants.

Kidney transplants can come from a cadaver or a living related donor. In most cases, the native kidneys are left in place and the donor kidney is implanted into either iliac fossa. Finally, the urinary tract is reconstructed. Urine is produced almost immediately.

Heart transplants are among the most common of all organ transplants. Orthotopic transplantation is the most common. Table 28-2 presents a summary of graft terminology. Heart transplantation requires the patient to be placed on cardiopulmonary bypass.

The donor heart is implanted by anastomosis of the left and right atria. After the surgical procedure, the patient is weaned off cardiopulmonary bypass.

Liver transplants are indicated for individuals with end-stage liver disease. In these transplants, which are also orthotopic, time is valuable because of the poor viability of the transplanted organ. Correct matching in terms of size is also important because a liver that is too large will compress the diaphragm and cause pulmonary complications. Anastomosis of the new liver involves the hepatic artery, inferior and superior venae cavae, the portal vein, and the biliary tract.

Pancreas transplantation offers normoglycemic states in type I diabetic patients. In pancreas transplantation, the native pancreas is left in place. The transplanted pancreas consists of a pancreatic segment (tail or body) or the whole pancreas. The donor pancreas is often placed in the right iliac fossa, and venous drainage is anastomosed into the common iliac vein and arterial blood supply comes from the common iliac artery. The exocrine duct is connected to the bladder for urinary excretion of pancreatic enzymes. Finally, pancreatic rejection is very difficult to detect, but much research is being done to improve detection.

TABLE 28-1. HISTORICAL OVERVIEW OF TRANSPLANTATION

1905	Development of vascular suture techniques
1933	First kidney transplant attempted
1954	First successful kidney transplant
1960	Development of tissue typing
1962	Azathioprine used as single immunosuppressive agent
1963	First liver transplant attempted
1963	Steroids with azathioprine found to have synergistic effects
1966	First segmental pancreas transplant attempted
1967	First successful liver transplant
1967	First successful orthotopic heart transplant
1968	First human heart-lung transplant attempted
1970	Cyclophosphamide tried as a substitute for azathioprine
1974	First clinical heterotopic heart transplant
1978	Clinical trials of cyclosporine initiated
1982	First successful heart-lung transplant
1983	Cyclosporine approved by the FDA
1983	Clinical trials of OKT3 (muromonab-CD3) initiated
1987	OKT3 approved by the FDA
1989	Clinical trials of FK-506 (tacrolimus) initiated
1990	Clinical trials of RS-61443 (mycophenolate) initiated

FDA, Food and Drug Administration.

In addition to the individual transplants discussed, heart-lung and kidney-pancreas transplants are also performed. The kidney-pancreas transplant success rate is nearly 90%. This success is due in part to careful nursing care.

All allotransplantations are at risk for graft rejection, which is triggered when specific cells of the transplant recipient, namely, T and B lymphocytes, recognize foreign antigens. The main antigens

TABLE 28-2. GRAFT TERMINOLOGY

Nomenclature	Definition
Autograft	A transplant of an organ taken from the recipient
Isograft	A transplant of an organ taken from a genetically identical donor
Allograft	A transplant of an organ from a genetically different donor of the same species
Xenograft	A transplant of an organ from a donor of a different species
Heterotopic transplant	A donor organ grafted into an ectopic position on the recipient's native organ, which is left in place
Orthotopic transplant	A donor organ placed at the site from which the recipient's native organ has been removed, with near normal anatomic reconstruction

involved in triggering rejection are coded for by a group of genes known as the major histocompatibility complex (MHC). These antigens define the "foreign" nature of one individual to another within the same species. In humans, the MHC complex is known as the human leukocyte antigen (HLA) system. The function of the HLA system in the nontransplant setting is to present antigens as fragments of foreign proteins that can be recognized by T lymphocytes. In the transplant setting, HLA molecules can initiate graft rejection through either humoral or cellular mechanisms. Humoral rejection occurs if the recipient has circulating antibodies specific to the donor's HLA from prior exposure (i.e., blood transfusion, previous transplant, or pregnancy) or if after transplantation, the recipient develops antibodies specific to the donor's HLA. The antibodies then bind to the donor's recognized foreign antigens, activating the complement cascade and leading to cell lysis. The blood group antigens of the ABO system, though not part of the HLA system, may also trigger this form of humoral rejection.

Cellular rejection is the more common type of rejection after organ transplants. Mediated by T lymphocytes, it results from their activation and proliferation after exposure to donor MHC molecules.

Graft rejection can be classified into four types: hyperacute (occurring within minutes after the transplanted organ is reperfused and due to the presence of preformed antibodies), accelerated (seen within the first few days after transplantation and involving both cellular and antibody-mediated injury), acute (seen within days to a few months after transplantation and predominantly a cell-mediated process), and chronic (occurring months to years after transplantation and due to immune and nonimmune responses). The incidence of acute graft rejection has declined due to advances in immunosuppressive therapy, yet chronic rejection is an increasingly common problem.

A knowledge base of immunosuppressive therapy and the response of the patient are helpful in providing nursing care. Table 28-3 outlines options for immunosuppression after transplantation, which have broadened significantly, involving a variety of drug combinations and protocols. All transplant recipients must take immunosuppressive medications to try to prevent rejection of their new organ. Immunosuppressive agents are usually used in combination therapy rather than as monotherapy. Two types of immunosuppression are recognized: *induction immunosuppression,* which is the administration of agents immediately after transplantation to

TABLE 28-3. IMMUNOSUPPRESSIVE AGENTS BY CLASSIFICATION

Immunophilin binders
    Calcineurin inhibitors
        Cyclosporine
        Tacrolimus (FK-506)
    Noninhibitors of calcineurin
        Sirolimus (rapamycin)
Antimetabolites
    Inhibitors of de novo purine synthesis
        Azathioprine
        MMF
    Inhibitors of de novo pyrimidine synthesis
        Leflunomide
Biologic immunosuppression
    Polyclonal antibodies
        ATGAM
        Antithymocyte Globulin rabbit (thymoglobulin)
    Monoclonal antibodies
        OKT3
        Daclizumab (IL-2R)
Others
    Deoxyspergualin
    Corticosteroids

ATGAM, antithymocyte gamma globulin; IL-2R, interleukin-2 receptor; MMF, mycophenolate mofetil; OKT3, anti-CD3 monoclonal antibody.

induce immunosuppression, and *maintenance immuno-suppression*, which involves the administration of agents to maintain immunosuppression once recipients have recovered from the surgical procedure. Common agents used for immunosuppression therapy include corticosteroids, azathioprine, cyclosporine, and tacrolimus (FK-506), among others, and a number of biologic agents including polyclonal and monoclonal antibodies.

Corticosteroids were the first immunosuppressive agents used in solid-organ transplants. Even today, low-dose prednisone remains a cornerstone of immunosuppressive therapy. These immunosuppressive drugs act to suppress antibody and complement binding as well as to reduce the synthesis of important immunomodulating cytokines. Side effects include hypertension, glucose intolerance, hyperlipidemia, and weight gain. Although steroids remain an integral part of most immunosuppressive protocols and are often the first-line agents in the treatment of acute rejection, concerns about side effects has contributed to a shift in withdrawing steroids from long-term maintenance protocols.

Antimetabolites such as azathioprine or mycophenolate are key in antirejection therapy. Azathioprine's immunosuppressive effects come from its inhibitory effects on the proliferation of T lymphocytes. A decrease in immunoglobulin antibody synthesis also

reduces antigen recognition. Side effects include myelosuppression, leukopenia, thrombocytopenia, and anemia. Hepatotoxicity has been reported in several cases. Azathioprine is used as an adjunctive component of immunosuppressive drug regimens.

Mycophenolate inhibits both T and B lymphocytes dependent pathways for proliferation. Mycophenolate is an inhibitor of inosine monophosphate dehydrogenase (IMPDH) which inhibits de novo guanosine nucleotide synthesis. Adverse effects associated with this drug include headache, gastrointestinal distress, hypertension, infections, and lipid and glucose abnormalities.

Cyclosporine is a cyclic endecapeptide with immunosuppressive activity. It primarily affects the T-cell immune response by blocking the production of interleukin-2 (IL-2). This drug has significantly reduced solid-organ rejection. Side effects include nephrotoxicity, hypertension, glucose intolerance, hyperkalemia, neurotoxicity, and hyperlipidemia. Careful monitoring of cyclosporine drug levels can help to reduce some of the side effects.

Tacrolimus (FK-506) is a macrolide that inhibits T-cell function by preventing the synthesis of IL-2 and other important cytokines. Tacrolimus has a very similar mechanism of action as cyclosporine but is 100 times more potent. Commonly reported side effects include nausea, vomiting, insomnia, tremors, and hyperesthesias of the feet. It also causes nephrotoxicity and hyperkalemia. Because of its lower incidence of adverse effects compared to cyclosporine, tacrolimus has supplanted the use of cyclosporine in many transplant centers.

Since the 1960s, polyclonal antibodies have been used in transplantation to reduce the number and function of lymphocytes in order to prevent rejection and to treat acute rejection episodes. Monoclonal antibodies (such as OKT3) are used to target specific subsets of cells to work at different stages of the immune response. A number of different monoclonal antibodies (MABs) are currently under development or have recently been approved for use in clinical transplantation.

OKT3 was the first MAB approved for use in organ transplantation. Early studies proved OKT3 to be successful in steroid-resistant rejection in kidney transplants. Further studies have shown similar success in the transplantation of the heart, lung, liver, and pancreas. Commonly, OKT3 is used to treat episodes of severe acute rejection. It binds to the CD3 receptor on T lymphocytes, causing an inactivation of CD3 cells. Side effects reported are fever, chills, nausea, vomiting, pulmonary edema, and hypotension. Anti-OKT3 antibodies have been noted in some patients.

Two MABs—basiliximab and dacluzimab—are currently approved for targeting of the IL-2 receptor in order to reduce the proliferation of cytotoxic T cells. Alemtuzumab, an MAB directed against the CD52 antigen found on B and T cells, has been used more recently, usually as an induction agent. Additional MABs are currently under development; their testing and future use will provide additional agents for posttransplant immunosuppression therapy.

29

Life-Threatening Coagulopathies

EDITORS' NOTE

Hematology and immunology comprise approximately 2% (two to four questions) of the PCCN exam. The exam is likely to focus on life-threatening coagulopathies, so expect one to three questions on this content.

DISSEMINATED INTRAVASCULAR COAGULATION

Disseminated intravascular coagulation (DIC) is a state of hypercoagulability which is triggered by activation of the clotting cascade with resultant generation of excess thrombin, deposition of fibrin in the microcirculation, and activation of the fibrinolytic system. It is not a specific disease but rather an acquired disorder that occurs in a wide variety of clinical disorders. Although many diseases can be complicated by DIC, it is most frequently associated with massive trauma, infection, sepsis, metastatic malignancy, and obstetric syndromes (abruptio placentae, amniotic fluid embolism, retained fetus, second-trimester abortion).

Pathophysiology

Regardless of the cause, specific pathophysiologic signs occur in DIC. The common denominator is the release of procoagulants into the circulatory system. Free hemoglobin, cancer tissue fragments, amniotic fluid, and bacterial toxins are some of the procoagulants that may activate the clotting cascade. Activation of the cascade results in diffuse intravascular fibrin formation. Fibrin is then deposited in the microcirculation.

With the clotting of the capillaries, blood is shunted to the arteriovenous anastomoses. This shunting causes the capillary tissue to use anaerobic metabolism. With the production of lactic and pyruvic waste products and blood stagnation in the microcirculation, acidemia develops.

Three procoagulant factors develop in capillary blood as a result of the DIC disease process. Acidosis acts as a strong procoagulant along with the "normal" procoagulants in the blood. The third factor is the concentration of procoagulants, which increases secondary to the stagnation of blood. All of these processes result in massive sequestration of clotted blood in the capillaries (Fig. 29-1).

DIC develops rapidly, so that coagulating factors are depleted in the microcirculation faster than the clotting factors can be replenished. Without circulating coagulant factors, hemostasis cannot be maintained (Fig. 29-2) and the patient begins to bleed.

Etiology

Many factors may precipitate DIC, including multiple trauma, crush injuries, hemorrhagic shock, malignant hypertension, incompatible blood transfusion, any and all cancers, burns, and coronary bypass surgery. Disseminated intravascular coagulation does not occur in isolation; it is always a sequela to some initiating event. All the major physiologic anticoagulants including antithrombin III, protein C, and tissue factor pathway inhibitor appear to be affected in DIC. The systemic formation of fibrin results from increased generation of thrombin and the simultaneous suppression of anticoagulation and delayed removal of fibrin due to impaired fibrinolysis.

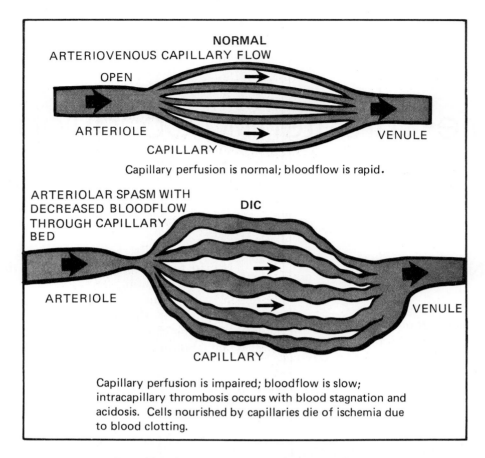

Figure 29-1. Sequestration of clotted blood in the capillaries.

Clinical Presentation

In most cases of DIC, arterial hypotension occurs secondary to the arteriovenous anastomoses. The anastomoses are caused by arterial vasoconstriction of the precapillary sphincter and vasodilatation of the capillaries.

Bleeding occurs after injections or venipunctures, from incisions, in the mucosa of the mouth, in the respiratory system, in the gastrointestinal system, and in the genitourinary system. It is common for several of these systems to be bleeding simultaneously; rarely is only one system involved.

Despite the complete depletion of circulating fibrinogen, some circulating thrombin still exists since fibrinogen is not present to convert it to fibrin. Activation of the clotting process produces thrombin and thereby fibrin. Fibrin and thrombin convert plasminogen to plasmin. Antithrombins (especially antithrombin III) destroy thrombin function. In DIC, thrombin production exceeds antithrombin III production and thereby promotes uncontrolled coagulation.

The initiation of fibrinolysis results in the dissolution of clots and degrades fibrin into its fractions, which further adds to the bleeding. Laboratory results suggestive of DIC include a decreased platelet count and fibrinogen level; a prolonged prothrombin time/international ratio (PT/INR), partial thromboplastin time (PTT), and activated partial thromboplastin time (aPTT); and an increased fibrin degradation products (FDP) and D-dimer.

Pulmonary compromise may require intubation. Following the trend of arterial blood gases (ABGs) and observing for signs and symptoms of hypoxemia will show when suctioning and/or mechanical ventilation is indicated.

Monitor fluid balance, especially if the patient receives multiple blood transfusions and other fluids or if the patient has another preexisting disease.

Skin care to preserve skin integrity is very important. Care must be taken to treat the patient very gently and to maintain good body alignment with adequate support. Sufficient but not excessive pressure is applied to sites of intramuscular injection or

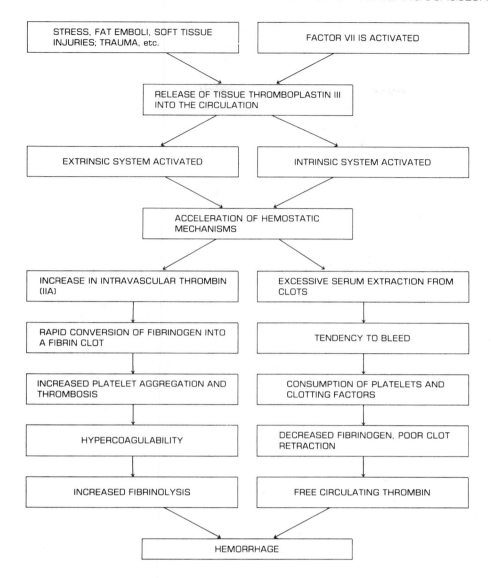

Figure 29-2. Alteration of the coagulation process in DIC.

venipuncture by laboratory personnel to prevent hematoma formation.

Petechiae are pinpoint, flat lesions that appear as reddish purple spots on the skin, buccal mucosa, and conjuctivae. Purpura is characterized by reddish brown spots usually evidencing the presence of fluid. Ecchymoses are black and blue bruises.

Psychosocial support is extremely important to decrease the anxiety of the patient, who is aware and frightened by all the lost blood and the flurry of activity around him or her. Very brief explanations should be given; for example, "I'm giving you some medicine through the vein to help stop your bleeding." Providing an explanation of DIC in terms that the

patient and family can understand will help to decrease anxiety and foster positive relationships among all parties.

Treatment

The primary treatment of DIC is to treat the underlying disease, which is easier said than done in the face of hemorrhaging. Disseminated intravascular coagulation can cause life-threatening hemorrhage and measures to control bleeding or thrombosis may require emergency measures. Treatment will vary with the clinical presentation. Patients with bleeding may require blood products, including fresh frozen plasma (FFP), to replace depleted clotting factors and platelets to correct thrombocytopenia. Platelets may be transfused if counts are less than 5000 to 10,000/mm^3, especially with active bleeding or hemorrhage. FFP is used to replenish coagulation factors and antithrombotic factors, although these are only temporizing measures. In some situations, infusion with antithrombin may be necessary.

It is necessary to replace the clotting factors so that the serum will be converted back to plasma. At the same time, the effects of thrombin must be stopped. Also at the same time, correction of acidosis, hypotension, hypovolemia, and hypoxia must be attempted since these four conditions act as procoagulants, causing continued utilization/depletion of clotting factors. Vitamin K (formation of prothrombin) and folic acid (thrombocytopenia) are administered to correct these deficiencies.

The use of heparin remains controversial because it is difficult to assess its effectiveness. Heparin neutralizes free circulating thrombin by combining with antithrombin III, which inactivates the thrombin. Heparin functions as an anticoagulant to prevent further thrombus formation in the microcirculatory system. (It does not alter the thrombi already formed.) Heparin prevents the activation of factor X. Heparin also inhibits platelet aggregation.

Caution: If used, heparin should be given intravenously, not subcutaneously. Factors affecting subcutaneous heparin include the absorption rate, which is dependent on the amount injected, the depth of injection, body temperature, and cardiovascular status. If a hematoma develops at the injection site, absorption is markedly altered. The amount of heparin needed may be too great for subcutaneous administration. The delay in reaching a therapeutic blood level may be too long with subcutaneous administration.

After heparin therapy is started, whole blood, FFP, and/or platelet transfusions are administered.

Complications

Prognosis varies depending on the underlying disorder. Disseminated intravascular coagulation may become an exsanguinating hemorrhage. Death is not uncommon.

Nursing Interventions

Assessment of patients at high risk for DIC includes looking for the development of petechiae, purpura, and ecchymoses. Oozing of blood from injection sites, intravenous lines, and invasive monitoring lines may indicate the onset of DIC.

Cardiac status must be monitored for dysrhythmias secondary to acidosis, hypovolemia, hypervolemia, and electrolyte imbalances. Early recognition and treatment of dysrhythmias may prevent progression to more serious dysrhythmias. The patient may need to be transferred to a critical care unit if unstable. Renal problems can develop as a consequence of fluid overload, fluid depletion, and hypotension. The oliguric or anuric patient cannot eliminate heparin adequately, so the dose must be titrated to match the patient's utilization and excretion of the drug.

Monitor the amount of bleeding and identify the system involved. All drainage should be tested for blood. Observe for frank bleeding.

Watch for signs of thrombus formation. If thrombi develop, the symptoms will vary according to the system involved. The kidneys are most often involved (oliguria or anuria).

Intracranial bleeding may be identified by an altered level of consciousness; orientation to person, place, and time; pupil reactions; and extremity movement. These must be checked frequently. Any change will indicate a possible bleed.

Avoid infection. The DIC patient is at high risk for infection, primarily because of all the entry ports for bacteria. Development of a fever is an indication to culture blood, urine, sputum, and any other drainage. If the bacteria are identified, appropriate antibiotics are started.

THROMBOTIC THROMBOCYTOPENIC PURPURA

Thrombotic thrombocytopenic purpura (TTP) can cause multisystem complications during the acute phase. It is a rare disorder with a poor prognosis; however, the survival rate is improving. It is characterized by thrombocytopenia, hemolytic anemia, fever, neurologic complications, and renal failure.

The etiology is unknown, but TTP appears to involve a deficiency of a von Willebrand factor–cleaving protease, ADAMTS13; in some cases, it is due to an antibody directed against the protease. The condition is occasionally precipitated by estrogen use, pregnancy, drugs (quinine, ticlopidine), or infections; TTP can also occur as a complication of bone marrow transplantation or the use of cyclosporine or tacrolimus. It tends to affect women more often than men and usually has an onset at about 40 years of age.

The pathophysiology of TTP includes widespread deposition of platelet microthromboli that occlude the arteries and capillaries. This is especially evident in the brain, bone marrow, and kidneys. The result is bleeding and petechiae.

Treatment of TTP is aimed at managing the manifestations of the syndrome, including severe thrombocytopenia and hemolytic anemia. The use of plasmapheresis, corticosteroids, and immunosuppression has been effective, and splenectomy may prevent subsequent relapses. The patient may need transfer to the critical care unit if unstable.

IDIOPATHIC THROMBOCYTOPENIA PURPURA

Idiopathic thrombocytopenia purpura (ITP) is defined as thrombocytopenia that occurs without any specific cause; however, many cases are due to an autoimmune response with antibodies against platelets developing. Idiopathic thrombocytopenia purpura is also known as immune thrombocytopenia purpura or immune-mediated thrombocytopenia purpura. It is usually chronic in adults and is more frequent in women. Symptoms of ITP include the development of bruising and petechiae, usually on the extremities, or bleeding from the nostrils or gums (especially when the platelet count is <20,000/mm^3). Bleeding time is prolonged but a normal bleeding time does not exclude the diagnosis. The diagnosis is often one of exclusion.

Treatment of ITP is generally indicated for a platelet count <20,000/mm^3 and a level <10,000/mm^3 is a potential medical emergency as the patient is at risk for spontaneous bleeding as well as subarachnoid or intracerebral hemorrhage if moderate head trauma were to occur. Treatment may include intravenous steroids (methylprednisolone or prednisone), intravenous immunoglobulin, thrombopoietin receptor agonists to simulate platelet production, or platelet infusion.

HEPARIN-INDUCED THROMBOCYTOPENIA

Heparin-induced thrombocytopenia (HIT) is due to an immune response that occurs as a result of heparin administration, either unfractionated or

low molecular weight. It has been designated as the most frequent drug-induced immune-mediated type of thrombocytopenia. It is estimated that up to 8% of patients receiving heparin will develop the antibody associated with HIT and 1% to 5% will progress to develop HIT with thrombocytopenia. In HIT, the platelet count falls below the normal range (<150,000/mm^3) within 5 to 14 days after heparin administration to ranges around 50,000 to 80,000/mm^3. Patients at higher risk for developing HIT include those status postcardiovascular surgery, orthopedic surgery, and general surgery. In HIT, the immune system forms antibodies against heparin and results in platelet activation and blood clot formation resulting in a decreased platelet count and a predisposition to thrombosis. All formulations of heparin (including low molecular weight heparins) should be avoided including flushes or heparin-coated catheters when HIT is suspected or confirmed. Alternative anticoagulation using direct-thrombin inhibitors such as argatroban, lepirudin, or bivaliruding should be used in patients with HIT.

The diagnosis of HIT is often made by measuring the platelet count and platelet factor 4 (PF4) antibody levels. The thrombocytopenia that occurs with HIT is often self-limited and is generally not low enough to lead to an increased risk of bleeding. The PF4 antibody that causes HIT will usually disappear after approximately 3 months and heparin therapy may be considered for new clots if the PF4 antibody test is negative.

Monitoring the patient for bleeding and minimizing bleeding risks are areas of focus for nursing care for both ITP and HIT.

BIBLIOGRAPHY

American Association of Allergy, Asthma, and Immunology. Media resources: Position statement 26. The use of epinephrine in the treatment of anaphylaxis. http://www.aaaai.org/media/resources/academy_statements/advocacy_statements/ps26.as p. Accessed 8/10/2010.

Aplastic Anemia & MDS International Foundation. P.O. Box 613, Annapolis, MD 21404-0613. (800) 747–2820 or (410) 867–0242. http://www.aplastic.org. Accessed 10/10/2010.

Cooney, M. G. (2006). Heparin-induced thrombocytopenia: advanced in diagnosis and treatment *Critical Care Nurse, 6*(26), 30–36.

Coyer, S. M., & Lash, A.A. (2008). Pathophysiology of anemia and nursing care implications MedSurg Nursing; http://findarticles.com/p/articles/mi_m0FSS/is_2_17/ai_ n25410188/. Accessed 9/20/2010.

Dressler, D. K. (2009). Death by clot: Acute coronary syndromes, ischemic stroke, pulmonary embolism, and disseminated intravascular coagulation. *Advanced Critical Care, 20*(2), 166–176.

Dressler, D. K. (2010). Hematology and immune systems. In M. Chulay, & S. M. Burns (Eds.). *AACN essentials of progressive care nursing* (pp. 283–294). New York, NY: McGraw-Hill.

Fauci, A. S., & Lane H. C. Human immunodeficiency virus disease: AIDS and related disorders. *Harrison's Online*. New York, NY: McGraw-Hill. Accessed 9/10/2010.

Feied, C., & Handler, J. A. Thrombolytic therapy. E-Medicine. http://www.emedicine.com/emerg/topic831. htm. Accessed 9/10/2010.

Gaspard, K. J. (2009). Disorders of red blood cells. In C. M. Porth, & G. (Eds.). *Pathophysiology: Concepts of altered health states* (8th ed.). Philadelphia, PA: Wolters Kluwer Health.

Glass, M., & Spitrey, J. (2009). Heparin-induced thrombocytopenia: Your questions answered. *Advanced Critical Care, 20*(1), 5–11.

Harrison's Online. Clinical immunology; hematology; disorders of hemostasis [online]. www. harrisonsonline. com. Accessed 9/12/2010.

Hirsch, J., Guyatt, G., Albers, G. W., Harrington, R., Schunemann, H. J. (2008). Antithrombotic and thrombolytic therapy. ACCP Guidelines. *Chest, 133*, 71S–105S.

Hoffman, F. M., Nelson, B. J., Drangstveit, M.B., Flynn, B. M., Watercott, E. A., Zirbes, J. M. (2006). Caring for transplant recipients in a nontransplant setting. *Critical Care Nurse, 26*, 53–73.

James, S. H. (2009). Hematology pharmacology: Anticoagulant, antiplatelet, and procoagulant agents in practice. *Advanced Critical Care, 20*(2), 177–192.

Katz, E. A. (2009). Blood transfusion: Friend or foe. *Advanced Critical Care, 20*(2), 155–163.

Leukemia & Lymphoma Society. 1311 Mamaroneck Ave., White Plains, NY 10605. (914) 949–5213. http://www.leukemia-lymphoma. org

McCraw, B., & Lyon D. E. (2008). Diagnosing disseminated intravascular coagulopathy in acute promyelocytic leukemia. Clinical *Journal of Oncology Nursing, 12,* 717–720.

Medline Plus Health Information. Anaphylaxis. National Institutes of Health (online). http://www.nlm. nih. gov/medlineplus/ency/article/000844.htm. Accessed 9/10/2010.

Munro, N. (2009). Hematologic complications of critical illness: Anemia, neutropenia, thrombocytopenia, and more. *Advanced Critical Care, 20,* 145–154.

Nabili, S. Anemia. http://www.medicinenet.com/anemia/article.htm. Accessed 9/20/2010.

Patel, P. Acute kidney failure. Available at http://www.nlm.nih.gov/medlineplus/ency/article/000501.html. Accessed 9/12/2010.

Raab, M. S., Podar, K., Breitkreutz, I., Richardson, P. G., Anderson, K. C. (2009). Multiple myeloma. *Lancet, 374,* 324–39.

Salinitri, F., Berlie, H., Desai, N. (2009). Pharmacotherapeutic blood pressure management in a chronic kidney disease patient. *Advanced Critical Care, 20,* 205–213.

Sarkodee-Adoo, C.Understanding Anemia—The Basics. http://www.webmd.com/a-to-z-guides/understanding-anemia-basics. Accessed 9/10/2010.

Silverman, M. A. Idiopathic thrombocytopenia purpura. *EMedicine* 2009. http://emedicine.medscape.com/article/779545. Accessed 9/5/2010.

Wilson, J. F. Anemias. Encyclopedia of Nursing & Allied Health. http://www.enotes.com/nursing-encyclopedia/anemias. Accessed 9/15/2010.

PART IV

Immunology and Hematology Practice Exam

1. Which of the following components of the white blood cell count makes up the largest percentage of the differential?
   (A) Segmented neutrophils
   (B) Band neutrophils
   (C) Monocytes
   (D) Lymphocytes

2. A 71-year-old man is admitted to your unit with recurrent pneumonia. Since the pneumonia was present before, which of the following types of cells would have the ability to remember the *Haemophilus* antigen from a prior infection?
   (A) Segmented neutrophils
   (B) Band neutrophils
   (C) Lymphocytes
   (D) Eosinophils

3. Which of the following types of cells produce antibodies?
   (A) Segmented neutrophils
   (B) Monocytes
   (C) B lymphocytes through plasma cells
   (D) Reticuloendothelial cells

4. Common side effects of antibiotic therapy include which of the following?
   (A) Potential bone marrow suppression
   (B) Reduction in normal bacterial flora and bleeding tendencies
   (C) Development of resistance to antibiotics and reduction in normal bacterial flora
   (D) Development of resistance and hypercoagulation

Questions 5 and 6 refer to the following scenario:

A 64-year-old woman is in your unit after a hepatic resection for cancer. During her second postoperative day, she complains of generalized discomfort with no change in incisional pain. She feels warm to the touch and her vital signs indicate the following:

Blood pressure	96/56 mm Hg
Pulse	115
Respiratory rate	28
Temperature	39°C

Lung sounds include scattered crackles throughout both lungs. Pulmonary artery catheter readings provide the following information:

PaO_2	74
$PaCO_2$	35
pH	7.32
FIO_2	0.40

5. Based on the preceding information, which condition is possibly developing?
   (A) Sepsis
   (B) Congestive heart failure (CHF)
   (C) Pneumonia
   (D) Acute respiratory distress syndrome (ARDS)

6. Which treatment would most likely be instituted based on the preceding information?
   (A) Mechanical ventilation
   (B) Amphotericin B and fluid bolus
   (C) Fluid bolus and triple antibiotics
   (D) Amphotericin B and fluid restriction

7. Which is the first response in coagulation following trauma to a blood vessel?
   (A) Vasoconstriction
   (B) Platelet aggregation
   (C) Fibrin formation
   (D) Thrombin formation

8. Which electrolyte is an integral part of the coagulation process?
   (A) Sodium
   (B) Potassium
   (C) Magnesium
   (D) Calcium

9. Which of the following characterizes disseminated intravascular clotting?
   (A) Decreased prothrombin time
   (B) Increased levels of fibrinogen degradation products
   (C) Antithrombin formation
   (D) Platelet proliferation

10. A patient admitted with a diagnosis of pulmonary embolism is to receive a thrombolytic agent. Which of the following is NOT considered a thrombolytic medication?
    (A) Tissue plasminogen activator (tPA)
    (B) Urokinase
    (C) Streptokinase
    (D) Heparin

11. Which test is best employed to assess the effectiveness of heparin therapy?
    (A) Partial thromboplastin time (PTT)
    (B) Prothrombin time (PT)
    (C) Platelet levels
    (D) Bleeding time

12. The thrombolytic effect of plasmin is due to which action?
    (A) Prevention of platelet aggregation
    (B) Blocking of the intrinsic pathway
    (C) Breaking down of fibrin
    (D) Ionization of calcium

13. Which of the following tests is used to diagnose a hemolytic transfusion reaction?
    (A) Coombs' test
    (B) Prothrombin time (PT)
    (C) Activated partial thromboplastin time (aPTT)
    (D) Fibrinogen level

14. The extrinsic pathway for coagulation is initiated by which mechanism?
    (A) Irregularity of the blood vessel wall
    (B) Presence of atherosclerotic plaques, causing increased turbulent blood flow
    (C) Exposure to interstitial tissue following trauma to the blood vessel
    (D) Introduction of an extrinsic substance into the blood

15. What is the first stage in the coagulation process?
    (A) Conversion of plasminogen to plasmin
    (B) Conversion of fibrinogen to fibrin
    (C) Activation of thrombin
    (D) Activation of thromboplastin

16. Tissue plasminogen activator (tPA) has potential advantages over streptokinase. What are these potential advantages?
    (A) It is clot-specific as opposed to systemic and is less expensive.
    (B) It is clot-specific as opposed to systemic and has a shorter half-life.
    (C) It is less expensive and has a shorter half-life.
    (D) All of the above.

17. Nursing care of the patient receiving thrombolytic therapy includes which of the following?
    (A) Avoiding intramuscular injections and using a soft toothbrush
    (B) Avoiding intramuscular injections and using oximetry rather than blood gas studies for Sao_2 determination
    (C) Using a soft toothbrush and using oximetry rather than blood gas studies for Sao_2 determination
    (D) All of the above

Immunology and Hematology
Practice Exam

Practice Fill-Ins

1. _____

2. _____

3. _____

4. _____

5. _____

6. _____

7. _____

8. _____

9. _____

10. _____

11. _____

12. _____

13. _____

14. _____

15. _____

16. _____

17. _____

1. __A__	6. __C__	11. __A__	16. __B__
2. __C__	7. __A__	12. __C__	17. __D__
3. __C__	8. __D__	13. __A__	
4. __C__	9. __B__	14. __C__	
5. __A__	10. __D__	15. __D__	

V

NEUROLOGY

Ruth M. Kleinpell
Mary Kay Bader

30

Anatomy and Physiology of the Nervous System

EDITORS' NOTE

Perhaps the questions on the PCCN exam that most often give nurses problems are those on neurologic principles. The difficulty in understanding these concepts can be traced to the complexity of central and autonomic nervous system dysfunction. The neurologic aspect of the PCCN exam does not require that you be knowledgeable about every potential disturbance of the nervous system; rather the primary focus is on problems commonly seen in general nursing practice. This focus makes preparing for the neurologic aspect of the PCCN exam more manageable.

In its present format, about 5% of the PCCN exam is devoted to neurologic concepts. The key aspects covered in the exam include increased intracranial pressure, stroke, intracranial hemorrhage, and seizure disorders. Supplemental content including arteriovenous malformation, aneurysm, hydrocephalus, neuromuscular disorders including muscular dystrophy, Guillain-Barré syndrome, myasthenia gravis, and space-occupying lesions are also reviewed in this chapter in order to provide a comprehensive neurologic review. By studying the chapters in Part V, seeking out patients with neurologic conditions, and practicing neurologic assessments and tests during your clinical practice, you will become well prepared for the neurologic part of the PCCN exam.

ANATOMY

It is customary to divide the nervous system into three segments to facilitate comprehension of the system and its dysfunctions. The three segments are the central nervous system ([CNS]—composed of the brain and spinal cord), the peripheral nervous system (composed of the cranial, spinal, and peripheral nerves), and the autonomic nervous system (composed of the sympathetic and parasympathetic systems).

Extracerebral Structures

Extracerebral structures include the scalp, skull, and meninges. These structures provide protection to the brain.

Scalp

The letters in the term *SCALP* form a mnemonic for remembering the cranial coverings (Fig. 30-1). "SCA" stands for the single layer of skin and cutaneous and adipose tissue that contains blood vessels. Because these vessels cannot contract, a scalp laceration bleeds more than an identical cut elsewhere on the body. "L" stands for the dense, fibrous, *l*igament-like layer called the galea aponeurotica. This layer helps to absorb the forces of external trauma. "P" stands for the *p*ericranium, which contains fewer bone-forming elements than the periosteum.

Skull

The bony calvarium (skull) comprises eight bones fused to form a solid, nondistensible unit. The cranium, which is the skull minus the mandible, is hollow and has a volume of 1400 to 1500 mL. It consists of an outer and an inner layer of regular bone and a middle layer, called the diploë (or diploic space), which is spongy and lightweight. This provides protection to the brain without being heavy.

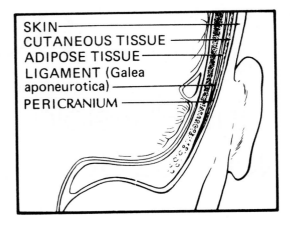

Figure 30-1. Layers of the scalp.

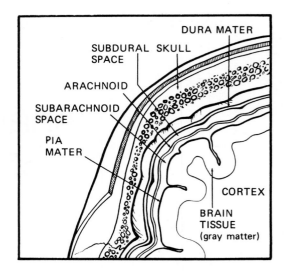

Figure 30-3. Meninges.

The bones comprising the cranium are the frontal (single), occipital (single), and pairs of parietal, temporal, sphenoid, and ethmoid bones (Fig. 30-2). The main function of the bony calvarium is to protect the brain from external forces. The bones formed during fetal life do not completely fuse until the infant is about 18 to 24 months of age. The fusion of these bones forms three landmarks. The coronal suture is the fusion of the frontal and parietal bones. The sagittal suture is the fusion of the two parietal bones. The lambdoid suture is the fusion of the parietal bones and the occipital bone.

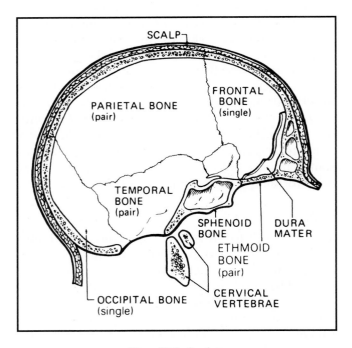

Figure 30-2. Cranium.

The internal surface of the cranium has three distinct ridges on it that serve to divide the brain into anterior, middle, and posterior segments called fossae (plural; singular is *fossa*).

Meninges

The three membranes covering the entire brain surface, the spinal cord, and the spinal canal below the cord are the meninges (Fig. 30-3). The mnemonic "PAD" may help you to remember the meningeal coverings and their purpose: the *p*ia mater, *a*rachnoid, and *d*ura mater are the meningeal layers, and they absorb shocks from sudden movements or trauma; they literally "PAD" the brain.

Starting from the brain itself, the first meningeal layer is the pia mater. The pia mater is contiguous with the brain's surface and its convolutions.

The arachnoid layer of the meninges is a delicate, avascular membrane between the dura and pia mater. It looks much like a lacy spider web with projections onto the pia mater. The space between the arachnoid layer and pia mater, the subarachnoid space, contains many cerebral arteries and veins, which are bathed by cerebrospinal fluid (CSF). The arachnoid membrane also has projections into the venous sinuses called arachnoid villi, which allow for the reabsorption of CSF from the subarachnoid space to the venous system. The subarachnoid space enlarges at the base of the brain to form the subarachnoid cisterns.

The outermost layer of the meninges is the dura mater. It is actually two layers of tough fibrous membrane that protect the underlying cortical matter.

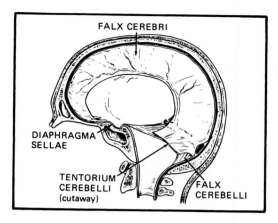

Figure 30-4. Sagittal section showing processes formed by the inner layer of the dura mater.

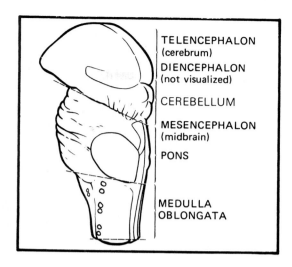

Figure 30-5. Gross anatomic sections of the brain.

The outermost layer forms the periosteum of the cranial cavity. The inner layer is lined with flat cells and contains arteries and veins. Between the two layers are clefts, which form the dural venous sinuses. The inner layer also gives rise to several folds, which divide the cranial cavity into compartments. There are four important compartments of this kind: the falx cerebri (separating the cerebral hemispheres); the falx cerebelli (separating the right and left cerebellar hemispheres); the tentorium cerebelli (separating the cerebral hemispheres from the cerebellum); and the diaphragma sellae, which forms a tent-like covering, or roof, over the pituitary gland (which sits in a part of the bony skull called the sella turcica) (Fig. 30-4). These compartmental dividers are significant anatomic landmarks in the brain. The extradural space, also called the epidural space, is a potential space between the inner table of the skull and the outermost meningeal layer, the dura mater. This potential space may become real when an individual experiencing a blow to the head develops an epidural hematoma. Epidural hematomas commonly result from a laceration of the middle meningeal artery in association with a skull fracture at the parietotemporal junction.

Another potential space, the subdural space, lies between the dura mater and the arachnoid. This is the site of subdural hematomas. This type of hematoma is most often venous in origin and results from tearing of the bridging dural veins.

Central Nervous System

The brain is made up of nervous tissue that fills up the cranial vault. It weighs about 3 lb in the adult male. Although it is an integrated unit, the brain is divided into three major sections: the cerebrum (cerebral hemispheres, white matter fibers, limbic system, basal ganglia, diencephalon); the midbrain; and the hindbrain (pons, medulla, and cerebellum) (Fig. 30-5).

Cerebrum

The cerebrum is contained in the anterior and middle fossae of the cranium. The left and right cerebral hemispheres are incompletely separated by a deep medial longitudinal fissure, called the falx cerebri, formed by the sagittal folds of the dura mater. The two cerebral hemispheres are joined by the corpus callosum (Fig. 30-6). It provides a path for fibers to cross

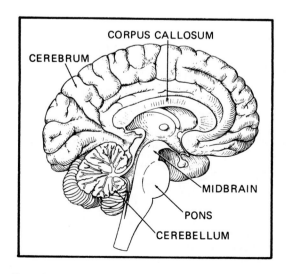

Figure 30-6. Midsagittal section showing the corpus callosum.

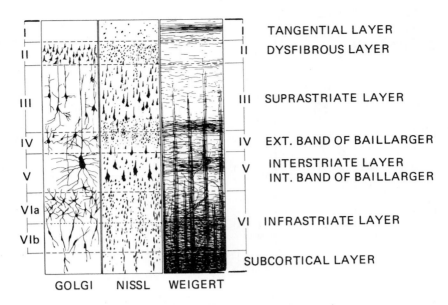

Figure 30-7. Six layers of the cerebral cortex.

from one hemisphere to the other. Each hemisphere has a lateral ventricle. These two hemispheres together are sometimes referred to as the telencephalon.

The cerebral surface is covered with convolutions, which give rise to gyri (raised portions) and sulci or fissures (depressions in the surface). The cerebral surface is about six cells deep and called the cerebral cortex. It normally appears to be gray in color; thus, these six layers (Fig. 30-7) are called gray matter. The cerebral cortex is estimated to contain 14 billion nerve cells.

From a lateral view, two fissures divide each hemisphere (Fig. 30-8). The lateral fissure (also

called the fissure of Sylvius) divides the temporal lobe from the parietal and frontal lobes. This area contains the primary auditory center. The central sulcus, also known as the fissure of Rolando, divides the frontal lobe from the parietal lobe. Immediately in front of the central sulcus is the precentral gyrus, which is the primary motor area. Immediately posterior to the central sulcus is the postcentral gyrus, which is the primary sensory cortical area.

In looking at pictures of the brain's surface that do not show the cerebellum, one can imagine the brain as a boxing glove. The thumb of the boxing glove always points toward the brain's frontal area. For descriptive purposes, the lateral surface of the hemisphere is divided into four lobes. The frontal lobe (approximately the anterior one-third of the hemisphere) is the portion that is anterior to the central sulcus and above the lateral fissure. The frontal lobe is responsible for voluntary motor function and higher mental functions such as judgment and foresight, affect, personality, inhibition, abstract thinking, and motor speech (dominant hemisphere). The parietal lobe extends from the central sulcus to the parietooccipital fissure. This lobe is responsible for sensory function, sensory association, and higher level processing of general sensory modalities. The occipital lobe is that part lying behind, or caudal to, an arbitrary line drawn from the parietooccipital fissure to the preoccipital notch. The function of the occipital lobe is visual reception and visual association.

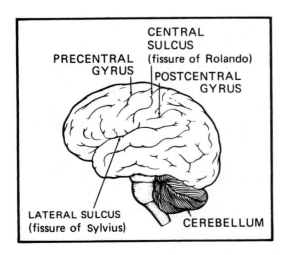

Figure 30-8. Fissures, sulci, and gyri dividing the cerebral hemisphere.

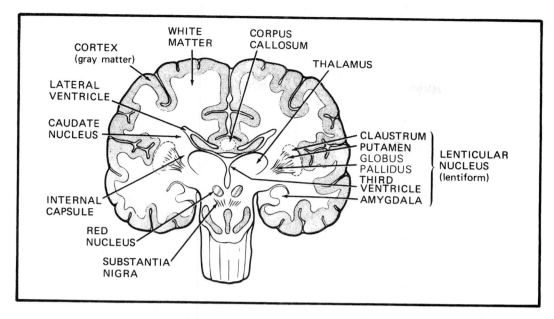

Figure 30-9. Coronal section of the brain showing internal parts of basal ganglia of the telencephalon.

The temporal lobes are located under the lateral fissures of Sylvius. The temporal lobes are each divided into a primary auditory receptive area (in dominant hemisphere), a secondary auditory association area, and a tertiary visual association area.

The basal ganglia, or basal nuclei, are also part of the telencephalon. The basal ganglia include the caudate nucleus, putamen, globus pallidus, claustrum, subthalamic nucleus, and substantia nigra (Fig. 30-9).

Specific functions of the brain segments are listed in Table 30-1.

TABLE 30-1. FUNCTIONS OF SPECIFIC BRAIN STRUCTURES

Structure	Function
Cerebrum (divided into cerebral hemispheres)	Governs all sensory and motor thought and learning; analyzes, associates, integrates, and stores information
Cerebral cortex (four lobes)	
Frontal lobe	Motor function; motor speech area; controls morals, values, emotions, and judgment
Parietal lobe	Integrates general sensation; governs discrimination; interprets pain, touch, temperature, and pressure
Temporal lobe	Auditory center; sensory speech center
Occipital lobe	Visual area
Basal ganglia	Central motor movement
Thalamus (diencephalon)	Screens and relays sensory impulses to cortex; lowest level of crude conscious awareness
Hypothalamus (diencephalon)	Regulates autonomic nervous system, stress response, sleep, appetite, body temperature, water balance, and emotions
Midbrain (mesencephalon)	Motor condition, conjugates eye movements
Pons	Contains projection tracts between spinal cord, medulla, and brain
Medulla oblongata	Contains all afferent and efferent tracts, most pyramidal tracts, and cardiac, respiratory, vasomotor, and vomiting centers
Cerebellum	Connected by cerebellar peduncles to other parts of CNS; coordinates muscle movement, posture, equilibrium, and muscle tone
Limbic system	Regulation of some visceral activities; some function in emotional personality

CNS, central nervous system.

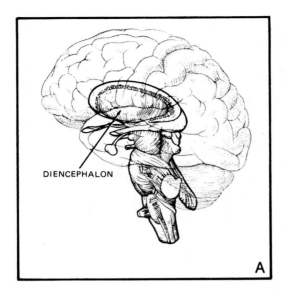

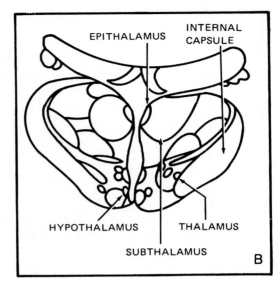

Figure 30-10. Position of the diencephalon (**A**) and the internal components of the diencephalon (**B**).

Diencephalon

The diencephalon is composed of the thalamus, epithalamus, subthalamus, and hypothalamus (Fig. 30-10). It is a paired structure with a thin fluid space between the two sides. The thalamus is the largest structure in the diencephalon; it integrates all body sensations except smell. It is also the major relay area for all neuronal impulses. The hypothalamus connects with the limbic system, thalamus, mesencephalon, and hypophysis (pituitary gland). The hypothalamus has neural as well as endocrine functions. It is responsible for the production of antidiuretic hormone (ADH) and oxytocin as well as influencing body temperature, water balance, and the intake of food.

Midbrain

The midbrain is also known as the mesencephalon. Located between the diencephalon and the pons, it contains the major motor nerves for eye movement, carries impulses down from the cerebrum, and controls the wakefulness of the brain through the reticular activating system (Fig. 30-11). Reticular-activating system (RAS) fibers connect with the thalamus, cerebral cortex, cerebellum, and spinal cord. They contain nuclei of the third and fourth cranial nerves.

Hindbrain

Pons. The pons is situated between the midbrain and the medulla oblongata. It forms a bridge (thus, its name from the Latin word for bridge)

between the cerebellar hemispheres and contains the neurons for sensory input and motor output for the face. It contains nuclei of the fifth, sixth, seventh, and eighth cranial nerves. The pons in conjunction with the medulla controls the rate and length of respirations.

Medulla Oblongata. The medulla oblongata is located between the pons and spinal cord. It is the structure that marks the change between the spinal

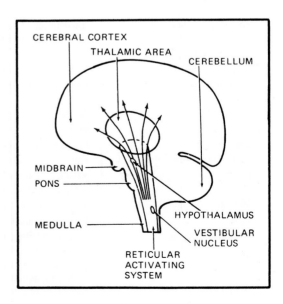

Figure 30-11. Reticular activating system.

cord and the brain itself. The corticospinal tracts, which mediate voluntary motor function, descend through the medulla, where they decussate in the lower medulla. They are responsible for specific symptoms of dysfunction occurring ipsilaterally (same side as the lesion or injury) or contralaterally (opposite side).

Collectively, the mesencephalon, pons, and medulla oblongata constitute the brainstem. Regulation of respiratory rhythm, rate, and strength of heartbeat and blood vessel diameter are controlled by the medulla. The nuclei for reflex activities such as coughing, sneezing, swallowing, and vomiting and the ninth to twelfth cranial nerves are found here.

Cerebellum. The cerebellum is situated in the posterior fossa of the cranial cavity. It is separated from the cerebrum by dura mater folds forming the tentorium cerebelli. The cerebral hemispheres are above the tentorium cerebelli and are thus supratentorial structures. The two cerebellar hemispheres are connected to each other by a structure called the vermis. They are connected to the brainstem by cerebellar peduncles. There are three cerebellar peduncles (Fig. 30-12). The superior cerebellar peduncles send impulses from the cerebellum to the thalamus. The middle cerebellar peduncles receive cerebral cortex information from nuclei in the pons. The inferior cerebellar peduncles receive impulses that reveal body and extremity positions.

The gray matter and the white matter compose the cerebellum. The cerebellum receives input from the brainstem and spinal cord nuclei, whose axons project to the cerebellar cortex. These tracts carry excitatory impulses to cerebellar cortex.

Equilibrium, posture, muscle tone, and ultimately muscle coordination are mediated by the cerebellum.

Circulation and Formation of Cerebrospinal Fluid

Four ventricles (cavities) are involved in the cerebrospinal fluid (CSF) system (Fig. 30-13). The largest two are the lateral ventricles, which are located in the cerebral hemispheres. The lateral ventricles are connected to the third ventricle via the interventricular foramen, or the foramen of Monro. The cerebral aqueduct of Sylvius exits from the floor of the third ventricle. This channel passes down through the brainstem to the fourth ventricle, which is continuous with the central canal of the spinal cord. The CSF is synthesized at approximately 20 mL/h by the choroid plexus. This is an area of modified epithelial cells covering tufts of capillaries found in all ventricles but predominating in the anterior

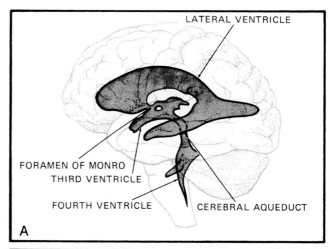

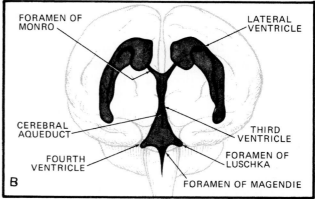

Figure 30-13. Lateral **(A)** and anterior **(B)** views of the ventricular system of the brain.

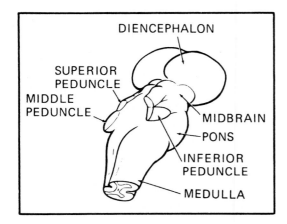

Figure 30-12. Cerebellar peduncles.

segment of the lateral ventricles. It is a clear, color-less liquid having a few cells, some protein, glucose, and a large amount of sodium chloride.

The foramen of Monro allows the CSF to leave the lateral ventricles and flow into the third ventricle. Obstruction at this point will produce hydrocephalus. The most common site of obstructive hydrocephalus occurs in the aqueduct of Sylvius at or above the fourth ventricle, obstruction at the foramen of Monro, or at the outlets of the fourth ventricle. From the third ventricle, CSF flows through the aqueduct of Sylvius into the fourth ventricle. Foramina of Luschka and Magendie direct the CSF from the fourth ventricle into the cisterns and subarachnoid space.

After circulating (in the subarachnoid space) over the entire brain and spinal cord, the CSF is reabsorbed by the arachnoid villi in dural sinuses and by pacchionian bodies found in the superior sagittal sinus.

The CSF "cushions" the brain and spinal cord to protect them from colliding with the cranium and vertebrae in response to moving forces. The CSF also reduces the gravitational weight of the brain. To a limited extent, the CSF adjusts to changes in the intracranial vault's pressure and volume. If the pressure or volume in the vault increases, more CSF will be absorbed and/or pushed into the spinal canal in an attempt to maintain normal pressure. Normally, 125 to 150 mL of CSF is in the ventricles and the subarachnoid space. An average of 500 mL of CSF is produced in a 24-h period, or approximately 22 mL/h. The CSF also participates in the exchange of nutrients and waste material between the blood and the cells of the CNS.

Cerebral Blood Supply

The brain is supplied with oxygenated blood from two arterial systems: the carotid arteries and the vertebral arteries. The common carotid arteries bifurcate, forming the external and internal carotid arteries. As a reserve to these two systems, the circle of Willis helps to provide adequate circulation through its anastomoses. The circle of Willis anastomoses are between the two vertebral arteries and the two carotid arteries (Fig. 30-14). The internal carotid carries about two-thirds of the blood that flows to the brain. The right and left vertebral arteries branch off the subclavian arteries. They pass through the foramen magnum as they enter the skull.

External Cerebral Blood Supply. The external carotid arteries feed the external face, head, and

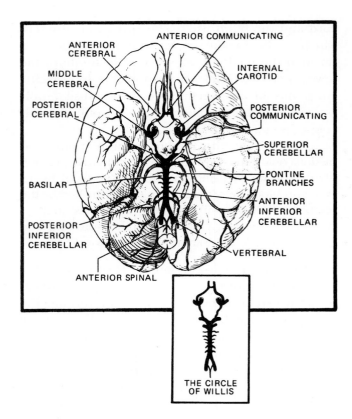

Figure 30-14. Circle of Willis.

neck. The external carotid arteries bifurcate and form the occipital, temporal, and maxillary arteries. The occipital arteries supply the posterior fossa. The temporal arteries supply the temporal region. The maxillary arteries form the middle meningeal arteries, which supply the anterior, middle, and posterior portions of the meninges and the fossae. While not a part of cerebral circulation, the external carotid artery and its branches may be used as a collateral channel to supplement cerebral circulation in the individual with cerebrovascular disease.

Internal Cerebral Blood Supply. On entering the skull, the internal carotid artery follows the carotid groove upward through the cavernous sinus and the sphenoid bone and into the circle of Willis at the base of the brain. Before this, smaller vessels originate, one of which is the ophthalmic artery. Temporary blockage of this vessel by microemboli may cause fleeting monocular blindness (amaurosis fugax).

Each internal carotid artery bifurcates to form a number of major branches, including the posterior communicating artery, anterior cerebral artery, anterior choroidal artery, and middle cerebral artery. The anterior communicating artery connects the left and right anterior cerebral arteries, forming a bridge to join the right and left anterior circulation. This bridge creates the front portion of the circle of Willis. The posterior communicating artery connects the internal carotid artery to the posterior cerebral artery and joins the anterior to the posterior circulation of the brain. These communicating arteries do not supply any part of the brain directly, but some are collateral channels helping to form the back portion of the circle of Willis.

The vertebral arteries enter the posterior fossa and join to form the basilar artery. The basilar artery gives off a number of major branches, including the superior cerebellar arteries and the anterior inferior cerebellar arteries, and bifurcates to form the posterior cerebral arteries. The superior cerebellar arteries supply the pons, midbrain, and cerebellum. The anteroinferior cerebellar arteries feed the cerebellum and the pons. The posterior cerebral arteries supply the posterior one-third of the cerebrum as well as parts of the midbrain and choroid plexus of third and fourth ventricles. Some of these arteries anastomose with each other to form the circle of Willis. They are the anterior cerebral artery, the anterior communicating artery, the posterior communicating arteries, and the posterior cerebral arteries. All of these arteries are involved in supplying blood to the anterior two-thirds of the cerebrum.

Only about 50% of all individuals have a "classic" circle of Willis. The most common difference is that the posterior communicating artery is not present and the posterior cerebral artery comes directly from the internal carotid artery.

Veins run parallel with many of the arteries. The middle meningeal arteries are special in that the veins that accompany these arteries are positioned between the arteries and the bones of the cranium. This helps protect the middle meningeal artery, which is frequently torn in skull fractures of the temporal bones.

As there is an internal and external arterial blood supply, there is a corresponding internal and external venous return system. Many of the veins are important in aneurysms and as surgical landmarks. The veins that drain the dura mater and diploë of the skull (external) empty into the venous sinuses, which are located between the layers of the dura mater. Internal cerebral veins also empty into venous sinuses.

Venous sinuses are lined with epithelium; they have no valves and no muscles in their walls. The sinuses connect with emissary veins, which in turn connect with external cranial veins that empty into the internal jugular veins. The superior sagittal sinus receives venous blood from the superior cerebral veins. The inferior sagittal sinus receives venous blood from the veins of the medial cerebral hemisphere. The straight sinus receives venous blood from the internal cerebral veins. There are many other sinuses that receive venous blood from other areas of the brain.

Components of Nervous Tissue

There are two main types of cells in the brain: neurons (Fig. 30-15) and neuroglia (glial cells). The neuron is the functioning unit of the nervous system;

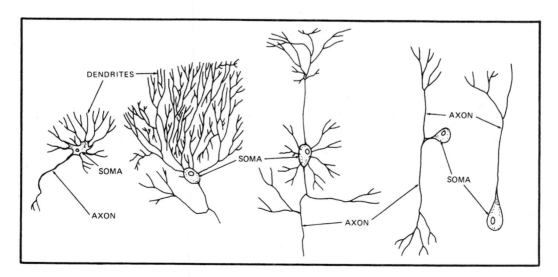

Figure 30-15. Various shapes of neurons and neuroglia.

its job is to transmit impulses. There are more than 10 billion neurons in the CNS and three-fourths of them are in the cerebral cortex.

Neurons are categorized in two ways: by the direction of impulse flow and/or by the number of processes emanating from the neuronal cell's body. Neurons that transmit impulses to the spinal cord or brain are afferent sensory neurons. Those transmitting impulses away from the brain or spinal cord are called efferent motor neurons. Interneurons transmit impulses from sensory neurons to motor neurons. The mnemonic "SAME" can help you to remember the direction and type of neuron: "SA" stands for sensory afferent and "ME" stands for motor efferent.

Neurons will be one of three types, according to the number of processes that exist. Unipolar neurons have one process coming from the cell body. After a short distance, this one process will split to form one axon and one dendrite (typical of both cranial and spinal nerves). Bipolar neurons have one axon and one dendrite coming from the cell body (rod and cone cells of the optic system to the CNS). Multipolar neurons have one axon and multiple dendrites (typical of motor neurons).

Regardless of the category of neurons, they all have certain unique structures unique to neurons (Fig. 30-16); that is, axons, dendrites, neurofibrils, Nissl's bodies, myelin, neurilemma, and nodes of Ranvier.

The cell body of a neuron is called a soma, or perikaryon. It contains a nucleus and many cytoplasmic organelles. The axon originates from a thickened area of the soma called an axon hillock. The axon transmits impulses away from the soma. There is one axon per neuron. Dendrites are short processes that transmit impulses to the soma. Multipolar neurons have many dendrites. The branching of dendritic processes is termed arborization, since the processes resemble tree branches. Neurofibrils are thin, thread-like fibers forming a network in the cytoplasm. Nissl's bodies specialize in protein synthesis with RNA to maintain and regenerate the neuronal processes.

Myelin is a protein-lipid compound that covers some axons. In the CNS, myelin is produced by oligodendrocytes. In the peripheral nervous system, myelin is produced by Schwann's cells. Myelin covers axons of nerve cells in between the nodes of Ranvier. The nodes of Ranvier are bare spots at regular intervals that speed the conduction of impulses.

The neurilemma is an outer coating of the neurons outside of the CNS. The neurilemma encompasses all structures, even myelin. It is the neurilemma that provides for the regeneration of peripheral nerves. Since the neurilemma is not found on neurons of the brain and spinal cord, these neurons cannot regenerate.

Neurons require an extensive support system to maintain optimal function. The neuroglia are responsible for this support system (Fig. 30-17). Neuroglia are composed of glial cells, and they outnumber the neurons by 10 to 1. Four types of specific cells compose the glial support system.

1. Astrocytes are star-shaped cells that form the actual tissue support system. Astrocytes, which may be made up of protoplasmic or fibrous tissue, constitute part of the blood-brain barrier by sending foot-like processes to the blood vessels.
2. Microglia are tiny cells that lie quiescent until nervous tissue is damaged. Because of their origin, microglia are part of the reticuloendothelial cell system. They wander in and out of the CNS in response to need. When damage occurs, the microglia mobilize and travel to the damaged tissue. They enlarge and phagocytize the debris.
3. Oligodendroglia help support the nervous tissue, but their primary function is the original formation of myelin in the CNS during fetal, neonatal, and early childhood years. Once the myelin has been formed, the oligodendroglia cannot form it again.
4. The ependyma is composed of special glial cells found lining the ventricles of the brain and the central canal of the spinal cord.

The spinal cord is the second part of the CNS. It is examined in Chap. 34.

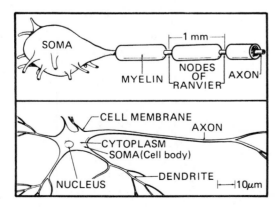

Figure 30-16. Schematic diagram of neuronal structures.

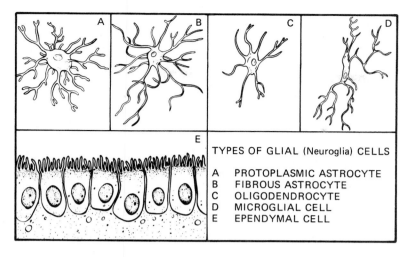

Figure 30-17. Types of glial cells (neuroglia).

Peripheral Nervous System

The peripheral nerves, the spinal nerves, and the cranial nerves form the peripheral nervous system. There are 31 pairs of spinal nerves and 12 pairs of cranial nerves.

The 31 pairs of spinal nerves are numbered in relation to the vertebral level at which they emerge from the spinal cord. Spinal nerves do not attach directly to the spinal cord. Instead, they attach to a short anterior (ventral, motor) root and a short posterior (dorsal, sensory) root (Fig. 30-18). The posterior root has a bulge called the spinal ganglion, which consists of neuronal cell bodies. There are 8 cervical, 12 thoracic, 5 lumbar, 5 sacral, and 1 coccygeal pairs of spinal ganglia.

Peripheral nerves often encompass more than one spinal nerve root. The sciatic nerve is a good example. It includes all the spinal nerve roots in the sacrum.

Spinal Nerve Fibers

The spinal nerves are composed of four types of nerve fibers:

1. Motor fibers, which originate in the ventral (anterior) horn of the spinal cord, with efferent fibers relaying motor impulses from the CNS to peripheral skeletal muscles.
2. Sensory fibers, which originate in the dorsal (posterior) horn of the spinal cord, with afferent fibers relaying sensory impulses from organs and muscles to the CNS.

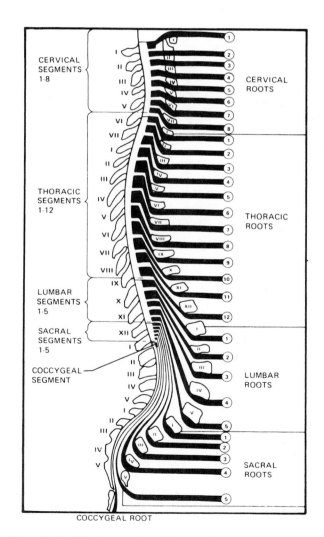

Figure 30-18. Spinal nerve roots and their attachment to the spinal cord.

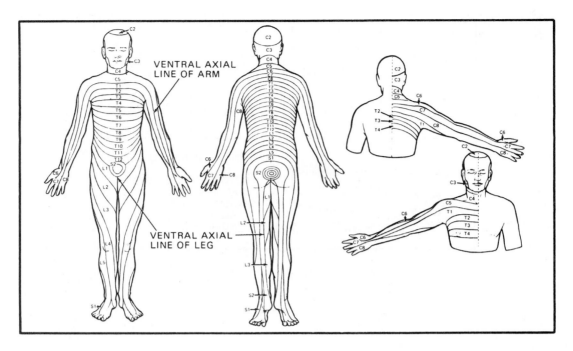

Figure 30-19. Dermatomes.

3. Meningeal fibers, which transmit sensory and vasomotor innervation to the spinal meninges.
4. Autonomic fibers, which are considered separately further on.

Dermatomes

Each spinal nerve's dorsal root innervates a specific portion of skin. These skin regions are called dermatomes (Fig. 30-19). They are clinically important in identifying areas of spinal cord injury.

Plexuses

The spinal nerves interweave in three areas called the cervical, brachial, and lumbosacral plexuses (Fig. 30-20). The cervical plexus involves spinal nerves C1 to C4. It sends motor impulses to neck muscles and the diaphragm and receives sensory impulses from the neck and head. The brachial plexus is composed of spinal nerves C4 to C8 and T1. It innervates the arms. The lumbosacral plexus is formed by spinal nerves L1 to L5 and S1 to S3. This plexus innervates the legs.

Cranial Nerves

Twelve pairs of cranial nerves complete the peripheral nervous system. Three pairs of cranial nerves are totally sensory, five pairs are totally motor, and four pairs are combined sensorimotor. The origins of the

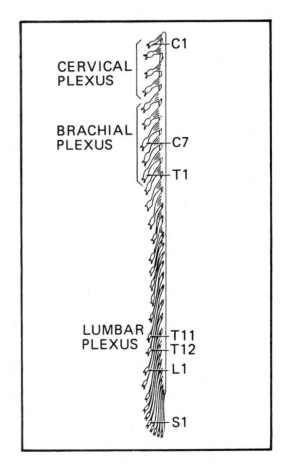

Figure 30-20. The three spinal nerve plexuses.

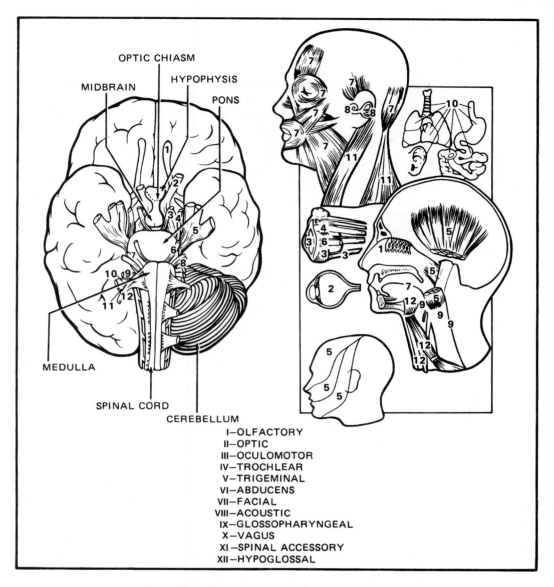

OPTIC CHIASM
MIDBRAIN
HYPOPHYSIS
PONS

MEDULLA
SPINAL CORD
CEREBELLUM

I—OLFACTORY
II—OPTIC
III—OCULOMOTOR
IV—TROCHLEAR
V—TRIGEMINAL
VI—ABDUCENS
VII—FACIAL
VIII—ACOUSTIC
IX—GLOSSOPHARYNGEAL
X—VAGUS
XI—SPINAL ACCESSORY
XII—HYPOGLOSSAL

Figure 30-21. Origins of the cranial nerves.

nerves are seen in Fig. 30-21. By convention, the cranial nerves are numbered by roman numerals as well as being named.

The cranial nerves are summarized in Table 30-2. The following mnemonic may help to keep them in order: *On Old Olympus' Towering Tops, A Finn And German Viewed Some Hops* (olfactory, optic, oculomotor; trochlear, trigeminal; abducens; facial; acoustic; glossopharyngeal; vagus; spinal accessory; hypoglossal).

Autonomic Nervous System

The sympathetic nervous system and the parasympathetic nervous system together form the autonomic nervous system. Technically, the autonomic nervous system is part of the peripheral nervous system. However, it seems easier to understand the autonomic nervous system if it is looked at as a separate system.

The sympathetic nervous system releases norepinephrine, which stimulates and prepares the body for "fight, fright, or flight." Norepinephrine and epinephrine are categorized as adrenergic chemicals (hormones). Fibers originating in the thoracic and lumbar areas form the peripheral sympathetic nervous system division.

The parasympathetic nervous system releases acetylcholine, which is categorized as a cholinergic chemical (hormone). In reality, the parasympathetic

TABLE 30-2. SUMMARY OF CRANIAL NERVES

Number	Name	Major Functions
I	Olfactory	Sense of smell
II	Optic	Central and peripheral vision
III	Oculomotor	Eye movement; elevation of upper eyelid; pupil constriction
IV	Trochlear	Downward and inward eye movement
V	Trigeminal	Touch, pain, temperature; jaw and eye muscle proprioception; mastication
VI	Abducens	Abduction of the eye
VII	Facial	Close eyelid, muscles of facial expression; secretion by glands of mouth and eyes; taste (anterior two-thirds of tongue)
VIII	Acoustic Vestibular branch	Equilibrium
	Cochlear branch	Hearing
IX	Glossopharyngeal	Movement of pharyngeal muscles; secretion by parotid glands; pharyngeal and posterior tongue sensation
X	Vagus	Pharyngeal and laryngeal movement; visceral activities; pharyngeal and laryngeal sensation; taste
XI	Spinal accessory	Pharyngeal, sternocleidomastoid, and trapezius movement
XII	Hypoglossal	Tongue movement

system is an antagonist to the sympathetic system and mediates or slows body responses when the "fight, fright, or flight" situation no longer exists. Fibers originating in the cranial and sacral areas form the peripheral parasympathetic nervous system division. Atropine is an example of a parasympathetic blocker.

Nerve Structures of the Autonomic Nervous System

The sympathetic nervous system has a chain of ganglia situated on both sides of the vertebrae (Fig. 30-22). Nerve fibers between the spinal cord and the ganglia are termed preganglionic fibers (or axons). The nerve fibers between the ganglia and visceral end organ are called postganglionic fibers (or axons). The norepinephrine that is released to maintain body functions is not easily or rapidly neutralized, so the effect is sustained for a period of time. The sympathetic system may be referred to as the thoracolumbar system, since major ganglia arise in the thoracic and lumbar regions.

The parasympathetic nervous system does not have a chain of ganglia next to the vertebral column. The preganglionic fibers (or axons) originate in the brain and sacrum (Fig. 30-23). These axons are long, allowing them to reach specific organs. Ganglia are found adjacent to or within specific organs. Postganglionic fibers (or axons) are, therefore, short. The chemical released by the parasympathetic system, acetylcholine, is rapidly neutralized by cholinesterase. Because of this, the parasympathetic effect is brief and must be renewed fairly regularly to counter the sympathetic stimulation. This system may be referred to as the craniosacral system, since the preganglionic fibers arise from certain cranial nerves and in the sacral spinal cord.

Neural Cell Depolarization and Repolarization

Depolarization and repolarization of the nerve cell follow the same principles as depolarization and repolarization of the cardiac cell.

Depolarization

The neuron in a resting state (resting membrane potential [RMP]) is positively charged outside the cell membrane and negatively charged on the inner surface of the cell membrane. When the cell is stimulated, sodium rapidly enters the cell and potassium leaves the cell. This produces a positive ionic charge at the entry site and decreases the RMP. This positive ionic charge is transmitted along the length of the neuron and is termed a wave of depolarization.

Repolarization

As soon as potassium reenters the cell and sodium leaves it, the resting state of the cell is reestablished.

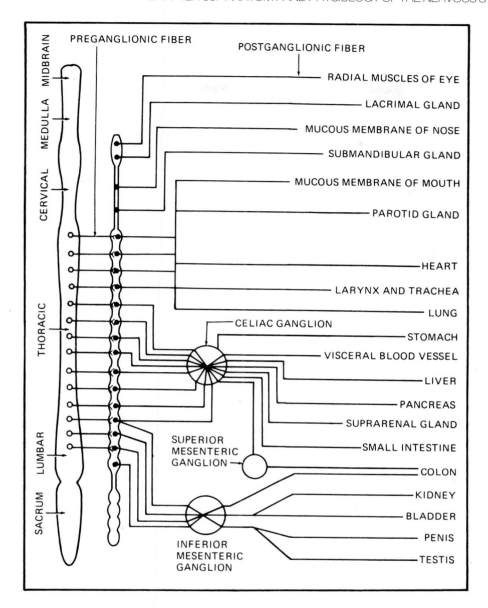

Figure 30-22. Ganglia of the sympathetic nervous system.

This is called repolarization. A specific mechanism exists to force the sodium ions that entered the cell's cytoplasm back into the extracellular fluid. This is termed the sodium pump. Without the sodium pump, ion homeostasis could not be preserved. At the same time, a potassium pump exists to maintain potassium ion homeostasis by forcing potassium ions back into the cell.

An action potential occurs when an ionic charge on one side of the membrane is different from an ionic charge on the other. Depolarization occurs when a stimulus is strong enough (threshold) to alter the cell membrane's permeability to sodium, allowing a change in the ionic charge. (Sodium ions enter and potassium ions leave the cell's interior.) Once an action potential exists and a stimulus of threshold-level magnitude occurs, the neuron totally depolarizes, following the all-or-none principle. It depolarizes in its entirety or else it does not depolarize at all. As with the cardiac cell, the neuron has a complete refractory period during which it is repolarizing and cannot be stimulated. Also, like the cardiac cell, the neuron has a relative refractory period. During this period, it can be stimulated (or excited), but only when the stimulus is at a threshold level.

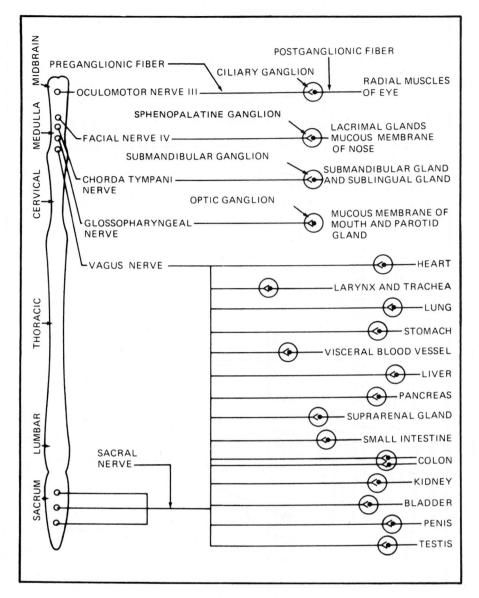

Figure 30-23. Ganglionic fibers of the parasympathetic nervous system.

Two terms are important in relation to action potentials. *Summation* refers to repetitive, accumulated discharges that eventually reach threshold level (much like placing building blocks one on top of the other until the top is reached). *Facilitation* is an increase in every subsequent neuronal stimulus even though the stimulus remains below threshold levels. No action potential occurs in facilitation. An action potential does occur in summation.

The rapid velocity at which the impulse is conducted is due in part to the neuron's structure (Fig. 30-24) and the size of the nerve fiber. Myelin is a protective, lipid insulation of the neuron that is nonconductive. This prevents an easy flow of ions

into the nerve fiber. The myelin sheath is segmented. At specified intervals, the myelin sheath is totally absent. These noninsulated points are called nodes of Ranvier. Ions flow easily around the nerve

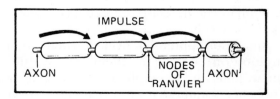

Figure 30-24. Nodes of Ranvier providing saltatory conduction.

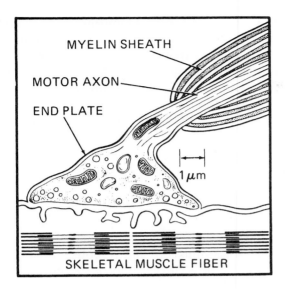

Figure 30-25. Chemical synapse.

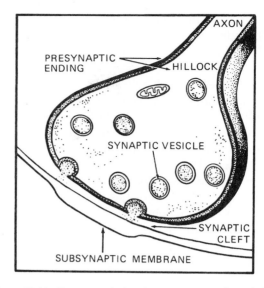

Figure 30-26. Neuromuscular junction or neuromuscular end plate.

fiber at these nodes. The action potential on myelinated nerve fibers jumps from one node to the next. This is called saltatory conduction and is far faster than conduction in an unmyelinated fiber. In unmyelinated fibers, the impulse must travel the entire length of the neuron.

Chemical Synapses

A synapse is a point of junction but not of contact between one neuron and another, a muscle cell, or a gland cell. Synapses differ in shape and size but function similarly in transmitting impulses.

The neuron's axon enlarges at its end, forming a synaptic knob. This knob may be called a terminal button or a presynaptic terminal (Fig. 30-25). The synaptic knob contains vesicles filled with specific neurotransmitter chemicals. When the axonal knob is stimulated, these chemicals are released. The presynaptic terminal is separated from the postsynaptic side by a minute space termed the synaptic cleft. The postsynaptic membrane is slightly thicker at the synaptic cleft than elsewhere and is termed the subsynaptic membrane. The extra thickness is thought to be due to an increased number of receptor sites for the neurotransmitter.

When the axons of a motor neuron synapse with skeletal muscle, the presynaptic terminal (synaptic knob) is called a neuromuscular junction or a neuromuscular end plate (Fig. 30-26). At this specific synapse, the presynaptic terminal looks like a plate. The neuromuscular junction is the only synapse specifically named.

Neurotransmitters

Acetylcholine

Acetylcholine is the neurotransmitter chemical found in the vesicles of neuromuscular junctions and in the parasympathetic system. Acetylcholine is the primary neurotransmitter of the peripheral nervous system. As the action potential in the axon reaches the neuromuscular junction, the neuromuscular junction is stimulated to release the chemical in its vesicles. The chemical diffuses across the synaptic cleft, coming in contact with receptors on the postsynaptic membrane. Acetylcholine acts on the postsynaptic membrane briefly before it is neutralized by the enzyme acetylcholinesterase (ACH). The milliseconds during which acetylcholine is in contact with the postsynaptic membrane are enough to propagate conduction of an impulse. The enzyme is found in abundance in skeletal muscles and blood, so it very rapidly breaks down acetylcholine into acetic acid and choline. This rapid degradation of acetylcholine ensures that only one action potential occurs at a time at the receptor sites on the postsynaptic membrane. The end products (acetic acid and choline) are resynthesized in the synaptic vesicles for use again.

The end result of the release of acetylcholine at many peripheral synapses is muscular contraction. The amount of acetylcholine released is determined in part by the diffusion of calcium ions into the presynaptic terminal. Calcium ions are necessary for depolarization at other peripheral synapses, so it is assumed that calcium plays a similar role at all chemical synapses.

Acetylcholine is a cholinergic neurotransmitter. It is thought that more cholinergic synapses exist in the CNS, but they have not been positively identified.

Monoamines

The monoamines that have been identified as neurotransmitters in the CNS include the catecholamines dopamine, norepinephrine, and epinephrine and the indolamine serotonin. Catecholamines are produced in the brain and in the sympathetic ganglia from their amino acid precursor tyrosine. Serotonin is produced in the brain and other tissues from the amino acid tryptophan. The activity of the monoamine neurotransmitters in the synaptic cleft is limited by their reuptake into the presynaptic ending, where they are recycled into vesicles for future release.

Dopamine

Dopamine is a precursor of epinephrine and norepinephrine. Dopamine acts as an inhibitory chemical transmitter and is among the most important chemicals involved in basal ganglionic functions (acetylcholine is the other important transmitter in basal ganglionic functions). Dopamine is decreased in the brains of patients with parkinsonism. It may play a role in eating, drinking, and sexual behavior.

Epinephrine and Norepinephrine

Epinephrine and norepinephrine are found in adrenergic fibers of the sympathetic nervous system. In the CNS, norepinephrine cell bodies are confined to the brainstem, but their axons extend to all parts of the CNS. Epinephrine neurons are restricted to the lower brainstem.

Like dopamine, norepinephrine has been found to have inhibitory influences on postsynaptic neurons. Little is known of the action of epinephrine as a central neurotransmitter. Within the sympathetic nervous system, epinephrine and norepinephrine are found in adrenergic fibers. They are responsible for exerting a generalized "fight, flight, or fright" response.

Serotonin

Serotonin is also a monoamine chemical. It is an inhibitory transmitter and is linked to slow-wave sleep patterns. Although it has been suggested that serotonin plays a physiologic role in sleep, psychotic states, pain transmission, and response to hallucinogenic drugs, little is known about its specific functions.

Gamma-aminobutyric Acid

Gamma-aminobutyric acid (GABA) is a neutral amino acid that has an inhibitory effect on synaptic function. It is found in the CNS.

Reflexes

A reflex is a stereotypical reaction of the CNS to specific sensory stimuli. There are two types of reflexes: monosynaptic and polysynaptic.

Monosynaptic Reflex Arc

This constitutes the simplest reflex in the body and is depicted in Fig. 30-27. Inside every group of muscles is a structure called a muscle spindle, which is made up of small fibers bound together by afferent sensory

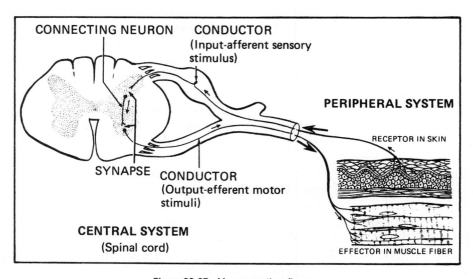

Figure 30-27. Monosynaptic reflex arc.

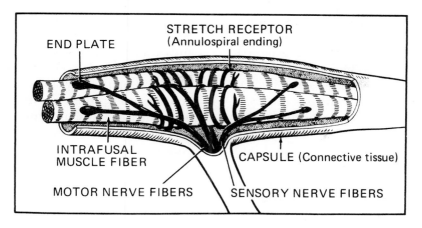

Figure 30-28. Muscle spindle.

fibers (Fig. 30-28). As a muscle spindle is stretched, an action potential develops and a sensory impulse travels to the dorsal root ganglion. From the ganglion the impulse enters the spinal cord. In the gray matter (unmyelinated) of the spinal cord, the impulse synapses with interneurons in the anterior portion of the cord. These interneurons have efferent (motor) fibers that leave the spinal cord through the anterior (ventral) root. The efferent fibers carry an impulse back to the original muscle. The muscle contracts upon receiving this impulse.

The monosynaptic reflex arc is more important in research than in practice. However, the muscle stretch reflex (knee jerk) is the one most commonly tested.

Polysynaptic Reflex Arc

The withdrawal reflex is a common example of the polysynaptic reflex (Fig. 30-29). Afferent nerve fibers in the peripheral muscles are excited, producing an impulse. This impulse enters the spinal cord via a dorsal root ganglion. This excited neuron will synapse with appropriate interneurons within the gray matter of the spinal cord.

The interneurons in the anterior (ventral) horn emerge from the spinal cord through efferent (motor) fibers. These fibers transmit the motor impulse to the original muscle that produced the sensory impulse. The muscle then contracts. There are literally hundreds of interneurons with which the impulse could and does synapse; thus, the name polysynaptic reflex arc.

When impulses effect a muscular contraction, other impulses must negate the function of opposing muscle groups. For the knee to bend, extensor muscles must be inhibited and flexor muscles concurrently excited. This is termed the law of reciprocal innervation.

Metabolism in the Brain

Both white matter (myelinated) and gray matter (unmyelinated) have the same metabolic needs.

The cerebral need for oxygen does not decrease in a resting state. Even though it weighs only about

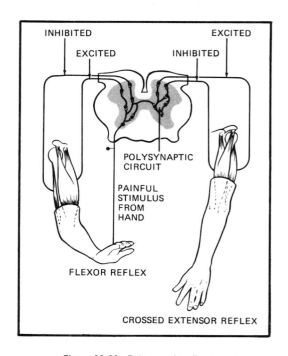

Figure 30-29. Polysynaptic reflex arc.

3 lb (2% of the body weight), brain tissue requires about 20% of the body's oxygen supply. The brain needs a constant supply of oxygen and is unable to store oxygen for future use. The energy necessary for the brain's metabolic functions is obtained from the oxidation of glucose. All oxidative reactions require oxygen. Hypoxia may occur without irreversible anoxic injury to brain cells. If the anoxic state lasts 4 min or more at normal body temperature, cerebral neurons are destroyed. Once destroyed, cerebral neurons cannot regenerate. The area of the brain most sensitive to hypoxia is the telencephalon, particularly the hippocampus, which is most likely to be damaged by small amounts of decreased oxygen. Since the cerebral cortex is only six layers (cells) deep (Fig. 30-7), the entire cerebral cortex, especially layer four, is very sensitive to decreases in oxygen. Damage here results in a condition termed laminar cortical necrosis.

The brainstem is the area most resistant to hypoxic damage. If hypoxia occurs in this area beyond the 4- to 5-min limit, irreversible coma or a persistent vegetative state usually develops.

Nutritional Needs

The extensive, continuous activity of the brain results in very high metabolic energy needs. Glucose, a carbohydrate, is the main source of energy (adenosine triphosphate [ATP]) for cellular activity. Glucose and oxygen are essential for reestablishing electrochemical gradients for impulse transmission, for the synthesis of neurotransmitters, and for maintaining cellular integrity. If the cerebral glucose level is less than 70 mg/100 mL, confusion results. With a glucose level of less than 20 mg/100 mL, coma develops, followed by death if there is no treatment. Whereas hypoglycemia causes confusion, coma, and death, hyperglycemia does not appear to have a direct influence on nervous system functions. Certain vitamins are essential in adequate amounts to ensure normal CNS functions.

Vitamin B_1 (thiamine) is important in the Krebs' cycle of energy production. Insufficient B_1, common in alcoholics, causes the Wernicke-Korsakoff syndrome, which in late stages causes cerebellar degeneration.

The function of vitamin B_{12} is not understood. However, insufficient B_{12} results in a gradual degeneration of the brain, optic nerves, spinal cord (especially posterior and lateral columns), and dorsal root entry zone of the peripheral nerves. Degeneration often starts with the spinal cord. Pernicious anemia is the dominant systemic disease of vitamin B_{12} deficiency. A deficiency is also present in alcoholism and other malnutritional states.

Pyridoxine is a coenzyme that participates in many enzymatic reactions in the CNS. Pyridoxine deficiencies produce polyneuropathies, seborrheic dermatitis, glossitis, and conjunctivitis.

Nicotinic acid is needed for synthesis of coenzymes. Insufficient nicotinic acid results in altered mentation, leading to coma, extrapyramidal rigidity, and tremors of the extremities. This form of encephalopathy seems to be becoming nonexistent in the United States. There may be a relationship between inadequate nicotinic acid and pellagra.

Circulatory Needs

The brain needs a more continuous supply of oxygenated blood, even during sleep, than any other organ because the brain's needs are never decreased. The cerebral blood flow (CBF) is the cerebral perfusion pressure (CPP) divided by cerebrovascular resistance, the difference between mean arterial (systemic) pressure (MAP) and intracranial pressure (ICP) (CPP = MAP − ICP). The size of the cerebrovascular system, activity, disease, fever, injury, and other factors determine the actual amount of blood needed at any given time.

Autoregulation. Hypercapnia ($PaCO_2$ >45 mm Hg) and to a lesser extent hypoxia (PaO_2 <60 mm Hg) will cause an arteriolar dilatation of the cerebral arteries, thus increasing the amount of blood flowing into the brain regardless of the actual amount needed. This may cause an increase in ICP that the healthy brain can accommodate but that an injured or diseased brain may not be able to accommodate. The brain has its own autoregulatory mechanism, which functions mainly by increasing (constricting arteries) resistance to blood flow or by decreasing (dilatation of arteries) resistance to blood flow, thus altering the diameter of the vessels. Autoregulation maintains constant blood flow over a range of perfusion pressures. The limits of autoregulation are generally thought to be an MAP between 50 and 150 mm Hg. This system works well until the ICP increases beyond a certain unknown point, when compensatory mechanisms fail. Hypocapnia ($PaCO_2$ <35 mm Hg) causes arteriolar constriction of the cerebral arteries and may be harmful to the brain due to a decrease in delivery of oxygenated blood. Balancing the $PaCO_2$ is imperative in optimizing CBF.

Increases in ICP will result in a decrease in blood perfusion to the brain because of compression of the arteries, veins, and brain mass as a whole.

Blood-Brain Barrier

A barrier is known to exist between the blood and brain, which controls the diffusion of substances from the blood into the extracellular fluid or CSF of the brain. The location and structure of this carrier is thought to be related to the "tight junctions" of cerebral endothelial cells. The permeability of cerebral capillaries and the choroid plexus controls the movement of specific substances.

Water, oxygen, glucose, and carbon dioxide move quickly through the blood-brain barrier. Other substances either move slowly or not at all across the barrier. This control determines the level of metabolism, ionic composition, and homeostasis of cerebral tissue.

In addition to a blood-brain barrier, there is a blood-CSF barrier. This barrier functions like the blood-brain barrier in controlling the composition of the CSF. This is a vitally important function because substances in the CSF are rapidly absorbed into the interstitial brain fluid.

Intracranial Pressure

In this chapter, the concepts of intracranial pressure are covered. Expect one to three questions on the PCCN exam to refer to the contents of this chapter.

The concepts of intracranial pressure (ICP) are fundamental to caring for any acute care neurology patient. Whether patients have sustained a severe traumatic brain injury, experienced a stroke, brain tumors, hemorrhage, hydrocephalus, or undergone a craniotomy, the pathophysiologic changes may lead to cerebral edema and increased ICP. An understanding of the dynamics of ICP and the prioritization of interventions to maintain perfusion are key to minimizing injury to the brain.

PHYSIOLOGY OF ICP

The volume of the cranial vault is about 80% brain tissue, 10% cerebrospinal fluid (CSF), and 10% intravascular fluid (blood). Together, these three components almost completely fill the cranial vault.

The adult cranial vault is nondistensible (it is bone), and the components of the vault are essentially noncompressible. Based on these tenets, a relationship between the vault and its contents is construed. The Monro-Kellie doctrine provides the framework for reviewing physiology and treatments for elevated ICP. The hypothesis states that brain tissue, blood volume, and CSF are balanced in a state of dynamic equilibrium. If an increase occurs in the relative volume of one component, such as CSF, the volume of one or more of the other components must decrease or an elevation in ICP will result. Within a very narrow range, the contents of the cranial vault can adjust to increases in ICP. When the limits of range and time are exceeded, the ICP rises precipitously.

Compensatory Mechanisms for ICP

Initial increases in the volume of the cranium are compensated for by two mechanisms, compression of the low-pressure venous system and the displacement of CSF.

1. A decrease in intravascular fluid (blood) occurs by compression of the low-pressure venous system. Intravascular volume is the most alterable of the three components of the cranium (brain tissue, CSF, and blood). There is a specific limit to the extent of compressibility. When this limit is exceeded, ICP rises.
2. Displacement of CSF is the compensatory mechanism for increasing ICP. As the ICP rises, CSF is displaced from the cranial vault into the spinal subarachnoid space. When maximal displacement of CSF has occurred, there is probably an increase in CSF absorption, which aids compensatory mechanisms.

These mechanisms function to keep the ICP constant. They function well when the ICP increases slowly. Even then, the mechanisms will lose their compensatory function at a certain point (variable with the individual). If the ICP rises rapidly, the compensatory mechanisms cannot function.

Intracranial Compliance

The brain's ability to adjust to increases in its contents refers to compliance. This is the relationship of change in volume for a given change in pressure. When the brain is compliant (compliance is high), increases in the volume of the content do not produce increases in ICP. When a state of noncompliance occurs (compliance is low), small increases in the contents of the cranial vault result in a large increase in ICP.

Intracranial pressure represents the ever-changing relationship between the brain, blood, and CSF inside the cranial vault. In adults, the normal ICP range is 5 to 15 mm Hg. An increase in ICP greater than 20 mm Hg is considered elevated and treatment measures are generally initiated at that level. Intracranial hypertension is defined as an ICP greater than 20 mm Hg that persists for 5 min or longer. The control of ICP elevations is an important aspect of the management of severe traumatic brain injury and other intracranial pathologies since sustained increases in ICP can result in decreases in the delivery of oxygenated blood to the brain as well as herniation and compression of the brain and brainstem. Without interventions to reduce the ICP, blood flow to the brain is compromised. The comprehension of blood-flow dynamics is essential to managing ICP.

Cerebral Blood flow

The brain requires approximately 50 mL/100 g/min of arterial blood flow. Decreases below 18 mL/100 g/min cause ischemia. If such conditions are not corrected, intracellular chaos will ensue, leading to edema and destruction of cells. Cerebral blood flow (CBF) is calculated by measuring the cerebral perfusion pressure (CPP) and dividing it by the cerebrovascular resistance. The CPP is used as a primary means to approximate the delivery of blood flow. CPP is the difference between the mean arterial pressure (MAP) and the mean ICP (CPP = MAP − ICP). In severe head injury, the minimal acceptable CPP is 50 to 70 mm Hg. When the CPP declines below this threshold, there is a risk that the cerebrovasculature will vasodilate, leading to worsening of ICP. The optimal or target CPP for patients should be individualized. Many factors influence the CBF besides the CPP. Autoregulation controls the CBF through many mechanisms. Globally, autoregulation maintains a constant CBF by vasodilating or vasoconstricting cerebral arteries normally during an MAP of 50 to 150 mm Hg despite increases or decreases in blood pressure. The CBF is altered due to metabolic changes in arterial carbon dioxide (CO_2) and oxygen (O_2). When $PaCO_2$ is high, vasodilation occurs, while a low $PaCO_2$ causes vasoconstriction of the cerebral arteries. A PaO_2 below 50 mm Hg leads to vasodilation. In addition, the blood's pH influences the CBF, with acidosis causing vasodilation and alkalosis causing vasoconstriction. All of these influences contribute to the delivery of blood to the cranium. By keeping the ICP low, an adequate CBF is promoted. With elevated ICP, the CBF is manipulated in an attempt to reduce blood volume and thus to decrease ICP.

CAUSES OF INCREASED ICP

A number of pathologies can potentially increase ICP. Remember that the contents of the cranium include the brain, CSF, and blood. The volume of the brain can increase with tissue swelling from trauma, stroke, or surgical manipulation; mass lesions such as brain tumors; or bleeding into the parenchyma. Alteration in the amount of CSF inside the cranium is caused by obstruction of CSF pathways, inability to reabsorb CSF, or overproduction of CSF. Increase in the blood content in the cranium occurs as a result of tearing of arteries/veins, creating hematomas, impairment in venous drainage from the brain by compression of neck veins, positioning the head of bed flat, increased intrathoracic or intra-abdominal pressure, and in response to the injury where the CBF dramatically rises, creating hyperemia. Other pathologies may lead to increased ICP, such as hypoxic brain injury, electrolyte abnormalities, infectious disease processes, and toxins. When any of these etiologies occur, it is prudent to measure the pressure inside the cranial vault.

Intracranial Mass Lesions

Intracranial mass lesions include intracranial space-occupying lesions such as tumors or abscesses that occur within the cranium or skull, vascular lesions (e.g., thrombosis, emboli), and lesions due to trauma. The symptoms of intracranial mass lesions are caused by a combination of increased ICP (headache, vomiting, confusion, coma) and focal neurologic brain tissue damage (hemiparesis, aphasia). The most frequent presenting symptoms are headache, drowsiness, confusion, seizures, hemiparesis, or speech difficulties. The symptoms and findings depend largely on the specific location within the brain.

Intracerebral Hemorrhage. Hemorrhage may result from trauma such as skull fracture, penetrating injury (bullets), contrecoup decelerative forces, and systemic diseases such as leukemia and aplastic anemia. If the hemorrhage occurs in the internal capsule of the brain, paralysis results. If the hemorrhage occurs in the dominant hemisphere, dysfunction is variable, depending on the location of hemorrhage. Signs and symptoms include nausea, vomiting, dizziness, headache, signs of increasing ICP, and a contralateral hemiplegia. A delayed intracerebral hemorrhage may occur hours to days after a closed head injury.

Subarachnoid Hemorrhage. Symptoms usually include headache, dizziness, tinnitus, facial pain (pressure on the fifth cranial nerve), ptosis, a unilaterally dilated pupil, nuchal rigidity, and hemiparesis or hemiplegia.

Arteriovenous Malformation. Arteriovenous malformations (AVMs) are defects of the circulatory system that are believed to arise during fetal development. They can occur in various parts of the body and when occuring in the brain are called cerebral AVMs. An AVM occurs as a result of abnormal configurations of the arterial and venous circulation network in which capillaries are replaced by larger sized blood vessels called shunts. The result is that the very high pressure in the arteries is no longer dampened by the capillaries, and the veins now experience the same high pressure as the arteries, and this can result in intracerebral bleeding and a hemorrhagic stroke. Symptoms of AVM vary according to the location of the malformation and often include headache, weakness, aphasia, vertigo, or seizures. An AVM is typically treated with surgical repair, radiation, or embolization.

Hydrocephalus. Hydrocephalus results from an abnormal accumulation of CSF in the ventricles, or cavities, of the brain. Hydrocephalus can cause increased ICP, seizures, and mental disability.

Hydrocephalus is usually due to blockage of CSF outflow in the ventricles or in the subarachnoid space, or from impaired reabsorption or excessive CSF production. Other causes include congenital malformation blocking normal drainage of the fluid, or from complications of head injuries or infections.

There are two main classifications of hydrocephalus: communicating and noncommunicating (obstructive). Both forms can be either congenital or acquired.

Communicating hydrocephalus, also known as nonobstructive hydrocephalus, is caused by impaired CSF reabsorption in the absence of any CSF flow obstruction between the ventricles and subarachnoid space. Several conditions that may result in communicating hydrocephalus include subarachnoid/intraventricular hemorrhage, meningitis, and scarring or fibrosis of the subarachnoid space following infectious, inflammatory, or hemorrhagic events.

Normal-pressure hydrocephalus is a form of communicating hydrocephalus characterized by enlarged cerebral ventricles, with only intermittently elevated CSF pressure.

Noncommunicating hydrocephalus, or obstructive hydrocephalus, is caused by a CSF flow obstruction that prevents CSF from flowing into the subarachnoid space (either due to external compression or intraventricular mass lesions).

Hydrocephalus can result in signs of increased ICP including headaches, vomiting, nausea, papilledema, sleepiness, or coma. Sustained elevated ICP may result in uncal and/or cerebellar herniation, with resulting life-threatening brain stem compression.

The treatment of hydrocephalus is surgical and involves the placement of a ventriculostomy to drain the excess CSF fluid or a shunt to redirect the CSF into other body cavities, from where it can be reabsorbed. Most shunts drain the fluid into the peritoneal cavity (ventriculoperitoneal shunt), but alternative sites include the right atrium or pleural cavity (ventriculopleural shunt).

Other Nursing Interventions

The control of body temperature is imperative in neurologic disorders. Optimally, the temperature is maintained at 36°C to 37°C. Temperature elevations above 37°C should be avoided due to increase in oxygen consumption by the brain and worsening neurologic outcomes, especially in patients with head injuries and stroke.

Nursing activities should be spaced out to ensure adequate rest periods for the patient with increased ICP. Keeping the room quiet with low lighting ensures a decrease in stimulation. The use of familiar touch by family and purposeful touch by team members may decrease ICP. Avoid excessive coughing, as this could increase the ICP. Glucocorticoids may be used to decrease cerebral edema in patients with brain tumors. The use of glucocorticoids in patients with head injuries is usually not indicated.

Patients with intracranial pathology are at risk for or actually have increased ICP. Nursing activities and interventions can minimize the impact of these pathologies on the brain.

32

Acute Head Injuries and Craniotomies

EDITORS' NOTE

The primary focus of this chapter is on head injury and space-occupying lesions (brain tumors). The PCCN exam may include several questions on the content covered in this chapter.

INTRODUCTION TO HEAD INJURIES

Acute traumatic brain injuries (TBIs) are caused by blunt, penetrating, or blast mechanisms. They commonly occur as a result of motor vehicle accidents, falls, assaults, or sports injuries. The incidence of TBI is higher in men than women and higher in persons aged 15 to 24 years and those older than 75 years. They can be classified by severity using the Glasgow Coma Scale (GCS). Mild brain injury refers to patients with a GCS score of 13 to 15; moderate injury indicates a GCS score of 9 to 12, and patients with a score of 8 or less are categorized as having severe brain injury. The damage caused by the event produces a primary injury to the brain, blood vessels, cranial nerves, or supporting structures. Primary injury occurs due to the biomechanical effects of trauma on the brain and skull as a result of the initial injury. Injuries are categorized as focal and diffuse.

Focal injuries include cerebral contusions, coup-contrecoup injuries where injury occurs both at the side of impact and the contralateral side, brain lacerations, cranial nerve injuries, and tearing of arteries/veins in the brain. Arterial tears of the middle meningeal artery produce epidural hematomas. Tearing of the bridging cortical veins produces subdural hematomas. Tears of small vessels can produce traumatic subarachnoid hemorrhage. Diffuse injuries are produced by twisting and turning of the brain tissue at the time of injury and can result in axonal damage. Mild diffuse injuries are called cerebral concussions and result in a brief, less than 15 min, alteration in consciousness. Severe diffuse axonal injury produces profound coma and severe derangement of the axons, with cerebral swelling and ischemia. The impact to the brain extends beyond the primary event. In addition to the primary source of injury, cytotoxic processes such as release of calcium, excitatory amino acids, and oxygen-free radicals can cause progressive cellular damage for up to 6 h following the primary injury.

Following the primary event, the brain is susceptible to secondary brain injury, which is defined as any subsequent injury to the brain after the initial insult. Secondary brain injury can result from hypotension, hypoxia, hypocapnia, elevated intracranial pressure (ICP), infection, anemia, elevated temperature, electrolyte imbalances, or the biochemical changes initiated by the original trauma. The treatment of head injury is directed at recognizing and treating the primary injury produced by the traumatic event. It is also directed at preventing or minimizing secondary brain injury.

A focused neurologic examination establishes the level of consciousness and responses to stimulation or pain.

CLASSIFICATION OF INJURY

A TBI occurs as the result of blunt trauma (direct blow to the head) or from penetrating trauma (e.g., gunshot wound). Blunt injury occurs as a result of a number of factors including:

Deceleration: the head is moving and strikes a stationary object (e.g., stairs).

Acceleration: a moving object (e.g., hammer) strikes the head.

Acceleration-deceleration: the brain moves rapidly within the skull, resulting in a combination of injury-causing forces.

Rotation: twisting motion of the brain occurs within the skull, usually due to side impact.

Deformation/compression: Direct injury to the head changes the shape of the skull, resulting in compression of brain tissue.

Closed Head Injuries

In a closed head injury, the scalp is intact and there is no break in the skull bones. As described above, the injuries produced at the time of the event are classified as diffuse or focal primary injuries.

Diffuse Head Injury

Concussion. Blunt trauma to the head by an accelerative or decelerative force causes a stretch injury to the axons in the brain. This type of injury occurs along a continuum with diffuse axonal injury (DAI) on the severe end and concussion on the mild end. It is generally believed that the axons sustain a stretch injury in concussion. The two types of concussions are mild and classic concussion. Clinically, the duration of unconsciousness may alter the description of the injury, but the primary consideration is that of neurologic deficit. Cortical dysfunction (attention span and memory) occurs with mild concussion and results from a temporary axonal disturbance. There is no loss of consciousness. Momentary confusion and disorientation may be seen with post-traumatic amnesia (antegrade and retrograde). The patient with classic concussion will have recovered consciousness within 30 min. Persistent symptoms of confusion, dizziness, headache, and nausea may persist for days following the concussion.

Although the patient may appear to have recovered, postconcussive syndrome can develop. Postconcussive syndrome presents within weeks to 1 year later. The symptoms are headache, dizziness, irritability, emotional lability, fatigue, poor concentration, decreased attention span, memory difficulties, depression, and intellectual dysfunction.

Brainstem Injury. Brainstem injury is associated with other diffuse cerebral injury. An immediate loss of consciousness with pupillary changes and posturing will be seen. On examination, cranial nerve deficits and changes in vital functions, such as respiratory rate and rhythm, are present. These injuries are classified as diffuse axonal injuries.

Diffuse Axonal Injury. Diffuse axonal injury (DAI) is also known as diffuse neuronal injury or shearing injury. Damage to nerve fibers is produced by linear and rotational shear strains following high-speed deceleration injuries. The injury disconnects the cerebral hemispheres from the reticular activating system. A DAI is characterized by immediate coma. Mild DAI involves loss of consciousness lasting 6 to 24 h. Basal skull fractures are associated with moderate DAI. Severe DAI is seen with primary brainstem injuries. Such patients present with prolonged coma, increased ICP, hypertension, and fever. Prognosis is poor.

Focal Head Injury

Contusion. Owing to accelerative or decelerative blunt trauma forces to the head, the cerebral cortex may bruise. These forces propel the brain against the rigid cranium (the coup force). With initial impact, the brain is then rotated or thrown back in the opposite direction (the contrecoup force), as shown in Fig. 32-1. This trauma invariably results in cerebral bruising and edema. Most susceptible to bruising are the inferior frontal and temporal lobes. Contusions are visible on computed tomography (CT) or magnetic resonance imaging (MRI) of the brain. The contusions may not appear for 6 to 24 h after the event.

If the forces are strong enough, lacerations and scattered intracerebral hemorrhages may occur. These usually occur along the axis line of the coup and contrecoup forces. Mild contusions will clear as the bruising and edema resolve, leaving no neurologic deficit. Temporal lobe contusions carry a great risk of swelling and brain herniation. Some patients present with a period of lucidity, which is followed by rapid deterioration and death without surgical intervention. Severe contusions that do not resolve, as indicated by continuing coma, indicate that the original bruising and/or lacerations caused a necrosis of brain tissue (possibly secondary to prolonged cerebral hypoxia at the injury sites).

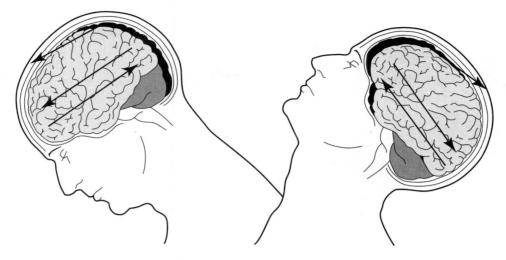

Figure 32-1. Coup and contracoup forces.

Acute Epidural Hematoma. Epidural hematomas are true neurosurgical emergencies. They occur at the time of the injury (Fig. 32-2) and are usually associated with a temporal or parietal skull fracture with laceration of the middle meningeal artery (and often vein). There is usually a loss of consciousness, which may be followed by a brief period (up to 4 to 6 h) of lucidity, followed by increasing restlessness, agitation, and confusion progressing to coma in one-third of patients. During the lucid period, nausea and vomiting often occur. Other signs may include ipsilateral oculomotor paralysis and seizures, contralateral hemiparesis/hemiplegia, and positive Babinski's

reflexes. As the hematoma increases in size, uncal herniation is the most common type to occur.

In one type of epidural hematoma, the linear fracture occurs across the sagittal sinus or the transverse sinus. In this instance, venous blood oozes into the area above the dura mater, producing a venous epidural hematoma. Symptoms may be delayed for several days.

Subdural Hematomas. Subdural hematomas are the most common type and have the highest mortality rate. There are three types of subdural hematomas: acute, subacute, and chronic forms. Subdural hematomas develop from bleeding in the subdural space between the dura mater and the arachnoid.

In the acute subdural hematoma (Fig. 32-3), symptoms occur usually within hours to several days. Acute subdural hematomas usually present with signs of increasing ICP, decreasing loss of consciousness (LOC), and ipsilateral oculomotor paralysis with contralateral hemiparesis. The signs and symptoms are those of a rapidly expanding mass lesion.

From 48 h to 2 weeks after the initial injury a subacute subdural hematoma may develop, requiring surgery. A steady decline in level of responsiveness indicates a potential subacute hematoma. Symptoms include headaches, slowness in thinking, confusion, and sometimes agitation. These symptoms progressively worsen.

In the chronic subdural hematoma, a period of weeks may follow the low-impact injury before symptoms occur, generally in the elderly. Symptoms include changes in personality, confusion, occasional headaches, problems walking, incontinence,

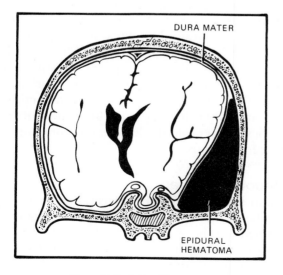

Figure 32-2. Epidural hematoma.

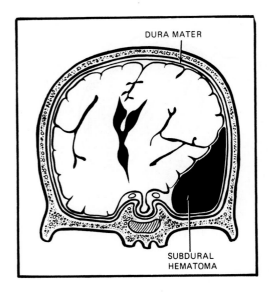

Figure 32-3. Subdural hematoma.

and rarely a seizure. The ICP may be normal, elevated, or decreased.

Subdural hematomas may occur spontaneously without any form of injury in patients on anticoagulant therapy or in those with clotting dysfunction. A CT scan will provide a diagnosis. Surgery is the treatment of choice.

Skull Fractures

Skull fractures are usually classified as linear, depressed, or basilar. A linear skull fracture that does not tear the dura mater will heal without treatment. If the linear fracture occurs over the temporal lobe and tears the dura (Fig. 32-4), there is a chance

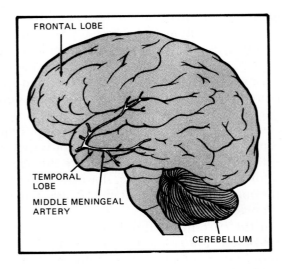

Figure 32-4. Linear skull fracture over the middle meningeal artery.

that the middle meningeal artery will also be torn. Such an injury constitutes a medical emergency, since the bleeding is arterial; this is commonly known as an acute epidural hematoma. The fracture may tear the dura mater over a venous sinus, resulting in slow bleeding that causes a chronic (nonacute) epidural hematoma. A depressed skull fracture that is *not* depressed more than the thickness of the skull is usually just monitored. However, a depressed skull fracture greater than the thickness of the skull (usually <5 to 7 mm) requires surgery to relieve the compression. Assessment of the extent of brain injury is essential. If the dura is torn, bone fragments may have entered brain tissue, requiring removal within 24 h, and the chance of infection is greatly increased.

With a basilar skull fracture there is a high risk of injury to cranial nerves, infection, and residual neurologic deficits due to coup and contrecoup forces (Fig. 32-5). Basilar fractures may occur in the anterior, middle, or posterior fossa. "Raccoon eyes" is a sign of bleeding into the paranasal sinuses and refers to ecchymosis developing around the eyes. Along with cerebrospinal fluid (CSF) draining from the nose (rhinorrhea), these signs indicate a basilar fracture in the anterior fossa. Draining of CSF from the ear canal (otorrhea) is a sign of a middle fossa basilar skull fracture. A temporal or basilar fracture in the posterior fossa is indicated by Battle's sign, an area of ecchymosis over the mastoid projection. Other symptoms of basilar fracture include tinnitus, facial paralysis, hearing difficulty, nystagmus, and conjugate deviation of gaze.

Patients with rhinorrhea will complain of a salty taste as the CSF drains into the pharynx. Caution the patient against blowing the nose, and avoid suctioning or nasal packing if rhinorrhea is present. Otorrhea can be tested for glucose. (Laboratory testing is more accurate than glucose testing sticks.) If glucose is present, the drainage is CSF. The "halo sign," a yellow ring that appears around bloody drainage on a nose or ear pad, is another indication of CSF leakage. The goal is early detection of intracranial fluid leakage and prevention of infection. Severe neurologic deficits are common with basilar fractures.

Compound Injuries

Compound injuries involve a laceration of the scalp with a head injury or skull fracture. If there is a laceration with a head injury (depressed fracture), surgery is usually performed immediately because of the threat of infection.

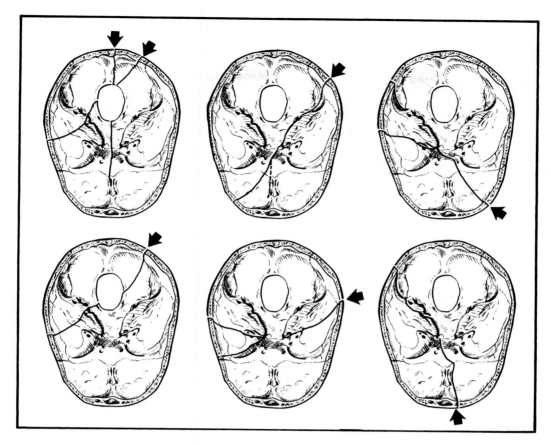

Figure 32-5. Coup forces of basilar skull fractures. Contrecoup forces go in the opposite direction along similar paths.

COMPLICATIONS OF HEAD INJURY

Closed Head Injuries

Complications of closed head injuries include cerebral edema (vasogenic and cytotoxic), hydrocephalus, seizures, increased ICP, diabetes insipidus, and residual neurologic deficits. Metabolic complications include respiratory insufficiency, infection, and systemic dysfunction as a result of associated trauma.

If the hypothalamus and/or pituitary gland is affected, diabetes insipidus will most likely occur. Biochemical stress ulcers are common and are frequently associated with electrolyte disturbances. Depending on the site and degree of injury, seizures may develop. Infections, both cerebrospinal and respiratory, are continuous threats.

DIAGNOSTIC TESTS AND FINDINGS

A CT scan is the primary diagnostic test in head injuries. It will reveal whether:

1. Air has entered the brain from fractures of the eye, mastoid, or sinuses.
2. Blood is present in brain tissue or in the ventricular system.
3. Blood is on the surface of the brain or in the basal cisterns.
4. Presence of cerebral edema and intracranial shift.
5. Ventricles are of normal size and in normal position.
6. The pineal gland has calcified and is in normal position.

Lumbar puncture is contraindicated in increased ICP and is rarely done in the diagnosis of head injuries.

Cerebral angiography or CT angiography is used if there is a suspicion of arterial dissection or the presence of a ruptured aneurysm or arteriovenous malformation (AVM).

Magnetic resonance imaging of the brain is obtained in more stable patients. Injuries to the brain parenchyma and the brainstem are more visible with MRI.

Arterial blood gases (ABGs) are helpful in determining the presence of hypoxia, hypocarbia, or hypercarbia. Electrolyte studies are done frequently, especially serum sodium and serum osmolarity, to monitor changes. Coagulation studies are done to monitor for the development of coagulopathy, which is detrimental to the brain-injured patient.

EXAMINATION OF THE PATIENT

Patients with acute head injuries may present along the neurologic continuum from awake to comatose. Prior to describing the interventions needed to care for the severe TBI patient, an overview of the neurologic examination applicable to all patients is presented.

Neurologic Examination

Mentation
There are five possible states or levels of consciousness. The definition and/or progression may differ in various institutions. It may be defined as follows:

1. Alert: The patient is oriented to person, place, and time.
2. Lethargic: The patient prefers to sleep and, when aroused, his or her degree of alertness or confusion is variable.
3. Obtunded: The patient can be aroused with minimal stimulation but will drift off to sleep quickly.
4. Stuporous: The patient is aroused only by constant, deep, and usually painful stimuli. The patient may respond by some attempt to withdraw, moaning, or exhibiting decerebrate or decorticate positioning.
5. Coma: The patient cannot be aroused.

The GCS (Table 32-1) is one of the standard methods used to identify a patient's level of consciousness (mentation) and determine his or her prognosis. The GCS measures both arousal and awareness. Eye opening is a measure of arousal. Verbal and best motor response are measures of awareness.

Cranial Nerves
Some of the 12 cranial nerves can be checked during routine patient care as well as during neurologic checks:

II: Optic nerve. Sensory limb of the pupillary light reflex. Visual acuity.

TABLE 32-1. GLASGOW COMA SCALE

Eye Opening (E)	Best Motor Response (M)	Verbal Response (V)
Spontaneous = 4	Obeys = 6	Oriented = 5
To speech = 3	Localizes = 5	Confused conversation = 4
To pain = 2	Withdraws = 4	Inappropriate words = 3
No response = 1	Abnormal Flexion = 3 Extension = 2	Incomprehensible sounds = 2 No response = 1
	No response = 1	

III: Oculomotor nerve. Motor limb of the pupillary light reflex; causes constriction of the pupil. Eyelid elevation. It controls four of the six eye muscles.

IV: Trochlear nerve. It turns the eye down and in.

The lowest score received has the worst prognosis.

V: Trigeminal nerve. Corneal sensation. Provides the sensory side of the arc for the corneal reflex. Sensation to the face. Muscles of mastication. *Note*: The seventh nerve (facial) provides the motor side of arc.

VI: Abducens nerve. It turns the eye out. This is the longest unprotected nerve in the brain.

VII: Facial nerve. Facial symmetry and movement and eyelid closure.

X: Vagus nerve. This controls palatal deviation. If the nerve is damaged, the uvula deviates away from the side of paralysis. In vagal nerve paralysis, there is ipsilateral paralysis of the palatal, pharyngeal, and laryngeal muscles. The soft palate at rest is usually lower on the affected side, and if the patient says "ah," it elevates on the intact side.

XI: (Spinal) Accessory nerve. It turns the head by use of the sternocleidomastoid muscles. It has some association with the upper trapezius muscles.

XII: Hypoglossal nerve. It controls tongue movement. If it is damaged, the patient cannot move the tongue from side to side, and tongue protrusion results in deviation toward the side of nerve damage.

Motor Function
Check to determine whether the patient moves all extremities voluntarily *and* equally. Note a one-sided

weakness. If muscle weakness is suspected, have the patient close his or her eyes and extend the arms directly in front. If there is a muscle weakness, there will be a drifting downward of the weakened extremity. Motor strength is measured using a scale from 0 to 5. Note any abnormal posturing of the arms or legs. Flexor posturing occurs when the arms flex up and inward. Extensor posturing occurs when the arms extend down with palms out and the feet extend downward.

Sensation

In trauma, patients may respond only to pain. In the awake neurologic patient, determine whether the patient has any numbness or tingling in the arms, legs, or face. Test sensation with the light touch of a cotton swab and pinprick with a pin. Additional assessment parameters in the head-injured patient include the following:

Scalp: Check for tears and/or swelling, which may indicate a subgaleal hematoma.

Face: Palpate the eye orbits, nose, teeth, maxilla, and mandible for facial fractures. Some facial fractures may cause leakage of CSF, and this would be an entry port for infection.

Ears: Blood in the external canal usually indicates a basal skull fracture.

Neck/Spine: Note any purple bruises over spinous processes. If the patient is awake, palpate the spinous processes to determine whether pain is present. *Note*: This should be done only by the physician with a team present to log-roll patient to the side, ensuring that the cervical spine is maintained in alignment.

Resuscitation Phase—ABCs (Airway, Breathing, and Circulation)

The ABCs of emergency care pertain to any patient presenting with an acute head injury. Multiple assessment and intervention priorities occur simultaneously. Patients presenting with a GCS of 3 to 8 require aggressive support of their ABCs. Always establish a patent airway, using extra care until the cross-table lateral radiographs confirm no neck fracture. Continually monitor the respiratory and cardiac systems to ensure early intervention in cases of dysfunction. Inadequate function of either system may result in the extension of neurologic impairment.

A brief focused neurologic examination, including LOC, is a key initial assessment in any neurologically impaired patient. The patient's pupils should be assessed and responses to stimulation noted. The secondary survey follows with an assessment of major organ systems.

Foley catheters and orogastric tubes are placed after the secondary survey is completed. Cervical spine precautions are paramount during this entire phase and maintained until the spine is cleared. The patient may require transfer to an intensive care unit setting if their condition becomes unstable.

NURSING INTERVENTIONS

The primary nursing intervention after assurance of a patent airway and the prevention of hypoxia is frequent neurologic assessment. Monitoring of vital signs and the maintenance of fluid balance and accurate intake/output records will help in evaluating treatment modalities aimed at stabilizing the patient. Standard procedures to prevent infections are employed.

33

Stroke and Intracranial Aneurysms

EDITORS' NOTE

In this chapter, the concept of cerebrovascular disturbance is covered. Common interruptions in cerebrovascular bloodflow may be the result of thrombosis, embolus, or hemorrhage. The PCCN exam will most likely have several questions on this content.

A stroke is a sudden focal or global neurologic deficit due to cerebrovascular disease. It is the most common cause of cerebral dysfunction in the United States.

STROKE

Etiology

Stroke is a leading cause of disability and is the third leading cause of death in the United States. A stroke is a neurologic event resulting from altered cerebral circulation, often due to either cellular ischemia/ infarction caused by a blockage of an artery feeding the brain or intracranial hemorrhage (ICH). Cerebral ischemia occurs as a result of reduced cerebral blood flow, which can last from several seconds to minutes. The end result of any interruption of oxygen to brain tissue for more than a few minutes is the death of those neurons not being oxygenated. Such a decrease in oxygen may be partial or complete. Symptoms due to an acute stroke can occur in about 10 s owing to hypoxia and energy depletion.

There are two main types of stroke: ischemic and hemorrhagic. Discrimination between the two is important as it influences the indicated treatment. Ischemic strokes account for 85% to 88% of all strokes. The vascular origin is from (1) a thrombotic or (2) embolic occlusion of a cerebral artery, resulting in an infarction. Hemorrhagic strokes are responsible for 12% to 15% of all strokes. These are caused by the spontaneous rupture of a vessel, leading to intracerebral or subarachnoid hemorrhage. Other causes of hemorrhage include brain tumors that bleed and uncontrolled anticoagulation. Risk factors include family history, hypertension, diabetes mellitus, smoking, atherosclerosis, atrial fibrillation and other cardioembolic sources, prior transient ischemic attack (TIA), advanced age, and trauma.

Clinical Presentation

Ischemic stroke results from decreased or disrupted blood flow. Embolic strokes (10% to 30% of ischemic strokes) present with sudden neurologic deficits occurring during periods of activity and are often due to cardiac events such as emboli from atrial fibrillation or acute myocardial infarction. In contrast, thrombotic strokes are due to atherosclerotic occlusion of a vessel and occur during periods of inactivity, often during sleep.

Any patient with sudden changes in neurologic functioning should be evaluated for a TIA or stroke. Specific symptomatology depends on location of the injury and the hemispheric dominance of the patient. The extent of the deficit is determined by which artery is occluded.

If the ischemic stroke occurs in the right cerebral hemisphere (usually the nondominant hemisphere), left-sided motor and sensory deficits occur such as autotopagnosia, and spatial-perceptual deficits resulting in apraxia can occur. Autotopagnosia is an inability to determine the position of parts of the body in relation to the rest of the body. Apraxia may be constructional or dressing. Constructional apraxia is the inability to complete the left half of a figure one is drawing or to arrange words in a correct manner, so that the patient may, for example, superimpose words. Usually a constructional apraxia will include the inability to complete the drawing of a picture (e.g., a clock). Dressing apraxia is the inability to dress oneself properly. Autotopagnosia, constructional apraxia, and dressing apraxia are common in right cerebral strokes. Neglect of the paralyzed side; impulsive, quick behavior; and poor judgment of one's abilities and limitations occur with right cerebral strokes.

Left cerebral hemispheric (dominant hemisphere) strokes are associated with right-sided motor and sensory impairment and aphasia. Expressive aphasia is the inability to express oneself verbally and understandably. Receptive aphasia is loss of the ability to understand spoken or written words. Other deficits include dyslexia, acalcia, agraphia, and astereognosis. Astereognosis occurs when the patient, with eyes closed, is unable to identify a common object placed in his or her hand.

In addition, these strokes tend to cause finger agnosia (inability to identify a finger being touched) and right-left disorientation. Behavior is slow, cautious, and disorganized. Regardless of which hemisphere is involved in a stroke, such patients tend to have a reduced memory span, are emotionally labile, and have spasticity of the affected extremities. Some patients will have anosognosia, which is the denial of a neurologic deficit such as hemiplegia. Anosognosia differs from a psychologic denial state.

Cerebral hemorrhage results in an abrupt and rapid onset of neurologic deficits including severe headache, nuchal rigidity, hemiparesis to posturing, cranial nerve deficits, stupor, and coma. The severity of symptoms depends on the size and location of the hemorrhage.

Diagnosis

The diagnosis of stroke is usually made on the basis of history, clinical symptoms, and diagnostic tests. In the case of ischemic stroke, the history frequently reveals transient ischemic attacks (TIAs), reversible ischemic neurologic deficits (RIND), and possibly "small" strokes in the past. In hemorrhagic strokes, there is usually no prodromal warning signs of the impending hemorrhage.

To differentiate between the two types of stroke, it will help to obtain a rapid computed tomographic (CT) scan within 25 min of the patient's arrival. Patients presenting within the first hours of ischemic stroke will generally have a negative CT scan of the brain. In some instances, an "MCA" sign, or white

clot visible in the middle cerebral artery (MCA), will be seen in MCA occlusions. Patients presenting 12 to 24 h after a stroke onset will have ischemic changes on CT, which will reveal decreased density in ischemic and infarcted areas. Hemorrhage on CT shows up as an increased white-appearing density. A magnetic resonance imaging (MRI) study can differentiate between the presence of an infarction, hemorrhage, the presence of a clot, or dissection of a vessel wall. Cerebral angiography may show vessel occlusion, vasospasm, arteriovenous malformations, and aneurysms.

Medical Treatment

Stroke patients presenting to a hospital are considered emergent cases. Rapid identification, triage, and diagnosis are imperative.

If the patient has had an ischemic stroke, treatment options depend on the time from symptom onset as well as a number of other factors. In patients presenting within 4.5 h of symptom onset, thrombolytic therapy (with tissue plasminogen activator [tPA]) should be considered as a treatment option if the patient meets inclusion criteria and has no exclusions. If tPA is given, the systolic blood pressure is maintained <185 mm Hg and the diastolic <110 mm Hg. Patients receiving tPA must be closely monitored with vital signs and neurologic checks every 15 min for 2 h, every 30 min for 6 h, and every hour for 16 h. These patients are usually admitted to the ICU, where cardiac/respiratory monitoring as well as close neurologic observation occur. Other interventions are listed in the following paragraph.

In patients unable to receive tPA due to time (>4.5 h from symptom onset) or a contraindication, there are other interventions that should be considered. Aspirin therapy used within 48 h of onset of symptoms has been demonstrated to reduce risk and mortality. Life-long antiplatelet therapy with aspirin, aspirin plus dipyridamole, ticlopidine, or clopidogrel must be considered in the absence of contraindications. The maintenance of cerebral perfusion pressure is an important component of treatment; blood pressure control is usually not instituted unless it is >220 mm Hg systolic or >120 mm Hg diastolic, as even minor decreases in blood pressure can affect the recovery of the area of ischemic penumbra.

Drugs of choice in stroke include labetalol and nicardipine. Antithrombotic therapy with heparin may be considered if an embolic etiology is suspected but is considered risky owing to the greater potential for cerebral hemorrhage. The use of statins (e.g., atorvastatin) following ischemic stroke has shown to reduce the incidence of repeat events.

Hemorrhagic stroke patients usually present with an altered level of consciousness. Depending on the location of the bleed, the intensity of care will vary. Following a large ICH in the dominant hemisphere, discussions with the family take place to determine the extent of care based on the probable outcome. If the ICH is in the nondominant hemisphere or there is a smaller one in the dominant hemisphere, then treatment options are discussed with the family.

Nursing Interventions

To some extent nursing interventions (and patient complications) depend on the type and site of a stroke, the patient's age, his or her general health, and the extent of neurologic deficit.

Priorities with regard to the patient with an ischemic stroke include the maintenance or restoration of cerebral perfusion, maintenance of life support, prevention of further injury or escalation of the life-threatening problem, and preservation of motor function, speech, and cognition to the greatest possible extent. Early dysphagia screening (decreased or absent gag) lowers the risk of aspiration and resultant pneumonia. The patient should be NPO (nothing by mouth) until the swallowing screen is done. Accurate systematic monitoring and assessment neurologic status will identify extensions of deficits that may be treatable. Nursing assessment should include level of consciousness and pupil size and reactivity; change in motor function and/or cranial nerve function; signs and symptoms of increased intracranial pressure (ICP), seizure, or hydrocephalus; and analysis of arterial blood gases (ABGs) and laboratory studies. Some centers utilize the National Institutes of Health Stroke Scale to assess the stroke patient. Communication with the patient is achieved in any way possible—through writing, pictures, gestures, and so on. Different aphasias make this task difficult. Generally, patients with left hemispheric stroke respond to visual images and gestures, while those with right hemispheric stroke respond to verbal cues. The latter patients usually suffer from left-sided neglect; therefore, call lights and other important aids should be placed on the right side of the bed.

Care priorities that apply to both types of stroke patients include glucose and temperature control as well as the prevention of deep venous thrombosis (DVT). Glucose levels are monitored closely. If the blood glucose exceeds 140 mg/dL, an insulin protocol is used to decrease glucose to a normal glycemic level. The patient's body temperature is maintained 36°C to 37°C. An increase in temperature of 1°C should be treated with Tylenol and cooling measures as indicated. It is imperative to prevent DVT through the use of sequential compression devices on the legs and/or the use of low molecular weight heparin.

Other important measures include turning, positioning, skin care, fluid and nutritional intake, emotional support, and early implementation of rehabilitation.

INTRACRANIAL ANEURYSMS

An aneurysm is a congenital, developmental, or traumatic defect in the muscle layer of arteries, normally occurring at points of bifurcation. (Recall that there are three layers in the arterial wall: the inner endothelial layer [the intima], a middle smooth muscle layer [the media], and an outer layer of connective tissue [the adventitia].)

Pathophysiology

The congenital weakness of the arterial wall results in a gradual "ballooning out" of that segment of the artery over a period of years. When vascular pressure rises to a sufficient (unknown) pressure, the weakened ballooning segment of the artery bursts.

Location, Incidence, and Etiology

Most cerebral aneurysms develop in the anterior arteries of the circle of Willis. Aneurysms are rare in children and teenagers and most common in middle-aged persons. Slightly more women than men develop aneurysms. Some 10% to 20% of patients with aneurysms have more than one (may be found on same or opposite side).

Etiologic risk factors include hypertension (present in a majority of cases) and smoking. Diseases such as Ehlers-Danlos syndrome, coarctation of the aorta, and polycystic kidneys put individuals at risk. No specific precipitating factors are present in all patients. Congenital anomalies account for some aneurysms and others occur for unknown reasons.

Clinical Presentation

Aneurysms are commonly asymptomatic until a bleed occurs. The exception is a very large aneurysm, which may cause symptoms related to pressure against surrounding tissues. The signs and symptoms of an unruptured cerebral aneurysm are dependent on its size and rate of growth and can range from no symptoms for a small aneurysm to loss of feeling in the face or visual changes with a larger aneurysm. Symptoms that may be experienced immediately after an aneurysm ruptures include sudden and unusually severe headache, nausea, vision impairment, vomiting, and loss of consciousness. Severe headache (unlike any other headaches) occurs as the aneurysm starts to bleed. Unconsciousness may occur and be transient or sustained secondary to ischemia and/or necrosis of brain tissue. Nausea and vomiting are common. Other neurologic deficits include numbness, aphasia, and hemiparesis.

Nuchal rigidity, photophobia, diplopia, Kernig's sign (inability to fully extend leg when the thigh is flexed at a 90-degree angle to the abdomen), Brudzinski's sign (involuntary adduction and flexion of legs when neck is flexed), and headache are common because of meningeal irritation. All these signs except diplopia are sometimes grouped together under the term *meningismus*.

Diagnosis

Initial evaluation includes a CT scan of the brain without contrast. If subarachnoid blood is present on CT, either a CT angiogram or cerebral angiogram is done. This may reveal the presence of aneurysms. A lumbar puncture is performed occasionally but not as often as in years past. Elevated cerebrospinal fluid (CSF) pressure, elevated protein levels, elevated red blood cells and oxyhemoglobin, decreased glucose, and grossly bloody CSF indicate hemorrhage in the subarachnoid space.

Classification of Clinical State following Aneurysmal Rupture

Aneurysms may be placed in one of five categories (grades). These are summarized in Table 33-1. If patients can be stabilized in grades I through V, they may be candidates for surgical intervention or coiling.

Prognosis

The prognosis depends on the site and severity of the bleed. Persistent coma beyond 2 days is a poor sign. Bleeding may recur as the original clot that formed around the bleed is absorbed (or lysed). This usually occurs between the seventh and eleventh day after the original bleed and carries a poor prognosis. The risk of rebleeding has decreased dramatically with early obliteration of the aneurysm through surgery or coiling. Cerebral vasospasm results in cerebral ischemia. Vasospasm is commonly seen on days 4 and 14 postbleed. Marked cerebral edema and/or the development of hydrocephalus places the patient at greater risk for a poor outcome.

Nursing Implications

If an aneurysm is diagnosed prior to a bleed, surgery may be performed to prevent a bleed depending on the size and location of the aneurysm. If an aneurysmal bleed has occurred and the patient has stabilized, surgery may be performed, as indicated. Conventional therapy for aneurysms includes clipping or endovascular techniques such as stenting and coil implantation. The decision to surgically clip

TABLE 33-1. GRADES OF ANEURYSMS

Symptom	Grade I	Grade II	Grade III	Grade IV	Grade V
Level of consciousness	Alert	Decreased	Confused	Unresponsive	Moribund
Headache	Slight	Mild to severe	Severe	—	—
Nuchal rigidity	Slight	Yes	Yes	—	—
Vasospasm	—	—	—	May be present	May be present
Decerebrate posturing	—	—	—	—	Yes

—, absent.

versus coil is based on site, shape, and condition of the patient.

Surgery may consist of one of several procedures:

1. Clipping of the aneurysm is probably the oldest and the most frequent surgical treatment (Fig. 33-1). If the aneurysm is extremely large, clipping may not be possible.

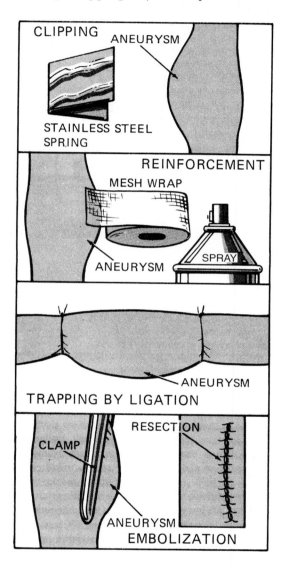

Figure 33-1. Surgical treatment of aneurysms.

2. Endovascular coiling of the aneurysm is done by a neurointerventionalist.
3. Reinforcing the arterial wall at the site of the aneurysm by wrapping some of the new mesh materials (strips of muscle, gauze, or plastic) around it may prevent further enlargement or rupture (Fig. 33-1). Care must be taken not to decrease the arterial lumen, especially if atherosclerotic disease is present.
4. Trapping the aneurysm by ligating it proximally and distally may be the procedure of choice if the aneurysm is large (Fig. 33-1).
5. Embolization of the aneurysmal clot may be performed once the patient is stabilized, especially if the clot is impinging on important structures (Fig. 33-1).

If the aneurysm cannot be reached and/or surgical risk of one of the above procedures is extremely high, the common carotid artery may be clamped. Prior to this procedure, angiography must demonstrate that vascular perfusion of the involved hemisphere is adequate from the opposite side.

Postoperative Nursing Interventions

Following occlusion of the aneurysm, nursing priorities include monitoring for neurologic changes. After aneurysm repair, the patient needs to be monitored for complications including seizures, cerebral edema, hydrocephalus, vasospasm, and hyponatremia. Systemic support is provided, including glycemic control, nutritional support, maintenance of normothermia, and deep venous thrombosis (DVT) prevention. Skin care and range of motion to all four extremities are important. Consultation with occupational, speech-language, and physical therapists takes place following stabilization. As progressive care nursing involves caring for patients during acute illness as well as planning for discharge needs, care of the neurologic patient often involves multidisciplinary team-focused care addressing rehabilitation needs.

34

The Vertebrae and Spinal Cord

EDITORS' NOTE

In this chapter, anatomy, physiology, and concepts of spinal cord dysfunction are reviewed. The PCCN exam usually has several questions on dysfunction or trauma associated with the spinal cord. This chapter should provide you with the essential information necessary to address content from the exam on the spinal cord. Again, keep in mind that anatomic and physiologic questions are usually not asked directly on the PCCN exam. Focus your studying on the function of the cord and the clinical conditions that stem from cord injury/dysfunction.

VERTEBRAL COLUMN

The spinal cord is protected and housed by the vertebrae. The vertebral column comprises a total of 33 vertebrae: 7 cervical, 12 thoracic, 5 lumbar, 5 sacral fused, and 4 fused as the coccygeal segment.

The body of a typical vertebra (Fig. 34-1) is the solid portion that lies anteriorly. Opposite the vertebral body is the spinous process (the bony segment felt down the back). Projecting laterally from each side of each vertebra are the transverse processes. The lamina is the curved portion of bone joining the transverse processes to the spinous process. The vertebrae may be fractured in the same way that other bones in the body are. The most common fractures of the vertebral column are vertebral body compression fractures. Between the vertebral body and the spinous process is the spinal foramen, the cavity through which the spinal cord passes.

Cervical Vertebrae

The seven cervical vertebrae are the smallest. Unique to the first six cervical vertebrae is the foramen transversarium. This foramen allows for passage of the vertebral arteries through the six vertebral bones. Figure 34-2 shows the atlas (C1), which articulates with the occipital bone and the axis (C2). The axis has an odontoid process (the only vertebra that does), which permits the atlas to articulate directly and provides rotation of the head. Trauma to the odontoid process may result in one of three fracture types and is rarely associated with cord injury. Hangman's fracture occurs when there has been a bilateral pedicle fracture of C2. The fracture causes separation of C2, C3, and their respective posterior elements. A common fracture to C1 is a Jefferson fracture, where there is disruption of the posterior and anterior arches; this rarely causes a neurologic deficit.

Thoracic Vertebrae

The 12 thoracic vertebrae (Fig. 34-3) have points of attachment for the ribs to help support the chest musculature.

Lumbar Vertebrae

The five lumbar vertebrae (Fig. 34-4) are the largest; they support the back muscles. Their vertebral disks are the most frequently herniated.

Sacral Vertebrae

The five sacral vertebrae (Fig. 34-5) are fused to form the sacrum, a frequent point of low back pain.

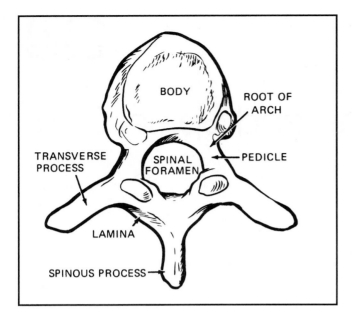

Figure 34-1. Typical vertebra.

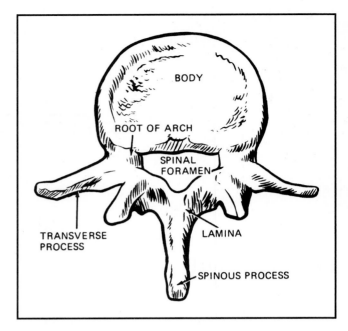

Figure 34-3. Thoracic vertebra.

Coccygeal Vertebrae

Depending on the individual, four vertebrae are fused to form the coccyx (Fig. 34-5).

INTERVERTEBRAL DISKS

Between each of the lumbar, thoracic, and cervical vertebrae excluding the atlas and axis is an intervertebral disk. These fibrocartilaginous disks absorb shock and reduce the pressure between one vertebra and another. The outer portion of the disk is called the annulus fibrosus. The center portion of the disk is a gelatinous material called the nucleus pulposus. Unexpected movement and/or force may

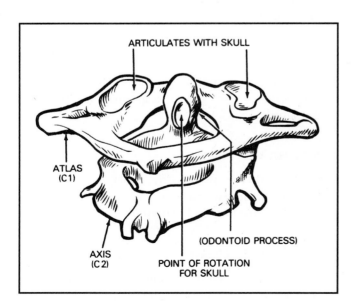

Figure 34-2. Articulation of C1 and C2 vertebrae.

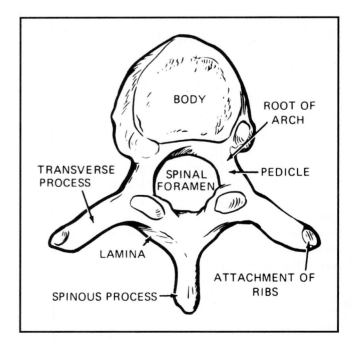

Figure 34-4. Lumbar vertebra.

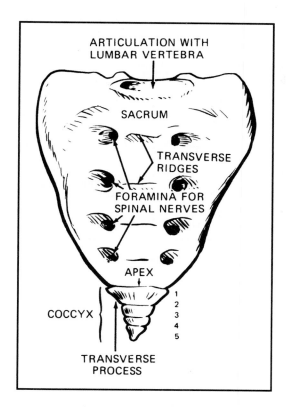

Figure 34-5. Sacral vertebrae and coccyx.

LIGAMENTS

A series of ligaments support the vertebral column. The anterior and posterior ligamentous structures support the vertebral column and help support the spinal cord. The series of ligaments that join various segments of the vertebral column give it stability. Disruption of the ligaments can lead to instability and movement of the bony structures of the vertebral column into the spinal cord.

Unfortunately, it is very common for the spinal cord to be damaged by extreme hyperextension, hyperflexion, and rotational or axial loading forces (Fig. 34-6). Damage may occur with or without fracture of the vertebrae.

SPINAL CORD

The spinal cord is the second major component of the central nervous system (the brain is the other) and is vital for life.

The spinal cord (Fig. 34-7) is continuous with the medulla oblongata in the brainstem. It is located in the spinal canal and is protected by the vertebral column. The cord is some 25 cm shorter than the vertebral column. Within the vertebral column, the spinal cord extends from the foramen magnum to the first to second lumbar vertebrae. Its tapered end is called the conus medullaris. The filum terminale is a group of fibers extending from the conus

"rupture" the disk, forcing the nucleus pulposus out of position. When out of position, the disk may impinge on the spinal canal, the spinal cord, or the emerging spinal nerves.

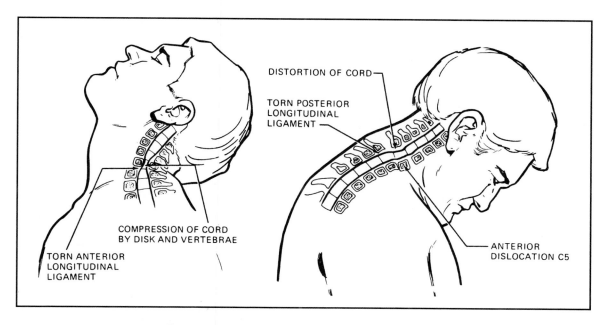

Figure 34-6. Hyperextension and hyperflexion of the spinal cord.

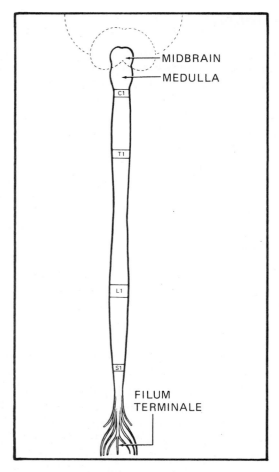

Figure 34-7. Spinal cord.

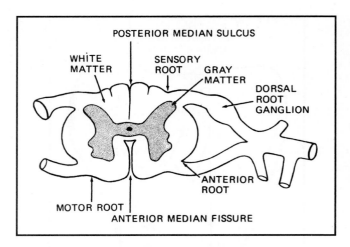

Figure 34-8. Gray and white matter of the spinal cord (cross section).

medullaris at the level of L1 to L2 to the first coccygeal vertebra.

Structure of the Spinal Cord

The spinal cord is surrounded by the same meninges that encase the brain. Between the L1 and S2 vertebrae, the arachnoid membrane enlarges somewhat to form the space known as the lumbar cistern, which is used for lumbar punctures. The spinal cord has a minute cavity in its center known as the central canal. It is an extension of the fourth ventricle and contains cerebrospinal fluid (CSF).

The spinal cord is composed of both white (myelinated) and gray (unmyelinated) tissue. The gray matter appears (with a little imagination) to be shaped like an H, which is surrounded by white matter (Fig. 34-8). The amount of gray matter varies with its location in the vertebral column. A mnemonic may help distinguish white/gray matter and myelinated/

unmyelinated fibers. The fourth letter of gray is "Y," as is the fourth letter of unmyelinated. So gray matter is unmyelinated fibers.

Gray matter is composed of nerve cells and unmyelinated fibers arranged in three columns (Fig. 34-9). The anterior gray columns are also known as the anterior horns. They contain cell bodies of efferent (motor) fibers. The middle gray columns, known as the lateral columns, contain preganglionic fibers of the autonomic nervous system. The lateral columns are largest in the upper cervical, thoracic, and midsacral regions. The posterior columns, also known as the posterior horns, contain cell bodies of afferent (sensory) fibers.

The white matter (myelinated) is arranged in three columns called the anterior, lateral, and posterior funiculi (Fig. 34-10). Within these columns are ascending (sensory) and descending (motor) tracts termed fasciculi (Fig. 34-11).

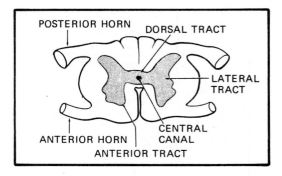

Figure 34-9. Columns (tracts) of gray matter in the spinal cord (cross section).

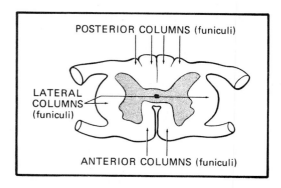

Figure 34-10. Funiculi of white matter in the spinal cord.

The significant ascending tracts are the fasciculus gracilis, fasciculus cuneatus, lateral spinothalamic tract, anterior spinothalamic tract, dorsal and ventral spinocerebellar tracts, and spinotectal tract. These tracts carry sensory impulses.

The significant descending tracts (Fig. 34-11) are the rubrospinal tract, ventral and lateral corticospinal tracts, and tectospinal tract. These carry motor impulses.

Lower motor neurons are spinal and cranial motor neurons that directly innervate muscles.

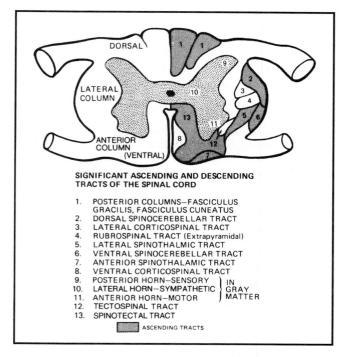

Figure 34-11. Significant ascending and descending tracts of the spinal cord. The left half of the picture is a mirror image of the right half.

Lesions cause flaccid paralysis, muscular atrophy, and absence of reflex responses. Upper motor neurons in the brain and spinal cord activate lower motor neurons. Lesions cause spastic paralysis and hyperactive reflexes.

Spinal Cord Injuries

Spinal cord injuries (SCIs) are more and more common and are mainly a result of automobile accidents, assaults involving gunshot wounds and other personal violence, falls, and sports-related injuries such as diving accidents and contact sport accidents. Over 80% of individuals with SCIs are male and two-thirds of all injuries occur in persons younger than 30 years. Over 50% of SCIs involve the cervical region of the spinal cord. These injuries cause varying degrees of motor and sensory loss below the level of injury. Similar to brain injury, deficits are due to both the initial impact (primary injury) and ongoing physiologic changes (secondary injury).

Hyperflexion injuries usually accompany head-on collisions and result in a sudden deceleration type of force. This type of injury results in flexion of the neck and disruption of the posterior ligaments and compression of the anterior vertebral column. Hyperextension injuries are associated with rear-end collisions. The force produced throws the neck backward, causing disruption of the anterior ligaments and compression of the posterior vertebral column. Rotational forces produce lateral rotation of the vertebral column, disrupting the ligaments and producing instability of the column. Axial loading injuries are associated with diving mishaps where force is exerted onto the spinal column. Burst fractures of the body and disruption of the posterior bony segments of the column occur. Penetrating forces cause an array of injuries due to penetration through bone, ligaments, meninges, and spinal cord. The end result of these forces are fractures of the bones, disruption of ligaments, and damage to the fragile spinal cord.

Damage to the spinal cord can be characterized as concussion, contusion, laceration, transaction, hemorrhage, or damage to the blood vessels supplying the spinal cord. Concussion causes temporary loss of function. Contusion is bruising of the spinal cord that includes bleeding into the spinal cord, subsequent edema, and possible neuronal death from compression due to edema or tissue damage. Laceration occurs when a tear in the spinal cord occurs that results in permanent injury. Contusion, edema, and cord compression can be seen with a laceration. Transsection is a severing of the spinal cord resulting in complete loss of function below the level of injury. Hemorrhage is bleeding that occurs in and around the spinal cord and can result in edema and cord compression. Damage to the blood vessels that supply the spinal cord can result in ischemia and infarction.

Spinal cord injuries can also be categorized as stable (ligaments are intact preventing movement of the vertebral bodies and bones into the spinal canal) or unstable (ligaments are disrupted and allow the vertebral bodies and bones to move, possibly injuring the spinal cord). Injuries may be classified according to the injury to the vertebral column. Such injuries include simple fracture, compression fracture, comminuted fracture, teardrop fracture, dislocation, subluxation, and fracture/dislocation. Injuries may also be classified in relation to the specific level of injury. These injuries are summarized in Table 34-1.

Disruption of the ligaments causing vertebral movement into the spinal canal, fractures of the vertebra, and/or disruption of the disks may injure the fragile spinal cord. An SCI often results in fractures and compression of the vertebrae, which then crush and result in axonal injury. Spinal cord injuries are classified as either complete or incomplete. A complete injury involves a total lack of sensory and motor function below the level of injury. In an incomplete injury, some motor or sensory function is maintained below the injury.

Additional complications that may result from an SCI are respiratory impairment (inability to breathe without a ventilator to diminished thoracic cavity excursion limiting tidal volume and cough reflex), inability to regulate blood pressure, variability in heart rate, reduced control of body temperature, an inability to sweat below the level of injury, skin breakdown due to loss of sensation, deep vein thrombus/pulmonary emboli, increased susceptibility to respiratory disease, sexual dysfunction, urine/bowel dysfunction, hypertrophic ossification, autonomic dysreflexia, and chronic pain. The psychologic impact of SCI includes depression, perceived altered body image, anxiety, and lack of independence.

Classification of SCIs

The severity of an injury depends on the level of the spinal cord that is affected. Tetraplegia (quadriplegia) results from injuries to the spinal cord in the cervical (neck) region, with associated loss of muscle strength in all four extremities. Paraplegia results from injuries to the spinal cord in the thoracic or lumbar areas, resulting in paralysis of the legs and lower body. A complete SCI produces total loss of all motor and sensory function below the level of injury. Nearly 50% of all SCIs are complete. The level of injury may be cervical, thoracic, or lumbar. The cervical injury is the most common.

Incomplete cord lesion involvement (or partial transection) leaves some tracts intact. The degree of

TABLE 34-1. CLASSIFICATION OF INJURY ACCORDING TO SPECIFIC VERTEBRAL LEVEL

Injury Level	Intact Function	Lost Function
Below L2	Mixed motor/sensory, depending on intact nerve fibers	Mixed motor/sensory; possibly bladder, bowels, and sexual functioning
T1 to L1 or L2	Arm function	Loss of intercostal muscles, leg functions; bladder, bowels, and sexual functioning
C7, C8	Arm movement include deltoids, biceps, and triceps muscles, head rotation, respiration	No intrinsic muscles of hand; no other function retained + above
C6, C7	Biceps muscle, head rotation, respiration	No triceps; no other function retained
C5, C6	Gross arm movement, head rotation, diaphragmatic respiration	No other function retained
C4, C5	Head rotation, diaphragmatic respiration	No other function intact
C3, C4	Head rotation	No other function intact (many die)
C1, C2	None	Poor prognosis

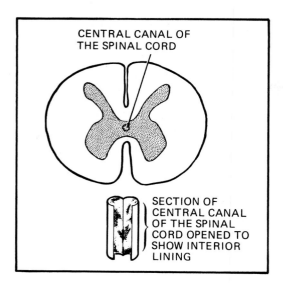

Figure 34-12. Central cord syndrome.

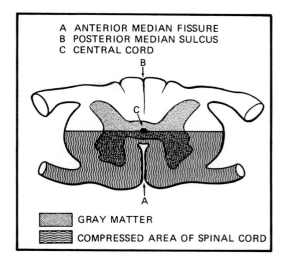

Figure 34-13. Anterior cord syndrome.

sensorimotor loss is variable depending on the level of lesion. There are a number of incomplete lesions.

When the damage is in the cervical central cord, it is termed central cord syndrome, which is characterized by microscopic hemorrhage and edema of the central cord (Fig. 34-12). There is motor weakness in both the upper and lower extremities, but the weakness is much greater in the upper extremities than the lower. Sensory dysfunction varies according to the site of injury or lesion but is generally more pronounced in the upper extremities. Reflexes in the lower extremities may be hyperactive temporarily. This syndrome is frequently due to hyperextension of an osteoarthritic spine. It is the most common type of cord injury when there is no overt fracture or dislocation. The extent of recovery depends on the resolution of edema and the intactness of the spinal cord tracts. As improvement occurs, it proceeds from proximal to distal parts.

Anterior cord syndrome is characterized by injury resulting in an acute compression of the anterior portion of the spinal cord, often a flexion injury (Fig. 34-13). Compression is usually caused by a disk or bony fragment. It may also be caused by the actual destruction of the anterior cord by an anterior spinal artery occlusion (thrombus). Symptoms include immediate anterior paralysis, which is complete from the injury or compression down. Hypesthesia (decreased sensation) and hypalgesia (decreased pain sensation) occur below the level of injury. Since the posterior cord tracts are not injured, there are sensations of touch, position, vibration, proprioception, and motion. If the syndrome is caused by the

compression of the anterior cord from bony fragments, surgical decompression is indicated.

The Brown-Séquard syndrome is due to transection or lesion of one-half of the spinal cord (Fig. 34-14). There is loss of motor function (paralysis) and position and vibratory sense as well as vasomotor paralysis on the same side (ipsilateral) and below the hemisection. On the opposite (contralateral) side of the hemisection, there is loss of pain and temperature sensation below the level of the lesion or hemisection.

The conus medullaris syndrome is compression of the last segment of the spinal cord. There is loss of bowel, bladder, and sexual function.

The cauda equina syndrome is caused by injury to the nerve roots below L1. There is motor loss to

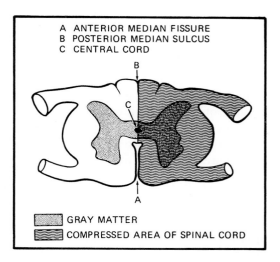

Figure 34-14. The Brown-Séquard syndrome.

the lower extremities, variable sensory loss, and are-flexive bowel and bladder.

When the spinal cord has sustained an injury, various pathophysiologic processes follow the injury. Injury to the spinal cord produces edema and reduction in blood flow to the cord. The ischemia that ensues is followed by a number of intracellular changes leading to cell death. Two other pathologic processes may accompany SCI. SCIs are frequently associated with trauma to the head or other systems. Disease states may relate specifically to the spinal cord—for example, tumor, arteriovenous malformations, and infections. In these instances, treatment of the underlying condition may result in improvement in spinal cord function.

Prevention of Complications

Respiratory System. Cervical injury or fracture may disrupt the diaphragm leading to diminished or absent respiratory function. Injury or fracture above C5 presents special problems in that total respiratory function is lost. Hypoventilation almost always occurs with diaphragmatic respirations because there is a decrease in vital capacity and tidal volume.

Since cervical fractures or severe injuries cause paralysis of the abdominal and frequently intercostal musculature, the patient is unable to cough effectively enough to remove secretions; this leads to atelectasis and pneumonia. Respiratory failure is the leading cause of death in the patient with SCI.

Cardiovascular System. Any cord transection above the level of T5 abolishes the influence of the sympathetic nervous system. If bradycardia occurs, appropriate medications (atropine) to increase the heart rate and avoid hypoxia may be necessary.

With the abolition of the influence of the sympathetic nervous system, vasodilatation occurs, decreasing venous return of blood to the heart. This decreases cardiac output, and hypotension can result. Intravenous fluids may resolve the problem, but close monitoring of vital signs is required.

Because of the loss of vascular tone, the patient is at risk for deep venous thrombosis (DVT). Sequential compression devices and/or low molecular weight heparin are used to reduce the risk of DVT.

Renal System. Urinary retention is a common development in acute spinal injuries and spinal shock. The bladder is hyperirritable. There is a loss of inhibition of reflex from the brain. Consequently, the patient will void small amounts of urine frequently. In spite of this, the bladder becomes distended since this is actually urinary retention with overflow. Urinary retention increases the chance of infection. In addition, urinary calculi are likely to develop in a distended bladder that is retaining urine. Continuous catheterization may be indicated in the early phase.

Gastrointestinal System. If the cord transection has occurred above T5, the loss of sympathetic innervation may lead to the development of an ileus or gastric distention. Intermittent suctioning by means of a nasogastric or orogastric tube may relieve the gastric distention, and standard treatment may be used for an ileus. A common occurrence in the past has been the development of biochemical stress ulcers due to excessive release of hydrochloric acid in the stomach. An H_2 antagonist is frequently used to prevent the occurrence of these ulcers during the initial extreme body stress. Because of the absence of clinical signs, any intra-abdominal bleeding that occurs will be difficult to diagnose. There will be no pain, tenderness, guarding, or other signs or symptoms. Continued hypotension in spite of vigorous treatment is suspicious. Expanding girth of the abdomen may be ascertainable, but not always.

If the rectum is not emptied on a regular basis, the patient may develop fecal impaction. Therefore, a bowel regimen is instituted as soon as possible with chemical stimulant agents and digital stimulation on a regular schedule. Nutritional support is instituted parenterally at first, followed by a transition to oral or enteral when peristalsis resumes.

Musculoskeletal System. The integrity of the patient's skin is of primary importance. Denervated skin can deteriorate very quickly, leading to major, life-threatening infection. Turning the patient every 1 to 2 h will relieve skin pressure points. In addition, meticulous skin care is required with frequent inspection to identify reddened areas or early stage of skin compression. A certain degree of muscle atrophy will occur during the flaccid paralysis stage, whereas contractures tend to occur during the spastic paralysis stage.

Poikilothermy is the adjustment of the body temperature toward room temperature. This occurs in these injuries because the interruption of the sympathetic nervous system prevents its temperature-controlling fibers from sending impulses that will reach the hypothalamus. Keep the patient normothermic.

Metabolic Needs. Correcting an existing acid-base disturbance and maintaining acid-base balance will promote the function of other body systems. Recall that nasogastric suctioning may lead to alkalosis, and decreased perfusion may lead to acidosis. Electrolytes must be monitored until a normal diet is resumed and suctioning has been discontinued. A positive nitrogen balance and a high-protein diet will help to prevent skin breakdown and infections and also to decrease the rate of muscle atrophy.

Nursing Interventions

The goal of nursing care is to prevent secondary injury and complication postinjury, prevent commonly occurring infections such as pneumonia and urinary tract infection, and begin planning for the patient's return home.

Cardiovascular monitoring of dysrhythmias and hypotension is essential. The dysrhythmias that occur may require standard treatment or only continued close monitoring. Hypotension is often controlled with intravenous administration of fluids, which requires that the nurse monitor the patient for the development of pulmonary edema.

The prevention of extension of cord injury is the next major nursing responsibility. If traction is employed, the rope knots should be taped, weights hanging freely, and traction lines kept straight or as positioned by the physician. Sensorimotor assessment should be done with monitoring of vital signs.

The common renal problem after vertebral and cord injury above the sacral level is urinary retention. A Foley catheter is often used in the early stages of the injury. If a Foley catheter is not inserted, intermittent catheterization is needed to ensure that an excessive urinary volume is not retained in the bladder, leading to further problems.

Gastrointestinal interventions include initial drainage of the stomach contents followed by intermittent suction by nasogastric tube, since gastric distention occurs and acid secretions are increased in the first few days. Contents suctioned should be routinely monitored for blood since biochemical stress ulcers may occur.

The patient's musculoskeletal needs include proper body alignment, support of bony prominences to prevent skin breakdown, and frequent turning (unless rotational bed therapy is used) to promote circulation and induce comfort. During the flaccid paralysis stage, extremities should be maintained in a functional position. During the spastic stage of the paralysis, medications and some physiotherapy may help control the spasms. Assessment should include motor testing every 4 h (0 = no movement, 5 = having movement with resistance). Prevention of thrombus formation is important and may include passive range of motion or use of antithrombic devices.

The patient's metabolic needs are initially met with intravenous fluids. As soon as he or she is stabilized, tube feedings are often started. Depending on the site of the injury and the residual deficits, the patient may be able to start oral feedings relatively soon after the injury. Rarely is hyperalimentation used unless protracted treatment of multiple trauma is required. The patient should be weighed on admission and then at least weekly. Multidisciplinary care addressing the patient's rehabilitation needs will also be a focus of progressive care nursing for the neurologic patient with a spinal cord injury.

Encephalopathies and Coma

EDITORS' NOTE

The concepts covered in this chapter are supplemental to the PCCN exam and are provided for a comprehensive review.

ENCEPHALOPATHIES

Encephalopathy is a term used for any diffuse disease of the brain that alters brain function or structure. It is the result of any disease that changes the structures of the brain or its functions. There are a number of different causes, including infectious diseases (bovine spongiform encephalopathy, Reye's syndrome, Lyme disease), thiamine deficiency (Wernicke's encephalopathy), abnormal metabolic or mitochondrial dysfunction, exposure to toxic chemicals, liver dysfunction (cirrhosis), hypertension (hypertensive encephalopathy), and hypoxia ischemia (hypoxic encephalopathy). The hallmark of encephalopathy is an altered mental state. Clinical signs usually involve progressive loss of memory, changes in cognition, problems concentrating, depressed level of consciousness to complete loss of consciousness, myoclonus, tremor, muscle atrophy and weakness, dysphagia, aphasia, and nystagmus. If an infectious agent is the cause, other symptoms include fever and headache. If the infection affects the limbic area of the brain, personality and behavioral changes, delirium, and mental status changes can occur.

Changes in level of consciousness occur for three reasons:

1. Reduction in oxygen delivery
2. Reduction in blood glucose
3. Reduction in cerebral perfusion pressure

COMA (AROUSAL DEFICIT)

A coma is a profound state of unconsciousness and the severity and mode of onset of coma depends on the underlying cause. Level of consciousness is differentiated into two components: arousal and awareness. Alterations in arousal reflect changes in the state of wakefulness, while alterations in awareness reflect changes in the content and quality of interactions. A change in the level of consciousness is considered the most important indicator of neurologic alteration. Decreased alertness and responsiveness represent a continuum that ranges from drowsiness to stupor (patient can be awakened only by vigorous stimuli) to coma, a deep sleep–like state from which the patient cannot be aroused. Table 35-1 outlines the terms used to describe level of consciousness. Two general types of pathologic processes lead to coma: (1) conditions that widely and directly depress the function of the cerebral hemispheres and (2) conditions that depress or destroy brainstem-activating mechanisms. Common to all impairments is a reduction in either cerebral metabolism or cerebral blood flow.

Three categories of disease are important in the aforementioned pathologic processes that lead to coma:

1. A supratentorial mass lesion will encroach on deep diencephalic structures, compressing or destroying the ascending reticular activating system.
2. A subtentorial mass or destructive lesion may directly damage the central core of the brainstem.
3. Metabolic disorders may lead to generalized interruption of brain function.

Coma does not occur as a result of focal injury or ischemia in a specific lobe; it occurs only when both cerebral hemispheres or brainstem divisions

TABLE 35-1. DEFINITIONS FOR TERMS DESCRIBING LEVEL OF CONSCIOUSNESS

Term	Definition
Alert	Awake and fully conscious and responsive
Drowsy	Sleepy but easily aroused and maintains alertness for brief periods
Confused	Disoriented to time, place, or person; may also exhibit agitation, restlessness, or irritability
Lethargic	Oriented but has sluggish response time for speech, motor, or cognitive activities
Obtunded	Arousable with stimulation; responds verbally or follows simple commands with stimulation
Stupor	Arousable only with vigorous stimulation
Comatose	Deep sleep–like state from which the patient cannot be aroused even with repeated noxious stimuli

Source: Adapted from Mahanes D. Neurologic System In: Chulay M, Burns S, eds. *AACN Essentials of Critical Care Nursing.* New York: McGraw-Hill; 2010. With permission.

are dysfunctional. The major catastrophe of coma is death due to brain herniation.

HERNIATION SYNDROMES

Herniation is the result of increased intracranial pressure (ICP) beyond compensatory levels. The rapid increase in size of a hematoma, tumor, or cerebral edema may cause the movement of brain tissue from an area of the cranium where it is normally located. The brain tissue is not evenly distributed, and unless the change is corrected rapidly, the impingement on blood flow and compression of brain tissue will cause ischemia and permanent

damage. This shift of tissue or protrusion through an abnormal opening is called herniation; it occurs from an area of greater pressure into an area of lower pressure. The most common type of brain herniation occurs when a portion of the temporal lobe is displaced (uncal herniation), resulting in compression of cranial nerve III, the midbrain, and posterior cerebral artery.

Stages of Herniation

There are four distinct stages of central herniation: (1) the early diencephalic stage, (2) the late diencephalic stage, (3) the mesencephalon–upper pons stage, and (4) the lower pons–upper medulla stage.

There are three stages of uncal herniation: (1) the uncal syndrome–early-third cranial-nerve stage, (2) the uncal syndrome–late-third cranial-nerve stage, and (3) the lower pons–upper medulla stage.

Monitoring Parameters

Specific parameters that indicate impending or active herniation can be monitored. Serial computed tomography (CT) or magnetic resonance imaging (MRI) can identify pathophysiology and significant changes.

In central herniation, the parameters are a decrease in the level of consciousness, pupillary function (small pupils to fixed, nonreactive midposition pupils to dilated, fixed, nonreactive pupils), respiratory pattern (Cheyne-Stokes respirations, central

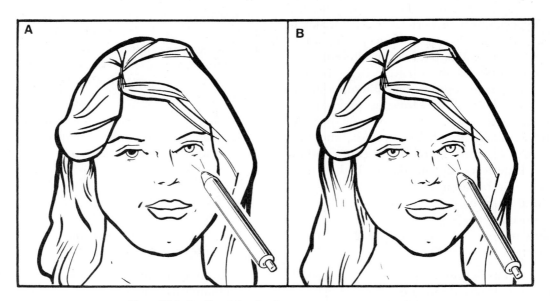

Figure 35-1. Pupillary light reflex (**A**) and consensual light reflex (**B**).

neurogenic hyperventilation, ataxic breathing patterns, and apnea), oculocephalic and oculovestibular responses (intact to disconjugate doll's eyes to no response), motor responses (localizes to pain to flexor/extensor posturing to quadriparesis), loss of cough and gag reflex, and deteriorating vital signs (bradycardia and widening pulse pressure on blood pressure monitoring).

In uncal herniation, altered level of consciousness, contralateral hemiparesis, unequal pupillary response, and unilateral third cranial nerve palsy are early important signs. Late signs include changes in respiration (central neurogenic hyperventilation or Cheyne-Stokes pattern), ipsilateral/nonreactive pupil, disconjugate oculocephalic reflex, and the presence of flexor/extensor posturing.

Parameter Norms and Testing Methods

Level of consciousness is explained in Chap. 32 and is not discussed again here.

Pupillary function is controlled by both sympathetic and parasympathetic tracts. These tracts are not easily affected by metabolic states. Therefore, the presence or absence of an equal pupillary light reflex is the single most important factor in differentiating metabolic from structural (neurologic) coma. The pupillary light reflex (Fig. 35-1) is best tested in a darkened room. In a normal state, the pupil will constrict when a light beam is directed into it. Normally, there is also a consensual response; that is, the pupil *not* having a light beam directed into it will constrict with the eye being tested.

Awareness of the significance of neurological changes is important for progressive care nurses as these changes may occur into the recovery period from an acute injury. Monitoring for vital sign changes, level of consciousness changes, and alterations in physical assessment parameters such as pupillary changes are important in detecting neurologic changes.

36

Meningitis, Muscular Dystrophy, and Myasthenia Gravis

EDITORS' NOTE

In this chapter, we address the concepts of infectious diseases of the neurologic system. This information is supplemental. It will be useful to have a basic understanding of these conditions, although it is unlikely that they will appear on the PCCN exam.

MENINGITIS

Meningitis is an acute infection of the pia and arachnoid membrane surrounding the brain and spinal cord. Because the pia and arachnoid space are communicating structures, meningitis is always a cerebrospinal infection.

Pathophysiology

A bacterial, viral, or fungal pathogenic organism gains access to the pia-subarachnoid space after gaining entrance to the central nervous system through local invasion of tissue or the bloodstream. After crossing the blood-brain barrier, it invades and causes an inflammatory reaction in the pia and arachnoid, in the cerebrospinal fluid (CSF), and in the ventricles of the brain. There is no host defense in the CSF allowing for rapid duplication of the pathogen. The first response is hyperemia of the meningeal vessels, followed by the infiltration of neutrophils into the subarachnoid space. An exudate forms and very quickly enlarges, covering the base of the brain and extending through the subarachnoid space and into the sheaths of cranial and spinal nerves. Polymorphonuclear neutrophils (PMNs) attempt to control the invading pathogen. Within a few days, leukocytes and histiocytes increase in number in an attempt to "wall off" the exudate from the pathogen or its toxins. Toward the end of the second week, the cellular exudate has formed two layers. The outer layer, which lies directly under the arachnoid membrane, is composed of PMNs and fibrin. The inner layer, which lies next to the pia, is composed of lymphocytes, plasma cells, and macrophages.

With appropriate drug therapy to destroy the pathogen, these two layers begin to resolve. The outer cellular layer against the arachnoid disappears. If the infection is arrested quickly enough, the inner layer will also disappear. However, if the infection lasts for several weeks, the inner layer, which contains fibrin, forms a permanent fibrous structure over the meninges. This produces a thickened, often cloudy arachnoid membrane and causes adhesions between the pia and arachnoid membranes.

The adhesions and prior inflammation result in the congestion of tissues and blood vessels. A degeneration of nerve cells follows, eventually resulting in congestion of adjacent brain tissue. This causes cortical irritation and increased intracranial pressure (ICP). Cerebral edema may lead to hydrocephalus. If uninterrupted, a progression of vasculitis with cortical necrosis, petechial hemorrhage within the brain, hydrocephalus, and cranial nerve damage occurs.

Etiology

Organisms obtain access to the subarachnoid space through penetrating head injuries, basal skull fractures with a torn dura mater, ICP monitoring, cranial surgery, mastoiditis, acute otitis media, lumbar punctures, injury to the paranasal sinuses, septic emboli, and sepsis. The infecting organism may be fungal, viral, or bacterial. Eighty percent of all cases of bacterial meningitis are caused by *Streptococcus pneumoniae*, *Neisseria meningitidis*, and *Haemophilus influenzae*. Other Gram-positive bacteria include *Diplococcus pneumoniae*. Gram-negative bacteria include *Klebsiella*, *Escherichia coli*, and *Pseudomonas*. After neurologic surgery, *Staphylococcus aureus* or *S. epidermidis* is a common bacterial contaminant. In children, it is *H. influenzae*. Other bacteria include *Streptococcus*, *Pneumococcus*, and, occasionally, *Mycobacterium tuberculosis*. The outcome of bacterial meningitis depends on early and aggressive treatment. Viral causes of meningitis include enteroviruses, arboviruses, and herpesviruses. Viral meningitis is commonly referred to as aseptic meningitis. Fungal meningitis is primarily caused by *Cryptococcus neoformans*.

Clinical Signs and Symptoms

Suspect meningitis if a fever, severe headache, and nuchal rigidity (resistance to flexion of the neck) exist. Positive Kernig's and Brudzinski's signs, photophobia, decreased sensorium, and signs of increased ICP are common. Kernig's sign is the inability to fully extend the leg at the knee when the leg is flexed at the hip. Brudzinski's sign is the involuntary adduction and flexion of the legs with attempts to flex the neck. With meningitis, a headache becomes progressively worse and is accompanied by nausea, vomiting, irritability, confusion, and seizures. Dysfunction of cranial nerves II through VIII may be present. Papilledema is more likely with brain abscess, subdural empyema, and venous sinus occlusion. Changes in vital signs occur with brainstem pressure. If the causative organism is the meningococcus, a petechial skin rash is common in 50% of cases. The rash progresses to purple blotches.

Diagnosis

A major diagnostic tool is examination of the CSF. Variations in the CSF depend on the causative organism. Levels of CSF protein are usually elevated; more so in bacterial than in viral cases. A decreased CSF glucose level is common in bacterial meningitis but may be normal in viral meningitis. In bacterial meningitis, the CSF appears purulent and turbid. It may be the same or clear in viral meningitis. The predominant cell in the CSF is the PMN.

Cultures of blood, sputum, and nasopharyngeal secretions are performed to identify the causative organism.

Radiographs of the skull may demonstrate infected sinuses. Computed tomographic (CT) scans are usually normal in uncomplicated meningitis. In other cases, CT may reveal evidence of increased ICP.

Nursing Interventions

Rapid identification of the patient with meningitis is imperative. Make sure that airway and breathing are adequate. Intravenous lines are started and blood cultures obtained. Antibiotics are administered based on the suspected organism. Respiratory isolation precautions will protect the staff and visitors but need not be continued past 24 to 48 h after the institution of antibiotic therapy.

Body temperature can be controlled by the administration of antipyretic drugs as indicated, use of a hypothermia blanket, and environmental temperature change.

Headache is usually treated with analgesics. A darkened, quiet room will help both the headache and photophobia. Avoid sudden quick movements.

Seizure precautions should be initiated. If seizures occur, anticonvulsant medication is indicated. Documentation of progression, limb involvement, and duration of the seizures will help determine an effective medication regimen.

Monitoring of electrolyte levels, especially sodium, is essential. Standard nursing procedures for these types of complications are followed.

MUSCULAR DYSTROPHY

Muscular dystrophy refers to a group of genetic, inherited muscle diseases that lead to muscle weakness. Muscular dystrophies are characterized by progressive skeletal muscle weakness, defects in muscle proteins, and the death of muscle cells and tissue.

The main symptoms of muscular dystrophy include progressive muscle weakness, poor balance, frequent falls, calf pain, decreased range of movement, drooping eyelids (ptosis), and difficulty walking. The diagnosis of muscular dystrophy is based on the results of a muscle biopsy. In some cases, a DNA blood test may be all that is needed.

A physical examination and the patient's medical history will help determine the type of muscular dystrophy as specific muscle groups are affected by different types of muscular dystrophy.

There is no specific treatment and no known cure for muscular dystrophy; the goal of treatment is to control symptoms. As inactivity (such as bed rest and even sitting for long periods) can worsen the disease, physical therapy and occupational therapy may be helpful. Physical therapy is aimed at preventing contractures and maintaining muscle tone. Orthopedic appliances such as braces can be used to improve mobility. Surgery on the spine or legs may be indicated in some cases to improve function. The cardiac problems that occur with Emery-Dreifuss muscular dystrophy and myotonic muscular dystrophy may require a pacemaker.

The main focus of nursing interventions is on maximizing functional status during acute illness by promoting mobility and activities of daily living.

MYASTHENIA GRAVIS AND CRISIS

Myasthenia gravis (MG) is an autoimmune-mediated neuromuscular disorder caused by a decrease in the number of available acetylcholine receptors at the neuromuscular junction. It is a chronic disorder of neuromuscular transmission resulting in weakness with exercise and the improvement of strength with rest.

Pathophysiology

Three theories have been proposed with regard to the pathophysiology of MG. Acetylcholine is released at nerve terminals and combines at the postsynaptic muscle membrane, producing an electrochemical reaction resulting in muscle contraction. In MG, either there are too few postsynaptic receptor sites for the amount of acetylcholine released to bind with and thus to provide for a full muscular contraction, so there is not enough acetylcholine released to cause full muscle contraction, or acetylcholinesterase degrades the acetylcholine before sufficient amounts can cause a full muscle contraction.

Etiology

How the autoimmune response in MG is initiated is not completely understood. The most prevalent hypothesis is that MG is an autoimmune process that damages the postsynaptic membrane. A statistically significant number of cases are associated with thymoma and thymic hyperplasia. This is substantiated by the finding of serum antibodies produced by sensitized lymphocytes or thymocytes, which block the action of acetylcholine and the production of immune bodies by the thymus.

Occurrence

MG occurs in from 1:10,000 to 1:50,000 persons. It may occur at any age but is rarely seen in persons younger than 10 years or those older than 70 years. Peak occurrence is in the 20- to 30-year age range. Below 40 years, the ratio of occurrence in women to men is 3:1; above 40 years, it is 1:1.

Clinical Signs, Symptoms, and Course

MG is characterized by fatigability of voluntary muscle groups with repeated use. Pathognomonic signs of MG include uneven drooping of the eyelids, a smile that resembles a snarl, a drooping lower jaw that must be supported by the hand, and a partially immobile mouth with the corners turned downward. However, few patients are first seen with these signs. In more than 90% of the cases, the eyebrows and extraocular muscles are involved, accompanied by weakness in eye closure. Ptosis and diplopia are common. The next most commonly affected muscles exhibiting symptoms are those of facial expression, mastication, swallowing, and speaking (dysarthria). Hoarseness occurs after only a few minutes of talking. Neck flexor and extensor muscles, the shoulder girdle, and hip flexors are less frequently involved. There is usually no sensory disturbance.

The course of MG is variable. Remission may occur for no discernible reason in fewer than half the cases and usually does not last longer than 1 to 2 months. The prognosis has improved as a result of advances in treatment, and most myasthenic patients can be successfully managed with proper therapy.

Associated Conditions

Approximately 15% of patients have a tumor of the thymus. There is an increasing incidence of tumors in older men. Thyroiditis, thyrotoxicosis, lupus erythematosus, and rheumatoid arthritis occur more often than statistically expected. A pregnancy may make the disease worse or better or may have no effect. Close to 15% of children born to myasthenic mothers exhibit symptoms of the disease. These symptoms are usually transient and resolve within 1 to 12 weeks.

Diagnosis

A history of an increasing muscular fatigability that improves with rest is a common characteristic of MG. Various laboratory tests can be used to aid in the diagnosis, including fatigue on repetitive electrical stimulation, single-fiber electromyographic testing, elevated serum acetylcholine-R antibody titers, and radiographic evidence of thymus enlargement on CT or magnetic resonance imaging (MRI). However, anticholinesterase tests are to be considered conclusive.

Treatment

The most useful treatments include anticholinesterase medications, immunosuppressive agents, thymectomy, and plasmapheresis or intravenous immunoglobulin. The major objective of therapy is to improve neuromuscular transmission and prevent complications. Early thymectomy may be employed.

Neuromuscular transmission is improved by administration of anticholinesterase drugs. Pyridostigmine bromide is a popular choice. If pyridostigmine bromide is not adequate to establish control of neuromuscular transmission, neostigmine is used. Prednisone has become an adjunctive drug of choice. It is extremely important to medicate the patient on schedule and to document carefully the patient's muscular response. The medication should be taken with a snack to prevent abdominal cramps and diarrhea. The major difference between pyridostigmine bromide and neostigmine is their duration of action. Pyridostigmine has a 4-h effect; neostigmine, 2-h. Fasciculation and increased weakness occurring 50 min after administration of drug is a sign of toxicity and should be reported immediately. Steroids may decrease the amount of anticholinesterase drug required to control myasthenic symptoms. Immunosuppression using glucocorticoids, azathioprine and other drugs is effective in nearly all patients with MG. Glucocorticoids and cyclosporine generally produce clinical improvement within a period of 1 to 3 months.

Nursing Interventions

A major nursing intervention is to maintain adequate ventilation in spite of a weak cough, an inability to clear secretions, and an increased likelihood of aspiration.

Prevention of aspiration, infection from any source, and emotional support of the patient are very important.

Specific drugs that impair neuromuscular transmission must be avoided. The aminoglycoside antibiotics and true mycin drugs are contraindicated. Such drugs include polymyxin, neomycin, streptomycin, tobramycin, amikacin, and gentamicin.

Quinidine, procainamide, morphine sulfate, and sedatives will aggravate muscle weakness.

Nursing education concerning the importance of taking prescribed medications on schedule is extremely important since an early or late dosage may immediately affect muscle strength. Regulation of daily living habits to avoid fatigue and provide rest must be tailored to the patient's lifestyle as much as possible. While immunosuppression therapy is gradually reduced, usually treatment for months or years may be needed, and close monitoring for side effects is required.

Complications: Myasthenic or Cholinergic Crisis?

Myasthenic and cholinergic crises both have extreme weakness as the predominant symptom. Myasthenic crisis is caused by insufficient drug dose. Cholinergic crisis is due to an overdose of drugs and is signaled by increased salivation and sweating. An impending cholinergic crisis can be detected by noting constricted pupils; 2 mm is the maximum constriction that should be allowed before intervention. To distinguish between these crises, an edrophonium bromide test is performed with a ventilator on standby. If the patient becomes weaker, a cholinergic (overdose) crisis exists. Treatment is to discontinue anticholinesterase drugs. After 72 h, drug therapy is usually restarted in small increments. Atropine (an anticholinergic drug) may control symptoms but may also block important symptoms of anticholinesterase overdose.

Myasthenic crisis is established by muscular improvement with the edrophonium bromide test. Anticholinesterase drugs are given and repeated as needed. Steroids are usually avoided during a crisis. Monitoring, assessment, and the documentation of muscular strength and oxygenation are continued throughout the crisis. Muscle assessment may include presence of the gag reflex, voice quality, swallowing difficulty, ptosis on upward gaze, diplopia on lateral gaze, and the ability to do deep knee bends, raise arms above head, rise from chair, or lift the head off the bed. Identification of the precipitating cause is important to treat and/or correct the cause. The most common cause of myasthenic crisis is infection. Other causes include heat exposure, emotional upset, surgery, thyroid disease, pregnancy, menses, hypokalemia, and drugs that block the neuromuscular junction. With advances in treatment, however, crisis rarely occurs in properly managed patients.

37

Seizures and Status Epilepticus

EDITORS' NOTE

In this chapter, concepts are covered that address the PCCN exam items of seizures and status epilepticus. You can expect several questions on this content.

SEIZURES

A seizure is a symptom of paroxysmal electrical discharges in the brain, resulting in autonomic, sensory, and/or motor dysfunction. Seizures may be associated with infection, trauma, tumors, cerebrovascular disease, genetic or congenital defects, or metabolic dysfunction. A seizure may also be related to a temporary condition, such as exposure to drugs, withdrawal from certain drugs, or abnormal levels of sodium or glucose in the blood. Seizures can cause involuntary changes in body movement or function, sensation, awareness, or behavior. A seizure can last from a few seconds to status epilepticus, a continuous seizure that will not stop without intervention. If seizures are recurrent and transient, the condition is classified as epilepsy. The term *convulsion* refers to the musculoskeletal contractions accompanying a seizure. A seizure lasting longer than 5 min is considered a medical emergency.

Classification

Seizures are classified according to whether the source of the seizure within the brain is localized (*partial* or *focal* onset seizures) or distributed (*generalized* seizures). Partial seizures are further divided as to the extent to which consciousness is affected (*simple partial* seizures and *complex partial* seizures). Partial seizures are usually associated with structural brain abnormalities and the seizure activity is restricted to discrete areas of the cerebral cortex. Generalized seizures involve diffuse regions of the brain simultaneously and can result from cellular, biochemical, or structural abnormalities. There are three main types of seizures: partial seizures, generalized seizures, and unclassified seizures. Table 37-1 gives a classification of seizures.

Partial Seizures

Partial seizures are of three types: simple, complex, and partial secondarily generalizing to generalized tonic-clonic seizure. Simple partial seizures are not associated with a loss of consciousness. The hyperactivity is focused in one area of the brain and does not spread to the other hemisphere. Seizures that initiate in one area and spread to a larger area of the same hemisphere are known as complex partial seizures. In complex partial seizures, loss of consciousness may initiate or be a sequela of the seizure. Both simple partial and complex partial seizures may evolve into tonic-clonic seizures.

Generalized Seizures

Generalized seizures are characterized by loss of consciousness with involvement of both cerebral hemispheres. They include absence, myoclonic, clonic, tonic, tonic-clonic, and atonic seizures.

Unclassified Seizures

Unclassified epileptic seizures include all seizures for which there are insufficient data as to cause or effect to classify them as partial or generalized seizures. Neonatal seizures are an example of this type of seizure.

TABLE 37-1. CLASSIFICATION OF SEIZURES

Partial seizures
   Simple partial seizure
   Complex partial seizure
   Partial seizure secondarily generalizing to generalized tonic–clonic
     seizure
Generalized seizures
   Absence seizure
   Myoclonic seizure
   Clonic seizure
   Tonic seizure
   Tonic-clonic seizure
   Atonic seizure
Unclassified epileptic seizures

Pathophysiology

It is unknown whether seizures occur as a result of increased neuronal excitability or a decreased neuronal inhibitory force. Focal neurons appear to be unusually sensitive to acetylcholine and possibly to deficits in specific neurotransmitters. Altered cell permeability and/or alteration in electrolytes may have a role in seizure activity. It is logical to assume that an electrical threshold for seizures exists in all persons. Factors thought to lower the electrical threshold of neurons include fever, fatigue, altered electrolyte-fluid balance, stress, emotional distress, and/or pregnancy. Regardless of these factors, the hyperexcited neurons become hyperactive. As these localized neuronal discharges become more intense, the hyperirritability spreads synaptically to adjacent neurons. In many instances, the entire brain is involved. When only one hemisphere is involved, consciousness is preserved. When both cerebral hemispheres are involved, there is usually a loss of consciousness. There are exceptions, however. In the case of bilateral simple partial seizures, loss of consciousness does not occur. Also, in complex partial seizures, consciousness may be altered but is not lost, since the seizures occur in the limbic system (even though it is bilateral).

Clinical Presentations

Simple Partial (Focal) Motor Seizures

These seizures were previously known as jacksonian seizures. The focal point is in the motor strip (the prerolandic gyrus). The typical seizure starts with a twitching of the fingers or toes or around the lips on one side of the body. The muscle movement becomes more severe and spreads (marches) by involving more muscle groups until one side of the body is totally involved. Consciousness is maintained unless the motor seizure becomes generalized and spreads to the remainder of the body.

Simple Partial (Focal) Sensory Seizures

These seizures may be described by the patient as a numbness, tingling, or "pins and needles" sensation. If the causative lesion is in the sensory strip between the frontal and parietal lobes (the postrolandic gyrus), the seizure may progress like a motor seizure. Visual sensations usually indicate an occipital lobe lesion. Auditory sensations are most commonly a buzzing or ringing in the ears. Auditory sensations are often accompanied by olfactory symptoms and dizziness. This indicates a temporal lobe lesion.

Complex Partial Psychomotor Seizures

An aura often precedes a seizure. The aura includes complex visceral and/or perceptual hallucinations. The patient appears to be awake but is in an unresponsive state. Simple or elaborate behavior patterns known as automatisms may be carried out during the seizure. These robot-like behavior patterns can include such behaviors as lip smacking, blinking, or picking at clothes. There may be motor activities such as wandering, running, or a jerking if the seizures are in the frontal lobe area. The average seizure lasts about 5 min. Attempts to interrupt the behavior pattern often precipitate violence. The seizure may end abruptly with the patient having complete amnesia, or the patient may have a period of headache, confusion, or sleepiness.

Tonic-Clonic (Grand Mal) Seizures

A peculiar sensation or feeling known as a (prodromal) aura may occur at the beginning of a seizure. An aura also accompanies complex partial seizures. For those who do experience an aura, it is almost always the same sensation or feeling. As consciousness is lost, the patient falls (if upright). The body becomes rigid. As air is forced from the lungs, the patient may emit a high-pitched, loud cry. The jaws become locked and the tongue is often caught between the clenched teeth. Pupils dilate and are nonreactive. Apnea results in cyanosis. Bladder incontinence is common. This tonic phase of the grand mal seizure lasts 10 to 20 s.

The clonic phase of the grand mal seizure is a period of violent, rhythmic, symmetric, alternating contraction and relaxation involving the entire body. Increased salivation, mixed with blood if the tongue has been bitten, results in "frothing" at the mouth. The patient is tachycardic, profusely diaphoretic, and apneic. The tonic and clonic phases last 1 to 5 min.

In the postictal phase, the seizure subsides, the patient resumes breathing, cyanosis clears, and the pupils react. The patient should be bagged with a high volume of oxygen during this stage to help compensate for the period of apnea. The patient is fatigued, has a headache, is sleepy and confused, and may have amnesia of the entire seizure excepting the aura. A residual neurologic deficit (Todd's paralysis) may continue for several hours.

Absence (Petit Mal) Seizures

These are generalized seizures that consist of frequent episodes of loss of consciousness termed absences. The absences last 10 to 15 s and are characterized by the cessation of motor activity, stopping speech in midsentence, and/or staring into space. During the seizure, the child (it is rarely seen in children >12 years) may twitch his or her lips or the lips may droop. The eyes may roll upward. There is no change in muscle tone. The patient may stagger or stumble but rarely falls. Absence seizures are benign neurologically; however, they may interfere with classroom learning.

Bilateral Myoclonus (Myoclonic Seizures)

These seizures are characterized by sudden, violent contractions of muscle groups. They may be generalized or focal and symmetric (both sides) or asymmetric (one side). Loss of consciousness is unusual in certain types of myoclonic seizure activity. The seizures may consist of a single jerking movement or intermittent periods of active seizure or be present in varying degrees all of the waking time. The seizures are absent during sleep, being precipitated by stimulation and intensified with intentional movement.

Atonic (Akinetic) Seizures

These may occur by themselves or in cases of absence seizures. There is a sudden, brief loss of muscle tone with or without a loss of consciousness. The child with such seizures falls often and may be labeled clumsy or awkward. Akinetic seizures may cloud the picture of absence seizures. These seizures often result from serious neurologic disease that cannot be treated.

Etiology of Epilepsy

Multiple causes of epilepsy are known. The most common is the abrupt cessation of antiepileptic drugs or other chronic sedative medications. Other causes include trauma, tumor, injuries (both perinatal and postnatal), central nervous system (CNS) infections, and cerebrovascular disease, including arteriovenous malformations. Metabolic and toxic disorders may cause seizures. The role of genetics and heredity is controversial at this time. In a large number of cases, the cause is unknown. These cases are termed idiopathic epilepsy.

Diagnosis of Epilepsy

Epilepsy is a common chronic neurologic disorder characterized by recurrent unprovoked seizures. These seizures are transient signs and/or symptoms of abnormal, excessive, or synchronous neuronal activity in the brain. The patient's history of seizure activity (duration, frequency, intensity, and progression) is among the most useful tools in establishing a diagnosis. The family should be asked for their observations and their knowledge of participating factors if the patient is unable to provide them. Past medical history should be closely examined for previous seizures, head injury, or other illness. Physical examination, laboratory studies, radiologic studies, and electroencephalograms (EEGs) may reveal factors supporting a diagnosis of epilepsy, or the studies may all be within normal limits.

Nursing Interventions and Complications

There are five major areas of nursing intervention for the patient having seizures:

1. Protecting the patient from injury is a priority. Remove objects from the immediate environment that might cause injury. Stay with the patient during the seizure. Bed rails should be up and padded and the bed placed in low position. The patient should not be restrained, but efforts to protect the patient's head from injury are appropriate (e.g., if a seizure occurs with the patient out of bed, a pillow may be placed under the head or a nurse may cradle—*not* restrain—the patient's head to protect it). *Nothing* should ever be used to pry open the patient's mouth, nor should anything be forced into the mouth during a seizure. Damage to the mouth and tongue occurs at the start of a seizure and only more damage will result by forcing objects into the mouth.

2. The observation and recording of seizure patterns with a video camera may help to identify the seizure focus. When surface EEG electrodes are insufficient, an implanted grid for

EEG monitoring may be used to locate the lesion. Data collected include precipitating factors, presence and type of aura, duration of unconsciousness, the pattern and progression of seizure activity, body parts involved (generalized or one-sided), incontinence, postictal activity, and, if monitored, EEG data.

3. Assessment of the respiratory system is extremely important. The danger in a tonic-clonic seizure is that the patient's respiratory status will be compromised during the tonic phase. The respiratory status may be further compromised by aspiration. Oxygen and suction should be at the bedside. The patient should be turned to the side to protect the airway after the seizure and be allowed to sleep.

4. Administration of medication on a regular basis and the evaluation of its effectiveness in controlling seizures as well as the psychologic effects on the patient are important actions and assessments. Teaching the patient the beneficial effects of following the prescribed medication regimen and identifying and overcoming patient objections may result in better patient adherence in the future.

5. The promotion of physical and mental health may sharply curtail the number of seizures. Regular routines for eating, sleeping, and physical activity should be established. Alcohol, stress, and fatigue tend to precipitate seizure activity. Modification of these factors will alter the seizure pattern. The patient should be instructed to take showers and avoid baths owing to the potential for seizure activity.

Treatment of Epilepsy

The treatment of a seizure disorder is almost always multimodal and includes treatment of underlying conditions, avoidance of precipitating factors, and suppression of recurrent seizures by prophylactic therapy with antiepileptic medications or surgery. If seizures are the result of tumor, infection, or metabolic dysfunction, correcting the underlying cause is the goal of therapy. In a majority of cases, an underlying cause may not be identifiable or be amenable to curative therapy. Antiepileptic drug therapy is used for the management of recurrent seizures of unknown etiology or a known cause that cannot be reversed. It is preferable to use a single drug to achieve control of seizure activity. Common drugs include phenytoin sodium, phenobarbital, primidone, ethosuximide, clonazepam, carbamazepine, valproic acid, and lamotrigine. Adjunctive therapeutic agents include topiramate, zonisamide, gabapentin, levetiracetam, and tiagabine. Established agents such as phenytoin, valproic acid, carbamazepine, and ethosuximide are generally used as first-line therapy. Most of the newer drugs are used as add-on or alternative therapy. For the therapeutic serum level of these drugs, their affinity for specific types of seizures, and their side effects, the reader is referred to any standard pharmacology text.

If drug therapy is ineffective and seizures are intractable and deny the patient a normal life, surgery may be performed. After identifying the specific epileptic focus and the patient's dominant hemisphere, a temporal lobectomy, extratemporal resection, or hemispherectomy may be done. Seizures may continue for a period after the surgery; therefore, the patient's medication is continued for approximately a year. Palliative surgery to restrict seizure spread includes partial or complete callosotomy. The patient must continue on antiepileptic medication following palliative surgery.

STATUS EPILEPTICUS

Status epilepticus is described as a seizure or series of seizures lasting longer than 30 min. Status epilepticus is a medical emergency and has an overall mortality of 20% to 30%. The state of status epilepticus is present when seizures follow each other so closely that a state of consciousness is not recovered between seizures. Status epilepticus may be partial or generalized in origin. An EEG is necessary to determine the type or, in the patient in coma, the presence of seizures.

Etiology

Inadequate dosage of antiepileptic medication in a known epileptic is a common precipitating factor. Other factors include sudden withdrawal of antiepileptic drugs and other sedative drugs, hyponatremia, fever, intercurrent infection (commonly in the CNS), cerebrovascular disease, and cerebral hypoxia, anoxia, and edema. Progressive neurologic diseases such as brain tumors and subdural hematoma may cause status epilepticus. A common triad of causes consists of alcohol abuse, drug abuse, and sleep deprivation. Head trauma or pregnancy (preeclamptic state) may precipitate status epilepticus. Metabolic causes include hypoglycemia, hyponatremia, hypocalcemia, uremia, and electrolyte imbalances.

Incidence and Prognosis

Approximately 6% of known epileptics will develop status epilepticus. Almost 50% of the cases of status epilepticus occur in known epileptics. Approximately 10% of patients in status epilepticus will die. Death is commonly due to respiratory and metabolic acidosis, hypoxemia, hypoglycemia, hyperthermia, electrolyte disturbances, and/or renal failure.

Pathophysiology

The pathophysiology is the same as that of epilepsy; however, in status epilepticus the seizures are almost continuous. The rapidly repeating tonic-clonic seizures lead to hypoxemia (patients are apneic during such seizures) and cerebral anoxia. The increased metabolic activity of the brain causes hypoglycemia and hyperthermia. Hypoxemia, hypoglycemia, and hyperthermia may themselves precipitate seizure activity, resulting in a vicious cycle.

Clinical Presentation

There are three variants in the clinical picture of status epilepticus:

1. Generalized tonic-clonic status epilepticus is a life-threatening emergency. These seizures are the most common and occur without a period of consciousness between seizures.
2. The second most common presentation is partial status epilepticus, termed epilepsia partialis continua. Focal motor seizures occur continuously or regularly. Consciousness is usually maintained unless generalization occurs. Complex partial status epilepticus presents as a prolonged confusional state followed by postictal confusion and sleepiness.
3. Absence status epilepticus patients may exhibit as many as 200 to 300 "absences" per day. This nonconvulsive state is difficult to differentiate from complex partial status epilepticus.

Electrical status occurs in every type of status and is not a distinct type. It is always associated with some clinical abnormality. The EEG shows continuous epileptic activity.

Treatment

The goal of therapy is to restore physiologic homeostasis and to stop the seizures by correcting the underlying cause. The first step in treatment is to ensure a patent airway and maintain breathing and circulation. The second step is to draw blood for antiepileptic drug levels, toxicology screen, glucose, electrolytes, calcium, magnesium, creatinine, blood urea nitrogen, complete blood count with differential, liver profile, arterial blood gases (ABGs), and creatine phosphokinase and to establish an intravenous line. Thiamine 100 mg intravenously is administered prior to 50% glucose 50 mL intravenously if alcoholism or hypoglycemia is suspected. The third step is to administer medications to stop seizure activity.

Benzodiazepines such as lorazepam given intravenously are often the drugs of choice in spite of their potential for suppressing respirations. Fast-acting antiepilepsy drugs very quickly enter and quickly leave the brain. But these very properties often make benzodiazepines a poor choice for long-term management of status epilepticus.

Phenytoin is given intravenously. It must be injected slowly (50 mg/min), and cardiac monitoring is essential for early intervention in the event that a dysrhythmia develops. Bradycardia and hypotension are especially common in patients older than age 40. Phenytoin requires 15 to 20 min to peak in brain tissue, and it remains in brain tissue over a long period. Fosphenytoin is a prodrug of phenytoin that can be given at a faster rate (150 mg/min) and less likely to cause harm to peripheral veins.

If seizures persist after 30 min, there is a high probability that acute CNS disease is causing them. Phenobarbital may be tried. A slow intravenous injection is recommended (50 to 100 mg/min). Respiratory depression and hypotension may develop. Phenobarbital and diazepam should not be administered concurrently. If benzodiazepines are used to stop seizures, phenytoin is given simultaneously to block recurrence of the seizures. A combination of benzodiazepines and barbiturate may cause respiratory depression and hypotension.

Lidocaine as a 20% solution in normal saline may be tried. In some medical centers general anesthesia (barbiturate coma) is administered to a depth of EEG silence when other drugs have failed. Pharmacologic neuromuscular blockade will not stop brain electrical activity but will stop movement. Surgical excision of epileptic foci that have not responded to medical therapy is being used with increasing effectiveness. Vagal nerve stimulation for intractable partial and secondarily generalizing seizures is also used for selected cases.

Nursing Interventions

An initial priority of seizure management for nursing care is maintaining patient safety. Maintaining a patent airway and providing adequate oxygenation are additionally important. Observation of the seizure type, duration, precipitating factors, along with any focal neurologic deficits, is essential. An intravenous line should be maintained. Electroencephalographic monitoring, continuous pulse oximetry, and blood pressure monitoring are indicated in patients with prolonged seizures. Cardiac drugs should be available as cardiac monitoring may reveal dysrhythmias. Hyperthermia is often treated with a hypothermia blanket. Because hypoglycemia can induce seizure activity, a glucose level should be checked. Fluid and electrolyte balance is monitored. Neurologic status is monitored closely.

BIBLIOGRAPHY

Adams, H. P, del Zoppo, G., Alberts, M. J., Bhatt, D. L., Brass, L., Furlan, A., . . . Wijdicks, E. F. (2007). Guidelines for the early management of adults with ischemic stroke. *Stroke, 38*, 1655–1711.

American Association of Neuroscience Nursing. (2006). *Guide to the care of the patient with craniotomy post brain-tumor resection.* Glenview, IL: American Association of Nurse Anesthetists.

American Association of Neuroscience Nursing. (2007a). *Care of the patient with aneurysmal subarachnoid hemorrhage.* Glenview, IL: American Association of Nurse Anesthetists.

American Association of Neuroscience Nursing. (2007b). *Guide to the care of the patient with seizure.* 2nd ed. Glenview, IL: American Association of Nurse Anesthetists.

American Association of Neuroscience Nursing. (2007c). *Cervical spine surgery: A guide to preoperative and postoperative patient care.* Glenview, IL: American Association of Nurse Anesthetists.

American Association of Neuroscience Nursing. (2008a). *Guide to the care of the hospitalized patient with ischemic stroke* (2nd ed.). Glenview, IL: American Association of Nurse Anesthetists.

American Association of Neuroscience Nursing. (2008b). *Nursing Management of adults with severe traumatic brain injury.* Glenview, IL: American Association of Nurse Anesthetists.

American Heart Association Guidelines for Management of Aneurysmal Subarachnoid Hemorrhage. Available at http://www.americanheart.org/presenter.jhtml?identifier=1192. Accessed 9/22/2010

American Association of Critical-Care Nurses, AANN, & American Association of Critical-Care Nurses. (2009). *AACN protocols for practice: monitoring neuroscience patients.* Sudbury, MA: Jones & Bartlett.

Arif., H., & Hirsch, L. J. (2008). Treatment of status epilepticus. *Seminars in Neurology 28*, 342–354.

Bederson, J. B., Connolly, E. S., Batjer, H. H., Dacey, R. G., Dion, J. E., Diringer, M. N., . . . Rosenwasser, R. H. (2009). Guidelines for the management of aneurismal subarachnoid hemorrhage: A statement for healthcare professionals from a special writing group of the stroke council, American Heart Association. *Stroke, 40*, 994–1025.

Brain Attack Coalition. TPA Stroke Study Group Guidelines. Administration of rt-PA to Acute Ischemic Stroke Patients. Available at http://www.stroke-site.org/guidelines/tpa_guidelines.html. Accessed 9/2/2010

Brain Trauma Foundation (2007). Guidelines for the management of severe traumatic brain injury. *Journal of Neurotrauma, 24*(Suppl 1), S1–S106.

Bratton, S. L., et al. (2007). Guidelines for the management of severe traumatic brain injury. VI. Indications for intracranial pressure monitoring. *Journal of Neurotrauma, 24*(Suppl 1), S37–S44.

Bratton, S. L., et al. (2007). Guidelines for the management of severe traumatic brain injury. VII. Intracranial pressure monitoring technology. *Journal of Neurotrauma, 24*(Suppl 1), S45–S54.

Bratton, S. L., et al. (2007). Guidelines for the management of severe traumatic brain injury. IX. Cerebral perfusion thresholds. *Journal of Neurotrauma, 24*(Suppl 1), S59–S64.

Bratton, S. L., et al. (2007). Guidelines for the management of severe traumatic brain injury. VI. Intracranial pressure thresholds. *Journal of Neurotrauma, 24*(Suppl 1), S55–S58.

Broderick, J., Connolly, S., Feldman, E., Hanley, D., Kase, C., Krieger, D., . . . Zuccarello, M. (2007). Guidelines for the management of spontaneous intracerebral hemorrhage in adults. *Stroke, 38*, 2001–2023.

Burns. T. M. (2008). Guillain-Barré syndrome. *Seminars in Neurology, 28*, 152–167.

Castera, F. M., Depew, J. S., & Moran, J. L. (2009). Neurological critical care. In J. J Wyckoff, D. Houghton, C. T. LePage (eds.). *Critical care* (pp. 139–245). Springer Publishing, New York.

Crippen, D. W. Head trauma. Emedicine. Available at http://www.emedicine.com/med/topic2820.htm. Accessed 9/2/2010

Eaton, J. D., Saver, J. L., Abers, G. W., Alberts, M. J., Chaturvedi, S., Feldmann, E., . . . Sacco, R. L. (2009). Definition and duration of transient ischemic attack. *Stroke, 40*, 2276–2293.

Foldvary-Schaefer, N., & Wyllie, E. (2007). Epilepsy. In C. G. Goetz (Ed.). *Textbook of clinical neurology.* (3rd ed.). Philadelphia, PA: Saunders Elsevier.

Frizzell, J. P. (2005). Acute stroke: pathophysiology, diagnosis and treatment. *American Association of Critical Care Nurses Clinical Issues. 16*, 421–440.

Hickey, J. V. (2008). *The clinical practice of neurological and neurosurgical nursing* (6th ed.). Philadelphia, PA: Wolters Kluwer Health/Lippincott Williams & Wilkins.

Hinkle, J. (2005). An update on transient ischemic attacks. *Journal of Neuroscience Nurses, 37*, 243–248.

Holland, N. J., & Madonna M. (2005). Nursing grand rounds: Multiple sclerosis. *Journal of Neuroscience Nurses, 37,* 15–19.

Luke, A. M. (2009). Critical care management of the patient with elevated intracranial pressure. *Critical Care Alert, 9,* 44–47.

Mahanes, D. (2010). Advanced neurologic concepts. In M. Chulay & S., Burns (Eds.). *AACN essentials of critical care nursing* (pp. 261–282). New York, NY: McGraw-Hill.

National Institute of Neurological Disorders and Stroke. Spinal Cord Injury Information. Available at http://www.ninds.nih.gov/disorders/sci/sci.htm. Accessed 8/22/2009.

National Institute of Neurological Disorders and Stroke. Cerebral Aneurysm Fact Sheet, Available at http://www.ninds.nih.gov/disorders/cerebral_aneurysm/detail_cerebral_aneurysm.htm. Accessed 8/20/2010.

Pass, M. (2008). Central nervous system infections. In E. Barker(Ed). *Neuroscience nursing: A spectrum of care* (3rd ed.). St. Louis, MO: Mosby.

Pugh, S., Mathiesen, C., Meighan, M., Summers, D., Zrelak, P. (2008). *Guide to the care of the hospitalized patient with ischemic stroke:* AANA *clinical practice guideline* (2nd ed.). Glenview, IL: American Association of Neuroscience Nurses.

Spenser, S. S. (2007). Seizures and epilepsy. In L. Goldman & D. Ausiello (Eds.) *Cecil Medicine* (23rd ed.). Philadelphia, PA: Saunders Elsevier.

Summers, D., Leonard, A., Wentworth, D., Saver, J. L., Simpson, J., Spilker, J. A., . . . Mitchell, P. H. Comprehensive overview of nursing and interdisciplinary care of the acute ischemic stroke patient. A scientific statement from the American Heart Association. *Stroke, 40,* 2911–2944.

Tunkel, A. R. Glaser, C. A, Block, K. C, Sejvar, J. J., Marra, C. M., Roos, K. L., . . . Whitley, R. J. (2008). The management of encephalitis: clinical practice guidelines by the Infectious Diseases Society of America. *Clinical Infectious Diseases, 47,* 303–327.

Neurology Practice Exam

1. Which meningeal layer lies closest to the brain?
   (A) Pia mater
   (B) Dura mater
   (C) Arachnoid
   (D) Subarachnoid

2. Which cerebral component is responsible for reabsorbing cerebrospinal fluid (CSF)?
   (A) Lateral ventricle
   (B) Dura mater
   (C) Arachnoid villi
   (D) Subarachnoid cisterns

3. Which meningeal layer lies closest to the skull?
   (A) Pia mater
   (B) Dura mater
   (C) Arachnoid
   (D) Subarachnoid

4. Which structure separates the left and right cerebral hemispheres?
   (A) Dura mater
   (B) Subarachnoid space
   (C) Fissure of Rolando
   (D) Falx cerebri

5. An injury to the temporal lobe would cause disturbances in which sensory component?
   (A) Sight
   (B) Hearing
   (C) Spatial orientation
   (D) Taste

6. A patient in your unit has suffered frontal head injuries from a motor vehicle accident. Which type of impairment may result from injury to the frontal lobe?
   (A) Loss of sensation
   (B) Loss of vision

   (C) Alterations in hearing
   (D) Alterations in personality

7. Neurohumoral control of respiration is located in which structure(s)?
   (A) Pons and medulla
   (B) Diencephalon
   (C) Reticular-activating system
   (D) Basal ganglia

8. The primary function of the cerebellum includes which of the following?
   (A) Thought integration
   (B) Maintenance of personality characteristics
   (C) Sight
   (D) Maintenance of equilibrium and muscle coordination

9. Obstruction of the foramen of Monro would produce which condition?
   (A) Ipsilateral dilatation of the pupils
   (B) Hydrocephalus
   (C) Hemiparesis
   (D) Compression of the third cranial nerve

10. Which of the following corresponds most closely to the primary purpose of the CSF?
    (A) Transport of oxygen to the brain
    (B) Manufacture of neurotransmitters
    (C) Cushioning the brain and spinal column
    (D) Maintenance of cerebral perfusion pressures

11. Which area of the brain is responsible for voluntary motor function?
    (A) Parietal lobe
    (B) Frontal lobe
    (C) Occipital lobe
    (D) Temporal lobe

12. The parietal lobe is responsible for which function?
    (A) Temperature regulation
    (B) Sensory integration
    (C) Motor function
    (D) Vision

13. Which artery or arteries are responsible for anterior circulation to the brain?
    (A) External carotid
    (B) Internal carotid
    (C) Basilar
    (D) Vertebral

14. Which area of the brain is most sensitive to hypoxia?
    (A) Brainstem
    (B) Cerebral cortex
    (C) Cerebellum
    (D) Subarachnoid villi

15. Which statement most accurately describes the circle of Willis?
    (A) It is located in the cerebrum.
    (B) It helps provide adequate circulation through its anastomosis.
    (C) It is responsible for sleep and wakefulness.
    (D) It is part of the brainstem.

16. Signs of acute subdural hematoma appear during what time frame after an injury?
    (A) 2 to 3 days
    (B) 1 week
    (C) Up to 2 weeks
    (D) More than 2 weeks

17. All of the following are symptoms of a basilar skull fracture but one. Which symptom is NOT indicative of a basilar skull fracture?
    (A) Rhinorrhea and otorrhea
    (B) Battle's sign, raccoon eyes
    (C) Tinnitus, nystagmus, and hearing difficulty
    (D) Loss of consciousness and dilated pupils

18. Which of the following can cause an epidural hematoma?
    (A) Skull fracture lacerating the middle meningeal artery
    (B) Rupture of an intracranial aneurysm
    (C) Infectious meningitis
    (D) Cerebral edema

19. Where are intracranial aneurysms most commonly found?
    (A) External carotid arteries
    (B) Anterior cerebral circulation
    (C) Common carotid arteries
    (D) Posterior cerebral circulation including the vertebrobasilar arteries

20. A 28-year-old man is admitted to the ICU with a diagnosis of closed head injury. The nurse should be aware of which potential complications?
    (A) Hypotension
    (B) Respiratory alkalosis
    (C) Tremors
    (D) Cerebral edema

21. Which of the following is a common risk factor associated with aneurysmal subarachnoid hemorrhage?
    (A) Cerebral edema
    (B) Hypertension
    (C) Prolonged hypotensive episodes
    (D) Valsalva's maneuvers

22. What percentage of total body oxygen consumption is accounted for by the brain?
    (A) 2% to 5%
    (B) 5% to 10%
    (C) 10% to 15%
    (D) 20%

23. How much of a reserve of oxygen exists in the brain?
    (A) 100 mL
    (B) 225 mL
    (C) 450 mL
    (D) None

24. Of the following factors, which does NOT play a role in maintaining consciousness?
    (A) Cerebral perfusion pressure
    (B) Oxygen transport level
    (C) Adequate blood glucose level
    (D) Normal serum potassium level

25. Initial assessment of the neurologically impaired patient should include measurement of which of the following?
    (A) Level of consciousness
    (B) Pupillary eye movement
    (C) Deep tendon reflexes
    (D) Brainstem reflexes

26. A fixed and dilated pupil indicates compression of which cranial nerve?
    (A) I
    (B) II
    (C) III
    (D) IV

27. Which structure or structures are parts of the supratentorial space?
    (A) Cerebellum
    (B) Pons
    (C) Cerebral hemispheres
    (D) Medulla

28. Which of the following is a common complication of a ruptured intracranial aneurysm?
    (A) Hypotension due to hypovolemia
    (B) Cardiac dysrhythmias
    (C) Acid-base disturbances
    (D) Vasospasm of cerebral arteries

29. Signs and symptoms of meningeal irritation include all of the following EXCEPT:
    (A) Nuchal rigidity and headache
    (B) Kernig's and Brudzinski's signs
    (C) Aphasia and paresis
    (D) Photophobia

30. Which of the following is an early sign of increased ICP?
    (A) Dilated pupils
    (B) Respiratory depression
    (C) Papilledema
    (D) Depressed level of consciousness

31. Nursing interventions for the patient having seizures include all of the following EXCEPT:
    (A) Protecting the patient from injury
    (B) Observing and recording seizure patterns
    (C) Administering anticonvulsive drugs such as phenytoin (Dilantin)
    (D) Restraining the patient

32. The nurse should be aware of the characteristics of psychomotor seizures. Which of the following statements regarding psychomotor seizures is true?
    (A) They are psychologic in origin.
    (B) The patient usually becomes unconscious.
    (C) They involve repetitive behavioral patterns.
    (D) They involve acts of random violence.

33. The most important treatment for the patient in status epilepticus is:
    (A) Maintenance of ventilation or respiratory support
    (B) Administration of diazepam
    (C) Administration of glucose
    (D) Administration of phenytoin

34. Pathophysiologic consequences of status epilepticus include all of the following except one. Which of the following consequences is NOT associated with status epilepticus?

35.
    (A) Hypoxemia
    (B) Hypoglycemia
    (C) Hyperthermia
    (D) Hypothermia

35. Which of the following organisms is the most common cause of bacterial meningitis in adults?
    (A) Meningococcus
    (B) *Haemophilus influenzae*
    (C) *Streptococcus pneumoniae*
    (D) Pneumococcus

36. Clinical signs and symptoms of meningitis include all of the following EXCEPT:
    (A) Positive Kernig's and Brudzinski's signs
    (B) Headache and photophobia
    (C) Hemiparesis and atrophy of muscles
    (D) Photophobia and seizures

37. What is the reason that even a nonmalignant brain tumor may have dangerous consequences?
    (A) Nonmalignant brain tumors can convert into malignant tumors.
    (B) Brain tumors can secrete exogenous catecholamines.
    (C) The mass in the brain can distort the ability to sense normal balance.
    (D) Any mass will increase the ICP because of the cranial structure's lack of distensibility.

38. Which substrate does the brain depend on most heavily for nutritional needs?
    (A) Fats
    (B) Proteins
    (C) Carbohydrates
    (D) Neurotransmitters

39. A patient with cerebrospinal rhinorrhea would benefit most from which of the following?
    (A) Assistance with nasal packing to tamponade the leak
    (B) Insertion of a nasogastric tube to aspirate swallowed CSF
    (C) Testing of the CSF with litmus paper to determine the origin of the fluid
    (D) Administration of prophylactic antibiotics

40. A normal consensual light reflex indicates proper functioning of which two cranial nerves?
    (A) Abducens and acoustic
    (B) Ophthalmic and hypoglossal
    (C) Optic and oculomotor
    (D) Trochlear and vagal

41. Which function is primarily regulated by the occipital lobe?

(A) Speech
(B) Vision
(C) Coordination
(D) Respiration

42. Meningeal irritation is indicated by which of the following signs?
(A) Nuchal rigidity
(B) Homan's sign
(C) Positive extensor plantar (Babinski's) reflex
(D) Flaccid paralysis

Questions 43 and 44 refer to the following scenario:

A 72-year-old woman is admitted to the unit following a fall at home. Her daughter explains that her mother tried to stand after dinner and immediately fell. Currently she is awake but unable to move her left side. She is able to talk and is alert and oriented. Admission vital signs are as follows:

Blood pressure	176/110 mm Hg
Pulse	62
Respiratory rate	16
Temperature	36.8°C

Pupils are equal and reactive; eye movements are normal. The patient states that she has been healthy and has never "needed to see a doctor."

43. Based on the preceding information, which condition is likely to be developing?
(A) Left-sided cerebrovascular accident (CVA)
(B) Internal carotid vasospasm
(C) Right-sided CVA
(D) External carotid obstruction

44. Which neurologic test would be most helpful in establishing the diagnosis in this patient?
(A) CT scan
(B) Cold-water caloric test
(C) Oculocephalic testing
(D) Electroencephalogram (EEG)

Questions 45 and 46 refer to the following scenario:

A 24-year-old woman is admitted to your unit following a fall from a horse. After the fall, the horse kicked her in the temporal region of the head. She is admitted to the unit directly from the emergency department. She is unresponsive except to deep, painful stimuli. CT scans of the head reveal a temporal skull fracture. The following data are available:

Blood pressure	170/90 mm Hg
Pulse	56
Respiratory rate	10

45. Based on the preceding information, which condition is likely to be developing?
(A) Epidural hematoma
(B) Subdural hematoma
(C) Obstructive hydrocephalus
(D) Contrecoup head injury

46. Which treatment would be indicated based on the preceding data?
(A) Increasing the ventilator rate
(B) Placement of an ICP monitor
(C) Immediate craniotomy
(D) Mannitol infusion

47. Which type of head injury typically produces rapid clinical deterioration?
(A) Subdural hematoma
(B) Depressed skull fracture without displacement
(C) Epidural hematoma
(D) Subarachnoid hematoma

48. Which test is the most diagnostic for identifying head injuries?
(A) Cranial roentgenogram
(B) Lumbar puncture
(C) CT scan
(D) Positron emission tomography (PET) scan

49. A 69-year-old man has a cardiopulmonary arrest and is brought to your unit. Which of the following medications, if given previously, would interfere with an assessment of pupillary response?
(A) Atropine and procainamide
(B) Amiodarone
(C) Lidocaine
(D) Atropine and epinephrine

Questions 50 and 51 refer to the following scenario:

A 43-year-old man is admitted to your unit with complaints of severe headache, pain in the neck on flexion, and sensitivity to light. He has no specific muscle weakness or sensory deficits but does have a positive Kernig's sign. Vital signs are as follows:

Blood pressure	142/84 mm Hg
Pulse	118
Respiratory rate	30
Temperature	40°C

50. Based on the preceding information, which condition is likely to be developing?
(A) Meningitis
(B) Intracerebral bleeding
(C) Myasthenia gravis
(D) Subarachnoid bleeding

51. Which treatment would most likely be instituted?
    (A) Craniotomy
    (B) Administration of anticholinesterase agents
    (C) Insertion of a ventricular drain to reduce the increased ICP
    (D) Administration of antibiotics

52. Which of the following best describes Kernig's sign?
    (A) Muscle spasms in the arm upon occlusion with a blood pressure cuff
    (B) Twitching of the face upon tapping the cheek
    (C) Inability to flex the neck
    (D) Inability to extend the leg when the thigh is flexed to the abdomen

53. Brudzinski's sign is best described by which of the following definitions?

    (A) Adduction and flexion of the legs with neck flexion
    (B) Pain in the neck upon raising the arms above shoulder level
    (C) Temporary flaccid paralysis after neck compression
    (D) Development of superficial muscle tremors after repetitive reflex testing

54. If a patient develops a grand mal (tonic-clonic) seizure, which initial nursing action should take place?
    (A) Forcing of an airway into the mouth
    (B) Protecting the patient from injury
    (C) Starting oxygen therapy
    (D) Placing a padded tongue blade into the mouth

Neurology Practice Exam

Practice Fill-Ins

1. _____	15. _____	29. _____	43. _____
2. _____	16. _____	30. _____	44. _____
3. _____	17. _____	31. _____	45. _____
4. _____	18. _____	32. _____	46. _____
5. _____	19. _____	33. _____	47. _____
6. _____	20. _____	34. _____	48. _____
7. _____	21. _____	35. _____	49. _____
8. _____	22. _____	36. _____	50. _____
9. _____	23. _____	37. _____	51. _____
10. _____	24. _____	38. _____	52. _____
11. _____	25. _____	39. _____	53. _____
12. _____	26. _____	40. _____	54. _____
13. _____	27. _____	41. _____	
14. _____	28. _____	42. _____	

PART V

Neurology Practice Exam

Answers

1.	A	15.	B	29.	C	43.	C
2.	C	16.	A	30.	D	44.	A
3.	B	17.	D	31.	D	45.	A
4.	D	18.	A	32.	C	46.	C
5.	B	19.	B	33.	A	47.	C
6.	D	20.	D	34.	D	48.	C
7.	A	21.	B	35.	B	49.	D
8.	D	22.	D	36.	C	50.	A
9.	B	23.	D	37.	D	51.	D
10.	C	24.	D	38.	C	52.	D
11.	B	25.	A	39.	D	53.	A
12.	B	26.	C	40.	C	54.	B
13.	B	27.	C	41.	B		
14.	B	28.	D	42.	A		

VI

GASTROENTEROLOGY

....

Donna Prentice

VI

GASTROENTEROLOGY

38

Anatomy and Physiology of the Gastrointestinal System

EDITORS' NOTE

This chapter provides a good review of the general anatomy and physiology of gastrointestinal function.

Few, if any, questions from this chapter will be included on the PCCN exam. Use this chapter to strengthen your overall understanding of gastrointestinal anatomy and physiology. Questions related to nutrition are likely to be on the exam.

The process of digestion and absorption of nutrients requires an intact, healthy epithelial lining in the gastrointestinal (GI) tract that is able to resist the effects of its own digestive secretions. It must move materials through the GI tract at a rate that facilitates absorption, and it requires the presence of enzymes for the digestion and absorption of nutrients.

In this system, enzymes and hormones are produced, vitamins are synthesized and stored, and food is broken down and then reconstituted. Nutrients, vitamins, minerals, electrolytes, and water enter the body through the GI tract. Catalysts and reactants play a role, some of which are recycled and used again. Finally, wastes are collected and eliminated. The two main functions of the GI tract can be summarized as the absorption of nutritional elements and the elimination of waste products.

UPPER GASTROINTESTINAL SYSTEM

Oral Cavity (Mouth)

The oral cavity consists of the lips, cheeks, teeth, gums, tongue, palate, and salivary glands. Its main functions include ingestion, mastication, salivation, and the first phase of swallowing (deglutition).

The salivary glands' total daily secretion is between 1.0 and 1.5 L of saliva. Saliva is secreted in the mouth. The salivary glands consist of the parotid, submaxillary, sublingual, and buccal glands. Saliva has three functions. The first function is protection and lubrication. Saliva is rich in mucus, which serves to protect the oral mucosa and to coat the food as it passes through the mouth, pharynx, and esophagus. The sublingual and buccal glands produce only mucous types of secretions. The second function of saliva is its protective antimicrobial action. The saliva not only cleanses the mouth but also, because of the enzyme lysosome that it contains, has an antibacterial action. Third, saliva contains ptyalin and amylase, which initiate the digestion of dietary starches.

Secretions from the salivary glands are primarily regulated by the autonomic nervous system. Parasympathetic stimulation decreases flow. These nuclei are controlled mainly by taste impulses and tactile sensory impulses from the mouth.

Tongue

The tongue is a mass of striated and skeletal muscles that is covered by a mucous membrane. It is a highly mobile muscular and tactile organ that plays an important part in articulate speech. It is also necessary to the digestive tract, being involved in mastication and swallowing as well as being the chief organ of taste. The surface of the tongue and its side edges are covered with papillae containing the taste buds, which are highly specialized nerve endings. A perfectly dry tongue cannot taste, and the sense itself is limited to four discriminations: bitter, sweet, salty, and sour. Many of the finer sensations attributed to taste are actually received by the sense of smell.

Swallowing is initiated when a bolus of food is pushed backward by the tongue into the pharynx, a voluntary act. The bolus stimulates swallowing receptor areas located in the pharynx, transmitting impulses to the medulla oblongata via the trigeminal nerve. The autonomic nervous system is activated, and a series of pharyngeal, laryngeal, and esophageal contractions result from transmission via the glossopharyngeal and vagus nerves.

Pharynx

The pharynx connects the oral cavity to the esophagus. The pharyngeal walls are composed of longitudinal and circular striated muscle fibers that surround the fibrous tissues involved in deglutition. The pharynx is divided into three sections: nasopharynx, oropharynx, and laryngeal pharynx.

Esophagus

The pharynx ends at the level of the sixth cervical vertebra to become the esophagus. The total length of the esophagus is about 25 cm (10 in.). The upper one-fifth lies in the neck; the lower four-fifths lie in the thorax. It is located posterior to the trachea and is capable of altering its own size.

Three cellular layers compose the wall of the esophagus. The innermost layer of cells is the mucosal layer, made up of squamous epithelium. The middle layer is muscle arranged circularly around the lumen. The upper one-third of this middle layer is skeletal (striated) muscle controlled directly by nerves from the brain; the remainder is smooth muscle that is only indirectly controlled by the central nervous system through the effects of the autonomic nervous system on the intramural plexus. The outermost layer of cells forms longitudinal muscle fibers.

When food is pushed from the pharynx through the hypopharyngeal sphincter into the esophagus, the propulsion continues throughout the length of the esophagus via peristaltic waves controlled by a vagal response. These peristaltic waves often exert as much as 50 to 70 cm H_2O of pressure. The peristaltic waves move the food bolus down the esophagus, through the gastroesophageal sphincter, and into the stomach. Food normally passes from the mouth through the esophagus and into the stomach in about 7 s.

Two sphincters keep food boluses from moving in and out of the esophagus. The hypopharyngeal sphincter, at the superior end of the esophagus,

opens to allow food to enter the esophagus from the pharynx. When the hypopharyngeal sphincter is relaxed, it is closed as a result of passive elastic tension. When the skeletal muscles contract, the sphincter opens and a bolus of food may enter the esophagus, creating a peristaltic wave that advances the food through the esophagus. The sphincter may also open during vomiting to allow the food to be regurgitated.

The gastroesophageal sphincter, also known as the cardiac sphincter, functions in the same way as the hypopharyngeal sphincter. The gastroesophageal sphincter controls food boluses leaving the esophagus and entering the stomach. It opens as peristaltic waves travel along the esophagus to allow the bolus of food to enter and closes to prevent a reflux of food and acid. Achalasia is a functional obstruction of the esophagus where the lower esophageal sphincter does not relax, resulting in nonperistaltic, spasm-like contractions. Achalasia results from damage to the innervation of the smooth muscles in the esophagus.

A condition known as reflux may occur as a result of inappropriate relaxation of the gastroesophageal sphincter. It may occur in a variety of conditions, such as pregnancy, obesity, excess caffeine and tobacco intake, hiatal hernia, and some medication ingestions. Treatment of the problem may help relieve the sensation of chest pain. Dietary changes may also relieve discomfort.

The opening in the diaphragm that allows passage of the esophagus is the esophageal hiatus. As soon as the esophagus passes through the opening, it almost immediately enters the stomach. If this opening becomes enlarged, the stomach usually bulges into it. This condition is termed a hiatal hernia.

No enzymes are secreted in the esophagus. The esophagus secretes only mucus, which protects the mucosa from excoriation from food that is in its most abrasive form.

Stomach

The stomach is the most dilated portion of the digestive tract and has an average capacity of about 1 L. It is located in the epigastric, umbilical, and left hypochondriac regions of the abdomen. It is subject to considerable variation in shape and size, but an average stomach is J shaped in general outline and has a maximum length of about 25 cm (10 in.) and a maximum breadth of about 14 cm (3 in.).

The stomach is generally described as having three sections: the fundus, the body, and the pylorus (Fig. 38-1). The upper lateral border of the stomach is

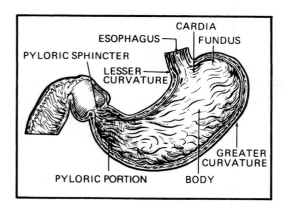

Figure 38-1. Divisions and curvatures of the stomach.

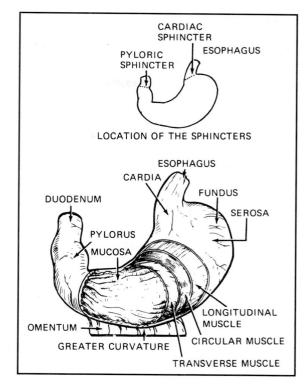

Figure 38-2. Layers of the stomach wall.

called the lesser curvature. The lesser curvature carries downward the line of the right border of the esophagus; throughout most of its extent, it is nearly vertical. The lower lateral border is called the greater curvature. The greater curvature is subject to considerable variation in length and position, depending on the condition of the stomach at the time of examination.

Openings of the Stomach
As the esophagus nears the stomach, it thickens; circular muscles ring the distal end just as it passes into the stomach. These thickened circular muscles form the cardiac sphincter.

The pyloric sphincter has the same anatomic structure and the same physiologic function as the cardiac sphincter. The pyloric sphincter controls the opening at the distal end of the stomach into the duodenum. It lies 3 cm to the right of the midline and about 5 cm below the tip of the sternum. The sphincter is slightly open most of the time, permitting fluids to be squirted out but preventing the escape of solids.

Layers of the Stomach
The stomach wall is composed of three muscular layers: the outer layer, consisting of longitudinal muscle fibers; the middle layer, consisting of circular fibers; and the innermost third layer, consisting of transverse (oblique) fibers (Fig. 38-2).

The gastric mucosa lines the interior of the stomach. The mucous membrane is thick and velvety, having a honeycomb appearance. In the body and the pyloric end, the muscularis mucosa is thrown into folds or ridges called rugae. These allow for distention.

The interior mucosa of the stomach has a layer called the submucosa, which is composed of blood and lymph vessels and connective and fibrous tissue.

Visceral peritoneum covers the exterior of the stomach and consists of tissue that "hangs" in a double layer from the greater curvature of the stomach to cover the anterior side of abdominal viscera. This is the greater omentum (Fig. 38-3).

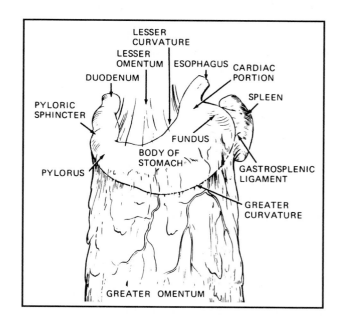

Figure 38-3. Greater omentum.

Gastric Glands

Glands are present throughout the GI tract to secrete chemicals that mix with the food and digest it. These secretions are of two types: (1) mucus, which protects the wall of the GI tract and liquefies the stomach contents, and (2) enzymes and allied substances, which break the large chemical compounds of the food into simple compounds.

Mucus is secreted by every portion of the GI tract. It contains a large amount of mucoprotein that is resistant to almost all digestive juices. Mucus also lubricates the passage of food along the mucosa, and it forms a thin film everywhere to prevent the food and hydrochloric acid from excoriating the mucosa. It is amphoteric, which means that it is capable of neutralizing either acids or bases. All of these properties make mucus an excellent substance for protecting the mucosa from physical damage and preventing digestion of the wall of the gut by the digestive juices.

A number of substances—such as aspirin, bile salts, ethyl alcohol, and acetic acid—have been shown to alter ion influxes and potential differences across gastric mucosa; these changes have been interpreted as a reflection of damage to the gastric mucosa. How these substances disrupt the gastric mucosa is not known. Possibly active ion transport is inhibited or metabolic processes are altered, thus leading to changes in the permeability of the mucosa and predisposing a person to destruction of mucosal cells (ulcer formation).

The proximal portion of the stomach, the cardia, receives the bolus of food from the esophagus. This stimulates gastric glands to secrete lipase, pepsin, the intrinsic factor, mucus, hydrochloric acid, and gastrone (which inhibits the secretion of the acids), collectively known as gastric juice. The mucosa of the stomach contains few gastric glands at the fundus, many glands in the body, and fewer glands at the antral (pyloric) portion of the body.

Gastric glands are tubular. The narrow neck of each gland opens into the stomach. Chief cells in the gastric gland's neck have two functions: to secrete mucus and to regenerate cells both for the glands themselves and for the intestinal surface epithelial tissue. Argentaffin cells are present in the tissues of the gastric glands. These cells contain granules thought to be the origin of serotonin.

The fundus (blind end of the gland) has parietal (oxyntic) cells that secrete hydrochloric acid, water, and the intrinsic factor. Hydrochloric acid is an enzyme involved in the digestion of proteins. It also activates other enzymes in the stomach for digestion and kills bacteria. The secretion of hydrochloric acid may be increased by four endogenous substances: histamine, gastrin, calcium, and acetylcholine. Atropine, a muscarinic antagonist, may block hydrochloric acid secretion caused by acetylcholine. Cimetidine, ranitidine, nizatidine, and famotidine, which are histamine H_2 receptor antagonists, block histamine-induced secretion of hydrochloric acid.

The intrinsic factor from the parietal cell is a mucoprotein that is essential for the absorption of vitamin B_{12}. Once released from the parietal cells, the intrinsic factor adheres to epithelial cells in the ileum. If the ileum is surgically resected, exogenous B_{12} must be taken for life.

Zymogenic (chief) cells found in the body of a gastric gland secrete pepsinogen, an inactive proteolytic enzyme. The hydrochloric acid activates the pepsinogen to form pepsin, an enzyme that begins the digestion of proteins by splitting amino acid bonds.

The pyloric (antral) portion of the stomach has increased depth, size, and muscle and secretes mucus and pepsinogen. The hormone gastrin, a large polypeptide, is secreted from G cells in the antral mucosa and is absorbed into the bloodstream. This hormone then passes by way of the blood to the fundic glands of the stomach and causes them to secrete a strongly acidic gastric juice. The acid, in turn, greatly aids in the digestion of the meats that first initiated the gastrin mechanism. In this way, the stomach helps to tailor-make the secretion to fit the particular type of food eaten.

Gastric Motility

The rugae allow for great distention of the stomach without increasing pressure (Laplace's law), which may be termed a receptive relaxation phenomenon. This may allow for stomach contents to approach 6 to 7 L before peristaltic contractions are initiated.

Factors affecting gastric motility include quantity of contents, pH of contents, the degree of mixing and peristalsis that has occurred, and the capacity of the duodenum to accept chyme from the stomach.

Usually, the fundus of the stomach is stimulated to initiate oscillations (mild "mixing waves") when about 1 L of food is in the stomach, but there may be considerably more food present. These mixing waves occur approximately once every 20 s. When the food (bolus) is digested to the chyme state, it is ready for passage into the duodenum.

However, mixing waves alone are unable to achieve this. If no other influences are functional, malabsorption will occur. To help the conversion of food boluses to chyme, the mixing waves help the hormones and acids to mix with the food. As the peristaltic contractions move toward the antral (pyloric) portion of the stomach, they become very strong in order to force the chyme into the duodenum. A pH of 1 to 3 is obtained by the hormone gastrin, stimulating the release of hydrochloric acid into the chyme and also stimulating peristaltic contractions, which will occur at a rate of about 3 per minute.

The enterogastric reflex (which causes lower gastrin and acid secretion) will delay the progression of chyme. This reflex is under vagal influence. It is stimulated by the degree of distention of the duodenum, by the presence of any degree of irritation of the duodenal mucosa, and by the osmolality, acidity, and degree of emulsification of the chyme.

Chyme must be of the proper consistency and acidity, and the duodenum must be receptive for the strong antral peristaltic contractions to force the chyme through the pyloric valve. The small size of the pyloric sphincter opening results in little chyme entering the duodenum. Most of the chyme is squirted back toward the body of the stomach as the pyloric valve relaxes and closes. This is an important action in the mixing of the chyme.

Gastric Emptying

The stomach empties at a rate proportional to the volume of its contents. The chemical composition of the chyme in the duodenum determines the rate and quantity of additional chyme entering the duodenum. The duodenum contains osmoreceptors, chemoreceptors, and baroreceptors (stretch receptors for volume distention) that influence duodenal activity. If the chyme has a high fat content upon entering the duodenum, a release of cholecystokinin occurs, inhibiting further release of chyme. High fat content is the factor most known for inhibiting gastric emptying. Secretin may also be released to inhibit gastric emptying by inhibiting the gastrin mechanism.

Other factors—such as emotional depression, sadness, and pain (both physical and psychologic)—inhibit emptying of the stomach. An inadequate fluid intake will also retard emptying of the stomach because a large quantity of liquid is necessary to turn fat, protein, and carbohydrates into chyme.

Normally about 2 L of gastric juices (primarily hydrochloric acid) is secreted per day. The pH is 1 to 3. This acidity and its resultant irritation affect gastric emptying by decreasing it. Inadequate protein breakdown and hypertonicity of the chyme will also slow gastric emptying.

Factors increasing gastric motility include aggression, increased volume of chyme, and fluids. The more liquid the stomach chyme is, the greater will be the ease of emptying.

Control of Gastric Secretions

Gastric secretions may be controlled through autonomic nervous system functions, by hormonal alterations, and/or through baroreceptors.

The control of the gastric secretions, specifically hydrochloric acid, may be broken down into three phases: cephalic, gastric, and intestinal. These three phases follow the path of food and then of chyme through the alimentary tract. When the stomach is at rest, normal secretion occurs at a rate of about 0.5 mL/min. This is known as the basal rate. With food in the stomach, the rate of secretion increases to about 3 mL/min.

Cephalic Phase. The parasympathetic nervous system controls the first phase of regulation of gastric secretion via the vagus nerve. The sight, smell, taste, or thought of food is sufficient to stimulate the release of hydrochloric acid in preparation for the expected arrival of food boluses. In addition to pleasant thoughts of food, hunger, hypoglycemia, and anger will also stimulate the secretion of hydrochloric acid.

Vagal control is decreased by certain drugs (especially the anticholinergic drugs), hyperglycemia, and duodenal distention. A vagotomy may eliminate the cephalic phase.

Gastric Phase. This second phase of control over gastric secretion begins when food actually enters the stomach. The predominant regulatory mechanism in this phase is hormonal. Gastrin is the major hormone; it increases acid secretion from the oxyntic cells. It is stimulated by antral distention, secretion of pepsinogen, and an alkaline pH in the stomach. This phase has a negative feedback effect: as hydrochloric acid is released in response to gastrin, the stomach contents eventually become acid. When the number of hydrogen ions (acidity; pH of 2) is adequately high, gastrin secretion decreases.

Intestinal Phase. This phase begins when chyme enters the duodenum. Chyme entering the duodenum is more acid than that in the body of the stomach because as polypeptide fragments move from the body of the stomach to the antrum, they stimulate acid secretion by an unknown mechanism (but to a lesser extent than in the stomach).

When the chyme has a pH below 2.5, it is accepted more slowly into the duodenum. In the gastric phase, the chyme becomes more alkaline, so that it will move into the duodenum in the intestinal phase.

Fat in the duodenum stimulates the secretion of cholecystokinin, which directly decreases gastric motility. Of the food types leaving the stomach, carbohydrates are the most rapid, followed by protein and then fat.

Gastric Digestion

Gastric digestion includes carbohydrates, proteins, and fats. The stomach is a poor absorptive area of the GI tract. Only a few highly lipid-soluble substances, such as alcohol, can be absorbed in small quantities.

Carbohydrates. Digestion of starches really begins in the mouth with action of ptyalin and continues in the stomach by hydrolyzing carbohydrates into oligosaccharides.

Protein. The first stage of protein breakdown by proteolytic enzymes occurs in the stomach.

Fats. Digestion of fats in the stomach is minimal. The only action the stomach has on fats is by gastric peristalsis, which reduces the size of triglyceride droplets and facilitates contact with a lipase secreted by von Ebner's glands.

LOWER GASTROINTESTINAL SYSTEM

Small Intestine

The small intestine extends from the pyloric sphincter to the cecum. This 18- to 20-ft tube is divided into three segments. The first segment is the duodenum, which arises at the pyloric sphincter. It is a C-shaped segment about 10 in. long and ends at the ligament of Treitz. The middle segment, the jejunum, extends about 8 ft from the ligament of Treitz and has an alkaline pH (7.8). The third segment is the ileum, which is about 12 ft long. There is no distinct change from the jejunum to the ileum.

Layers of the Small Intestinal Wall

The small intestinal wall has the same layering as does the stomach. The wall of the intestine consists of a secreting and absorbing mucous membrane called the mucosa. It is composed of epithelial and columnar cells, smaller blood vessels, nerve fibers, plasma, and blood cells. The next layer is the muscularis mucosa. It is lined with areolar tissue (the submucosa). The submucosa contains larger blood vessels, connective tissue, nerves, ganglia, and lymphoid elements. The submucosa is covered with two smooth muscular coats, an outer longitudinal one and an inner circular one. The intestine also possesses still another coat since it is closely invested by peritoneum; this coat is the serous membrane (serosa) lining the walls of those cavities and reflected onto the walls of the tube.

The activity of GI smooth muscle is controlled by local, humoral, and neural influences. The rhythmic movements are integrated by an intramural network that lies between the two muscular layers of the intestine. This network has two layers of nerve fibers, a submucosal network (Meissner's plexus) and a second layer that lies between the circular and longitudinal layers of smooth muscle (the myenteric, or Auerbach's, plexus). The intramural network is responsible for many of the locally controlled movements that occur in the digestive tract. The afferent fibers of this system are located largely within the submucosal network and the motor fibers are within the myenteric plexus.

The intrinsic tone and rhythmic activity of the digestive tract can be modified by the autonomic nervous system. Generally, the parasympathetic nervous system increases GI activity, while the sympathetic nervous system slows its activity.

Ileocecal Valve

At the junction of the ileum and the cecum is the ileocecal valve. This valve controls the flow of contents into the cecum and allows no regurgitation of cecal contents into the ileum.

Villi of the Small Intestine

Villi (singular, *villus*) are the distinguishing characteristics of the small intestine (Fig. 38-4). These fingerlike projections into the lumen provide an extensive surface area. The villi and microvilli increase in absorptive capacity 600-fold, for a total surface area of about 250 m^2. An extraordinary number of villi project from the mucosa into the lumen of the small intestine. Each villus contains microvilli to actively absorb nutrients from the intestinal tract. Each villus also contains a lymph vessel and a dense capillary bed to aid in the absorption process. This lymph vessel is called a lacteal. Carbohydrates, fats, proteins, vitamins, and minerals are absorbed into the small bowel through the villi.

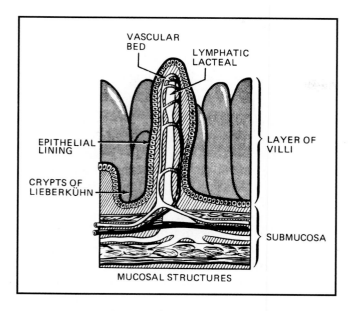

Figure 38-4. Structure of a villus (a lacteal).

Glands of the Small Intestine

The intestinal lumen is lined with simple, cuboidal, and columnar epithelial cells interspersed with goblet cells. The many goblet cells secrete mucus to protect the mucosa. The goblet cells decrease in numbers markedly toward the end of the ileum. Crypts of Lieberkühn (Fig. 38-5) are tubular glands found between the villi in the submucosa of the duodenum.

Absorptive and secreting cells have been identified but not differentiated in function. It is known

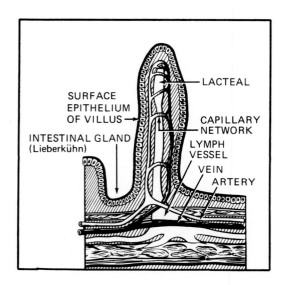

Figure 38-5. Crypts of Lieberkühn.

that the crypts of Lieberkühn are extremely mitotic and replace villous cells. The entire intestinal epithelial surface is replaced every 32 h.

Crypts of Lieberkühn are small pits found on the entire intestinal surface except in the area of Brunner's glands. The crypts of Lieberkühn secrete a watery fluid immediately absorbed by the villi. This supplies a carrier substance for absorption by villi as chyme contacts them. This secretion is controlled principally by local nervous reflexes.

Brunner's glands are mucus-secreting glands that are concentrated in the first portion of the duodenum, between the pylorus and the ampulla of Vater. The function of Brunner's glands is inhibited by the sympathetic nervous system. Lack of sufficient mucus may be related to the development site of peptic ulcers. Brunner's glands are thought to protect the duodenum from digestion by the gastric juices.

Peyer's patches are lymphoid follicles that lie in the mucosa and submucosa of the ileum. They participate in antibody synthesis and the body's immune responses.

The small bowel also secretes several hormones that enter the bloodstream and stimulate the pancreas to release its digestive secretions.

Movements of the Small Intestine

The presence of chyme in the small intestine stimulates baroreceptors that initiate a type of concentric contraction called segmentation. When the small intestine becomes distended, many constrictions occur either regularly or irregularly along the distended area. The constrictions then relax, but others occur at different points a few seconds later. Each contraction results in a segmentation of the chyme and moves the chyme forward about 1 to 2 cm. These segmenting contractions normally occur 7 to 12 times per minute. This helps to mix secretions of the small intestine with the chyme particles.

Propulsive contractions are called peristaltic contractions. They are elicited by distension of the intestine. Peristaltic contractions should be regularly spaced. The peristaltic waves (contractions) push the chyme slowly toward the colon. These waves are short and are found predominantly in the first portions of the duodenum and jejunum.

Distention of the small intestine activates the nerves to continue the contraction sequence, known as the myenteric reflex. As the chyme nears the large intestine, contractions in the ileum increase. As chyme reaches the end of the ileum and is ready to enter the colon, a gastroileal reflex is stimulated.

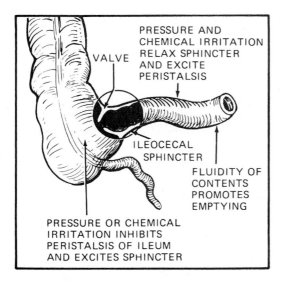

Figure 38-6. Gastroileal reflex.

The gastroileal reflex regulates the movement of chyme from the small intestine into the large intestine. Between the ileum and the cecum is the ileocecal valve, which is normally closed. The tissue immediately before the ileocecal valve is highly muscular, forming the ileocecal sphincter, and the flaps of the ileocecal valve (Fig. 38-6) extend into the cecum. The sphincter is normally contracted except after a meal, when it relaxes and allows chyme to move from the ileum into the cecum. Chyme is prevented from returning to the ileum during colonic contraction by the valve leaflets being floated out to close the ileocecal valve (in much the same way as the heart valves).

Absorption Mechanisms in the Small Intestine

Normally, absorption from the small intestine each day consists of several hundred grams of carbohydrates, 100 g or more of fat, 50 to 100 g of amino acids, 50 to 100 g of ions, and 8 or 9 L of water. Its absorptive capacity is much greater than this. There are five basic mechanisms for absorption in the small intestine: hydrolysis, nonionic movement, passive diffusion, facilitated diffusion, and active transport.

Hydrolysis. Hydrolysis is the chemical action of uniting compounds with water to split the compounds into simpler compounds. Enzymes and hormones act as catalysts in the process of hydrolysis. Catalysts speed up the process of hydrolysis. (Catalysts speed up a chemical reaction without entering into the reaction.)

Nonionic Movement. Nonionic transport allows substances to move freely in and out of cells with no need for energy or carrier substances. Such molecules include drugs and unconjugated bile salts.

Passive Diffusion. In passive diffusion, there is free movement of molecules based on a concentration gradient, primarily from an area of high concentration to an area of low concentration. Free fatty acids and water are molecules that move by passive diffusion.

Facilitated Diffusion. Facilitated diffusion may be defined as a process by which a carrier picks up an ion, crosses the cell membrane, liberates the ion inside the cell, and then returns outside to pick up another molecule (ion). This diffusion does not require energy, and ions cannot move alone against an electrochemical gradient.

Active Transport. For nutrients to be absorbed by active transport, energy (adenosine triphosphate [ATP]) is required. Ions such as Na^+ and K^+ and molecules such as proteins and glucose require active transport.

Nutrient Digestion and Absorption

Some 90% of nutrients and 50% of water and electrolytes are absorbed in the jejunum. Meticulous nutritional counseling and follow-up are important for patients who have undergone resection of the small bowel.

Carbohydrates. Carbohydrates enter the duodenum in the forms of starch, polysaccharides (complex sugars), disaccharides, and monosaccharides. The starch and polysaccharides are hydrolyzed under the influence of amylase to form maltose. Maltose and directly ingested disaccharides such as sucrose, lactose, and maltose are hydrolyzed by intestinal enzymes into simple sugars of monosaccharides, which are then absorbed into the bloodstream via the intestinal mucosa.

Approximately 350 g of carbohydrates is absorbed daily (60% starch, 30% sucrose, and 10% lactose). The three basic sugars are fructose, glucose, and galactose. Each of these basic sugars yields 4 kcal/g. Glucose and galactose are actively transported across the small intestinal wall into the blood. Fructose is transported by facilitated diffusion.

Proteins. Dietary proteins are first acted upon by enzymes called proteases. The principal proteases are pepsin (in the gastric secretion) and trypsin (in the pancreatic secretion). These enzymes catalyze the hydrolysis of the very large protein molecules into intermediate compounds (proteoses and peptones) and subsequently into amino acids. In the digestive sequence, protein is broken down into proteoses and peptones in the stomach. These simpler compounds are next broken down into polypeptides and then into amino acids in the small intestine.

Approximately 70 to 90 g of protein is absorbed daily, yielding 4 kcal/g. Of the amino acids, eight (isoleucine, leucine, lysine, methionine, phenylalanine, threonine, tryptophan, and valine) are essential. Amino acids are absorbed (primarily from the duodenum and jejunum) by active transport into the blood of the intestinal villi. This transport is carrier mediated and requires an expenditure of energy.

Fats. Before fats can be digested, they must be emulsified. This function is performed in the small intestine by bile, which is secreted by the liver and stored in the gallbladder.

The bile salts aggregate to form micelles. These micelles have a fatty core but are still stable in the intestines because the surfaces of the micelles are ionized, which is a property that promotes water solubility. The fatty acids and the glycerides become absorbed in the fatty portions of these micelles as they are split away from fat globules and are then carried from the fat globules to the intestinal epithelium, where absorption occurs.

The emulsification of ingested fat globules provides a greater contact area between the fat molecules and pancreatic lipase, which is the principal fat-digestive enzyme. The end products of fat digestion are glycerides, fatty acids, and glycerol. Some fatty acids and glycerol may be absorbed into the blood via the blood vessels found in the villi of the intestinal mucosa. However, most fatty acids and glycerides are absorbed into the lymphatic system via the lacteals of the intestinal villi.

Approximately 60 to 100 g of fat are absorbed daily, providing 9 kcal/g.

Electrolytes. Electrolytes are absorbed in all parts of the intestine by active transport.

Water. Approximately 8 to 9 L of water are absorbed from the intestine each day by both diffusion and osmosis.

Water-Soluble Vitamins. The water-soluble vitamins, vitamin C and B complex, are absorbed in all parts of the intestine through passive diffusion directly into the blood.

Fat-Soluble Vitamins. The fat-soluble vitamins, A, D, E, and K, are absorbed from the GI tract (mainly the jejunum) in the same way as lipids are. Once in the bloodstream, these vitamins are escorted by protein carriers because they are insoluble in water.

Calcium. The top portion of the duodenum is specialized for the absorption of calcium.

Iron. In the intestines, only about 10% of dietary iron is normally absorbed, but if the body's supply is diminished or if the need increases for any reason, absorption increases. This regulation is provided by a blood protein, transferrin, which captures iron from food and carries it to tissues throughout the body by active transport.

Large Intestine

The large intestine (colon) is 5 to 6 ft long and extends from the ileum to the anus. It is significantly different from the small intestine in that it contains no villi. The colon is 2.5 in. in diameter (larger than the small intestine) and has many sacculations (saclike segmentations) called haustra. The colon has three segments: the cecum, large intestine, and rectum. The colon is further subdivided into four sections: the ascending, transverse, descending, and sigmoid colons. The large intestine is mainly responsible for the absorption of water and some electrolytes and the elimination of waste products.

Cecum

The cecum is a blind-end sac (Fig. 38-7) into which the ileum empties its contents. The vermiform appendix is attached to the base of the cecum. The appendix has no known use and must be surgically removed if it becomes infected in order to prevent peritonitis.

Colon

Immediately above the cecum is the ascending colon, which passes upward to become the transverse colon at the right colic flexure (hepatic flexure). It then crosses the abdomen, where it is now called the transverse colon, and becomes the descending colon at the left colic flexure (splenic flexure). At the iliac crest, the descending colon arches backward to form the sigmoid colon (Fig. 38-7). The sigmoid colon is the portion of the colon that

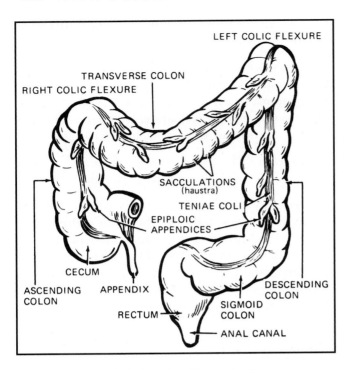

Figure 38-7. Large intestine (anterior view).

crosses from the left side to the midline to become the rectum (Fig. 38-7), which follows the curvature of the lower sacrum and coccyx.

Rectum and Anus. The rectum is about 7-in. long. The distal 1 to 2 in. is the anal canal (Fig. 38-8). Mucous membrane lines the rectum and is arranged in vertical rows called rectal columns. Each rectal column contains an artery and a vein. These veins

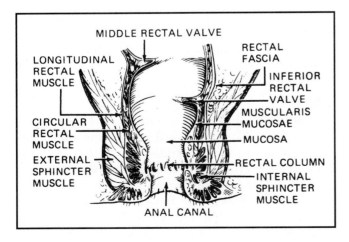

Figure 38-8. Section of the rectum.

frequently enlarge to form hemorrhoids. Two sphincters control the anus (the exterior opening of the rectum). The internal sphincter is composed of involuntary smooth muscle. The external sphincter is voluntary striated muscle.

Layers of the Colon Wall. Epithelial cells form the mucosa of the colon, which is actively involved with absorption of water and some electrolytes. The muscle layers here are different from those in the small intestine. The circular layer becomes somewhat spherical (Fig. 38-7), and the fibers of the longitudinal layer are evenly dispersed in three strips (called taenia coli) around the colon. This produces in sacculation, and the resulting pouches are the haustra.

Colonic Motility. The colon moves its contents slowly through the colon system to allow for fluid absorption, so that 800 to 900 mL of liquid chyme is absorbed along with nutrients. Thus, of the 1000 mL of chyme entering the colon, only 150 to 250 mL of fluid will be evacuated in the stool per day.

Mixing Movements in the Colon. Segmentation of chyme in the large intestine is caused by contraction of the inner muscle layer. There is a slow progress analward with segmentation in the colon. Mixing movements may also be called haustrations. As the circular segmenting contraction occurs, the taenia coli also contract. This provides for more surface contact of the contents to the lumeal wall for absorption.

Propulsive Movements in the Colon. The propulsive movements in the colon result from the haustral contractions, but they are insufficient to provide for the necessary expulsion of waste products. A mass movement occurs in response to an irritation or distention, usually in the transverse colon. These contractions, as a unit, force the entire mass of fecal material forward. A series of mass movements usually occur for up to 30 min and may then occur again in one-half to 1 full day.

Mass movements can cause increased colonic motility as a result of intense stimulation of the parasympathetic nervous system, irritation secondary to conditions such as ulcerative colitis, osmotic overload or simply distention, use of drugs such as morphine sulfate or magnesium sulfate, an increase in bile salts, bacterial endotoxins, and high-residual diets. Hypermotility results in diarrhea and may cause severe fluid loss and electrolyte imbalance.

Mass movements are inhibited by all of the anticholinergic drugs and by diets deficient in bulk. This may result in constipation, since the extra length of time in the large intestine allows for more fluid absorption.

Colonic Absorption. The colon may increase its absorption rate by threefold if threatened with large amounts of fluid. Most of the absorption in the colon occurs in its proximal half (the ascending and transverse colon). The distal colon functions principally for storage.

The mucosa of the large intestine has a very high capacity for active absorption of sodium, and the electrical potential created by the absorption of the sodium causes passive chloride absorption. The mucosa of the colon actively secretes both bicarbonate and potassium.

Bacteria. Bacterial action in the colon causes the formation of gases, which provide bulk and help to propel the feces. Bacteria are capable of digesting small amounts of cellulose, in this way providing a few calories of nutrition to the body each day. These organisms also synthesize some important nutritional factors such as vitamin K, thiamine, riboflavin, vitamin B_{12}, folic acid, biotin, and nicotinic acid. The main anaerobic bacterium in the colon is *Bacteroides fragilis*. The main aerobic bacterium is *Escherichia coli*.

Defecation. The stimulus to defecate is the distention of the rectal wall, resulting in the stimulation of the myenteric plexus. These nerves cause peristaltic waves in the rectum; the internal anal sphincter relaxes (receptive relaxation) and then the external anal sphincter relaxes, so that defecation will occur.

Approximately 150 g of feces is eliminated daily. Feces are three-fourths water and one-fourth solid matter. The organic constituents include undigested food residues, digestive secretions and enzymes, dead cells, bile pigments, and mucus. Some 30% of the mass consists of bacteria and another 30% is fat. The nature of the diet does not change the contents of the stool except for the amount of cellulose present. Stereobilinogen gives feces its brown color.

CHEMICAL MESSENGERS OF THE GI SYSTEM

The GI chemical messengers can act in one of three ways: under an endocrine stimulus, as a neurotransmitter, or as a neuroendocrine messenger.

An endocrine stimulus is a chemical substance formed in part of the body and carried to another part of the body to alter the functional activity or structure of that part. Examples are gastrin, secretin, gastric inhibitory hormone, insulin, and glucagon.

A neurotransmitter is any specific chemical agent released by a presynaptic cell upon excitation; it crosses the synapse to stimulate or inhibit the postsynaptic cell. Examples are vasoactive intestinal peptide, acetylcholine, norepinephrine, and serotonin.

A neuroendocrine messenger consists of cells that release a hormone into the circulating blood in response to a neural stimulus. An example is cholecystokinin.

BLOOD SUPPLY OF THE GI TRACT

Arterial Vascularization

The celiac artery, the superior mesenteric arteries, and the inferior mesenteric arteries all branch from the abdominal aorta. Figure 38-9 shows the arterial vascularization of the GI tract.

Venous Blood Return

The venous circulation of the GI system is unique in that the venous blood enters the portal vein system (Fig. 38-10). All blood from the GI tract enters the portal vein system, which empties into the liver sinusoids. This makes the portal system extremely important for filtering microorganisms and for synthesizing many enzymes and clotting factors needed by the body. The liver also removes various absorbed nutrients, especially glucose and proteins, from the blood and stores them for later use by the body. Generally, the vein corresponding by name to the artery drains the same areas supplied by the artery.

The portal vein drains into the liver sinusoids. These sinusoids join branches of the hepatic artery to form the hepatic vein. In turn, the hepatic veins drain blood from the portal vein and hepatic artery into the inferior vena cava.

INNERVATION OF THE GI SYSTEM

In comparison with the other body systems, the GI tract is unique in that it has its own separate intrinsic nervous system. The GI tract can be influenced by the autonomic nervous system.

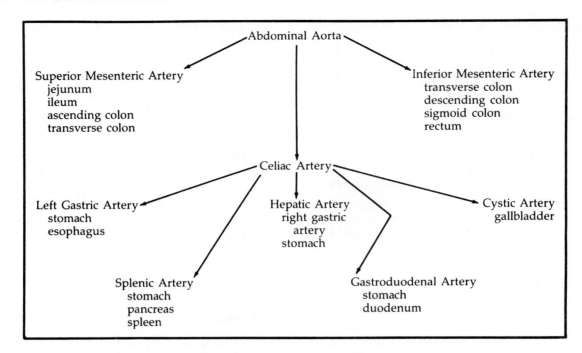

Figure 38-9. Arterial vascularization of the GI tract.

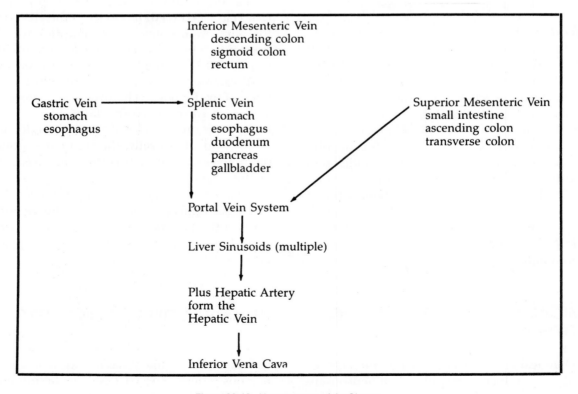

Figure 38-10. Venous return of the GI tract.

The intrinsic nervous system has two layers of neurons connected by specific fibers. The outer layer of neurons is called the myenteric plexus, or Auerbach's plexus. It is located between the longitudinal and circular muscle layers. The inner layer of neurons, called the submucosal plexus or Meissner's plexus, is located in the submucosa.

Generally, the myenteric plexus controls movement of the GI tract and the submucosal plexus (Meissner's plexus) controls the secretions of the GI tract and sensory function through impulses received by stretch receptors in both the GI wall and GI epithelium.

Stimulation of the myenteric plexus results in increasing motor tone of the GI wall and increasing intensity, rate, and speed of peristaltic waves. An increase in Meissner's plexus activity results in increasing secretions.

The extrinsic nerves of the autonomic nervous system can alter the effects of the GI system at specific points, or from the mouth to the stomach and then from the distal end of the colon to the anus. Parasympathetic supply for the gut is from the 10th cranial (vagus) and sacral nerves. Acetylcholine is the neurotransmitter from the postganglionic fiber. A few cranial parasympathetic fibers innervate the mouth and pharynx. Extensive parasympathetic innervation exists in the esophagus, stomach, pancreas, and first half of the large intestine. The sacral parasympathetic fibers innervate the distal half of the large intestine, especially the sigmoidal, rectal, and anal portions.

The sympathetic nervous system fibers flow along blood vessels of the entire gut. The sympathetic fibers to the GI tract originate in the spinal cord between segments T8 and L3. Its neurotransmitter, norepinephrine, inhibits GI tract activity. This causes effects opposite those of acetylcholine, the parasympathetic neurotransmitter. If the effects are strong enough, the sympathetic system can virtually halt activity of the GI tract.

ACCESSORY ORGANS OF DIGESTION

The accessory organs involved in making chyme suitable for nutrient absorption are the salivary glands, the pancreas, and the biliary system (liver and gallbladder).

Salivary Glands

There are three salivary glands: the parotid, the submandibular, and the sublingual (Fig. 38-11). All of the salivary glands are paired.

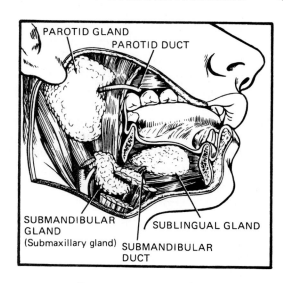

Figure 38-11. Salivary glands.

Hormones have no influence on the salivary glands. Salivary secretion is controlled by the superior and inferior salivatory nuclei located in the brainstem. Nervous stimuli of the glands occur from the thought, sight, and smell of food.

Pancreas

The pancreas is a soft, fish-shaped lobulated gland lying behind the stomach (Fig. 38-12). It is composed of three segments: the head, the body, and the tail.

The pancreas is both an endocrine and exocrine organ. The endocrine portion includes the secretion

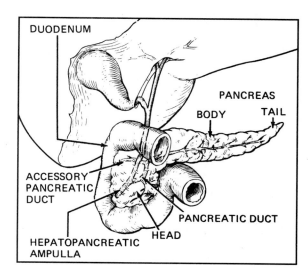

Figure 38-12. Pancreas.

of insulin from the beta cells and the secretion of glucagon from the alpha cells (see section, Chemical Messengers of the GI System above). The exocrine portion is related to the GI system and produces three enzymes whose release is controlled by two hormones produced in the small intestine.

The main pancreatic duct is the duct of Wirsung, which runs the whole length of the pancreas from left to right and joins the common bile duct on the right.

The exocrine function of the pancreas is composed of acinar glands, which are little sacs called alveoli. These cells are arranged around a small central lumen into which the cells drain the exocrine enzymes that they have synthesized. The central lumens drain into multiple ducts, which eventually drain into the main pancreatic duct. The ampulla of Vater (Fig. 38-13) is the short segment just before the common bile duct enters the duodenum.

The secretions of the acinar glands are digestive enzymes, water, and salts (sodium bicarbonate, sodium, and potassium). These colorless secretions total up to 1200 mL each day and are emptied into the upper portion of the small intestine 4 cm beyond the pylorus. They have a pH of 8.0 to 8.5. The pancreatic (acinar) fluid is composed of three major types of enzymes: amylytic, lipolytic, and proteolytic. At least 10% of the pancreatic enzymes must be present to prevent malabsorption. During illness or injury, the volume of pancreatic fluid usually decreases and the composition may change.

The amylytic enzyme is predominantly alpha-amylase, first encountered in the saliva. Alpha-amylase is responsible for the hydrolysis of carbohydrates. The end products of this process are glucose and maltose (a disaccharide of two glucose molecules). The difference between salivary and pancreatic amylase is that the latter is able to digest raw starches as well as cooked starches. Amylase also contains calcium and is excreted in the urine.

The lipolytic enzymes are pancreatic lipase and phospholipase A, which are important in the early stages of the digestion of fats. Lipase breaks down triglycerides to free fatty acids, glycerol, and monoglycerides. Bile salts are essential for this function. Phospholipase A hydrolyzes lecithin (a complex lipid) to lysolecithin.

Proteolytic enzymes are actually proenzymes; that is, they must be altered to become biochemically active. The three most important proteolytic proenzymes are trypsinogen, chymotrypsinogen, and procarboxypeptidase.

Trypsin is involved in the activation of all three proenzymes to enzymes. The proteases are secreted in an inactive form; otherwise, they would act on pancreatic tissue and cause destruction. Once in the intestine, intestinal enterokinase acts on trypsinogen, converting it to trypsin. Trypsin then acts on the other proteases to convert them to active enzymes. These enzymes break the amino acid bonds of protein chains, forming small polypeptides and single amino acids.

In addition to the digestive enzymes, pancreatic secretions contain large amounts of sodium bicarbonate, which reacts with the hydrochloric acid emptied into the duodenum in the chyme from the stomach to form sodium chloride and carbonic acid. The carbonic acid is absorbed into the blood and eliminated through the lungs as carbon dioxide. The net result is an increase in the quantity of sodium chloride, a neutral salt, in the intestine. Thus, pancreatic secretions neutralize the acidity of the chyme coming from the stomach. This is one of the most important functions of pancreatic secretion.

Two other important pancreatic enzymes are nuclease and deoxyribonuclease. These enzymes degrade nucleotides within DNA and RNA molecules into free mononucleotides.

Regulation of Pancreatic Secretions

The cells lining the acinar glands contain large amounts of carbonic anhydrase. The alkaline secretions (HCO_3^-) of the duct cells (cells lining the acinar glands) mix with the amylytic, lipolytic, and proteolytic enzymes prior to reaching the major pancreatic duct, the duct of Wirsung.

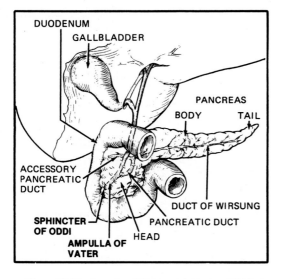

Figure 38-13. Ampulla of Vater and sphincter of Oddi.

Secretions of the pancreas are controlled by hormonal and neural factors. There are three phases of secretion: cephalic, gastric, and intestinal. The cephalic phase is activated by the same factors as in the cephalic state of the stomach and is mainly controlled by the vagus nerve (parasympathetic impulses). Stimulation of the vagus nerve (by thought, smell, taste, chewing, and swallowing of food) causes the secretory cells of the pancreas to secrete highly concentrated enzymes with minimal amounts of HCO_3^-. The quantity of fluid secreted, however, is usually so small that the enzymes remain in the ducts of the pancreas and later are floated into the intestinal tract by the copious secretion of fluid that follows secretin stimulation.

The gastric and intestinal phases are interrelated and controlled by two hormones, secretin and cholecystokinin. When the chyme is predominantly undigested proteins and fats, the pancreatic juice will be rich in enzymes. When the chyme is mainly acidic (low pH), the pancreatic juice will be rich in HCO_3^-. The secretion of cholecystokinin stimulates the enzyme-rich secretion of pancreatic juices; secretin stimulates the release of HCO_3^- and water-rich pancreatic juice. The pancreatic juices enter the duodenum along with the biliary system secretions at the sphincter of Oddi.

Biliary System

The biliary system is composed of the liver and gallbladder.

Liver

The liver is the single largest organ in the body, weighing 3 to 4 lb. It is located in the right upper quadrant of the abdomen, lying up against the right inferior diaphragm.

Gross Structure. The liver is divided into right and left lobes by the falciform ligament (Fig. 38-14). This ligament also attaches the liver to the abdominal wall and to the diaphragm. On the inferior liver surface is the quadrate lobe and on the posterior liver surface, the caudate lobe. Both the quadrate and caudate lobes are small. Most of the liver is covered by peritoneum.

Functional Unit. Each of the hepatic lobes is further divided into numerous lobules. The hepatic lobule is the functioning unit of the liver (Fig. 38-15). Each lobule has a hepatic artery, a portal vein, and a

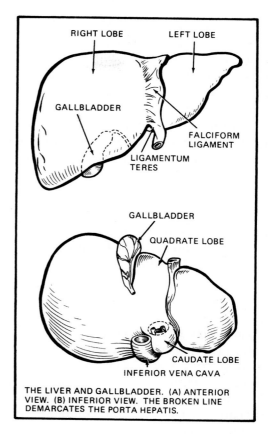

Figure 38-14. Divisions of the liver.

bile duct; these are known collectively as the portal triad. Between columns of epithelial cells are intralobular cavities called sinusoids. Each sinusoid is lined with Kupffer's cells, which are phagocytic cells.

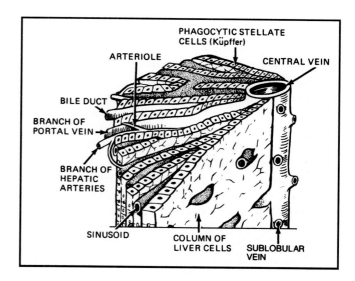

Figure 38-15. Liver lobule.

Blood Supply. Each sinusoid receives oxygenated blood from the hepatic arterioles and blood rich in metabolic precursors from the hepatic vein. The blood is filtered by the phagocytic Kupffer's cells. Products removed from the blood include amino acids, nutrients, sugars, and bacterial debris. Blood leaves the sinusoid by entering the vein of the central lobule. It then enters the hepatic veins and follows the normal venous circuit. Approximately 1500 mL of blood enters the liver each minute, making the liver one of the most vascular organs in the body.

Function. The role of the liver in digestion is to synthesize and transport bile pigments and bile salts for fat digestion. The liver cell, the hepatocyte, synthesizes bile (approximately 600 mL/day), which aids in the metabolism of carbohydrates, fats, and proteins. The bile is secreted into bile canaliculi (ducts), which branch and combine, eventually forming the right and left hepatic ducts. Immediately after leaving the liver, the right and left hepatic ducts merge to form the common hepatic duct. The hepatic ducts drain bile salts and the products of hemoglobin and drug metabolism.

The cystic duct of the gallbladder joins the common hepatic duct to form the common bile duct. The common bile duct joins the major pancreatic duct to form the ampulla of Vater just prior to entering the duodenum at the sphincter of Oddi.

The Kupffer cells of the liver sinusoids are typical reticuloendothelial cells. They are tissue macrophages that are capable of removing and phagocytizing old and defective blood cells, bacteria, and other foreign material from the portal blood as it flows through the sinusoid. This phagocytic action removes the colon bacilli and detoxifies harmful substances that filter into the blood from the intestine.

The liver eliminates bilirubin (by-product of the breakdown of hemoglobin) from the blood through urine and feces. Failure to eliminate bilirubin causes jaundice.

The liver is involved in the metabolism of many hormones by virtue of its role in hormone biotransformation, activation, and excretion. It is particularly involved in the metabolism of steroid hormones, such as the estrogens and progesterone, testosterone, glucocorticoids, and aldosterone. Steroid hormones are taken up from the circulation by the liver and then metabolized by hepatic enzymes. The steroid hormones directly influence many of the liver's biochemical and physiologic functions.

A major biochemical function of the liver is the detoxification and metabolism of drugs, vitamins, and hormones. Some compounds are metabolically converted to relatively inactive forms (steroid hormones), whereas others become more biologically active (vitamin D). Of prime importance in maintaining homeostasis and protecting the body against ingested toxins is the ability of the liver to metabolize and detoxify a wide variety of absorbed substances that reach it directly in the portal blood.

The liver is essential in the regulation of carbohydrate metabolism, since it directly receives from the portal circulation most of the ingested carbohydrates and then, by hormonal regulation, controls the concentration of blood glucose in the fed and fasting states. The liver stores glycogen through glycogenesis (glucose to glycogen) and breaks it down in a process called glycogenolysis (glycogen to glucose) as needed. It also synthesizes glucose from amino acids (gluconeogenesis), lactic acid, and glycerol.

The liver is involved in many aspects of lipid synthesis and metabolism. It is a major site of triglyceride, cholesterol, and phospholipid synthesis. It is involved in the formation of lipoproteins, the conversion of carbohydrates and proteins to fats, and the formation of ketones from fatty acids.

The liver's role in protein metabolism includes the deamination of proteins for glucose availability, the formation of urea from ammonia so it may be eliminated from the blood, and the synthesis of plasma proteins such as albumin, haptoglobin, transferrin, and alpha and beta globulins.

The liver is the site of synthesis of the blood-clotting proteins fibrinogen (factor I), prothrombin (factor II), and factors V, VII, and X. It also stores the fat-soluble vitamins (A, D, and K), vitamin B_{12}, iron, and copper.

Gallbladder

The gallbladder (Fig. 38-16) is a sac-like storage structure for bile.

Function. Bile is manufactured by the parenchymal cells (hepatocytes) of the liver and secreted by them into the bile canaliculi. The bile then travels to the hepatic duct, to the cystic duct, and then to the gallbladder for concentration (by as much as 12-fold) and storage. Upon stimulation, the gallbladder forces bile into the cystic duct, the common bile duct, and the duodenum. The adult gallbladder stores from 30 to 50 mL of bile. The major components of bile are bile acids, bile salts (sodium cholate and chenodeoxycholate), and pigments. The major pigment is mainly bilirubin. Other components include cholesterol, phospholipids (lecithin), alkaline phosphatase, electrolytes, and water.

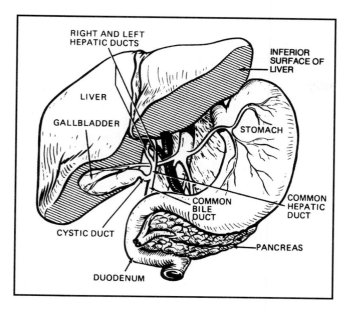

Figure 38-16. Location of the gallbladder.

Bile is responsible for the emulsification of fats and micelle formation. Inside the gallbladder, bile salts react with water, leaving a fat-soluble end to mix with cholesterol and/or lecithin. These formed particles are called micelles. Gallstones may form when the micelles become supersaturated with cholesterol. If bile salts are absent or diminished in the small intestine, normal fat digestion and absorption cannot occur. This results in fat malabsorption and steatorrhea (fatty stools). Most of the bile salts (approximately 80%) are reutilized by reabsorption in the ileum and enter the vascular system to be carried to the liver. The rest are excreted in the feces.

Bile pigments result from the degradation of hemoglobin. These pigments give the feces its brown color. Absence of bile pigments, as with obstructive jaundice, produces a whitish gray feces.

Normally, bile pigments do not form stones. However, in some diseases, there is an overconcentration of bile pigments, resulting in precipitation of bilirubinate stones. Most of gallstones (approximately 90%) are composed essentially of cholesterol.

Bilirubin is the main bile pigment. Once red blood cells have completed their 120-day sojourn through the circulatory system, they become fragile and rupture, releasing hemoglobin. The hemoglobin is phagocytized by cells of the reticuloendothelial system and thus split into heme and globin. It is from the heme ring that bile pigments are made. Bilirubin is the first pigment to be formed; however, it is soon reduced to free bilirubin and released into the plasma. Once in the plasma, free bilirubin combines quickly with plasma albumin and becomes protein-bound free (fat-soluble) bilirubin. It is also known as unconjugated, or indirect, bilirubin. Free bilirubin becomes conjugated (or direct) once it is absorbed into the hepatic ducts and combines with other substances. Conjugated bilirubin is now water soluble. Approximately 80% of protein becomes conjugated with glucuronide acid to form bilirubin glucuronide. Another 10% conjugates with sulfate to form bilirubin sulfate, and the remaining 10% conjugates with still other substances. In these three forms, bilirubin is excreted into the bile and passes through the bile ducts. From this point on, bilirubin is found in the plasma, intestinal contents, and urine.

A small amount of conjugated bilirubin formed by the hepatic cells escapes back into the plasma, creating a small portion of plasma bilirubin as conjugated rather than free. Most of the bilirubin passes into the intestines, where bacterial action produces urobilinogen. Some urobilinogen is reabsorbed by the portal blood and returned to the liver, which in turn reexcretes most of this urobilinogen back into the intestines. About 5% of this urobilinogen passes into the urine and is excreted as urobilin (oxidized urobilinogen). Urobilinogen oxidized in the feces becomes stereobilinogen.

Normally, the total plasma concentration of both the free and conjugated forms of bilirubin is approximately 0.5 mg/100 mL plasma. In normal subjects, almost all of the bilirubin in the plasma appears to be in the unconjugated form. The concentration of bilirubin in the plasma represents a balance between the rate of entry of the pigment into the plasma and the hepatic clearance of bilirubin.

With jaundice, plasma levels of both unconjugated (indirect) and conjugated (direct) bilirubin are measured. If there is either a marked increase in the rate of formation of bilirubin or a defect in any of the processes underlying the hepatic clearance of unconjugated bilirubin (e.g., liver cell dysfunction), conjugated bilirubin will accumulate in the plasma. In contrast, impairment to biliary flow either at a canalicular or bile ductular level (e.g., biliary tract obstruction) will cause reflux of conjugated bilirubin into the plasma.

Stimulation of the Gallbladder. The sphincter of Oddi opens upon vagal and hormonal stimulation. Vagal stimulation increases bile secretions through the sphincter of Oddi. The sphincter of Oddi in a normal state remains slightly opened, providing for a constant but minuscule amount of bile to enter the small intestine.

During normal digestion, the gallbladder contracts in response to the hormone cholecystokinin, pushing increasing amounts of bile through the sphincter of Oddi into the duodenum. The gallbladder does not contract when there is no stimulation by cholecystokinin (e.g., between meals or during starvation diets).

GUIDE TO GI ELEMENTS AND DIAGNOSTIC TESTS

Table 38-1 provides a quick reference to key chemical elements in the GI system. Tables 38-2 to 38-5 provide quick references to common GI diagnostic tests presented in the next several chapters.

EDITORS' NOTE

Under normal circumstances, human nutrition relies on a few key concepts. These concepts include minimal caloric needs (about 25 kcal/kg/day), minimal levels of substrate and vitamin ingestion, and ability of the GI system to process the food. The PCCN exam may have questions on nutritional concepts. This section is designed to provide enough information to cover the major current concepts of caloric need and substrate ingestion (GI processing of food has been covered) in order to provide sufficient material for the exam. This section is not a comprehensive review of nutritional concepts. Controversial practices not supported by research (e.g., reducing diarrhea from tube feedings) are not addressed.

NUTRITION

Caloric Needs

At rest, humans consume about 25 kcal/kg/day. A 70-kg man, for example, would consume 1750 kcal if he were on bed rest. During normal active states, the energy expended would increase to about 35 kcal/kg/day. Most acutely ill patients are near the rest phase of about 25 kcal/kg/day. Temperature elevations are the most common cause of increasing energy expenditure (and caloric needs). Temperature elevations will increase energy needs by about 10% for each degree centigrade of elevation.

Each patient should receive at least 25 kcal/kg/day (ideal body weight) for minimal nutritional support. There are many formulas to calculate (e.g., the Harris-Benedict equation) or measure energy expenditure and caloric needs (indirect calorimetry), but for the purpose of the PCCN exam, remember only the basic information on the approximate caloric needs of the critically ill. Formula calculations are problematic in the acutely ill and particular in the bariatric populations. Indirect calorimetry is the most accurate way to identify caloric need; however, this is difficult to accomplish in the acutely ill patient.

Substrates and nutrients are required in different degrees, depending on the person's condition. For example, proteins are typically given in levels of about 1 g/kg/day. Some patients may require more than this amount (postsurgical, burns); nitrogen balance studies may be performed to better determine specific protein needs. Protein deficits, such as albumin levels and total lymphocytes, are often used to assess the severity of malnutrition. Albumin levels <2.5 g/dL and lymphocytes below 1000 mm^3 indicate potential malnutrition. The PCCN exam, however, does not currently require in-depth knowledge regarding substrate, trace elements, or electrolyte concentrations as they relate to nutrition.

For the purpose of the PCCN exam, information regarding basic nutritional support methods may be required. Enteral feedings, including commonly used formulas such as Osmolite, Ensure, and Jevity, usually have about 1 kcal/mL. Proper nutrition for a 70-kg man would require 1750 mL of full-strength enteral feeding (based on 25 kcal/kg and 1750 mL of enteral feeding, which would equal 1750 kcal).

Some enteral preparations have increased caloric values. Pulmocare and Magnacal, for example, have about 2 kcal/mL. In addition, some formulas, such as Pulmocare, have a potential advantage in the higher lipid concentration and subsequent reduced production of carbon dioxide. The reduced carbon dioxide production in theory reduces the stimulation to breathe. Patients with difficulty weaning from mechanical ventilation may do better with a diet high in lipids as a consequence of a lessening of the drive to breathe.

Parenteral solutions have the ability to give higher levels of calories and substrates. For example, 50% dextrose (D50) can give 10 times the calories provided by D_5W, and 1 L of D50 can give about 1700 kcal, providing almost all the patient's caloric

TABLE 38-1. CHEMICAL ELEMENTS IN THE GASTROINTESTINAL TRACT

Chemical Messenger	Origin	Stimulus	Inhibitors	Action
Gastrin (endocrine)	G cells of gastric antrum, duodenal mucosa	Distention of stomach from food Presence of products from protein digestion, vagal stimulation, elevated blood levels of calcium and epinephrine	Acid in stomach	**Stimulates secretion of HCl and pepsin, growth of gastric mucosa,** relaxes ileocecal sphincter Promotes antral activity Stimulates parietal cells and chief cells
Secretin (endocrine)	Duodenal mucosa	Acid gastric contents entering the duodenum	Lack of acid gastric contents	Stimulates secretion of watery alkaline pancreatic fluid, stimulates pancreatic and hepatic HCO_3^-, augments action of cholecystokinin, decreases gastric acid secretion, stimulates secretion of pancreatic digestive enzymes, may inhibit gastric-emptying time
Cholecystokinin (neuroendocrine)	Duodenal mucosa	Products of protein and fat digestion entering the duodenum	Lack of stimulus	Stimulation of pancreatic enzyme secretion, stimulates gallbladder contraction caused by fat in the intestine, relaxation of the sphincter of Oddi, stimulation of pancreatic growth, inhibits gastric emptying, enhances insulin release, stimulates pepsin secretion, may weakly and selectively stimulate gastric acid secretion, stimulates motility of small bowel, augments secretion in stimulating secretion of alkaline pancreatic juice
Vasoactive intestinal peptide (neurotransmitter or neuropeptide)	Granules located in nerve terminals in the intestinal mucosa	Esophageal distention, intestinal distention, electrical vagal stimulation, intraduodenal fat or acid, serotonin, oxytocin, by intestinal ischemia	None known	Relaxation of smooth muscle, vasodilation and stimulation of pancreatic and intestinal secretion Stimulates insulin release, intestinal secretion of electrolytes and water, inhibits gastric acid secretion, dilates peripheral blood vessels and lowers blood pressure Mediator of lower esophageal sphincter relaxation and of internal and sphincter relaxation
Gastric inhibitory hormone (endocrine)	Duodenal and jejunal mucosa	Presence of glucose and fat in the duodenum, not affected by acid Released in response to bombesin and to betaadrenergic stimulation	Lack of stimulus	Enhances insulin release, may inhibit gastric secretion
Insulin (endocrine)	Beta cells of the islets of Langerhans in the pancreas	Presence of glucose in the gut and blood	Low glucose levels	Controls glucose metabolism in the body by controlling the entry of glucose into the fat and muscle cells, increases the quantities of amino acids available in the cells for synthesizing proteins, stimulates the formation of proteins by ribosomes, stimulates the formation of RNA in cells, presence of insulin causes the body to use carbohydrates as fat, in the absence of insulin, fatty acids are mobilized and used in place of carbohydrates
Glucagon (endocrine)	Alpha cells of the islets of Langerhans in the pancreas	Low glucose concentrations (as low as 60 mg/100 mL of blood), intense exercise, and/or starvation	Normal-to-high glucose concentrations (>60 mg/100 mL of blood)	Regulates blood glucose level, mobilizes glucose from the liver by glycogenolysis (breakdown of the glycogen to glucose), increases gluconeogenesis (conversion of proteins to glucose) by the liver—does this by mobilizing proteins from the tissues of the body and then promotes the uptake of amino acids into the liver as well as conversion of the amino acids into glucose

HCl, hydrochloride; RNA, ribonucleic acid.

TABLE 38-2. LIVER TESTS BASED ON DETOXIFICATION AND EXCRETORY FUNCTIONS

Type of Test	Associated Pathologies
Serum bilirubin (direct and indirect)	Increased indirect → hemolytic disorders Increased direct → liver or biliary tree disease, multiple blood transfusions, sepsis
Urine bilirubin	Indicates increased direct serum bilirubin and implies liver disease
Sodium sulfobromoph–thalein dye test	Indicates liver clearance function
Indocyanine green	Measures liver blood flow
Blood ammonia	Increased levels indicate hepatocellular disease and portal hypertension, detects hepatic encephalopathy
Serum bile acids	Sensitive to overall liver function

nutritional needs. Delivering early nutrition support therapy, primarily using the enteral route, is seen as a proactive therapeutic strategy that may reduce disease severity, diminish complications, decrease length of stay, and favorably impact patient outcome. Enteral feedings should be delayed if the patient is hemodynamically unstable on high-dose vasopressers or active resuscitation is in process. Both small bowel and gastric feeds are acceptable methods of enteral feeding. Small bowel feeds may be beneficial in patients that have repeated high gastric residual volumes or who are at increased risk of aspiration. Aspiration risks can be minimized with elevating the head of bed >30 degrees and switching to small bowel feeds when high residual volumes are encountered. Monitoring for aspiration with food dye or glucose testing on secretions are not reliable and not recommended. The use of protocols to advance enteral feeds are preferred to help patients achieve caloric goal. Complications of enteral feedings, such as diarrhea, may require a reduction in enteral volume or formula change. If the GI system is unable to process food, parenteral solutions could be employed as a supplement or replacement for enteral feedings. Patient's prior nutritional status and health are factors to consider when deciding

needs; 500 mL of a 20% lipid solution can give about 900 kcal (based on 9 kcal/g lipid and 20 g/dL in the 500 mL of lipids).

Enteral solutions are preferred and should be started as soon as possible based on the patient's

TABLE 38-3. TESTS THAT MEASURE BIOSYNTHETIC FUNCTION OF THE LIVER

Type of Test	Associated Pathologies
Albumin	Decreased levels may indicate chronic hepatocellular disorders, malnutrition, protein-losing enteropathy, inflammatory bowel disease, and nephrotic syndrome.
Serum globulins (serum protein electrophoresis)	Increased levels indicate chronic liver disease.
Coagulation factors Prothrombin time Partial thromboplastin time Fibrinogen	Elevated in hepatitis, cirrhosis, vitamin K deficiencies, malabsorption, obstructive jaundice, and treatment with broad-spectrum antibiotics.
Ceruloplasmin	Elevated values are seen with inflammatory diseases such as cholestatic disorders.
Ferritin	Low in iron deficiency, elevated in iron storage diseases such as hemochromatosis.
Alpha$_1$-fetoprotein	Elevated in hepatocellular carcinoma.
Serum Enzymes	
Aminotransferases ALT/SGPT AST/SGOT	Elevated levels indicate acute hepatocellular disease.
Alkaline phosphatase 5'-Nucleotidase GGT	Elevated in inflammation of the biliary tree.

ALT/SGPT, alanine transaminase/serum glutamate pyruvate transaminase; AST/SGOT, aspartate transaminase/serum glutamate oxaloacetate transaminase; GGT, gamma-glutamyltranspeptidase.

TABLE 38-4. TESTS USEFUL IN THE DIAGNOSIS OF MALABSORPTION

Type of Test	Associated Pathologies
Stool fat	Steatorrhea
Xylose absorption	Disorders affecting the mucosa of the proximal small intestine
Small intestinal biopsy	Value of the differential diagnosis of malabsorption
Schilling test for vitamin B_{12} absorption	Abnormal in disorders affecting the ileum such as regional enteritis and lymphomas
Secretin test	Used in the diagnosis of pancreatic insufficiency
Serum calcium, albumin, cholesterol, magnesium, and iron	Low level may be indicative of malabsorption
Serum carotenes, vitamin A, and prothrombin time	May indicate malabsorption of the fat-soluble vitamins
Breath tests (hydrogen and bile acid)	Abnormal hydrogen breath test indicates lactase deficiency. Abnormal bile acid breath test indicates bacterial overgrowth syndromes
Pancreatic Function Tests	
Amylase	Increased levels are associated with pancreatitis

TABLE 38-5. GASTROINTESTINAL AND RADIOLOGIC STUDIES

Upper GI series	Barium and/or gas is taken orally to show structural or functional problems of the esophagus and stomach. Barium is usually followed through the small bowel with radiographs to determine its rate of passage and look for structural abnormalities.
Lower GI series (barium enema)	The large colon is studied with barium and/or gas given per rectum. Sufficient barium and/or gas are given to distend the bowel and show any abnormalities in structure or a tumor.
Cholangiography	Oral cholangiography is based on the ability of the liver to extract from the blood a radiopaque dye that has been absorbed from the intestinal tract and then secrete it into bile. Indicates gallbladder disease.
	Intravenous cholangiography is based on the slow intravenous injection of a radiopaque dye, its extraction from blood by the liver, and then its rapid excretion into bile. Indicates cystic duct obstruction, most likely from gallstones.
Endoscopy (upper GI endoscopy, colonoscopy, proctosigmoidoscopy, and fiberoptic sigmoidoscopy)	Endoscopy is the visualization of the inside of a body cavity by means of a lighted tube. Useful in diagnosing mass lesions, ulcers, strictures, dyspepsia, heartburn, bleeding, or cancers. Also used for biopsies and removal of foreign objects. Being used widely therapeutically for sclerosing, polyp removal, heater probe therapy, and removal of gallstones from the common bile duct.
Percutaneous transhepatic cholangiography	Performed by inserting a long needle into the liver percutaneously and injecting radiopaque dye into the bile duct. Useful in diagnosing obstructive jaundice.
ERCP	The ampulla of Vater is cannulated through a side-viewing endoscope. A radiopaque dye is injected, and both the pancreatic and bile ducts can be visualized. Allows for diagnosing obstruction, malignancy, and inflammation. Endoscopic sphincterotomy and extraction of gallstones may also be performed.
Percutaneous liver biopsy	Puncture of the liver to diagnose hepatocellular disease, prolonged hepatitis, hepatomegaly, hepatic filling defects, fever, and staging of lymphoma.
Angiography	The femoral artery is entered with a large needle that is then exchanged with a catheter that is passed into the celiac artery or one of its branches (superior mesenteric or hepatic). The contrast medium is injected and films are taken. This procedure allows visualization of the visceral vessels to identify abnormalities of vascular structure and function, visualize masses, and note sites of bleeding.
Computed tomography	Noninvasive procedure used in identifying masses. Provides a three-dimensional image.
Ultrasound	Noninvasive procedure using sound waves to outline the pancreas, liver, gallbladder, and spleen. It will distinguish fluid from solid structures and will show an abscess or the volume of fluid present in ascites.
Esophageal manometry	Contractions generated by the esophageal wall are measured as luminal pressures. Useful in the evaluation of achalasia, diffuse spasm, scleroderma, and other motility disorders.
Hepatobiliary imaging	Noninvasive nuclear medicine scan allowing visualization of extra hepatic biliary system and hepatic takeup and excretion of isotope.
Tagged RBC scan	Noninvasive nuclear medicine scan used to gauge leakage of isotope-tagged RBCs in acute GI hemorrhage.
TIPS	Percutaneous creation of a shunt between the hepatic and portal veins within the liver followed by placement of an expandable stent in the tract created, performed by a transjugular route under radiologic guidance. It is done for the treatment of bleeding esophageal varices.

ERCP, Endoscopic retrograde cholangiopancreatography; RBC, red blood cell; TIFS, Transjugular intrahepatic portosystemic shunt.

when to begin parenteral nutrition. Careful glycemic control is required. Parenteral nutrition increases the patient's risk for infection, particularly fungemia. Frequent reassessment of the ablity to use the enteral route should be done. Because of their high osmolality, parenteral solutions must usually be administered into a central vein. Some parenteral preparations, such as $D_{10}W$ or lipids, can be given peripherally. A common practice is the mixing of all parenteral solutions in a single intravenous bag.

39

Gastrointestinal Hemorrhage and Esophageal Varices

EDITORS' NOTE

This chapter addresses concepts that may be tested on the PCCN exam. Review this material to help understand GI disturbances related to GI hemorrhage and to help with being able to perform a comprehensive GI exam and recognizing changes.

Hematemesis is gross vomiting of blood. The blood may be fresh, indicated by a bright red color, or old, having the appearance of coffee grounds, with a black color. If the blood is excreted in the stool, fresh blood will be maroon and may have clots. Old blood turns feces black (called melena). Hematochezia is the passage of bright red blood through the rectum. Bleeding from the stomach or small intestine is usually manifest as melena or maroon stools; bleeding from the colon produces maroon or bright red stools.

GASTROINTESTINAL HEMORRHAGE

Upper gastrointestinal (GI) hemorrhage is considered to be a bleed from the stomach or small intestine. Peptic ulcer disease (PUD), the most common cause of upper GI bleeding, refers to bleeding either from ulcers or from shallow erosions in the stomach, esophagus, or first part of the small intestine. Other causes of upper GI bleeding include esophagogastric varices, arteriovenous malformations, Mallory-Weiss tears, tumors, and Dieulafoy's lesion.

Lower GI hemorrhage is from a site distal to the ligament of Treitz in the distal portions of the small intestine and the colon. The causes of lower GI bleeding may be grouped into several categories: anatomic (diverticulosis), vascular (angiodysplasia, ischemic, radiation-induced), inflammatory (infectious, idiopathic), and neoplastic.

Pathophysiology

GI bleeding occurs when a break in the lining of the GI tract erodes arteries, arterioles, or veins. The more serious bleeding usually occurs when arteries are eroded; however, some venous bleeding, such as bleeding from esophageal varices associated with cirrhosis, can be just as catastrophic.

Etiology

Upper GI bleeding usually results from ulcers, erosions, acute mucosal tears, or esophageal varices. Ulcers are areas of breakdown in the wall of the GI tract that have significant depth. Erosions (e.g., gastritis, duodenitis, or esophagitis), which also represent areas of breakdown in the wall, are much more superficial than ulcers. Approximately 80% of the ulcers are in the duodenum, with duodenal ulcers often causing bleeding.

There are multiple causes of ulcers or erosions, including excessive acid production. Side effects of medicines (e.g., nonsteroidal anti-inflammatory drugs [NSAIDs and COX-2 inhibitors], aspirin, and clopidogrel), stress ulcers associated with surgery, severe burns, head trauma, sepsis, cardiac or respiratory failure, and alcohol use. Stress ulcers are usually thought to be from ischemia, since acid production is usually not increased. Primary ulcer prophylaxis with antisecretory agents such as H_2 receptor antagonists or proton pump inhibitors (PPIs) decreases the risk of stress-related mucosal damage and upper GI bleeding in high-risk patients. Another type of ulcer may be due to infection caused by the bacterium *Helicobacter pylori*.

Lower GI bleeding usually results from colon tumors (e.g., cancer), diverticuli (which are outpouchings of the colon wall), hemorrhoids, or abnormal jumbles of arteries and veins (arteriovenous malformations [AVMs]).

Clinical Presentation

The great majority of ulcers and erosions do not cause bleeding. Usually, the patient will present with recurring abdominal pain, which is usually burning or gnawing in character and is localized either below the xiphoid process, just inferior to the xiphoid in the epigastrium, or in the right upper quadrant of the abdomen. The pain is usually relieved by drinking milk or taking antacids and is usually worse between 30 min and 2 h after eating. Alcohol, aspirin, caffeine, and spicy foods often worsen the pain.

When GI bleeding does occur, it usually manifests itself either as vomiting of fresh blood, old blood that has been acted on by gastric juices ("coffee grounds"), or bloody bowel movements. A patient who has had a blood loss of less than 1 unit of blood, or 10% of the blood volume, usually will not have dizziness or orthostasis. A loss of more than 1 unit but less than 2 units (10% to 20% of the blood volume) is associated with dizziness and orthostasis. Bleeding of more than 2 units (20% of blood volume) is often associated with shock (hypotension, cold clammy skin, oliguria). Epigastric pain may or may not be present in GI bleeding. A slow bleed may produce only weakness, fatigue, and pallor.

Diagnosis

Diagnosis of the probable site of a bleed can usually be made from the history and physical examination. If blood with a coffee-grounds appearance or red blood is vomited, the site of bleeding is the esophagus, stomach, or duodenum. Maroon or red blood with or without clots passed from the rectum is usually indicative of a bleed from the colon, but a severe upper GI bleed can sometimes be manifest as passage of red blood through the rectum without vomiting of blood. Previous ulcer disease, alcohol, aspirin,

NSAID use, or liver disease can help determine the site of the bleed.

Passage of a nasogastric tube can sometimes be useful in assessing the site and severity of the bleed. Bright red blood indicates a more recent and usually a more severe bleed than the return of coffee-grounds appearing blood. However, for a variety of reasons, the nasogastric aspirate is far from perfect for assessing either the source or severity of the bleed.

Upper endoscopy is the best test for diagnosing and possibly treating an upper GI bleed. Endoscopy is highly sensitive and specific for locating and identifying bleeding lesions in the upper GI tract. In addition, once a bleeding lesion has been identified, therapeutic endoscopy can achieve acute hemostasis and prevent recurrent bleeding in most patients. Endoscopy involves passage of a long, flexible tube into the esophagus, stomach, and duodenum through which the physician can see the inside lining of the GI tract. Sometimes, however, bleeding is massive and a good examination with an endoscope is not possible. In such a case, angiography or a scan with tagged red blood cells (RBCs) can be used to locate the source of bleeding.

Bleeding from the colon is often diagnosed by a combination of colonoscopy and various radiologic studies, such as the tagged RBC or angiography. The etiology of lower GI bleeding is often difficult to determine because individual patients may have multiple lesions found at colonoscopy. Only when a lesion is witnessed to be actively bleeding can it be definitively considered the cause of bleeding.

Complications

The major complications of GI bleeding are from the hemodynamic effects. Hypotension can cause serious organ damage, including cerebral infarction or myocardial infarction, renal failure, and intestinal infarction. All of these can be prevented if fluid and/or blood resuscitation is given early enough after the onset of the bleed. Therefore, hemodynamic parameters must be carefully monitored.

Also, aspiration of blood can cause severe respiratory difficulties, especially in unconscious or semiconscious patients. The aspiration of GI contents predisposes patients to acute respiratory distress syndrome. Perforation and peritonitis occur very rarely.

Treatment

The most important aspect of treatment of GI bleeding is the maintenance of blood pressure and circulating blood volume. Assessment of hemodynamic stability and resuscitation as necessary are the critical early goals of therapy. This is accomplished by meticulous attention to pulse, blood pressure, and signs and symptoms of organ perfusion, such as urine output (at least 20 to 30 mL/h) and mental status. Serial hemoglobin and hematocrit determinations are made to decide whether and when transfusion of blood is indicated. Large-bore intravenous access should be attained for the possible transfusion of blood products and also fluids. The proper fluids to give to restore blood volume are isotonic solutions, such as normal saline or lactated Ringer's solution, or packed RBCs. After multiple red cell transfusions, fresh frozen plasma or platelet transfusions may also be needed.

Endoscopic therapy has become an important therapeutic modality. Several different types of endoscopic treatment for bleeding peptic ulcers have been described, including thermal coagulation, injection therapy, hemostatic clips, fibrin sealant (or glue), argon plasma coagulation, and combination therapy. An intravenous proton pump inhibitor (PPI) is started immediately even prior to endoscopic therapy. The major endoscopic predictors of persistent or recurrent bleeding include active bleeding during endoscopy, adherent clot, and/or a visible vessel.

Interventions such as surgery or angiography are indicated in patients who have active bleeding that is not stopped or slowed down significantly with endoscopic therapy. Radiologic therapy, usually by angiography and surgery, is sometimes needed to manage GI bleeding. Arterial GI bleeding can be controlled by angiography by the selective arterial infusion of vasoconstrictive drugs, by embolization of particulate matter into the bleeding artery, or by a combination of these techniques. Bowel ischemia and infarction can be complications of embolization.

Histamine-blocking agents such as famotidine, cimetidine, ranitidine, and sucralfate and other antacids are inferior choices to PPIs for healing ulcers and erosions. High-dose antisecretory therapy with an intravenous infusion of PPI such as pantoprazole or esomeprazole has significantly reduced the rate of rebleeding as compared to standard treatment in patients with bleeding ulcers. Antibiotic treatment is required if testing for *H. pylori* is positive.

Fortunately, between 80% and 90% of GI hemorrhages cease spontaneously. Patients whose bleeding ceases spontaneously usually do very well, while those who need aggressive therapy are more vulnerable to complications and the risk of death.

Classic guidelines for considering surgery are uncontrollable shock or rebleeding. With the introduction of newer endoscopic therapies, these recommendations may change. Types of surgery may include vagotomy, pyloroplasty, and oversewing or resection of the ulcer. For stress ulcers, total gastrectomy may be needed.

Nursing Intervention

Fluid and electrolyte balance and adequate nutrition are key objectives of nursing treatment. Nursing interventions for hypovolemic shock should also be implemented.

Blood studies should include a complete blood count, type, and cross match; electrolytes; blood urea nitrogen; and coagulation screen. Two large-bore (14- to 16-gauge) intravenous lines should be started for rapid fluid and blood replacement. If large peripheral access is not possible, the patient may need a large central venous catheter such as an introducer sheath.

Anticholinergic medications used to inhibit GI action may have side effects such as dizziness, rash, mild diarrhea, leukopenia, blurred vision, headache, and urinary retention. These medications, in addition to the action of antacids, work to increase gastric pH. They will not stop bleeding. The PPIs have antisecretory actions and may be administered intravenously or orally.

The most important role for the nurse is to monitor the patient's hemodynamic status and observe for signs of continued bleeding. Careful attention to vital signs will guide fluid and blood replacement. Assessment of cardiac and pulmonary status will detect signs of possible fluid overload from overly vigorous fluid and blood replacement, which may risk the development of pulmonary edema.

If an intra-arterial infusion of vasopressin is used, the patient must be monitored closely for bradycardia, hypotension, water intoxication, and post–vasopressin diuresis. Volume status and renal perfusion can be measured by urinary output, which should be measured at least hourly and should be greater than 30 mL/h. Tachydysrhythmias are constant potential complications requiring monitoring and intervention as indicated.

The patency of the nasogastric tube should be maintained to monitor a recurrence of the bleed. Repeated blood from the rectum, return of red blood from a nasogastric tube, or recurrent hematemesis is an indication of continuing or recurrent hemorrhage.

Emotional support of the patient and family will help reduce stress and facilitate cooperation. As the bleeding is brought under control, reassurance will decrease the patient's fear.

ESOPHAGEAL VARICES

Esophageal varices are dilated, engorged, tortuous veins usually seen in the mid to distal esophagus. Varices are usually seen in patients with cirrhosis of the liver. They result from increased pressure in the portal veins (the veins that drain the stomach and the small and large intestines). With severe cirrhosis, the blood can no longer pass through the fibrotic liver and finds alternate pathways through the veins in the distal esophagus. Being engorged, these veins are fragile and have a tendency to bleed, usually massively. Each episode of active variceal hemorrhage is associated with a 30% risk of mortality. In addition, survivors of an episode of active bleeding have a 70% risk of recurrent hemorrhage within a year of the bleeding episode. Other causes of esophageal varices are splenic, portal, or hepatic vein thrombosis.

Clinical Presentation

Most patients with bleeding esophageal varices have signs of cirrhosis. Jaundice and ascites are often present. Such patients also often have elevated liver function tests, such as bilirubin, lactic dehydrogenase (LDH), transaminases (serum glutamate oxaloacetate transaminase/aspartate aminotransferase [SGOT/AST], serum glutamate pyruvate transminase/alanine aminotransferase [SGPT/ALT]), alkaline phosphatase, and prothrombin time.

These patients usually bleed massively and painlessly, with signs of shock present. They often become disoriented or lapse into coma as a complication of the bleeding and underlying cirrhosis.

Diagnosis

Diagnosis usually requires endoscopy, since patients with cirrhosis are not always bleeding from varices; instead, bleeding may stem from ulcerations in the esophagus, stomach, or duodenum. The history, physical examination, and laboratory blood studies will be suggestive of cirrhosis.

Treatment

Treatment of esophageal varices is frustrating, as the bleeding is difficult to control and often recurs days to months after initial control has been achieved.

Initially, treatment includes control of shock and maintenance of the patient's cardiopulmonary status. Endotracheal intubation may be necessary to help prevent aspiration and protect the airway. The current treatment options include medications such as vasopressin or octreotide for acute management and nonselective beta blockers (propranolol or nadolol) for long-term prevention of rebleeding. Nonmedical therapy includes endoscopy, surgery, and transjugular intrahepatic portosystemic shunting (TIPS).

Medical Therapy

The use of prophylactic antibiotics in cirrhotic patients hospitalized for bleeding causes a reduction in infectious complications and may decrease mortality. Antibiotics may also reduce the risk of recurrent bleeding in hospitalized patients who have bled from esophageal varices. Typical agents utilized include ceftriaxone or fluoroquinolones.

Medical therapy of a continuous intravenous infusion of vasopressin is sometimes utilized. Vasopressin works by reducing portal venous pressure. The dosage is 0.4 to 1 unit/min. Vasopressin can achieve initial hemostasis in 60% to 80% of patients, but it has only marginal effects on early rebleeding episodes and does not improve survival from active variceal hemorrhage. Vasopressin can cause serious cardiac ischemia and should be used with caution in patients with coronary artery disease. For patients who are receiving intra-arterial vasopressin, cardiac monitoring and frequent neurologic assessments are performed because this drug is a very potent vasoconstrictor. The simultaneous use of intravenous nitroglycerin can decrease some of the cardiovascular risk posed by vasopressin.

Somatostatin inhibits the release of vasodilator hormones, such as glucagon, indirectly causing splanchnic vasoconstriction and decreased portal inflow. It has a very short half-life and disappears within minutes of a bolus infusion; octreotide is a long-acting analog of somatostatin and has supplanted the use of somatostatin in many centers. These agents lead to the achievement of hemostasis and to the prevention of early rebleeding; they may be superior to vasopressin because they have fewer side effects. Treatment with somatostatin or octreotide infusions, when used in addition to sclerotherapy, is superior to sclerotherapy alone or somatostatin alone for the prevention of early rebleeding, possibly also ensuring a better chance for survival. Typical duration of treatment is 3 to 5 days following initial presentation once hemostasis has been achieved.

Endoscopic Therapy

Endoscopic therapy is the definitive treatment for active variceal bleeding. Two forms of endoscopic treatment are available: sclerotherapy and variceal band ligation. Sclerotherapy consists of injecting a sclerosing, fibrosing agent into the bleeding vein through the endoscope. Such treatment is often effective, but it requires considerable expertise in the actively bleeding patient. Outcomes are improved when sclerotherapy is used in conjunction with somatostatin.

Variceal band ligation involves placing small elastic bands around varices. Clinical trials suggest an advantage of band ligation over sclerotherapy in the long term. Band ligation can also be used in patients who fail sclerotherapy. Complications of endoscopic therapy include local complications (bleeding, ulcers, stricture formation, dysmotility), regional complications (mediastinitis, esophageal perforation), and systemic complications (sepsis, aspiration).

Interventional Radiology (Transjugular Intrahepatic Portosystemic Shunt)

The transjugular intrahepatic portosystemic shunt (TIPS) is an interventional radiologic procedure that uses the normal vascular anatomy of the liver to create a shunt between the portal and systemic venous systems within the liver (Fig. 39-1). The procedure involves jugular vein access, hepatic vein sheath placement, and portal vein identification. A tract is made through the liver parenchyma between the hepatic and portal veins. The tract is then enlarged via balloon dilatation and a metallic stent is deployed, allowing blood to flow from the portal vein to the hepatic vein. In this way, portal hypertension is reduced, minimizing the incidence of variceal bleeding, and this procedure has resulted in a reduction of the mortality rate as compared with surgical shunt procedures. TIPS is the procedure of choice in patients who are poor risks for surgery. The principal cause of rebleeding after TIPS is the recurrence of

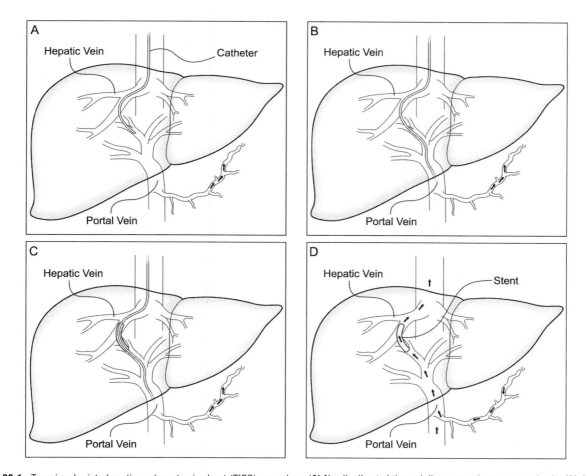

Figure 39-1. Transjugular intrahepatic portosystemic shunt (TIPS) procedure. **(A)** Needle directed through liver parenchyma to portal vein. **(B)** Guidewire passage. **(C)** Balloon dilatation. **(D)** Placement of stent.

portal hypertension. This may result from TIPS thrombosis, stent retraction and kinking, stent stenosis, or the development of right heart failure. Some 30% of TIPS patients will develop postshunt encephalopathy, as do patients undergoing the surgical portosystemic shunt procedure.

Surgical Therapy

Portosystemic shunt surgery, aimed at bypassing the liver to lower pressure in the varices, is usually effective in stopping bleeding but can carry a 50% higher mortality in acutely bleeding patients. Emergency portacaval shunts are more likely to thrombose than elective shunts. With the improvement in endoscopic therapy, the need for surgical intervention is declining.

Radiologic Therapy

Radiologic procedures, although available, are seldom used nowadays in the management of acute variceal hemorrhage.

Balloon Therapy

Balloon tamponade, using versions of the Sengstaken-Blakemore (SB) (Fig. 39-2), Minnesota, or Linton tube, is often effective in stopping acute bleeding. Unfortunately, there is a high incidence of rebleeding

once these tubes are removed. These tubes are placed through the nose or mouth into the stomach. They utilize balloons in the upper part of the stomach and/or esophagus to place pressure on the bleeding veins. The use of these tubes, however, is fraught with dangers. Aspiration of blood, occlusion of the airway, esophageal necrosis, and esophageal rupture are all potential complications. Balloon pressures must be monitored carefully to prevent or recognize these complications early.

Nursing Intervention

A primary objective of nursing intervention is to control the bleeding and prevent or reverse hypovolemic shock. Attention to the patient's hemodynamic status is crucial. Monitoring of electrolyte balance, fluid balance, and nutritional needs will enable early intervention if a problem appears imminent.

A patient with a balloon tamponade tube is continually observed for signs of asphyxiation or aspiration. These tubes can migrate and occlude the airway, or the patient may aspirate either blood or secretions into the lungs. Frequent suctioning of pharyngeal secretions is required. If suctioning does not improve the patient's respiratory status, check for breath sounds in the lungs. If no sounds are heard, most often the tube has slipped and is occluding the trachea. The nurse must immediately cut across all three tubes and remove the tube. For this emergency, scissors are often taped to the head of the bed. Many patients with a balloon tamponade tube will be prophylactically intubated to prevent airway occlusion. The mortality rate is high for this disease, approaching 30% for all patients with variceal bleeding despite optimal medical and nursing therapy.

LOWER GI BLEEDING

Etiology

The major causes of lower GI bleeding are diverticulosis, AVMs, hemorrhoids, and colonic polyps or tumors.

Diverticulosis

Colonic diverticulosis is the presence of outpouchings, usually multiple and most often in the left side of the colon. Diverticulosis is thought partially to result from a relative deficiency of fiber in the

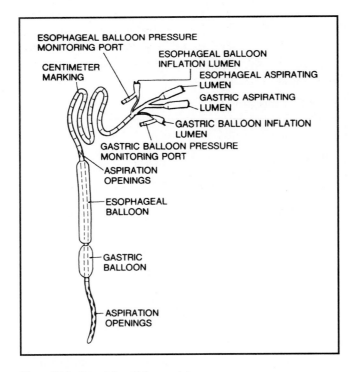

Figure 39-2. Sengstaken-Blakemore tube.

American diet. It is very common in the United States, with approximately one-third of persons older than 60 years being affected. It usually is asymptomatic, but the diverticuli can become infected and may bleed. The bleeding is usually painless and can be massive. The blood almost always appears red as it exits the rectum. Therapy again consists of supporting the patient's hemodynamic status via fluids and blood products. Most often such bleeding ceases spontaneously. Diagnosis is usually made by colonoscopy or barium enema examination. A barium enema has no role in an acutely bleeding patient. A nuclear medicine scan with tagged red cells detects bleeding that is occurring at a rate of 0.1 to 0.5 mL/min; it is more sensitive than angiography but less specific than either a positive endoscopic or angiographic examination. Radiologic therapy by angiography and intra-arterial infusion of vasopressin or embolization to decrease blood flow to the affected bowel is often effective but rarely needed. The advantage of angiography is that it does not require bowel preparation, and the resulting anatomic localization is accurate. Surgery in the form of partial colonic resection is sometimes necessary to control diverticular hemorrhage. At present, there is no effective endoscopic therapy for diverticulosis.

Arteriovenous Malformations

Arteriovenous malformations (AVMs), also called angiodysplasia, are closely packed tangles of arteries and veins that have a tendency to bleed. They are usually located on the right side of the colon but can be present anywhere in the colon, small intestine, or stomach. They are a very common cause of lower GI bleeding. Diagnosis is usually by colonoscopy, with bright red areas seen on the normally pink colon wall. They can also be noted by angiography but not by barium enema examination. Therapy is possible with endoscopic laser, thermal, or electrical coagulation using a small tube introduced through the colonoscope. Angiographic therapy with intra-arterial vasopressin infusion or embolization and surgical resection of the affected portion of the colon are also sometimes necessary. As with diverticulosis, bleeding usually ceases spontaneously. Initial therapy is aimed at stabilizing the patient's hemodynamic status.

Colon Polyps or Tumors

Colon tumors, such as cancer, or polyps, which are thought to be a premalignant growth, are usually asymptomatic. They often bleed, but usually very slowly. These lesions are slightly more likely than diverticuli or AVMs to produce pain with bleeding. Diagnosis is usually by colonoscopy or barium enema. Therapy is with either colonoscopic or surgical removal. As with any GI hemorrhage, initial therapy is aimed at stabilizing the patient hemodynamically.

Nursing Intervention

Nursing management of patients with lower GI bleeding is aimed at the assessment of hemodynamic status. Careful assessment of vital signs, signs of hypovolemic shock, blood cell counts, coagulation studies, and electrolytes should be done frequently. Fluid and electrolyte losses should be replaced. Patients receiving intra-arterial vasopressin should be monitored for cardiac and neurologic abnormalities.

40

Hepatitis, Cirrhosis, Hepatic Failure, and Acute Pancreatitis

EDITORS' NOTE

The content of this chapter will help you to understand hepatic and pancreatic diseases which will be part of the PCCN exam.

HEPATITIS

Viral hepatitis is hepatic inflammation caused by a variety of different viruses with a propensity to infect the liver. The major viruses have specific characteristics that help to differentiate the diseases that they cause. The four major groups of viruses causing viral hepatitis are hepatitis A, hepatitis B, hepatitis D (delta hepatitis), and hepatitis C.

Viruses Causing Hepatitis

Hepatitis A
Hepatitis A virus (HAV) is an RNA picornavirus that is excreted through the feces of infected individuals. It is spread through fecal-oral contact and is common in developing countries with poor sanitation. Poor hygienic practices facilitate the spread. Contaminated food and water have been associated with occasional epidemics. Good hand washing is highly effective in preventing transmission of HAV. It is a very common infection. The majority of patients who acquire the illness have had personal contact with an infected person. Hepatitis A is often misdiagnosed as a gastroenteritis. Immunity after

infection is lifelong. In adults with no prior immunization, the illness is more severe. The incidence of decline in the United States is related to vaccination.

The incubation period is between 15 and 50 days. There are two phases of symptoms. The prodromal phase, occurring 2 to 7 days before the icteric phase, consists of symptoms such as fatigue, malaise, nausea, vomiting, anorexia, fever, and right upper-quadrant pain. The icteric phase, usually lasting between 1 and 4 weeks, follows. The icteric phase symptoms consist of darkened urine, light stools, pruritus, and jaundice. A diffuse rash may be present.

The most profound changes are in the liver function tests. Transaminases (serum glutamate oxaloacetate transaminase/aspartate aminotransferase [SGOT/AST], serum glutamate pyruvate transminase/alanine aminotransferase [SGPT/ALT]) rise dramatically. Alkaline phosphatase also rises but usually not to a similar degree. Bilirubin levels can range from normal to markedly elevated. Bilirubinuria is often present. Leukopenia is often seen, as is a mild anemia. Stools can be light-colored, and steatorrhea may be present.

Patients are usually fully recovered within anywhere from 6 weeks to 3 months but may have vague symptoms for up to a year. Rarely, fulminant hepatic failure and death occur. Patients with underlying liver disease are more likely to develop fulminant hepatic failure from HAV. Mortality rates in large epidemics are approximately 15%. Hepatitis A usually has no progression to chronicity. It may serve as a trigger for autoimmune hepatitis in genetically susceptible individuals. The virus is excreted in the feces for up to 2 weeks before the icteric period and usually disappears prior to resolution of the clinical hepatitis. Patients with acute hepatitis A should be placed on universal precautions. Treatment is usually supportive since the disease is self-limiting in the majority of individuals.

The antibody response to HAV is the key to diagnosis. The virus elicits both an immunoglobulin M (IgM) and an IgG antibody response. HAV-IgM appears in the acute infection and persists for 2 to 6 months. Detection of HAV-IgM is, therefore, indicative of infection within the last 6 months. IgG also appears in acute infection but persists for years. Therefore, the presence of IgG indicates a recent or past infection and probably ensures lifelong immunity.

Vaccination for HAV infection has decreased the occurrence of hepatitis A and can also be used to prevent infection in exposed subjects. Vaccination for HAV infection has been recommended for patients with chronic liver disease because of the increased morbidity and mortality associated with acute HAV infection in such patients. Vaccination is also recommended for food workers. Immune serum globulin is recommended for close personal contacts of an infected person and in all those exposed to the food and water in an identified epidemic. This treatment has been shown to reduce the rate of infection in exposed subjects.

Hepatitis B

Hepatitis B virus (HBV) is a deoxyribonucleic acid (DNA) virus. It consists of a protein coat (known as the surface antigen [HBsAg]) and a core, which contains the double-stranded circular DNA, the e antigen (HBeAg), the core antigen (HBcAg), and the DNA polymerase. Each of these can be detected either in the liver itself or the circulating blood, and various antigens and antibodies have clinical relevance. HBsAg in the blood indicates either an acute or chronic continuing infection. Surface antibody (HBsAb), however, indicates a resolved infection. HBeAg is associated with a high risk of infectivity and correlates with ongoing viral synthesis. It usually appears transiently during an acute attack. E antibody (HBeAb) is a marker of low infectivity and persists for a few months after the acute infection resolves. HBcAg is not currently detectable, but core antibody (HBcAb) is. Immunoglobulin M HBcAb indicates either acute or chronic infection, and IgG HBcAb is usually a marker for a past, nonactive infection.

Hepatitis B is usually transmitted through blood, but it can also be transmitted through saliva and sperm. Hepatitis B is a global public health problem. Transmission of HBV varies by geographic location. Perinatal infection is the predominant mode of transmission in high-prevalence areas. In comparison, horizontal transmission, particularly in early childhood, accounts for most cases of chronic HBV infection in intermediate-prevalence areas, while unprotected sexual intercourse and intravenous drug use in adults are the major routes of spread in low-prevalence areas. The HBV used to be a common cause of transfusion-associated hepatitis, but with present serologic screening of donors, hepatitis B is only rarely transmitted through blood transfusions. The virus can survive outside the human body for a prolonged period; as a result, transmission via contaminated household articles such as toothbrushes, razors, and even toys may be possible. The risk of being infected with HBV by health-care workers has been eliminated with the introduction of the hepatitis B vaccine. The vaccination of infants, children, and adolescents further decreases the risk of transmission.

The incubation period for HBV infection is generally 6 to 9 weeks. The patient usually is infectious both 1 to 2 weeks before and during the icteric phase. A serum sickness prodrome may occur, with symptoms such as rash and arthralgias. The clinical course can vary between mild and severe or can be asymptomatic. Fulminant hepatic failure and death can result. Why hepatitis B has a fulminant course in some patients is not well understood. Symptoms and laboratory findings are similar to those for hepatitis A. The major difference between hepatitis A and hepatitis B is the possibility of chronicity in hepatitis B. The rate of progression from acute to chronic hepatitis B is primarily determined by the individual's age at infection. The younger the person is at time of infection, the greater the chance of developing a chronic HBV infection. Immunocompromised individuals are more likely to develop a chronic HBV infection. Although it is usually asymptomatic, this condition can lead to cirrhosis or hepatocellular carcinoma. Alcohol use in the presence of HBV infection has been associated with worsening liver disease and an increased risk of hepatocellular carcinoma.

Therapy for acute hepatitis B is supportive once the infection is established. Treatment should be delayed for 3 to 6 months in newly diagnosed HBeAg-positive patients with compensated liver disease to determine whether spontaneous HBeAg seroconversion will occur. Prevention of HBV infection is the main focus, as no effective therapy to eradicate the infection exists. There is now a very effective vaccine to prevent HBV infection that is composed of the surface antigen. Response to the vaccine and protection against infection are usually excellent. Vaccination is now a required neonatal procedure by the World

Health Organization. Catch-up vaccinations are indicated for high-risk groups. The cost of vaccination is the greatest limitation to implementation worldwide. The degree of elevation of the serum ALT is an important factor in deciding which patients with HBeAg should be treated since it will help predict risk of seroconversion. Treatment strategies for chronic HBV infection include interferon and antiviral therapies (lamivudine, adefovir, dipivoxil, and entecavir). Many new treatments are undergoing testing. Thus, an approach to the care of patients with HBV infection is evolving rapidly.

Persons exposed to hepatitis B, as in accidental needlesticks, should have their hepatitis serologies checked. If they are HBsAg- and HBsAb-negative, they should be given hepatitis B immune globulin (HBIG). In addition, the hepatitis B vaccine should be given. The HBIG needs to be given only once, but the vaccine should be given again in 1 and 6 months. If the HBsAb is positive, the person exposed is already immune, and neither HBIG nor the vaccine need be given. If the HBsAg is positive, the individual is already infected and should be evaluated for acute or chronic hepatitis. Blood and body fluid precautions (universal precautions) should be followed in dealing with infected individuals.

Hepatitis D

Hepatitis D virus, also called delta hepatitis virus, is a viral particle. It is a ribonucleic acid (RNA) virus that infects only patients with coexistent hepatitis B infection. Therefore, a patient may have both hepatitis D and hepatitis B but cannot have hepatitis D alone. It can superinfect patients with either acute or chronic hepatitis B.

Delta hepatitis is uncommon. When it is present with acute hepatitis B, it usually causes a much more severe clinical hepatitis. Delta hepatitis infection of patients with chronic hepatitis B usually results in an acute exacerbation or worsening of symptoms in addition to increases in liver function tests.

Because delta hepatitis requires infection with hepatitis B, the way to prevent infection is through immunization of groups at high risk of contracting hepatitis B. At present, there is no vaccine solely for hepatitis D. The only drug approved at present for the treatment of chronic hepatitis D is interferon alfa (IFN-α); however, the overall response to treatment is poor.

Hepatitis C

Hepatitis C virus (HCV), an RNA virus, can be detected by serology tests that show antibodies to HCV or molecular assays that detect or quantify HCV RNA. Chronic hepatitis C is the most common chronic liver disease and is the top reason for liver transplantation. Recurrence of HCV infection following liver transplantation is high. People at risk for HCV infection include intravenous drug users, individuals who received clotting factors before 1987 or received blood or organs before 1992, chronic hemodialysis patients, health-care workers who have been exposed by needlestick or mucosal exposure to HCV-positive blood, people with multiple sexual partners and/or human immunodeficiency virus (HIV) infection, and children born to HCV-positive women. There is debate over whether high-risk patients should be tested routinely. Rare epidemics from food or water sources have also been described. However, some cases have no risk factors.

The incubation period varies but is usually about 7 weeks. Many of the infections are asymptomatic; when they are symptomatic, the disease is usually mild. The clinical manifestations are the same as for a mild case of hepatitis A or B. Hepatitis C rarely causes fulminant hepatic failure (FHF). Anti-HCV enzyme-linked immunosorbent assay (ELISA) tests become positive as early as 8 weeks after exposure. A positive test does not discriminate between patients who cleared the infection and those who are chronically infected.

Although the initial clinical disease is usually mild, there is a high propensity for the infection to become chronic. It is estimated that 60% to 80% of acute infections, many of which are asymptomatic, lead to chronic hepatitis and sometimes to cirrhosis. Rates of developing chronic HCV infection after needlestick exposure may be less. Approximately 20% to 30% of those chronically infected will develop cirrhosis, and a percentage of these will develop hepatocellular carcinoma. There is currently no vaccine to prevent HCV infection. In addition, immune globulin is not effective as postexposure prophylaxis.

Hepatitis C antibody can detect chronic but not acute cases. Patients with chronic HAV infection should be vaccinated for HAV and HBV. Patients with chronic HCV infection who may require treatment show the presence of measurable HCV, a liver biopsy showing portal or bridging fibrosis, and at least moderate inflammation and necrosis; the majority of these patients have persistently elevated serum ALT values. The goal of therapy is to prevent the progression of liver disease. Success of treatment is determined largely by the achievement of a sustained virologic response; defined as undetectable HCV RNA level in the blood at the end of the treatment period and at 6 months after treatment ends. Treatment with the combination of interferon and ribavirin is used, but success rates are still low. These medications carry significant side effects related to treatment including depression, psychosis, asthenia, and hemolytic anemia. Risk of treatment must be weighed against risk of disease. Patients with decompensated cirrhosis should be referred for consideration of liver transplantation.

Hepatitis E

Hepatitis E virus (HEV), previously called non-A, non-B hepatitis, is a single-stranded RNA virus that causes a self-limited, enterically transmitted acute viral hepatitis. Contaminated water sources have been associated with large outbreaks. The clinical features of acute HEV infection are similar to HAV infection. Fulminant hepatic failure is more likely to develop in patients who are pregnant or who have preexisting liver disease. Diagnosis is based on detection of HEV in serum or feces by polymerase chain reaction (PCR) or by the detection of IgM antibodies to HEV. Treatment is largely supportive. Work is underway on an effective vaccine.

Nursing Interventions

Nursing priorities for hepatitis are aimed at reducing demands on the liver while promoting patient well-being, minimizing disturbance in self-concept due to communicability of disease, relieving symptoms and increasing patient comfort, promoting patient understanding of the disease process and rationale of treatment, and stressing the patient's awareness of potential complications such as hemorrhage, hepatic coma, and permanent liver damage.

Placing the patient on bed rest with good skin care, providing a quiet environment by possibly limiting visitors, pacing activities, and increasing activity as tolerated can help to prevent decreased mobility due to the lowered energy metabolism of the liver, activity restrictions, pain, and depression.

Nutritional monitoring is important because of anorexia, nausea, and vomiting from visceral reflexes that may reduce peristalsis. Bile stasis as well as altered absorption and metabolism of ingested foods may also produce these symptoms. Diet is ordered according to the patient's need and tolerance. A low-fat, high-carbohydrate diet is most palatable to the anorexic patient. Protein should be given in low quantities. Counsel the patient to avoid alcoholic beverages. Accurate records of intake and output may be necessary because of severe continuing vomiting and diarrhea. Adequate hydration with intravenous fluids may be necessary. Serum electrolytes must also be monitored.

Particular attention must be paid to the patient's self-concept. Annoying symptoms, confinement, isolation, and length of illness may lead to feelings of depression. Universal precautions should be observed by health-care workers with any patient contact. In addition, members of the health-care team should be aware of those patients with acute hepatitis. Allow times with the patient for listening. Offer diversional activities based on energy levels.

Assess the patient's level of understanding of the disease process and provide specific information regarding prevention and transmission of the disease. Contacts may receive gamma globulin; personal items should not be shared; strict handwashing and sanitizing of clothes, dishes, and toilet facilities are necessary. While liver enzymes are elevated, avoid mucous membrane contact; blood donations should be discouraged. Discuss the side effects of and dangers of taking over-the-counter drugs as well as prescribed medications. Emphasis should be placed on the importance of follow-up physical examination and laboratory evaluation.

CIRRHOSIS

Cirrhosis is the end stage of many types of liver disease. Basically, cirrhosis is defined as the abnormal fibrous regeneration of the liver, usually in response to chronic damage.

Types and Etiology

There are two major categories of cirrhosis, micronodular and macronodular. The distinction between the two is the size of the regenerating nodules. There are distinct causes under each category, but there can be overlap, with different diseases potentially causing either type. The morphologic classification system has a number of limitations, and morphology can change over time. Cirrhosis usually results in increased resistance to blood flow through the liver and failure of the hepatic cells to function properly.

Micronodular cirrhosis is the most common type, and alcoholism is the most common cause of this type of cirrhosis in the United States; however, for unexplained reasons, only a minority of alcoholics develop cirrhosis. Cirrhosis is very unusual with less than 5 years of alcohol abuse, demonstrating that chronic injury is usually necessary for cirrhosis to develop. Alcohol itself injures liver cells directly, but other factors influence the development of cirrhosis. Micronodular cirrhosis is also seen with cholestatic causes of cirrhosis and obstruction of hepatic venous outflow.

Macronodular cirrhosis results from any of a variety of causes. Chronic viral hepatitis is the most common cause of this type of cirrhosis worldwide. Other causes include other types of infection, biliary cirrhosis, iron or copper overload, autoimmune diseases, and idiopathic or cryptogenic cirrhosis. Nonalcoholic steatohepatitis (NASH) is a syndrome that develops in patients who are not alcoholic and causes liver damage that is histologically indistinguishable from alcoholic hepatitis. The following risk factors are associated with NASH: obesity, dyslipidemia, and glucose intolerance. All types of cirrhosis generally produce a firm, shrunken liver, although at times the liver can be enlarged. Fibrosis, or scarring, is prominent. Splenomegaly can also be present, especially in those with nonalcoholic causes of cirrhosis. The scarring causes resistance to normal blood flow through the liver. Loss of hepatocytes can result in hepatic failure.

Clinical Presentation

Usually, cirrhotic patients present with gastrointestinal bleeding (often massive), ascites, jaundice, or abnormalities detected on routine blood testing. They may experience weight loss, poor appetite, and a history of alcohol abuse. Some patients may have no obvious signs of cirrhosis.

Ascites, or the accumulation of fluid in the peritoneal cavity, is usually present in moderate to advanced cirrhosis. The patient notes increased abdominal girth, abdominal discomfort, and often pedal or ankle edema. A number of factors are involved in the formation of ascites, including (1) a low albumin level (the cirrhotic liver is often unable to make adequate albumin); (2) portal hypertension, resulting in leakage of fluid into the peritoneal cavity and poor fluid resorption; and (3) abnormal renal responses in cirrhosis, which lead to more fluid retention.

Endocrine changes can also be seen. Gynecomastia and testicular atrophy resulting from reduced testosterone levels are often seen in males, and menstrual irregularities are seen in females. Aldosterone and antidiuretic hormone levels are increased, causing peripheral edema and contributing to ascites formation.

Jaundice is also usually present in advanced cirrhosis. The eyes and skin generally assume a light to bright yellow discoloration as a consequence of elevated levels of bilirubin in the blood.

Other findings include a decreased or abnormal mentation, termed hepatic encephalopathy. This is often seen with an increased serum ammonia level and is caused by an accumulation of toxins that would normally be filtered by the liver. Asterixis (an abnormal flapping of the hands), a hyperkinetic circulation, cyanosis, fetor hepaticus, renal failure, easy bruising, and low platelet and red and white blood cell counts may be seen. Abnormal red clusters of blood vessels on the surface of the skin, termed spider angiomata, can also occur (Fig. 40-1).

Abnormalities in the serum concentrations of the hepatic transaminases (AST and ALT) and other enzymes (lactate dehydrogenase [LDH], alkaline phosphatase) are usually present. Abnormal coagulation tests (prothrombin and partial thromboplastin times) are often present since the diseased liver

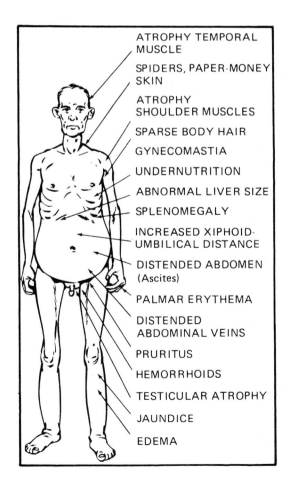

Figure 40-1. Signs of advanced cirrhosis.

TABLE 40-1. LABORATORY TESTS FOR CIRRHOSIS

Decreased Levels	Increased Levels
WBC	Globulin
Hemoglobin	Total bilirubin
Hematocrit	Alkaline phosphatase
Albumin	Transaminase
Serum sodium	Lactate dehydrogenase
Serum potassium	Urine bilirubin
Serum chloride	Fecal urobilinogen
Serum magnesium	Urine urobilinogen
Folic acid	Prothrombin time
	International normalized ratio

WBC, white blood cell.

frequently does not make sufficient clotting factors. Acidosis can occur either from shock or from the liver's inability to clear lactate from the blood.

Diagnosis

Abnormalities in the patient's physical examination and laboratory data (Table 40-1) suggest the diagnosis. Ultrasonography is routinely used during the evaluation of the cirrhotic patient. Surface nodularity and increased echogenicity with irregular-appearing areas are consistent with cirrhosis. Ultrasonography may be used as a screening test for hepatocellular carcinoma and portal hypertension. A liver biopsy is necessary to confirm the presence of cirrhosis and often determines the cause of the disease. Determination of the etiology of cirrhosis is important since it can determine treatment options for the patient and education of the family as well as predicting potential complications.

Treatment

At present, there is no satisfactory treatment to reverse advanced cirrhosis. Treatment is aimed at decreasing any further liver damage, as through the cessation of alcohol use, symptom management, prevention of complications, and evaluation for and timing of liver transplantation. Management of ascites consists of a low-sodium diet, spironolactone plus loop diuretics, and large-volume paracentesis for tense ascites. Protein restriction may be used in patients with encephalopathy, although there is little evidence to support this practice. Beta blockers can be used for the prevention of acute variceal bleeds. Vitamin K therapy may be used for the treatment of

coagulation abnormalities associated with vitamin K deficiencies. Prevention of hepatitis B by immunizing high-risk populations is probably the most important way to decrease the prevalence of cirrhosis worldwide. Patients with cirrhosis have a markedly increased risk of developing hepatocellular carcinoma (HCC).

Bacterial infection is a common complication of cirrhosis related to increased organism translocation from the gastrointestinal (GI) tract into the bloodstream. Patients with cirrhosis are at increased risk of sepsis. Assessment of ascites fluid for the presence of spontaneous bacterial peritonitis (SBP) helps in the early recognition and treatment of this devastating infection. Intravenous antibiotic treatment in conjunction with albumin has been shown to improve renal function in some patients with SBP. Hospitalized cirrhotic patients with GI bleeding have a decreased mortality if prophylactic treatment with antibiotics occurs. Patients with one episode of SBP should receive antimicrobial prophylaxis for life.

Liver transplantation, although costly and necessarily involving lifelong intense medical care, is an option for highly selected patients with cirrhosis. Often, patients die while waiting for liver transplantation, so the aggressive treatment of cirrhosis and prevention of complications is important. Survival in patients with cirrhosis is improving. The prediction of prognosis can be difficult since multiple variables are involved. There are models used to help predict survival. One helpful method of classification is the Childs-Pugh system (Table 40-2). The more recent method is called the Model for End-Stage Liver Disease (MELD). It uses the patient's values for serum bilirubin, serum creatinine, and the international

TABLE 40-2. CHILDS-PUGH CLASSIFICATION OF SEVERITY OF LIVER DISEASE

Parameter	Points Assigned		
	1	2	3
Ascites	Absent	Mild	Moderate
Bilirubin mg/dL	≤2	2–3	>3
Albumin g/dL	>3.5	2.8–3.5	<2.8
Prothrombin time Seconds over control	1–3	4–6	>6
INR	<1.7	1.8–2.3	>2.3
Encephalopathy	None	Grade 1–2	Grade 3–4
Total score/grade	5–6/grade A Grade A	7–9/grade B Grade B	10–15/grade C Grade C
1–2-year survival	100/85%	80/60%	45/35%

INR, international ratio.

TABLE 40-3. MELD

3-month mortality in hospitalized patients:

MELD Score	Mortality (%)
≥40	100
30–39	83
20–29	76
10–19	27
<10	4

normalized ratio (INR) for prothrombin time to predict survival (Table 40-3). The maximum MELD score is 40 so values >40 are changed to 40. If a patient has been dialyzed twice in the last 7 days, the creatinine will be given a value of 4 for their creatinine, and the last caveat is that any value less than 1 is given the value of 1.

Nursing Intervention

Monitor the neurologic status for behavior changes, increasing lethargy, and neuromuscular dysfunction such as asterixis. Provide a safe environment (three side rails up, bed in low position, low lighting) for patients who are not completely lucid. Avoid pharmacologic sedation despite restlessness and irritable states because of decreased drug clearance. Use verbal reassurance and family involvement.

Serum ammonia levels do not correlate to the degree of encephalopathy in most patients, but with an individual patient the levels can be trended to gauge the patient's response to treatment. Lactulose, a poorly absorbed sugar that decreases the bowel pH and increases ammonia excretion through the stool, may be ordered. If the patient does not respond to lactulose, then neomycin, a poorly absorbed antibiotic that destroys the normal flora of the large intestine, may be used.

Nutritional intervention is mandatory since poor nutrition is influential in the development and progression of cirrhosis. Tube feedings or total parenteral nutrition (TPN) may be necessary. Increasing protein (if there is no impending liver failure) may help to regenerate liver tissue if the disease is not too far advanced. Carbohydrates should be increased (up to 2000 to 3000 kcal/day) to sustain weight and spare the use of protein for healing. Vitamin supplements may be necessary.

Check the skin, gums, emesis, and stools often for bleeding and apply pressure at intramuscular sites. Notify the physician of the development of bleeding dyscrasias or an increase in bleeding. Help the patient to minimize trauma by avoiding the use of harsh toothbrushes, forceful nose blowing, and bodily injury.

Monitor fluid retention by weighing the patient daily. Check for dependent edema and maintain accurate intake and output records. Fluid and sodium restrictions may be necessary. Administer diuretics as required. Aldactone, an aldosterone antagonist, is most frequently used. Recommended diuresis is 1 L/day to prevent cardiovascular compromise and hypovolemic shock.

Paracentesis may be indicated in the patient with marked ascites. Paracentesis is generally not the initial treatment of ascites. If paracentesis is performed, note the amount of fluid removed, make sure that a specimen is sent for appropriate laboratory and microbiology tests, and closely monitor the patient for signs of shock.

Monitor respiratory status for signs of ineffective breathing patterns. General debilitated states place patients at risk for acquired infections. Pressure on the diaphragm due to ascites causes reduced lung volumes, and hypoxemia may occur. Semi-Fowler's or high-Fowler's positions may be necessary. Auscultate lung sounds and turn the patient every 2 h; also, have the patient breathe deeply and change his or her position at the same intervals. Additional laboratory tests to monitor include arterial blood gases (ABGs) and white blood cells (WBCs).

Skin breakdown, which is not uncommon, is due to edema and pruritus. Bathe the patient with moisturizing lotion, not soap. Turn the patient regularly (at least every 2 h), elevate heels, use pressure relieving bed surfaces, and ensure rest to prevent fatigue.

Educate the patient and family on the importance of proper diet, avoidance of alcohol, moderate exercise, and avoidance of any drugs (including over-the-counter medications), especially aspirin and acetaminophen, unless the physician approves their use.

HEPATIC FAILURE

Hepatic failure is the result of a very severe acute hepatitis, an advanced cirrhosis, or fatty liver. Causes of fatty liver include alcohol ingestion, starvation, obesity, diabetes mellitus, TPN, and the third trimester of pregnancy. Hepatic failure indicates failure of the liver to adequately perform either part or all of its functions.

Pathophysiology

Hepatocytes perform a variety of functions. The liver has a great deal of reserve, and it is estimated that 75% to 90% of normal liver cell function must be lost before liver failure occurs.

With hepatic failure, the liver is unable to adequately synthesize the plasma proteins. The most commonly deficient proteins are albumin and the coagulation factors. Inadequate albumin can lead to ascites and pedal edema. Deficient coagulation factors can lead to problems of easy bleeding or bruising.

Inability to metabolize substances that the liver normally breaks down leads to increased levels of potentially toxic chemicals in the blood. One of these potentially toxic agents is ammonia (NH_3). Increased levels are seen with mental status changes; that is, hepatic encephalopathy. Hepatic encephalopathy may be mild or may lead to full coma.

Etiology

Hepatic failure can be acute or may occur as the result of a chronic advancing cirrhosis. *Fulminant hepatic failure* (FHF) refers to the rapid development of severe acute liver injury with impaired synthetic function and encephalopathy in a person who previously had a normal liver or had well-compensated liver disease. Fulminant and subfulminant hepatic failure differ in their clinical features and prognosis. As an example, cerebral edema is common in fulminant disease and rare in chronic disease. In contrast, renal failure and portal hypertension are more frequently observed in patients with chronic hepatic failure. Fulminant hepatic failure can result from a wide variety of causes, of which viral or toxin-induced (particularly acetaminophen) hepatitis are the most common. Hepatitis B is more likely to produce FHF than hepatitis A or C. Vascular causes of FHF include portal vein thrombosis, hepatic vein thrombosis (Budd-Chiari syndrome), veno-occulsive disease, and ischemis hepatitis. Wilson's disease, acute fatty liver of pregnancy, and Reye's syndrome are examples of metabolic disorders which may cause FHF. Establishing the underlying cause of FHF is important since it will direct the treatment and determine the prognosis.

Various factors can precipitate hepatic failure in patients with cirrhosis. These include gastrointestinal bleeding, sedatives, chemical imbalances, dehydration, infections (especially spontaneous bacterial peritonitis), alcohol intake, and different anesthetics or surgeries, a portacaval shunt or transjugular intrahepatic portosystemic shunt (TIPS).

Clinical Presentation

Patients with FHF usually present with mental status changes, which can be subtle, such as mild confusion or a mild loss in short-term memory, or severe, resulting in coma. In mild changes, writing usually deteriorates (patient writes above and below the line) and the ability to concentrate diminishes. An abnormal flapping of the hands (asterixis) is usually present. Hepatic encephalopathy is a major complication of FHF.

Hepatic encephalopathy can be divided into five stages. Stage 1 is the early stage, with slurred speech, mild confusion, and disordered sleep. Stage 2 shows signs of moderate confusion and lethargy. Stage 3 involves marked confusion; the patient is incoherent with sleeping but the patient is still arousable. Stage 4 is frank coma. Stage 5 is very deep coma without response to any stimuli.

Diagnosis

Diagnosis of FHF is made by recognizing the presence of underlying liver disease and noting the changes in mental status or laboratory values stated previously. Specifically, liver function tests such as ALT, AST, bilirubin, alkaline phosphatase, albumin, prothrombin time, and partial thromboplastin time are abnormal. Hepatitis A, B, and C studies should be checked to exclude these three infections. The hemoglobin should be checked for signs of gastrointestinal hemorrhage, and the WBC count should be checked as a clue to the presence of infection or sepsis.

A computed tomographic (CT) scan of the brain is indicated in every patient with overt hepatic encephalopathy. This will rule out other clinical findings that may be the cause of the mental status changes (such as a subdural hematoma from trauma). Furthermore, the CT scan can demonstrate the presence of generalized or localized cerebral edema, which is a major concern in FHF.

Treatment

Patients with FHF are susceptible to a wide variety of complications in addition to encephalopathy. These include cerebral edema, renal failure, hypoglycemia, metabolic acidosis, sepsis, coagulopathy, and multiorgan failure. All patients with FHF should be managed in an intensive care unit at a facility capable of performing liver transplantation.

Hepatic encephalopathy is often amenable to therapy. The most important part of therapy is to reverse any precipitating factors. Treatment consists of changing the bacterial flora of the colon, thus decreasing the production of potentially toxic agents that are absorbed into the bloodstream. Lactulose and neomycin are the two most useful agents. Lactulose is usually well tolerated, and the dose should be titrated to achieve two to three soft stools per day. The oral route of administration is more convenient; however, enemas may be required if oral administration is not possible. Lactulose therapy in FHF is controversial and may not be as effective as in chronic hepatic disease. Oral therapy must be used with extreme caution in patients with rapidly deteriorating mental status related to aspiration risks. Rifaxamin is a newer minimally absorbed antimicrobial that has been shown to reduce episodes of hepatic encephalopathy and lead to reduced hospitalizations.

Cerebral edema develops in approximately 80% of FHF patients with grade 4 hepatic encephalopathy. The consequences of cerebral edema include elevated intracranial pressure (ICP) and brainstem herniation, which are the most common causes of death in FHF. Neurologic manifestations may include the classic Cushing's triad (hypertension, bradycardia, and irregular respirations), increased muscle tone, hyperreflexia, and altered pupillary responses. However, early in the course of FHF, these signs and symptoms may be absent or difficult to detect. Many centers will use invasive monitoring of ICP to help with early detection. The goal is to maintain cerebral perfusion pressure greater than 50 mm Hg and to keep the ICP below 20 mm Hg. Invasive ICP monitoring poses a risk of infection and bleeding. Careful titration of fluids must occur to avoid overhydration and the increase of cerebral edema. Maintaining a quiet environment and keeping the head of bed elevated $\geq$30 degrees, with the head in a midline position, and minimizing suctioning can help reduce ICP. Patients who develop elevated ICP may be treated with mannitol maintaining plasma osmolality between 310 and 325 mOsm/kg. Hyperventilation ($PaCO_2$ <25 mm Hg) can help to temporarily lower ICP; however, it may worsen cerebral ischemia. Pentobarbital coma may be used if other therapies fail to lower ICP.

Correcting electrolyte disturbances such as hypokalemia (hypokalemia increases renal ammonia production), protein restriction (oral protein intake should not exceed 70 g/day), and the treatment of GI hemorrhage are also important factors of therapy. Intravascular volume should be maintained, but care taken to avoid overhydration.

Hepatorenal syndrome is the development of acute renal failure in patients with advanced liver disease. It is the result of poor renal perfusion. Other causes of poor renal perfusion, such as hypovolemia, must be excluded. Hepatorenal syndrome is characterized by oliguria, a very low rate of sodium excretion, and a progressive rise in the plasma creatinine concentration. Hepatorenal syndrome carries a poor prognosis; however, it does reverse over time after successful liver transplantation. Every effort should be made to prevent the development of acute renal failure by maintaining adequate systemic blood pressure, identifying and treating infections, and avoiding nephrotoxic medication.

The only proven therapy to increase survival is orthotopic liver transplantation. Patients with FHF should be managed in an institution capable of performing liver transplantation.

Nursing Intervention

Frequent assessment of the FHF patient's neurologic status provides an index of response to therapy. Administer medications as ordered, avoiding sedatives and hepatotoxic drugs (e.g., acetaminophen, amino acids). If the patient is comatose, initiate eye care to prevent corneal abrasions.

Monitor intake and output, fluid status, and electrolyte status. Signs of anemia, infection, alkalosis (increasing serum HCO_3^-), melena, or hematemesis should be reported to the physician to provide an opportunity to prevent complications. Monitor glucose levels with bedside glucose measurements, as acute hypoglycemia can occur.

Replace dietary protein with calories from glucose. During recovery, introduce protein in very small increments (approximately 20 g at a time). Oral protein intake should not exceed 70 g/day in a patient with a history of hepatic encephalopathy. Administer nutrients through tube feedings or TPN.

Monitor respiratory status closely, especially during times of decreasing mental status. Maintain a patent airway and administer oxygen as needed.

Stop all nitrogen-containing drugs and administer neomycin and lactulose. Monitor all side effects of medications and decrease dosages as needed. Some 80% of patients will respond to lactulose therapy with improved mental status. Continuous administration of lactulose in patients with recurrent or subclinical encephalopathy is recommended. Patients with advanced encephalopathy who may not be able to protect their airway may need intubation before lactulose can be administered.

Prevention of infection and monitoring for signs of infection are essential in the care of patients with liver failure. Meticulous nursing care of central venous catheters, Foley catheters, and respiratory precautions to prevent nosocomial infections are crucial. Careful monitoring for signs of infection and careful collection of cultures are required. Prophylactic antibiotic therapy is not recommended and its use is controversial. Antibiotics may be considered if there is rapid progression of encephalopathy, refractory hypotension, and the presence of systemic inflammatory response syndrome.

Emotional support of the patient (if alert) and family with realistic reports of the patient's condition is appropriate and essential since the expected outcome is poor. Honest and open discussion of the end of life should take place.

ACUTE PANCREATITIS

Acute pancreatitis is an inflammatory disease of the pancreas that can result in enzymatic autodigestion of the pancreas. Local inflammation occurs; however, it will often trigger a systemic inflammatory response. The disease course will vary; it may be mild and self-limiting (70% to 80%) or, at the other extreme, acute and possibly necrotizing pancreatitis that may cause a severe systemic inflammatory response (20%).

Pathophysiology

Acute pancreatitis is thought to result from activation of pancreatic enzymes inside the pancreas itself. Normally, the enzymes are released from the pancreas in an inactive state and then activated by fluids present in the duodenum. These enzymes normally digest food products, breaking down nutrients into substituents that can be absorbed by the intestinal cells.

In acute pancreatitis, the enzymes are activated before they leave the pancreatic duct and enter the duodenum. It is postulated that an obstruction, usually temporary, leads to activation of these enzymes. Once activated, they are blocked from release into the duodenum, thus causing them to act on the pancreatic tissue and leading to potentially severe damage to the pancreas. The enzyme trypsin is important mainly in the activation of other pancreatic enzymes. The enzymes phospholipase A_2 and elastase are probably the most important causes of pancreatic damage. Elastase damages blood vessel walls, and phospholipase A_2 acts on acinar cell and fat cell membranes.

Severe edema, necrosis, and hemorrhage can occur in the pancreas and can spread to adjacent organs. Fat and pancreatic necrosis leads to an exudative phlegmon, or inflammatory mass, that induces hypoalbuminemia, and calcium sequestration can lead to a loss of ionized calcium.

Etiology

The two most common causes of pancreatitis are gallstones and alcohol, with alcohol being the most common cause. Most alcohol-related pancreatitis occurs in heavy drinkers. Alcohol has been shown experimentally to increase the protein content of pancreatic juice, and intraductal protein plugs have been noted to form. This intraductal obstruction has been postulated to lead to activation of pancreatic enzymes. Alcohol may also cause spasm of the sphincter of Oddi, increase of pressure in the pancreatic ductal system, and cause direct injury to the pancreas, leading to an inflammatory response. Likewise, gallstones in the distal common bile duct may block off the pancreatic duct, causing an obstruction that can lead to the reflux of bile into pancreatic ducts and hence pancreatitis. An increase in serum ALT is suggestive of gallstone pancreatitis.

There are many other, less common, causes of pancreatitis. Some examples include abdominal surgery, blunt trauma to the abdomen, hyperlipidemia (especially types I, IV, and V), hypercalcemia, certain drugs (such as azathioprine, sulfonamides, thiazide diuretics, estrogen, some HIV medications, and salicylates), ulcers in the stomach or duodenum, endoscopic retrograde cholangiopancreatography (ERCP), tumors, and certain infections. A considerable percentage of cases of acute pancreatitis do not have an identifiable cause (they are idiopathic).

Clinical Presentation

Pain is the universal symptom of acute pancreatitis. Usually, the pain is in the upper abdomen and radiates through to the back. The pain can be severe and is eased by sitting forward. Intense abdominal tenderness may be present, along with guarding and rebound tenderness in severe pancreatitis. The abdomen may also be distended, and bowel sounds may be decreased or absent, in an ileus pattern. Vomiting is often present, sometimes accompanied by fever, tachycardia, and hypotension. Pleural effusions, usually small, or atelectasis may be present. Severe necrotizing pancreatitis will be associated with clinical signs and symptoms of hypovolemic shock due to the massive sequestration of fluids within the peritoneum.

Four specific physical findings deserve mention. Grey Turner's sign (ecchymoses in the flanks) and

Cullen's sign (ecchymoses around the umbilicus) are due to hemorrhage and induration. These signs may appear within days to 1 to 2 weeks after the onset of hemorrhagic pancreatitis, but they are not specific to pancreatitis in general. Chvostek's sign (facial muscle twitching when the cheek is tapped) and Trousseau's sign (spasm of the hand when the blood pressure cuff is inflated over systolic blood pressure for greater than 3 min) are manifestations of hypocalcemia of any origin and may be present but are also not specific to pancreatitis.

Diagnosis

Diagnosis of acute pancreatitis is made by the clinical presentation discussed above and an elevated level of amylase or lipase, both pancreatic enzymes, on a serum sample (Table 40-4). The elevated serum amylase is the "gold standard" and will begin to rise during the first 24 h after onset of symptoms. Elevated serum amylase can also be found in other diseases and is not a marker of the severity of pancreatitis. Urinary amylase or a urinary amylase/creatinine ratio may also be elevated, but these measurements are rarely necessary. Liver function tests are often elevated, usually to a minor degree. Patients who are severely affected often have hypocalcemia, anemia, leukocytosis, hypoxemia, hypoalbuminemia, and hyperglycemia. Since the serum albumin is often low, following the ionized calcium is preferred over serum calcium.

Other diseases that can be confused with pancreatitis include cholecystitis, ulcers, and myocardial infarction. The measurement of amylase usually leads to the correct diagnosis.

Imaging Studies

Ultrasound can play a key role in identifying the presence of gallstones and compromise to the biliary tree. It can also identify pancreatic and peripancreatic fluid collections. Ultrasound provides limited visualization of the pancreas and cannot identify pancreatic cell necrosis.

The CT scan is the clinical standard for the diagnosis of acute pancreatitis. It is useful in estimating the size of the pancreas as well as identifying cysts, mass lesions, fluid collections, and abscesses. Contrast enhancement increases the quality of images but can also cause renal injury as a result of intravenous contrast and aspiration from oral contrast.

Magnetic resonance imaging (MRI) offers the best assessment of internal masses and fluid collections. Often, it can identify which lesion is drainable and which is solid. The difficulty of transporting a critically ill patient to MRI as well as safe ongoing monitoring of such a patient during the procedure are limitations to its more frequent use.

Approximately one-third of patients with acute pancreatitis have abnormalities visible on the chest radiograph, such as elevated hemidiaphragm, pleural effusions, basal atelectasis, pulmonary infiltrates, or acute respiratory distress syndrome (ARDS). Left-sided or bilateral pleural effusions suggest an increased risk of complications.

Complications

Severe acute pancreatitis is a serious, potentially fatal disease. Ranson's criteria can be used as a prognostic tool to identify patients at risk for complications, guide early therapy, and predict prognosis. This is done at hospital admission and at 48 h (Table 40-5).

TABLE 40-4. LABORATORY TESTS TO DIAGNOSE PANCREATITIS

Markedly elevated serum amylase levels, often >500 units.

Characteristically, amylase levels return to normal 3 to 5 days after the onset of pancreatitis.

Supportive laboratory values include the following:
1. Increased serum lipase levels
2. Low serum calcium (hypocalcemia)
3. WBC counts ranging from 8000 to 20,000/mm^3, with increased polymorphonuclear cells
4. Elevated glucose levels may be as high as 500–900 mg/100 mL
5. Serum amylase to serum lipase ratio > 2:1 (alcohol-induced pancreatitis)

WBC, white blood cell.

TABLE 40-5. RANSON'S CRITERIA FOR PANCREATITIS[a]

Zero Hour (Onset)	
Age	>55 years
WBC count	>16,000/mm^3
Serum glucose	>200 mg/dL
LDH	>350
AST	>250
48 hours	
Hematocrit	Fall by ≥10%
Blood urea nitrogen despite fluids	Increase by ≥5 mg/dL
Serum calcium	<8 mg/dL
P$_{AO_2}$	<60 mm Hg
Base deficit	>4 mEq/L
Fluid sequestration	>6000 mL

AST, aspartate aminotransferase; LDH, lactate dehydrogenase; WBC white blood cell.
[a]The presence of 1–3 criteria is associated with mild pancreatitis and <1% mortality. The mortality increases with 4 (6%), 5–6 (40%), and >6 (100%).

A rising C-reactive protein at 48 h can be another marker of severe pancreatitis.

Complications that can lead to major morbidity or mortality include hyperglycemia, hypocalcemia, renal failure, ARDS, infection, hypotension, blood coagulation disorders, abscess formation, fistula formation, and pancreatic pseudocyst formation. Early death associated with severe acute pancreatitis is related to multiple organ failure, whereas late deaths are associated with infections and the development of sepsis.

Treatment

Treatment of acute pancreatitis involves maintaining the cardiorespiratory status, placing the pancreas at rest, and careful observation and early treatment of any complications that may develop. Monitoring in an intensive care unit may be needed for more serious cases. Invasive or noninvasive hemodynamic monitoring is indicated to optimize intravascular blood volume. Mortality is often associated with cardiovascular compromise. The goal of treatment is to maintain perfusion and limit pancreatic injury by maintaining blood supply. Large amounts of fluid leak into the peritoneal and retroperitoneal space due to hypoalbuminemia (loss of oncotic pressure) and massive inflammation. As much as 12 L of fluid can leak and be sequestered. Aggressive fluid management and assessment of preload are essential. If a patient remains hypotensive despite fluid therapy, vasopressors may be required. Aggressive fluid replacement may lead to electrolyte abnormalities; hence, close monitoring and replacement of potassium, magnesium, and ionized calcium levels are necessary. Hyperglycemia is common; therefore, careful monitoring of blood glucose levels and insulin therapy may be required.

Abdominal pain is a hallmark of pancreatitis making pain management a high priority. Often, intravenous analgesia is required to control the pain. If the patient is awake enough to use a patient-controlled analgesia device, it should be used. There are no data to suggest that one type of analgesia versus another aggravates pancreatitis by increasing the sphincter of Oddi pressure.

Pulmonary complications can range from mild atelectasis to ARDS. Treatment is supportive based on level of need. As abdominal girth increases, greater restriction on respiration occurs; therefore, careful monitoring of ABGs, SpO$_2$, and respiratory effort is required.

The pancreas is placed at rest by strict adherence to an NPO (L. *nulla per os*, nothing by mouth) regimen and often by nasogastric (NG) suction (in the presence of ileus). Placing the patient on NPO may not decrease pancreatic secretion but will decrease pain. Somatostatin, which inhibits release of pancreatic polypeptides, may be used, but this is controversial since it has been reported to worsen pancreatitis in some patients. Nutritional support is important. When enteral feedings are used, they are given past the duodenum into jejunum to prevent stimulation of the pancreas. The benefit to enteral feeding is the maintenance of the intestinal mucosa and prevention of bacterial translocation. Total parenteral nutrition should be used only in patients who fail a trial of enteral feeding. Close attention to glycemic control must occur. H$_2$ blockers or proton-pump inhibitors may be given to prevent gastric hypersecretion and stress ulcers.

Fine-needle aspiration, guided by radiology, of peripancreatic and intra-abdominal fluid collections is necessary to guide antibiotic therapy. Antibiotic prophylaxis should be restricted to patients with substantial pancreatic necrosis. Drainage of fluid is the mainstay of therapy.

Patients who have severe acute pancreatitis as a result of gallstone obstruction should undergo therapy to relieve the obstruction. Endoscopic retrograde cholangiopancreatography (ERCP) should be done within 72 h of diagnosis. Patients who are not candidates for ERCP should have the obstruction relieved in another manner.

Surgery is rarely needed and indicated only acutely in necrotizing pancreatitis with documented infection where there is solid or semisolid material that cannot be drained percutaneously. Among the techniques used are surgical drainage of abscesses, pancreatic lavage, and subtotal or total pancreatectomy. These procedures carry high morbidity and mortality.

Nursing Intervention

In acute cases, pancreatitis is life threatening and requires both vigorous treatment and nursing care. All vital signs are checked at least hourly. Intake and output should be documented carefully. Insensible losses should be taken into account. Monitor laboratory values such as hematocrit and hemoglobin, blood urea nitrogen, serum protein, creatinine, blood glucose, and electrolytes. Frequent fingerstick glucose monitoring is necessary to monitor insulin therapy and maintain glycemic control.

Observe for muscular twitching, jerking, or irritability. Frequent vomiting and/or gastric suctioning may cause loss of electrolytes, with the possible development of tetany. Calcium is lost because it binds to the fatty acids and is lost in the stool.

Respiratory status is monitored by levels of arterial oxygen saturation and arterial blood gases as well as hourly auscultation of lungs for crackles, wheezes, and diminished breath sounds. Cardiac monitoring is essential to detect dysrhythmias, which are frequent with shock and/or electrolyte imbalances.

An NG tube is often inserted and connected to suction so as to decrease stimulation of the pancreas and reduce the risk of gastric aspiration when an ileus is present. Observe and record color, amount, and nature of NG drainage as well as pH and the presence of blood. Mouth and nose care should be given hourly, especially if anticholinergic drugs are administered.

Nutritional support is very important. Placement of a feeding tube will be necessary so that postduodenal enteral feeds can begin as soon as possible. Increases in serum amylase and lipase levels postfeeding will indicate that a patient is not tolerating enteral feeding and TPN may be required. The TPN should be administered in severe cases so as to not stimulate the gastrointestinal tract. Small amounts of clear liquids are allowed when the patient can tolerate the NG tube clamped. Eventually, a bland high-protein, high-carbohydrate, low-fat diet with frequent small meals is recommended.

Medicate the patient to alleviate pain. Use a pain scale to guide therapy. Observe for side effects of all medications, especially antibiotics.

Emotional support is very important because the pain is severe, the NG tube is uncomfortable, and the monitoring equipment increases apprehension.

41

Intestinal Infarction, Obstruction, Perforation, and Trauma

EDITORS' NOTE

This chapter addresses the areas of the PCCN exam on bowel infarction, obstruction, perforation, and trauma. Expect questions related to assessment and recognizing patient changes related to abdominal exam for these processes.

INTESTINAL INFARCTION

The intestinal tract receives a rich blood supply. Three major vascular trunks from the aorta supply the intestinal tract: the celiac axis and the superior and inferior mesenteric arteries. Since there is much collateral flow, gradual occlusion of even two of these three major trunks usually does not cause clinical difficulties. Up to 20% of cardiac output after meals is delivered to the intestinal tract.

Because of this rich collateral circulation, mesenteric or intestinal infarction is unusual. Many patients have extensive atherosclerosis of the aorta and intestinal branches, but few have ischemia or infarction.

Pathophysiology and Etiology

Mesenteric ischemia usually results from one of two processes. In the first process, termed occlusive, cardiac output is usually adequate, but an embolus can dislodge from either the heart or aorta and flow into the superior mesenteric artery, lodging a short distance from the aorta and totally occluding blood-flow in this area. Another cause could be an acute thrombosis in a vessel with atherosclerosis, much as one sees with coronary occlusion. The result from this sudden occlusion is infarction of part or all of the small intestine and possibly some of the colon. With this sudden occlusion, the collateral circulation is unable to compensate by increasing blood flow to the ischemic bowel.

The second major type, termed nonocclusive, is related to atherosclerosis of the intestinal vasculature. Already there is narrowing of the blood vessels, but in the normal state these narrowings are not clinically significant. When cardiac output or blood pressure is compromised—as in dehydration, myocardial infarction, atrial fibrillation, or shock from any cause—overall blood supply to the intestines may diminish below a critical level, at which point intestinal infarction can occur. In this type of infarction, the intestinal ischemia is secondary to an overall reduction in cardiac output. Vasospasm may also play a role in nonocclusive mesenteric ischemia.

Consequences of either type of ischemia in the intestines are similar. In milder cases, only the mucosa is affected, with sloughing of the mucosa, bleeding, and abdominal pain. With severe ischemia, the submucosal and muscular layers of the intestine can be involved. If the injury is severe, transmural bowel necrosis and perforation can occur. With transmural necrosis, peritonitis will result, and intestinal bacteria enter the bloodstream, causing sepsis. In these circumstances, the disease is usually fatal.

Clinical Presentation

Occlusive mesenteric ischemia usually presents dramatically. The patient often experiences the sudden onset of severe abdominal pain, usually located in the periumbilical area or the epigastrium. There is usually diaphoresis, and the patient prefers to sit up, being more uncomfortable when forced to lie still. The abdomen, in contrast to the impressive ill appearance of the patient, usually has little tenderness. Guarding, rigidity, and rebound tenderness are usually absent. Nausea and vomiting may be present. Signs of peritoneal inflammation will develop over time as bowel ischemia progresses. If diagnosis and treatment are delayed, peritonitis and intestinal perforation result.

Nonocclusive mesenteric infarction, in contrast, does not present dramatically. Often, the patient is hospitalized for other diseases. Intestinal infarction is usually preceded by a vague abdominal discomfort with few physical findings. Routine diagnostic studies undertaken for other causes of abdominal pain—such as plain abdominal films, ultrasound, and upper gastrointestinal (GI) series—are usually negative in the course of the disease. With continuing ischemia, infarction and death usually result.

A milder form of nonocclusive ischemia can affect the colon without affecting the small bowel. In these patients, the clinical presentation is similar, but they experience bloody diarrhea and mild crampy pain. These patients usually do not go on to full-thickness infarction, perforation, and death, unlike those whose ischemia involves the small intestine as well.

Diagnosis

In occlusive disease, when the diagnosis is considered and other causes such as perforated ulcer are excluded, the diagnosis can usually be confirmed at surgery or preoperatively by angiography. When a strong clinical suspicion of mesenteric ischemia exists, the patient should go directly to angiography. Angiography will reveal either an embolus or a thrombosis of the superior mesenteric artery, and surgery will reveal either ischemia or an infarcted small and possibly an infarcted large intestine.

Nonocclusive disease is usually more difficult to diagnose. Symptoms are not as dramatic, and usually an acute surgical abdomen is not present. Blood analysis often reveals a leukocytosis, increased amylase and lactate dehydrogenase, and decreased pH and bicarbonate, all of which are nonspecific abnormalities. Lactate levels will be increased, and although they are not specific to mesenteric ischemia, they can be trended to see patient's progress and response to therapy once the diagnosis has been made. A computed tomographic (CT) scan may reveal air in the bowel wall or mesenteric vasculature, and focal or segmental thickening of the bowel wall may be seen. The CT scan can help rule out other causes of acute abdominal pain. Magnetic resonance angiography (MRA) provides more detailed information about the mesenteric vessels. Plain abdominal radiographs are usually of little help. Findings on the plain film may be normal (25%), show distended loops of bowel, bowel wall thickening, or pneumatosis. Colonoscopy or sigmoidoscopy can help make the diagnosis of ischemic colitis. The colon will appear pale, cyanotic, with petechial bleeding, and/or ulcerations. In patients with pseudomembranous colitis, the colon will appear yellow with round plaques. Doppler ultrasound may show stenosis or occlusions. Unfortunately, diagnosis is usually made at autopsy, at which time bowel infarction can readily be appreciated. Diagnosis can also be made during exploratory laparotomy, but at this point the chances of survival are slim.

Treatment

The goal of treatment of intestinal infarction is to restore intestinal blood flow as quickly as possible. Treatment begins with adequate resuscitation and hemodynamic stabilization, hopefully to restore blood flow to the intestines, broad-spectrum antibiotics, avoiding vasoconstrictive agents, systemic anticoagulation (unless actively bleeding), and placement of a nasogastric tube for decompression.

The treatment of occlusive disease has classically been surgical. Embolectomy or thrombectomy with or without bypass is usually performed. Surgical therapy also provides the opportunity to resect any questionable areas of intestine and evaluate the extent of injury. Surgery should not be delayed if perforation is suspected.

Angiographic management allows for treatment with local infusion of thrombolytic (clot-dissolving) agents, intra-arterial vasodilators, angioplasty, placement of a stent, and/or embolectomy.

Thrombolytic therapy should be considered only in patients who can undergo angiography within 8 h of the onset of abdominal pain and who do not have clinical evidence of bowel necrosis or other contraindications to thrombolytic therapy. Management should also include prevention of future embolic events.

Primary therapy for patients with nonocclusive mesenteric ischemia involves the infusion of papaverine (a vasodilator) through the angiographic catheter and attempts to reverse the underlying condition that has led to splanchnic vasoconstriction. Surgery should be reserved for patients with peritoneal signs. However, the underlying circulatory abnormality of poor cardiac output or hypotension should first be corrected. Early laparotomy and resection of infarcted intestine are necessary in patients whose pain does not rapidly resolve with correction of the low-flow state or vasospasm. Often, the patient's abdominal wall is left open (see temporary closure under Abdominal Compartment Syndrome section later in the chapter), so that subsequent reoperations can be accomplished easily to assess areas of the bowel that were ischemic during the first operation. Often, the patient returns to the operating room 1 to 2 days after the initial surgery; possibly additional visits will be required. Postsurgical infusion of papaverine may be necessary.

Delay in diagnosis of either type of intestinal infarction is almost always associated with a fatal outcome. Even with the diagnosis made and surgical therapy performed in a timely manner, the mortality rate is high.

Nursing Intervention

Careful and astute assessment of patients with unexplained abdominal pain is the key to recognizing intestinal infarction. Monitor the type of pain and relieving factors.

Supportive management of patients with intestinal infarction includes nasogastric suction, appropriate fluid and electrolyte replacement, and administration of antibiotics after cultures have been obtained. Treatment of shock and metabolic acidosis should be managed with fluid therapy since alpha-stimulating amines can have an adverse effect on intestinal perfusion and precipitate renal failure by reducing blood flow to the kidneys. Positive inotropic agents such as dobutamine or milrinone may be used to augment a low cardiac output. The primary objective of initial management should be to prepare the patient for possible surgery before these complications arise. Since most patients with intestinal infarction require surgery, once intestinal stabilization is present and the patient has gone to surgery, the nurse must redirect interventions to postoperative surgical care. Such postoperative interventions are covered later in this chapter.

INTESTINAL OBSTRUCTION

Intestinal obstruction is among the most common indications for abdominal surgery. Obstruction is often seen in the adult population; the patient usually presents with crampy abdominal pain, vomiting, and decreased passage of stool or flatus. Intestinal obstruction is divided into gastroduodenal, proximal or distal small intestinal, and colonic.

Pathophysiology

Bowel obstruction often results in problems with fluid balance. Alteration in fluid balance is due to fluid trapped in the intestine and the reduced capacity to ingest and absorb fluids. Often, patients are profoundly dehydrated from decreased intake, vomiting, and fluid trapped in the intestinal loops. Serum chemical imbalances can occur, specifically with sodium, potassium, chloride, and bicarbonate.

Etiology

In adults, the most common cause of intestinal obstruction is adhesions from previous surgery. When the peritoneal cavity is explored, as in cholecystectomy or gastric surgery, fibrous bands often form between loops of intestine. Usually these fibrous bands, otherwise known as adhesions, are asymptomatic, but they can also obstruct different segments of the small intestine.

The other major causes of intestinal obstruction in adults are hernias, tumors, and ulcers. A loop of intestine can become incarcerated in a hernia, causing an obstruction. Tumors, usually of the colon, can grow, so that they completely block off the lumen of the colon and thus produce obstruction. Ulcers, usually in the distal stomach or duodenum, can also cause blockage from scarring and fibrosis.

Other, less common causes of obstruction include infections such as diverticulitis, abscesses, inflammation, ischemia, gallstones, and some congenital anomalies.

Clinical Presentation

The presentation of intestinal obstruction depends on the location and etiology of the bowel obstruction. In patients with a gastroduodenal or proximal small intestinal obstruction, vomiting and crampy epigastric pain are the major symptoms. The symptoms will occur early after the obstruction, usually within a few hours. However, if the obstruction is in the distal small intestine or colon, vague, crampy, periumbilical or diffuse abdominal pain is the initial symptom. Patients have vomiting usually hours to days after the start of the pain and may actually present for medical care before they have any vomiting at all.

Commonly, tachycardia and dizziness due to dehydration are present. Later symptoms include decreased bowel movements and passage of gas.

Examination often reveals a distended abdomen with hyperresonance or tympany on percussion, sounding like a kettledrum. Bowel sounds are usually increased and high pitched (tinkling), and the abdomen may be diffusely, although usually not severely, tender. There is usually no guarding or rebound tenderness. The fluid vomited may be yellow or green in proximal obstructions of the small bowel or darker and feculent smelling in obstructions of the distal small bowel or colon.

Diagnosis

Diagnosis is made on the basis of history, a careful physical examination, and routine abdominal radiographs. The radiographs will usually show dilated small bowel loops with air-fluid levels or a horizontal line above which air is seen. In patients with nonspecific plain radiographs, a CT scan can be helpful. A CT scan with oral contrast can simultaneously provide information about the presence, level, severity, and cause of obstruction. In addition, other abdominal pathology can be detected. In some cases, closed-loop or strangulating obstruction may be demonstrated. Surgery usually allows the diagnosis of the cause of the obstruction. Barium-contrast radiographic studies, either of the upper GI tract or via a barium enema, are sometimes used for diagnosis prior to surgical therapy. Abdominal ultrasound may also be used to diagnose a bowel obstruction.

Treatment

Treatment consists of correcting fluid and electrolyte imbalances. Intravenous fluids are given while carefully monitoring serum electrolyte concentrations, vital signs, and urine output. Passage of a nasogastric tube and applying suction to remove air and fluid can often reverse a small bowel obstruction due to adhesions and should be used in virtually all cases of either proximal or distal bowel obstruction. Decompression of the stomach will also help to improve the comfort level of the patient. Nonoperative management requires that bowel strangulation be ruled out. Surgery is often necessary to break the bands of adhesions in obstructions and is almost always necessary in obstructions from tumors. Approximately one-half to three-fourths of patients will require surgical intervention. If a hernia can be manually reduced, surgery may not be necessary. If bowel infarction or gangrene has occurred, intestinal resection and antibiotics are needed.

Nursing Intervention

Nursing interventions again are aimed at ensuring hemodynamic stability. Careful observation of fluid and electrolyte balances is of primary importance. Strict records of intake and output, daily weights, vital signs, and serum electrolyte concentrations are maintained.

Careful assessment of the patient's nutritional status must be done on a daily basis to prevent a catabolic state. Because the patient must have nothing by mouth, nutrition may need to be maintained by total parenteral nutrition (TPN) if surgery is delayed or the obstruction does not resolve within a reasonable length of time.

Because nasogastric suction is very important in relieving a bowel obstruction, patency must always be maintained. Note consistency, type, color, amount, and pH of drainage.

As in intestinal infarction, the primary objective of initial management should be to prepare the patient for possible surgery to relieve the obstruction. Refer to the Nursing Intervention section in the discussion of GI Surgery later in the chapter, for nursing interventions for the postoperative care of patients with bowel obstruction.

GI PERFORATION

Intestinal perforation is usually a catastrophic event. The patient will generally experience a sudden onset of abdominal pain and appear very ill. Perforations occur in the stomach, duodenum, appendix, or colon. Rarely, however, other areas of the GI tract can also perforate.

Pathophysiology

Perforation of the intestinal tract results in leakage of intestinal contents into the peritoneal cavity. If the stomach or duodenum perforates, ingested foodstuffs, acids, and enzymes leak into the peritoneal cavity. If the appendix or colon perforates, feces, which contain large amounts of bacteria, are released into the peritoneal cavity. All of these substances are irritating to the peritoneum and cause an intense inflammatory reaction, with leakage of fluid and pus into the peritoneal cavity. Fever and leukocytosis result, and severe pain is usually present when the peritoneum becomes inflamed.

Etiology

The most common cause of intestinal perforation in the United States is appendicitis. If diagnosed early, appendicitis usually will not cause perforation. If diagnosis is delayed, the inflamed appendix may rupture, causing either a diffuse or localized peritonitis. Other major causes of colonic perforation are colonic diverticulitis, which represents infection of outpouchings from the colon, or colonic tumors, which can perforate the bowel wall. The most common cause of gastric or duodenal perforation is ulcers. Small intestinal perforations rarely occur and are usually caused by tumors, congenital malformations, trauma, or ischemia.

Clinical Presentation

Patients usually present with the acute onset of abdominal pain, which is likely to begin in the periumbilical area and spread throughout the abdomen. The patient prefers to lie still, flat on the back, as movement usually accentuates the pain. The patient is often feverish, possibly tachycardic, and his or her respirations are shallow. Hypovolemia may be present and be manifest as hypotension. Hypovolemia is secondary to the exudation of fluid into the peritoneal cavity and its sequestration in the intestines due to an ileus. The patient is often diaphoretic and looks moderately ill. Abdominal examination often reveals a board-like abdomen with absent bowel sounds. Diffuse tenderness with muscle rigidity and rebound tenderness may be present. In the case of a local perforation that walls off, as occasionally occurs with a perforated appendix or gastric ulcer, the physical findings may be isolated to a certain area of the abdomen.

Diagnosis

Diagnosis is usually made by the history and physical examination. A leukocytosis with a left shift is usually present, and the hemoglobin may be falsely raised due to intravascular volume depletion. Serum electrolytes may be abnormal. A CT scan is the diagnostic tool of choice with accuracy rate of close to 95%. An ultrasonic Doppler can be used to detect appendicitis. Plain radiographs of the abdomen often reveal free air underneath the diaphragm on an upright abdominal or chest film. An ileus pattern is

often present. Diagnosis of the specific cause is usually made by exploratory laparotomy. In certain cases, either an upper GI series or colonic enema with a water-soluble contrast agent such as diatrizoate will show extravasation of the contrast agent, demonstrating an intestinal perforation.

Treatment

In the vast majority of cases, therapy consists of surgical repair of the intestinal perforation. In some walled-off perforations in poor-risk patients, conservative management may be attempted, with nasogastric suction, intravenous fluids, and parenteral broad-spectrum antibiotics. Prior to surgical therapy, the patient's hemodynamic status may need to be stabilized with intravenous fluids. Antibiotics should be given to treat the peritonitis. The overall prognosis depends on the time from the perforation to definitive therapy, underlying medical disorders, and any postsurgical complications. With prompt diagnosis and treatment, most patients will do well.

Nursing Intervention

Refer to the Nursing Interventions in the discussions of Intestinal Infarction and Intestinal Obstruction in this chapter.

GI SURGERY

Esophagus

The most common surgical procedures related to the esophagus are those for the treatment of esophageal carcinoma. This disease usually occurs in men older than 60 years. Cigarette smoking and alcohol intake are the two major risk factors. The carcinoma can be squamous or adenocarcinoma. Patients usually have dysphagia as the main symptom and a recent unexplained weight loss. At the time of diagnosis, the great majority of tumors have spread beyond the esophagus to the mediastinum, lymph nodes, liver, or pulmonary system. Esophageal tumors are often not curable by either surgery, radiation therapy, or chemotherapy.

Surgery is undertaken to either cure the disease or palliate symptoms. Unfortunately, surgery is not always possible. The usual surgical procedure is esophagogastrectomy with primary esophagealgastric anastomosis. The mortality rate associated with this procedure is anywhere from 2.8% to 17.0%. Another surgical procedure that was done more frequently in the past is primary esophagectomy with colonic interposition between the cervical esophagus and stomach. Radiation therapy is usually an effective palliative procedure for those who are not operable or have had a recurrence of their tumors. Current studies of chemotherapy do not show much benefit, but further studies of both chemotherapy and radiation therapy are in progress and have shown some success.

In Barrett's esophagus, an abnormal columnar epithelium replaces the stratified squamous epithelium that normally lines the distal esophagus. It is a consequence of chronic gastroesophageal reflux disease (GERD) and predisposes to the development of adenocarcinoma of the esophagus. Treatment is focused on decreasing the reflux with proton-pump inhibitors and H_2 blockers. Esophagectomy may be indicated in severe cases once dysplasia has developed.

Stomach

Gastric surgery is generally performed for ulcer disease, gastroesophageal reflux disease, neoplastic disease, and bariatric weight loss.

A number of different operations are performed for ulcer disease. One surgery is a vagotomy and pyloroplasty. The vagotomy (severing of the vagus nerve) results in decreased acid production because of the loss of vagally mediated gastric secretion. Pyloroplasty, or widening of the pyloric channel, is necessary to prevent gastric stasis. This surgery is generally associated with a low rate of ulcer recurrence, but a combination of vagotomy and antrectomy has an even lower recurrence rate. In this more complicated surgery, the distal half of the stomach is removed to decrease gastrin production; another stimulus to acid production. Another surgical treatment for ulcers is the highly selective vagotomy; also called the parietal cell or proximal gastric vagotomy. In this operation, the vagal branches to the proximal stomach, the fundus, and the body are severed. Because this is where acid secretion occurs, this surgery decreases acid production without affecting the motor activity of the distal stomach. This surgery, however, is technically more difficult to perform than the other two.

Gastroesophageal reflux of acid results in problems with esophagitis and esophageal strictures. Symptoms include heartburn, regurgitation, and dysphagia. Usually these conditions can be treated medically (proton-pump inhibitors, H_2 blockers), but some cases are refractory to conservative therapy. In such cases, surgery is necessary. Among the operations most commonly performed is the Nissen fundoplication. Fundoplication involves wrapping the fundus of the stomach around the lower esophagus and anchoring the distal esophagus in the abdominal cavity. This greatly reduces reflux of gastric juices into the esophagus, allowing the esophagitis to heal. Another procedure, done less commonly, involves the placement of a plastic ring around the distal esophagus to reduce reflux. This ring is called the Angelchik prosthesis.

Surgery for gastric neoplasms often takes many forms. Adenocarcinoma is the most common malignancy of the stomach. Symptoms often appear late, after spread has already occurred. In lesions that have not spread, the usual procedure is a subtotal gastrectomy, with removal of over half the stomach. Some tumors are large enough to require a total gastrectomy. In patients with tumors that have already metastasized, gastric bypass in the form of a gastrojejunostomy is often needed for palliation.

Obesity is a chronic disease with increasing prevalence. Class III obesity (body mass index >40 kg/m^2) has contributed to an increase in bariatric surgery. This complex disease with associated comorbidities (diabetes mellitus, obstructive sleep apnea, hyperlipidemia, hypertension) requires special management. Surgical options are considered after failed diet and exercise regimens. The surgical options include biliopancreatice diversion, jejunoileo bypass, vertical banded gastroplasty, adjustable gastric band, gastric bypass, and combinations of these procedures. Psychologic support with lifestyle modifications are a necessary part of the postoperative management since surgery is not a cure. Surgical complications can occur during three phases. Phase 1 (1 to 6 weeks) complications may include bleeding, leaking at operative site, pulmonary embolism, bowel perforation or obstruction, and/or wound infection. Phase 2 (7 to 12 weeks) includes vomiting, ulcerations at the surgical margins, and dumping syndrome. Dumping syndrome is nausea, diaphoresis, and diarrhea after eating foods high in refined sugar. Phase 3 (12 weeks to 12 months) complications may include cholelithiasis, small bowel obstruction, and/or band slippage. Bariatric patients require specialized equipment for optimal management of their care and close surgical/medical follow-up. A strong nutritional support team is necessary to guide patients through the dietary transitions postoperatively.

Small and Large Intestines

Surgery of the small intestine is usually performed for removal of tumors, treatment of hemorrhage, correction of intestinal herniation, or treatment of inflammatory bowel disease. Tumors of the small intestine are rare, and treatment usually involves simple resection of the tumor itself plus a limited margin of normal intestine on either end. Hemorrhage is also uncommon and usually results from arteriovenous malformations, which in most cases form in the colon and not the small intestine. Small intestinal herniation can be either internal or external. Internal herniation is associated with trapping of intestinal loops by adhesive bands that form as a result of previous abdominal surgery. The herniation is referred to as internal because it is within the peritoneal cavity. External herniation involves trapping of an intestinal loop outside the peritoneal cavity, as in inguinal, femoral, or ventral hernias. Surgical therapy of either type involves freeing the trapped loop of intestine and attempting to prevent its recurrence.

Surgery of the large intestine is usually performed for appendicitis, colonic carcinoma, diverticulitis, or lower GI bleeding.

Appendicitis

In western populations, appendicitis is probably the major cause of an acute abdomen. The appendix arises from the cecum and varies in length. The appendix can become inflamed, distended, and perforated. Appendicitis is thought to arise from an obstruction in the more proximal part of the appendix, with stasis and bacterial proliferation distally. The visceral peritoneum initially becomes inflamed, with resultant exudation of fluid and proteins. At this stage, pain is localized to the periumbilical area or right lower quadrant. As a response to the infection and inflammation, catecholamine is released, resulting in tachycardia and sweating. With further distention of the appendix and visceral peritoneal inflammation, inflammation of the adjacent parietal peritoneum results. This leads to the finding of localized involuntary abdominal musculature contractions; termed guarding. Rebound tenderness is often present in the right lower quadrant. With continuing obstruction and infection, the pus-filled appendix will perforate. With perforation, pus and bacteria are released into the peritoneal cavity. An intense inflammation of the peritoneum results, with increased abdominal tenderness. If the infection

is still isolated by loops of intestine to the right lower quadrant, the physical findings will be primarily in that site. If, however, the infected fluid spreads throughout the abdominal cavity, then diffuse direct tenderness, rigidity, and rebound tenderness of the abdomen result. At this stage, the intravascular blood volume will be low, the patient may be hypotensive, and urine output will fall. The patient will prefer to lie quietly in bed without moving, and his or her respirations are shallow. The temperature is usually elevated, as is the white blood cell (WBC) count, with a shift to more immature forms of neutrophils. The hemoglobin may be raised due to hemoconcentration.

Therapy of appendicitis is surgical after fluid and electrolyte resuscitation is initiated. If there has been no perforation, an appendectomy is performed and recovery is usually rapid. If free perforation has occurred, copious irrigation of the peritoneal cavity with an antibiotic solution is required in addition to the appendectomy. Usually the surgical wound must be left open to protect against wound infection. Time to recovery and length of hospitalization are usually greater than in patients without perforation.

Colonic Carcinoma

Colonic carcinoma is presently the second leading cause of cancer death in the United States. Unfortunately, symptoms often appear late in the disease, after spread beyond the colon has occurred, or are ignored by the patient and attributed to other causes. One example of the latter is rectal bleeding, which is often perceived by patients as resulting from hemorrhoids. However, rectal bleeding can also be from a polyp or tumor in the rectum or sigmoid; it should be evaluated by sigmoidoscopy and possibly by barium enema examination. Other possible symptoms of colon cancer include constipation, diarrhea, and colonic obstruction. All of these are results of either a partial or complete mechanical colonic obstruction. Colon cancer may not produce early symptoms, but one early sign can often be found. The presence of microscopic amounts of blood (occult blood) not visible to the naked eye can be noted in many cases of colon cancer. Occult blood can be discovered by card tests, such as Hemoccult. Tests are recommended annually for all individuals older than 50 years in the United States. Screening colonoscopy is also recommended for all people older than 50 years or 10 years prior to the age an immediate family member presented with colon cancer. If colon cancer is detected at an early stage, the likelihood of cure with surgical excision is excellent. However, if the tumor has spread, the chance of surgical cure is poor. Surgical excision involves removal of the tumor with wide margins of uninvolved intestine on either side and with resection of the areas of regional lymphatic drainage. Usually a permanent colostomy is not required except in carcinoma of the distal rectum.

Diverticulitis

Diverticulitis, often seen in the older population, is a common cause of abdominal pain in patients older than 50 years. It involves infection of one of the outpouchings of the colon. Patients may have anywhere from mild abdominal pain and tenderness to diffuse peritonitis from colonic perforation. Therapy is usually with antibiotics and bowel rest, but free perforation or abscess formation may mandate surgical exploration with performance of a temporary diverting colostomy.

Pancreas

Carcinoma of the pancreas is the fourth leading cause of cancer death in men and the fifth most common in women. It usually arises insidiously and is almost always incurable at the time of diagnosis. Risk factors for pancreatic cancer include cigarette smoking, certain dietary and environmental factors, and juvenile-onset diabetes mellitus.

Most patients with pancreatic cancer complain of vague, dull epigastric discomfort that may radiate through to the back. Insidious weight loss and anorexia are also present. Approximately one-fourth of patients have a palpable abdominal mass. The tumor can spread to the duodenum, liver, lymph nodes, and lungs and can impinge on the stomach. Other symptoms vary with the sites of metastases. If the tumor is compressing the stomach, gastric outlet obstruction and vomiting are common. If the bile duct is obstructed, jaundice, pruritus, and acholic stools can result. Diagnosis of pancreatic cancer is usually made by CT scan of the abdomen, followed by either percutaneous needle biopsy or surgical exploration.

Most cases of pancreatic cancer are not surgically curable. Those that are resectable require extensive, complicated surgery for attempted cure. The two major procedures undertaken are pancreaticoduodenectomy (Whipple's procedure) and total pancreatectomy. Whipple's procedure involves resection of the head of the pancreas along with contiguous structures. The gastric antrum, duodenal C loop, gallbladder, and lymph nodes are removed. A loop of jejunum is anastomosed to the tail of the pancreas, the stomach, and the common bile duct. The procedure is difficult, and surgical mortality (death within 30 days of surgery) is 5%. Major complications of the procedure have been leakage or hemorrhage at the site of pancreaticojejunostomy. Five-year survival of one large series of patients treated by Whipple's procedure for pancreatic cancer was 20%.

Total pancreatectomy is another option in pancreatic cancer. In this procedure, the same organs are removed as for Whipple's procedure but a pancreaticojejunostomy is not necessary since the whole pancreas is removed. This procedure is technically simpler to perform than Whipple's procedure. Metabolic management, however, is much more difficult.

Most surgical procedures for pancreatic cancer are palliative rather than curative. The aim is to treat or prevent obstruction of the common bile duct and gastric outlet. Therefore, anastomosis of the jejunum to either the gallbladder or common bile duct as well as gastrojejunostomy are most often done.

Nursing Intervention

Nursing priorities for patients undergoing GI surgery should include promoting an optimal physical condition preoperatively, alleviating psychosocial concerns, meeting nutritional needs, promoting proper GI functioning postoperatively, and preventing complications.

Preoperatively, the patient must ideally be hemodynamically stable, have fluid and electrolyte balances in normal limits, be in a reasonable nutritional state (not catabolic), and be emotionally prepared for the impending surgery.

Postoperatively, the first goal of therapy is to ensure hemodynamic and respiratory stability. Maintain an airway by ventilation or oxygen therapy and assess the pulmonary effects of anesthesia. If the patient is not intubated, make sure that he or she coughs and deep breathes every 2 h (instruct the patient on splinting the incision). Suction the endotracheal tube as needed and note the color, amount, and odor of the secretions. Monitor arterial blood gases (ABGs) and/or pulse oximetry values.

Assess vital signs at least every 15 min initially after surgery and progress to longer intervals as the patient's stability allows. Note urine output and maintain at least 30 mL/h. If the patient has hemodynamic monitoring, note hemodynamic measurements every hour initially and progress as stability allows. Assess intake and output every hour, and monitor serum electrolytes as available. Assess the type and amount of drainage from the nasogastric tube, from incision, and from the drainage tubes. Note any foul odor from any drainage. Assess for possible abdominal fluid accumulation or postoperative hemorrhage.

Maintain nutritional status by TPN if the patient will not tolerate oral or enteral intake within the first several days after surgery. The alimental route for nutrition is restricted because of cessation of peristalsis from intraoperative handling of intestines, anesthesia, and/or potassium loss, with resultant decreased smooth muscle contractility. If the patient is not able to eat, maintain the patency of the nasogastric tube and record the characteristics of any drainage. Once bowel sounds are present, clear liquids—progressing to full liquids and then to diets low in residue and high in protein, carbohydrates, and calories—may be initiated.

Maintain the integrity of the skin by providing pressure relief by turning as well as monitoring for signs and symptoms of infection. Assess vital signs frequently, noting increased pulse, tachypnea, and apprehension. Check dressing and wound frequently during the first 24 h for signs of bright blood or excessive incisional swelling. Note temperature elevations and elevated WBCs. Monitor for signs of peritonitis (rigidity, guarding, rebound tenderness, and the absence of bowel sounds).

Patients who have had pancreatic resections must have their blood glucose monitored closely. Glycemic control may be necessary with a continuous infusion of insulin.

Emotional support of the postoperative patient is important to both the patient and the family. This is particularly important for patients who have had ostomies placed. Maintain a reassuring, accepting environment and give the patient opportunities to express fears and anxieties regarding his or her altered self-concept.

GI TRAUMA

Blunt or Penetrating Abdominal Trauma

Since violence is common in our society, stab wounds and blunt injuries to the abdomen are increasingly seen in emergency departments, operating rooms, and intensive care units. Injury to the abdomen may occur from a blow to the abdomen in

an automobile accident, altercation, sports injury, or fall. These injuries may occur even though the abdominal wall is still intact. Other penetrating injuries, such as those from stab wounds, may appear superficial and unimportant, but they are often deep and may have lacerated several internal organs. Trauma of any kind is apt to cause bleeding or contusions and may open the bowel lumen, causing peritonitis. In closed abdominal wounds, the spleen, the kidneys, the duodenum, and the liver are injured in approximately that order of frequency; in stab wounds, the liver, stomach, and colon receive most of the injury because of their anterior location.

Diagnosis

Abdominal trauma may cause injury to the liver, spleen, pancreas, GI tract, spine, retroperitoneum, kidneys, and pelvic organs. Injuries to the spleen, liver, pancreas, and GI tract are the most difficult to diagnose by conventional radiologic methods. A CT scan has been shown to be beneficial for the early diagnosis and accurate evaluation of the extent of internal injuries following abdominal trauma. A CT scan is capable of detecting lacerations, subcapsular hematomas, and ruptures of all abdominal organs and, therefore, has advantages over organ-specific procedures. In addition, CT scans directly image even small amounts of intra-abdominal hemorrhage, which cannot be identified by other conventional imaging techniques.

At some institutions, a diagnostic peritoneal lavage or abdominal ultrasound are done as an emergency evaluation tool for the patients who have suffered trauma to the abdomen. These procedures can help determine which patients need laparotomy because of perforated viscera or lacerations of the liver or spleen. Angiography can be beneficial in assessing injury and in helping to manage bleeding with embolization.

Clinical Manifestations

If the injury is severe (especially with a significant blood loss), the patient may exhibit signs of hypovolemic shock (low blood pressure, shallow respirations, weak rapid pulse, and decreased urine output). The patient may have pain, depending on the site and extent of injury. A physical insult to the abdomen is apt to cause cessation of bowel motility. If there is colonic injury, there may be blood in the stool and possible signs of intestinal perforation or obstruction.

In blunt trauma, the pancreas is particularly susceptible to rupture where it passes over the spine; such injuries are often associated with duodenal rupture.

With trauma to the pancreas, pancreatitis often follows but is usually asymptomatic. Elevation of serum amylase is not a dependable sign. Traumatic pancreatitis is often recognized only during exploratory laparotomy for gunshot or stab wounds. However, in the nonpenetrating, blunt abdominal trauma, traumatic pancreatitis often goes unnoticed because of the protected retroperitoneal location of the pancreas. This unnoticed pancreatitis may lead to the development of a pseudocyst, a subdiaphragmatic abscess, or massive GI hemorrhage. The disease, regardless of whether it is diagnosed during a laparotomy, carries a 14% mortality rate.

Symptoms of liver and splenic injury are similar but vary in the side of tenderness. If blood loss is great enough, signs of shock will be present.

Treatment

Initial treatment is aimed at maintenance of the patient's hemodynamic status and prevention of shock by addressing the ABCs of resuscitation. Rapid intravenous fluid and blood replacement may be necessary. Antibiotics may be necessary to prevent peritonitis, especially for open, penetrating wounds. Monitor the patient's ongoing blood loss via serial hemoglobin and hematocrit measurements. Patients with liver or splenic lacerations may undergo arterial embolizations to preclude surgery.

Surgical intervention must readily be instituted for those who are hemodynamically unstable. Most of these patients will undergo exploratory laparotomy to repair or remove injured organs and surrounding tissue. Vigorous rinsing of the abdominal cavity with an antimicrobial solution is necessary if bowel perforation has occurred. Patients with closed injuries require astute observation for organ failure or hemorrhage necessitating surgical intervention. The abdomen may be left open in order to facilitate frequent returns to the operating room and to allow for abdominal swelling, thus decreasing the possibility of abdominal compartment syndrome.

Abdominal Compartment Syndrome

Abdominal compartment syndrome (ACS) occurs when intra-abdominal pressure (IAP) is abnormally high and associated with organ dysfunction. It is characterized by abdominal distention, elevated IAP, elevated airway pressure, and decreased renal function. Traditionally, it has been thought to occur primarily in trauma patients, but it is also seen in a wide variety of medical and surgical processes. This syndrome occurs in 5% to 33% of trauma patients and 38% of patients undergoing major abdominal surgery as well as approximately 8% of patients in medical intensive care. Massive volume resuscitation is the leading cause of ACS. The etiology of ACS in the nontrauma patient is generally related to an inflammatory process that initiates a vicious cycle of capillary leak, fluid sequestration, rising IAP, inadequate tissue perfusion, and lactic acidosis. Clinical abdominal assessment is unreliable. An IAP of 5 to 7 mm Hg in a critically ill adult is considered normal. Intra-abdominal hypertension (IAH) is defined as a sustained IAP ≥12 mm Hg. Acute IAH refers to elevation of the IAP that develops over a few hours and can lead to rapid development of ACS. Subacute IAH that develops over several days may also lead to ACS. Subacute IAH is usually seen in medical patients. As the pressure rises, the risk of ACS becomes greater. The absolute pressure number where ACS develops may vary, but values >20 mm Hg are strongly suggestive of ACS. Measurements of IAP can be done using intragastric, intracolonic, intravesical (bladder), or inferior vena cava catheters. The bladder pressure measurement is the easiest, minimally invasive, and accurate. Potentially every organ system can be affected. Cardiovascular effects include decreased venous return, low cardiac output, increased systemic vascular resistance (SVR), and elevated filling pressures. Pulmonary effects include increased airway pressures, hypoxia, and hypercarbia due to diaphragmatic compression. Renal perfusion is decreased due to renal vein compression, with resulting oliguria and acute renal failure. In addition, decreased blood flow to all intra-abdominal organs can occur, leading to their failure. Treatment of ACS is focused on relieving the pressure and reestablishing organ perfusion. A decompression laparotomy is performed. The abdomen is left open or with a temporary closure of artificial materials to the fascia, which will allow expansion of abdominal contents.

Nursing Intervention

Patients with abdominal injury must be carefully observed for coexisting cardiothoracic injury. Signs of pneumothorax, cardiac tamponade, cardiac rupture, and injuries to the aortic or pulmonary vasculature must be assessed.

Astute assessment of the patient's hemodynamic and respiratory status must be carried out continuously. Fluid and electrolyte replacements are given to counteract third spacing and hypovolemic shock. Anaerobic and aerobic coverage with antibiotics is initiated immediately. Ventilatory and oxygen support may be necessary.

A careful abdominal assessment is performed to evaluate injuries. The nurse must assess for rebound tenderness, muscle rigidity, anorexia, nausea, vomiting, abdominal distention, presence of bowel sounds, and pain. A nasogastric tube should be placed, and changes in drainage should be noticed.

Emotional support is important for the patient and family since GI trauma is usually quite unexpected and coping mechanisms are not readily available.

Other Trauma to the Gastrointestinal Tract

Caustic injury is usually produced by strong alkaline or acidic agents. The ingestion of caustic agents can initiate a progressive and devastating injury to the esophagus and stomach. Most caustic injuries are seen in patients who are very young, psychotic, alcoholic, or suicidal.

Acidic solutions usually cause immediate pain, and unless ingested intentionally, they are rapidly expelled. The alkali liquid solutions are often tasteless and odorless and thus are swallowed before protective reflexes can be elicited. Alkali solutions penetrate tissue more rapidly than acid solutions do and are more difficult to treat. Caustic injuries to the GI mucosa are classified pathologically in the same manner as skin burns.

Symptoms may be present, especially early after the ingestion. Edema, ulceration, or a white membrane may be present over the palate, uvula, and pharynx. Hoarseness, stridor, dysphagia, epigastric pain, emesis of tissue or blood, tachypnea, and shock may be present. Late symptoms include perforation of the stomach or esophagus, mediastinitis, and peritonitis.

Early treatment includes neutralization of the caustic agent. Acid injuries should be neutralized with large volumes of water or milk. Alkali injuries

occur so rapidly that even immediate attempts to neutralize them are likely to be unsuccessful; they should not be undertaken because of the exothermic properties of dilution and neutralization.

Resuscitation should immediately be instituted. Establishment of an airway, fluid and blood resuscitation, and GI rest (nothing by mouth [NPO]) should be first priorities.

Endoscopic evaluation should be performed once the patient is stable in order to evaluate the extent of the damage. If there is perforation, a thoracotomy or laparotomy may be done to repair injured organs.

The mortality rate after caustic ingestion is 1% to 3%. However, if the patient survives the acute effects of caustic ingestion, the reparative response can result in esophageal and gastric stenosis and an increased incidence of esophageal cancer.

Esophageal Perforation

The most common causes of esophageal perforation are medical tubes and instruments, forceful vomiting, and foreign bodies. Less frequent are perforations caused by gunshot wounds, necrotizing infections or tumors, and caustic agents.

Perforations are recognized by symptoms of respiratory distress; chest, neck, abdominal, and upper neck pain; and odynophagia. Subcutaneous crepitation, fever, shock, a mediastinal crunching sound with the heartbeat, leukocytosis, and radiographic abnormalities may also occur.

The most important determinants of survival are the size and location of the perforation and whether gross contamination outside the esophagus has occurred. Most causes of esophageal perforation are surgically managed to repair the perforation.

42

Management of the Patient with a Gastrointestinal Disturbance

EDITORS' NOTE

This chapter provides an overview of general nursing interventions for patients with any type of gastrointestinal disturbance, including the conditions previously discussed in Chaps. 39 through 41. Priority interventions include measures to maintain fluid and electrolyte balance, ensure adequate nutritional intake, maintain bowel elimination, maintain comfort, and prevent infection. The chapter concludes with a brief summary of physical assessment steps in assessing the gastrointestinal system.

INTERVENTIONS TO MAINTAIN FLUID AND ELECTROLYTE BALANCE

1. Maintenance of accurate intake and output. Include number, character, amount, and site of gastrointestinal (GI) fluid losses.
2. Monitoring of serum electrolytes per laboratory data. GI fluid losses through tube suction, ostomy drainage, diarrhea, and vomiting can cause losses of essential electrolytes, especially H^-, Cl^-, and K^+, and may produce alkalosis.
3. Correct use of GI tubes for decompression and diagnosis. Two types of tubes are used:
   a. Short tubes, used for the stomach and duodenum. Example: nasogastric tubes.
      i. Levin's (single-lumen tube).
      ii. Salem sump (double-lumen tube). This is the most widely used type because the second lumen, which is open to air, prevents the development of excessive negative pressure by bringing air into the cavity continuously. Low, intermittent levels of suction are used. The second port of the Salem sump (pigtail) must be placed above the patient's midline to prevent reflux into the pigtail. Commercially made antireflux valves are available.
   b. Long tubes. These are intended to extend the length of the small bowel. They come in 6- and 20-ft lengths.
      i. Miller-Abbott
      ii. Cantor
      iii. Harris' long tubes are threaded from the nose into the stomach and then through the pylorus, where the peristaltic activity of the bowel carries it to the desired area. If this does not occur, gravity or guidance under fluoroscopy may be used. Once the tube is in the correct location, it is taped securely in place to prevent further migration. With all of the GI tubes, the material aspirated should be noted for color, odor, and quantity.
4. Maintenance of blood volume during GI hemorrhage.
   a. Blood volume replacement as needed.
   b. Monitor hematocrit/hemoglobin every day and as needed during instability.
   c. Monitor amount, color, and area of bleeding.
   d. Administer oxygen therapy as needed. Pulse oximetry can be used to titrate oxygen therapy.

e. Monitor hemodynamic status.
f. Adminster crytalloid IV fluids as needed to maintain volume status.

5. Relief of nausea and vomiting.
   a. Monitor for distention; a nasogastric tube may be placed to decompress stomach.
   b. Monitor emesis for amount, color, frequency, and the presence of blood.
   c. Administer antiemetics.
   d. Place patient on side to prevent aspiration of vomitus.

INTERVENTIONS TO MAINTAIN NUTRITIONAL STATUS

Patients who are unable to eat must be fed enterally or parenterally. Normally, patients at rest require 25 kcal/kg/day (ideal body weight). The nurse should assess the calories given versus what is needed.

1. Evaluation of the patient's nutritional status.
   a. History taking.
      i. Medical history: Illness, surgery, GI disease, alcoholism, and so on.
      ii. Social history: Food storage and preparation facilities, finances, and education.
      iii. Drug history: Antibiotics, chemotherapy, anticonvulsants, an so on.
      iv. Diet history: 24-h recall.
   b. Anthropometric measures: Physical measurements that reflect growth and development compared with standards specific for sex and age. Compares body fat and skeletal muscle obtained through measurements of triceps skin fold, midarm circumference, and midarm muscle circumference.
   c. Types of protein and biochemical tests.
      i. Somatic protein (skeletal): Somatic protein is the protein of voluntary muscles. Indicators of somatic protein losses are low ideal body weight or usual body weight percentages, low fatfold thickness, negative nitrogen balance from nitrogen balance studies, and increased 24-h urinary creatinine.
      ii. Visceral protein: Visceral protein is the protein of the internal organs. Indicators of visceral protein losses are low total lymphocyte count (<1000), serum albumin (<3.5), and serum transferrin (<200 mg/dL).

d. Measurements of immune function: Various forms of protein malnutrition have been associated with depression of the immune system.
   i. Lymphocytes: White blood cells (WBCs) that defend against infection. Decrease in number as protein depletion occurs. Decrease for many other reasons also, so they are not nutrition specific.
   ii. Antigen skin testing: A test of the immune system's competence, in which an antigen is injected just under the skin. A reaction means that the immune system is working normally.

2. Enteral feeding administration: A person who has a functioning GI tract but is unable to eat enough food may be a candidate for tube feeding. Enteral feeding is preferred to parental feeding provided there is no contraindication to using the GI tract.
   a. Types of tubes: Silicone (Silastic) or polyurethane.
   b. Placement of tubes: Esophagostomy, gastrostomy, jejunostomy, nasogastric, and nasoenteric (nasoduodenal or nasojejunal).
   c. Tube feeding formulas: Selected after the client's needs have been identified.
      i. Polymeric formulas: These contain protein, carbohydrates, and fats of higher molecular weights. A person must be able to digest and absorb nutrients without difficulty to use this type of formula.
      ii. Monomeric formulas: These contain smaller molecules of protein, fat, and carbohydrates. They are "predigested" or elemental and are recommended for those who lack digestive capabilities or have a smaller than normal area for absorbing nutrients.
   d. Administration guidelines: Bolus feedings via gravity drip or continuous feedings via pump are used. Which method is preferred remains controversial. Generally, bolus feeds are given into the stomach and continuous feeds into the small intestine.
   e. Initial feedings:
      i. Check tube placement before feeding with radiographic verification.
      ii. Check residual amount in stomach. If >200 mL, notify physician and hold feeding.

iii. Check continuous drip rate every 1 to 2 h.

iv. Feeding should be at or slightly below body temperature. Cold formula may induce vasoconstriction, which reduces the flow of gastric digestive juices.

v. Monitor intake and output.

vi. Changing feeding bag and tubing every day.

vii. Monitor laboratory data, especially serum electrolytes.

viii. Flush tube with 50 to 100 mL of water before and after each feeding to maintain patency.

f. Complications:

i. Diarrhea: From bacterial contamination, lactose intolerance, hypertonic formulas, low serum albumin, or drug therapy.

ii. Dehydration: From excessive diarrhea, inadequate fluid intake, carbohydrate intolerance, or excessive protein intake.

iii. Aspiration pneumonia: From regurgitation of formula that is subsequently aspirated into the lungs or from displacement of feeding tube.

iv. Vomiting: From obstruction or delayed gastric emptying.

v. Nausea, cramps, distention: From obstruction, delayed gastric emptying, or intolerance to concentration or volume of formula.

vi. Increased glucose levels: From excess glucose loads.

3. Parental alimentation (hyperalimentation): If GI absorption and delivery of nutrients are inadequate, impossible for prolonged periods of time, or contraindicated, nourishment should be provided parenterally. Total parenteral nutrition (TPN) is done with a hypertonic mixture of dextrose, amino acids, electrolytes, vitamins, and trace minerals. It may be given peripherally (dextrose concentrations of <20% only) or through central veins.

a. Nutrient solutions: The concentration and quantity of the solution is gradually increased until a desired state is reached. A typical TPN solution contains 25% to 75% dextrose and 3.5% to 8.0% amino acids. One liter of a D50 solution provides about 1700 kcal daily. Electrolytes, vitamins, and trace minerals are added. The fluid may be concentrated if it is infused through a central line.

b. Lipid emulsions: Lipids supply 9 kcal/g, more than twice the energy supplied by 1 g of glucose. They are isotonic and prevent deficiencies of essential fatty acids.

c. Administration guidelines

i. Monitor serum electrolytes, albumin levels, and nitrogen balance studies. Increase TPN concentrations as nutritional status warrants.

ii. Monitor daily weight and daily intake and output.

iii. Monitor serum glucose every 4 to 6 h. It may be necessary to administer insulin. Monitor serum glucose every 1 to 2 h if patient is on an insulin infusion.

iv. Monitor infusion rate every 1 to 2 h. If the rate falls behind, monitor for hypoglycemia and spread whatever deficit has occurred over the next 24 h.

d. Complications

i. Infection or sepsis: Stringent aseptic technique must be maintained during catheter insertion and dressing changes.

ii. Thrombosis of great veins or embolism from the catheter: Remove catheter and start anticoagulation therapy if not contraindicated.

iii. Hyperosmolar nonketotic hyperglycemia: Discontinue TPN; give insulin, saline, and D_5W to replace free water.

iv. Hyperglycemia: Insulin therapy, slow rate.

v. Hypoglycemia: Check to make sure TPN has not been interrupted or the wrong concentration given.

vi. Electrolyte disturbances: Maintain appropriate concentrations.

INTERVENTIONS TO MAINTAIN BOWEL ELIMINATION STATUS

1. Diarrhea

a. Identify caustic factors.

b. Record color, amount, and frequency of stools.

c. Maintain intake and output to prevent dehydration.

    d. Monitor serum electrolytes.

    e. Check for blood in stools.

    f. Administer antidiarrheal medications to decrease intestinal motility if not contraindicated.

    g. Begin nutritional supplement.

    h. Protect skin with barrier creams or use a stool collection system.

2. Constipation

    a. Increase fluid intake if not contraindicated.

    b. Monitor time and consistency of stools.

    c. Administer laxative or enema if not contraindicated. Needed after barium studies.

INTERVENTIONS TO MAINTAIN COMFORT STATUS

1. Pain

    a. Observe for signs and location of pain; determine type and severity.

    b. Administer analgesics and monitor their effectiveness.

INTERVENTIONS TO PREVENT INFECTION

1. Monitor temperature and WBC counts.

2. Use full barrier precautions (sterile gown, sterile gloves, hat, mask, and large drapes) when placing central lines. Use aseptic technique for changing dressings and make sure that dressings remain intact.

3. Use universal standard precautions for blood and body fluids.

4. Assess sources of contamination. Culture infected drainage and blood.

5. Use good handwashing techniques to prevent cross contamination.

6. Elevate head of bed >30 degrees if not contraindicated to prevent aspiration.

7. Brush the patient's teeth every 12 h and use chlorhexidine oral rinse twice daily

PHYSICAL ASSESSMENT

Physical assessment of the GI system can be briefly summarized by following the steps listed below:

1. Begin the assessment with inspection of the abdomen. Do not begin palpation, particularly deep palpation, until the last phase of assessment. This will avoid any stimulation of the GI system and the initiation of painful stimuli.

2. Auscultation is the second phase of assessment. Bowel sounds are usually heard in all four abdominal quadrants. Observe for a change in sounds or bowel sound intensity and character. Bowel sounds are not always a reliable assessment tool owing to the transmission of sound throughout the abdomen.

3. Percussion is the third step in assessment. Usually, the GI tract has air present and will result in hearing a resonant or hyperresonant sound. Tympanic sounds can be heard in the stomach, although elsewhere these sounds may indicate an obstruction.

4. Palpation, both superficial and deep, is the last phase of assessment. The goal is to detect abnormal organ size, such as liver or spleen enlargement, and to determine whether pain is present in the abdomen.

BIBLIOGRAPHY

Banares, R., Albillos, A., Rincon, D., et al. (2002). Endoscopic treatment versus endoscopic plus pharmacologic treatment for acute variceal bleeding: A meta-analysis. *Hepatology, 35,* 609.

Barkun, A., Bardou, M., & Marshall, J. K. (2003). Consensus recommendations for managing patients with nonvariceal upper GI bleeding. *Annals of Internal Medicine, 139,* 843.

Belongia, E. A., Costa, J., Gareen, I. F., et al. (2008). NIH consensus development statement on management of Hepatitis B. *National Institutes of Health Consens State Science Statements, 25,* 1.

Blei. A. T. (2005). The pathophysiology of brain edema in acute liver failure. *Neurochemistry Inernational, 47,* 71.

Braga, M., Gianotti, L., Nespoli, L., et al. (2002). Nutritional approach in malnourished surgical patients: A prospective randomized study. *Archives of Surgery, 137,* 174.

Cardenas, A. (2005). Hepatorenal syndrome: A dreaded complication of end-stage liver disease. *American Journal of Gastroenterology, 100,* 460.

D'Amico, G., Pietrosi, G., Tarantino, I., et al. (2003). Emergency sclerotherapy versus vasoactive drugs for variceal bleeding in cirrhosis: A Cochrane meta-analysis. *Gastroenterology, 124,* 1277.

Demirpolat, G., Oran, I., Tamsel, S., et al. (2007). Acute mesenteric ischemia: Endovascular therapy. *Abdominal Imaging, 32,* 299.

Dhiman, R. K., Jain, S., Maheshwari, U., et al. (2007). Early indicators of prognosis in fluminant hepatic failure: An assessment of the model for end-stage liver disease (MELD) and Kings' College Hospital criteria. *Liver Transplantation, 13,* 814.

Fahy, B. G., Sheehy, A. M., & Coursen, D. B. (2009). Glucose control in the intensive care unit. *Critical Care Medicine, 37*(5), 1769–1776.

Forsmark, C. E., & Baillie, J. (2007). AGA institute technical review on acute pancreatitis. *Gastroenterology, 132.*

Garcia-Taso, G., Sanyal, A. J., Grace, N. D., et al. (2007). Prevention and management of gastroesophageal varices and variceal hemorrhage in cirrhosis. *Hepatology, 46,* 922.

Jacobs, R. J., Koff, R. S., & Meyerhoff, A. S. (2002). The cost-effectiveness of vaccinating chronic hepatitis C patients against hepatitis A. *American Journal of Gastroenterology, 97,* 427.

Jalan, R. (2005). Acute liver failure: Current management and future prospects. *Journal of Hepatology, 42,* S115.

Kanwal, F., Gralnek, I. M., Martin, P., et al. (2005). Treatment alternatives for chronic hepatitis B virus infection: A cost-effectiveness analysis. *Annal of Internal Medicine, 142,* 821.

Kouglas, P., Lau, D., El Sayed, H. F., et al. (2007). Determinants of mortality and treatment outcomes following surgical intervention for acute mesenteric ischemia. *Journal of Vascular Surgery, 46,* 467.

Krinsley, J. S. (2003). Association between hyperglycemia and increased hospital mortality in a heterogeneous population of critically ill patients. *Mayo Clinic Proceedings, 78,* 1471.

Lok, A. S. F., & McMahon, B. J. (2007). Chronic hepatitis B: AASLD practice guidelines. *Hepatology, 45*(2), 507.

Malbrain, M. L., Chiumello, D., Pelosi, P., et al. (2005). Incidence and prognosis of intraabdominal hypertension in a mixed population of critically ill patients: A multiple-center epidemiological study. *Critical Care Medicine, 33,* 315.

Marik, P. E., & Zaloga, G. P. (2001). Early enteral nutrition in acutely ill patients: A systematic review. *Critical Care Medicine, 29,* 2264.

Martindale, R. G., McClave, S. A., Vanek, V. W., et al. (2009). Guidelines for the provision and assessment of nutrition support therapy in the adult critically ill patient: Society of critical care medicine and American society for parenteral and enteral nutrition: Executive summary. *Critical Care Medicine, 37*(5), 1757.

Matheny, N. A., Schallom, L., Oliver, D. A., et al. (2008). Gastric residual volume and aspiration in critically ill patients receiving gastric feedings. *American Journal of Critical Care, 17*(6), 512.

McNelis, J., Marini ,C. P., Simms, H. H. (2003). Abdominal compartment syndrome: Clinical manifestations and predictive factors. *Current Opinion in Critical Care, 9,* 133.

Nathans, A. B., Curtis, J. R., Beale, R. J., et al. (2004). Management of critically ill patients with severe acute pancreatitis. *Critical Care Medicine, 32,* 2524–2536.

Nice Sugar Study Investigators. (2009). Intensive versus conventional glucose control in critically ill patients. *New England Journal of Medicine, 360*(13), 1283–1297.

Richards, C. F., & Mayberry, J. C. (2004). Initial management of the trauma patient. *Critical Care Clinics, 20,* 1.

Seef, L. B., & Hoofnagle, J. H. (2002). National Institutes of Health consensus development conference: Management of hepatitis C. *Hepatology,(Suppl 1),* S1.

Strader, D. B., Wright, T., Thomas, D. L., et al. (2004). Diagnosis, management, and treatment of hepatitis C. *Hepatology, 39,* 1147.

Stravitz, R. T. (2008). Critical management decisions in patients with acute liver failure. *Chest, 134,* 1092.

Suri, S., Gupta, S., Sudhakar, P. J., et al. (1999). Comparative evaluation of plain films, ultrasound and CT in the diagnosis of intestinal obstruction. *Acta Radiology, 40,* 422.

Swaroop, V. S., Chari, S. T., & Clain, J. E. (2004). Severe acute pancreatitis. *Journal of the American Medical Association, 291,* 2865.

Todd, S. R. (2004). Critical concepts in abdominal injury. *Critical Care Clinics, 20,* 119.

Tucker, O. N., Szomarwin, S., & Rosenthal, R. J. (2007). Nutritional consequences of weight-loss surgery. *Medical Clinics of North America, 91,* 499.

Van den Berghe, G., Wouters, P., Weekers, F., et al. (2001). Intensive insulin therapy in the surgical intensive care unit. *New England Journal of Medicine, 345,* 1359.

Van den Berghe, G., Wouters, P. J., Bouillon, R., et al. (2003). Outcome benefit of intensive insulin therapy in the critically ill: Insulin dose versus glycemic control. *Critical Care Medicine, 31,* 359.

Vogt, T. M., Wise M. E., Bell, B. P., et al. (2008). Declining hepatitis A mortality in the United States during the era of hepatitis A vaccination. *Journal of Infectious Diseases, 197,* 1282.

PART VI

Gastroenterology Practice Exam

1. Achalasia refers to which of the following?
   (A) Decreased production of trypsin
   (B) Increased backflow of gastric acid into the duodenum
   (C) Loss of peristaltic waves in the small intestine
   (D) Failure of the gastroesophageal sphincter

Questions 2 and 3 refer to the following scenario:

A 26-year-old man is admitted to your unit with complaint of chest pain unrelated to exercise. His pain is not relieved by rest. No electrocardiographic (ECG) changes are evident. His abdomen is soft to palpation and free of pain. His diet has been normal and he reports no change in his stool patterns. He reports no problems with swallowing.

2. Based on the preceding information, what is the likely origin of the problem?
   (A) Malfunction of the cardiac sphincter
   (B) Duodenal ulcer
   (C) Pyloric sphincter reflux
   (D) Myocardial ischemia

3. What treatment would most likely be instituted in this situation?
   (A) Esophageal resection via the thoracic approach
   (B) Antrectomy
   (C) Vagotomy
   (D) Diet change

4. A 44-year-old man had a gastrostomy tube (G tube) placed for nutritional support following diagnosis of a malabsorptive syndrome. He was discharged with the G tube in place. Several weeks later, he is admitted to your unit with complaint of disorientation. The family states that they have been irrigating and aspirating the G tube after his tube feedings. This irrigation of the G tube would most likely cause which disturbance?

   (A) Metabolic acidosis
   (B) Metabolic alkalosis
   (C) Respiratory alkalosis
   (D) Respiratory acidosis

5. The normal pH of the stomach falls within which of the following ranges?
   (A) 1 to 3
   (B) 4 to 6
   (C) 6 to 8
   (D) Over 8

6. Approximately how many calories are in a gram of protein?
   (A) 2 kcal
   (B) 4 kcal
   (C) 6 kcal
   (D) 9 kcal

7. D_5W has 5 g of glucose per 100 mL of solution. Approximately how many calories are in 1 L of D_5W?
   (A) 20 kcal
   (B) 200 kcal
   (C) 500 kcal
   (D) 2000 kcal

8. Which of the following enzymes is active in the digestion of proteins?
   (A) Amylase
   (B) Maltose
   (C) Lipase
   (D) Trypsin

9. Which of the following enzymes is active in the digestion of fats?
   (A) Amylase
   (B) Maltose
   (C) Lipase
   (D) Trypsin

10. Which of the following enzymes is active in the digestion of carbohydrates?
    (A) Amylase
    (B) Pepsin
    (C) Lipase
    (D) Trypsin

11. Emulsification (dispersion into small droplets) of fat occurs because of which substance?
    (A) Chyme
    (B) Lipase
    (C) Bile
    (D) Cholecystokinin

12. Following a gunshot wound to the abdomen, a 27-year-old man has a complete colectomy with creation of an ileostomy. What nursing measures will be necessary considering that the function of the large intestine has been eliminated?
    (A) Administration of proteolytic enzymes via tube feedings
    (B) Observation of intake and output since reabsorption of water will be diminished
    (C) Administration of proteolytic enzymes via tube feedings and administration of emulsifying agents
    (D) Observation of intake and output and administration of emulsifying agents

13. What is the primary function of the small intestine?
    (A) Absorption of nutrients
    (B) Reabsorption of water
    (C) Reabsorption of carbon dioxide
    (D) Acting as a reservoir for food

14. Increased colonic motility is produced by which of the following?
    (A) Parasympathetic stimulation
    (B) Sympathetic stimulation
    (C) Central nervous system stimulation
    (D) Increased fat content in the diet

15. Which drug would potentially decrease colonic motility?
    (A) Nifedipine
    (B) Atropine
    (C) Digitalis
    (D) Gentamicin

16. All venous blood from the intestines eventually drains into which vein?
    (A) Gastric
    (B) Superior mesenteric
    (C) Portal
    (D) Celiac

17. The portal vein empties into which structure?
    (A) Inferior vena cava
    (B) Liver
    (C) Large intestine
    (D) Bile duct

18. A duodenal feeding tube was placed by the RN on a prior shift. You want to check the placement of the tube in order to confirm that it is in the duodenum rather than the stomach. To check its position, you utilize a pH reading from aspirated tube contents. Which pH range would suggest a duodenal rather than a gastric location?
    (A) 1 to 3
    (B) 4 to 6
    (C) 6 to 8
    (D) Over 8

19. Which of the following are major functions of the liver?
    (A) Production of bile and synthesis of amino acids
    (B) Production of bile and gluconeogenesis
    (C) Synthesis of amino acids and gluconeogenesis
    (D) Production of bile, synthesis of amino acids, and gluconeogenesis

20. A 39-year-old woman presents with complaint of right lower-quadrant pain. Prior to performing an abdominal assessment, in what order should you consider performing the following assessment techniques?
    (A) Inspection, palpation, and auscultation
    (B) Palpation, auscultation, and inspection
    (C) Inspection, auscultation, and palpation
    (D) Auscultation, palpation, and inspection

21. Depression of overall protein stores is commonly monitored during a nutritional assessment. Which of the following are measured as part of the routine protein assessment during an analysis of nutritional status?
    (A) Total lymphocytes and albumin
    (B) Total lymphocytes and lactate
    (C) Albumin and lactate
    (D) Total lymphocytes, albumin, and lactate

22. A 76-year-old man is receiving tube feeding supplements consisting of Osmolite at 75 mL/h. Approximately how many calories are

being administered every 24 h based on this feeding rate?
(A) 1200 kcal
(B) 1800 kcal
(C) 2400 kcal
(D) 3000 kcal

23. Which of the following is thought to be the most common cause of stress ulcers?
(A) Ischemia
(B) Excessive acid production
(C) Mechanical injury
(D) Infections

24. Hydrogen-ion blocking agents, such as cimetidine (Tagamet) and ranitidine (Zantac), work by which of the following mechanisms?
(A) Decreasing gastric acid production
(B) Supplying a protective membrane against hydrochloric acid
(C) Increasing bicarbonate production
(D) Blocking the release of catabolic hydrogen enzymes

25. Which of the following treatments is NOT routinely indicated in the treatment of upper GI bleeding?
(A) Endoscopy with coagulation of bleeding site
(B) Fluid replacement with crystalloids
(C) Blood transfusions
(D) Iced lavage of the stomach

26. Esophageal varices are the result of increases in which of the following vascular parameters?
(A) Hepatic arterial pressure
(B) Hepatic venous pressure
(C) Portal venous pressure
(D) Superior iliac arterial pressure

27. Transjugular intrahepatic portosystemic shunt (TIPS) works to decrease bleeding from esophageal varices by which mechanism?
(A) Decreasing portal venous pressure
(B) Improving vena caval blood flow
(C) Improving production of clotting factors
(D) Decreasing blood return to the liver

28. A 61-year-old man is admitted to your unit with the diagnosis of upper GI bleeding. He has a history of alcohol abuse and prior GI bleeding. His abdomen is distended and his liver is enlarged. He does not complain of pain. His vomitus is bright red. Based on this information, which condition is most likely present?

(A) Diverticuli
(B) Esophageal varices
(C) Duodenal ulcers
(D) Colonic varices

29. Which of the following is NOT a common cause of lower GI bleeding?
(A) Diverticulosis
(B) Colon tumors
(C) Arteriovenous malformations
(D) Hepatic failure

30. Which of the following is NOT a treatment for an upper GI tract bleeding?
(A) Octreotide
(B) Endoscopy
(C) Colon resection
(D) Balloon tamponade

31. A 57-year-old man with the diagnosis of hepatitis A is admitted to your unit. He is also recovering from vascular surgery and has an open wound on his left lower leg. Which type of isolation is appropriate for this patient?
(A) Universal standard precautions
(B) Respiratory
(C) Wound
(D) Reverse

Questions 32 and 33 refer to the following scenario:

A 23-year-old woman is admitted to your unit after being found unresponsive by paramedics. She has no overt signs of injury or physical abuse. After starting an intravenous drip, you accidentally stick yourself with the same needle used for the venipuncture.

32. Based on the preceding information, to what type of hepatitis would you most likely be exposed after a needle stick injury?
(A) Hepatitis A
(B) Hepatitis B and hepatitis C
(C) Hepatitis D
(D) No risk of hepatitis acquisition

33. You and the patient receive appropriate serologic testing. Assuming you have had no prior exposure to hepatitis, initial treatment for you includes administration of which of the following?
(A) Hepatitis B immune globulin (HBIG) and vaccine if not HbsAb positive
(B) Hepatitis A immune globulin (HAIG)
(C) Interferon
(D) Hepatitis A vaccine

Questions 34 and 35 refer to the following scenario:

A 67-year-old man is admitted to your unit with complaints of generalized fatigue and weakness. His abdomen is distended due to ascites, producing shortness of breath. His liver is hard but not enlarged. You note spider angiomas on his chest and he has atrophied skeletal muscles. His sclerae are icteric. Vital signs are blood pressure 96/60 mm Hg, pulse 110, and respiratory rate 28.

34. Based on the preceding information, which condition is likely to be responsible for his symptoms?
    (A) Acute hepatitis
    (B) Cirrhosis
    (C) Esophageal varices
    (D) Hepatorenal syndrome

35. Which initial treatment would help relieve his respiratory distress from the ascites?
    (A) Placing the patient in a supine position
    (B) Endoscopy
    (C) Protein restriction in the diet
    (D) Administration of diuretics and sodium restriction

36. All of the following are nursing measures for the patient with acute hepatitis except one. Which one is NOT indicated in the patient with hepatitis?
    (A) Low-protein, high-carbohydrate diet
    (B) Monitoring of liver enzyme tests
    (C) Maximizing periods of rest
    (D) Avoiding periods of rest, initiating active exercise regimens

37. Asterixis is regarded as a sign of the development of which condition?
    (A) Left ventricular failure
    (B) Acute calcium disturbance
    (C) Hepatic encephalopathy
    (D) Seizures

Questions 38 and 39 refer to the following scenario:

A 53-year-old man is admitted to the unit with the diagnosis of cirrhosis. He is confused and disoriented. He has a "flapping" movement of both hands and has jaundiced skin. Laboratory values are as follows:

SGOT/AST	100
SGPT/ALT	88
Lactate dehydrogenase	250
Alkaline phosphatase	165
BUN	10
Creatinine	0.8

38. Based on the preceding information, which condition is likely to be developing and causing the behavioral changes?
    (A) Acute renal failure
    (B) Loss of cerebral perfusion pressure
    (C) Loss of cerebral glucose from hepatic failure
    (D) Hepatic encephalopathy

39. Which treatment would be utilized in the treatment of this patient?
    (A) Lactulose
    (B) High-protein diet
    (C) Glucose bolus
    (D) Vitamins D and B administration

Questions 40 and 41 refer to the following scenario:

A 76-year-old woman is admitted to your unit with vomiting, nausea, and diffuse abdominal pain. The vomitus has a fecal odor. She had a cholecystectomy in the past, but has been in good health until she developed the abdominal pain 2 days earlier. Her abdomen exhibits a hyperresonant sound on percussion, and she complains of tenderness to palpation. Laboratory data are normal.

40. Based on the preceding information, which condition is likely to be developing?
    (A) Bowel obstruction
    (B) Mesenteric artery occlusion
    (C) Pyloric stenosis
    (D) Obstruction of the pancreatic duct

41. Treatment for this condition most likely would include which of the following?
    (A) Endoscopy for pyloric valve repair
    (B) Endoscopy with embolectomy of the pancreatic head
    (C) Laparotomy with possible mesenteric embolectomy
    (D) Laparotomy for relief of obstruction

Questions 42 and 43 refer to the following scenario.

A 29-year-old man is admitted to your unit with complaint of generalized abdominal pain. His pain started on the previous day and became worse. It improved before worsening again on his morning of admission. His abdominal examination reveals diffuse tenderness and "board-like" rigidity, with the patient preferring not to move. An abdominal radiograph reveals free air under the diaphragm. Laboratory data reveal the following:

Na^+	141
K^+	4.2
Cl^-	99
HCO_3^-	25
Amylase	50
WBC	13,000

42. Based on the preceding information, which condition is likely to be present?
    (A) Pancreatitis
    (B) Obstruction of the superior mesenteric artery
    (C) Intestinal perforation
    (D) Cholecystitis

43. Which treatment is indicated for this condition?
    (A) Placement on an NPO regimen with GI suction
    (B) Analgesia with narcotics while waiting for the pain to subside
    (C) Upper and lower endoscopy to search for obstructions
    (D) Exploratory laparotomy

Gastroenterology Practice Exam

Practice Fill-Ins

1. _____	12. _____	23. _____	34. _____
2. _____	13. _____	24. _____	35. _____
3. _____	14. _____	25. _____	36. _____
4. _____	15. _____	26. _____	37. _____
5. _____	16. _____	27. _____	38. _____
6. _____	17. _____	28. _____	39. _____
7. _____	18. _____	29. _____	40. _____
8. _____	19. _____	30. _____	41. _____
9. _____	20. _____	31. _____	42. _____
10. _____	21. _____	32. _____	43. _____
11. _____	22. _____	33. _____	

PART IV

Gastroenterology Practice Exam

PART VI

Answers

1.	D	12.	B	23.	A	34.	B
2.	A	13.	A	24.	A	35.	D
3.	D	14.	A	25.	D	36.	D
4.	B	15.	B	26.	C	37.	C
5.	A	16.	C	27.	A	38.	D
6.	B	17.	B	28.	B	39.	A
7.	B	18.	C	29.	D	40.	A
8.	D	19.	D	30.	C	41.	D
9.	C	20.	C	31.	A	42.	C
10.	A	21.	A	32.	B	43.	D
11.	C	22.	B	33.	A		

VII

RENAL

Ruth M. Kleinpell

43

Anatomy and Physiology of the Renal System

EDITORS' NOTE

Renal patient care problems comprise approximately 5% (six to seven questions) of the PCCN exam. These questions cover three major areas: acute renal failure, electrolyte imbalances, and end-stage renal disease. The following chapters contain information necessary to address each of these areas.

This chapter provides the essential concepts of renal anatomy, information that probably is not addressed directly on the PCCN exam. Understanding the contents of this chapter will, however, prepare you to better appreciate the clinical situations addressed by the PCCN exam. As you review this chapter, do not focus on minute concepts but rather concentrate on general anatomic features relevant to renal concepts that might be addressed in clinical practice. Knowledge of the anatomy and physiology of the renal system will enable application of key concepts to the care of the progressive care patient with altered renal status.

ANATOMY

Kidney

Location

The kidneys lie in the retroperitoneal space on each side of the vertebrae, with the upper border between T11 on the right and T12 on the left. This difference in position results from the natural displacement of the right kidney by the liver. The lower border is at approximately L3. The posterior surfaces are protected by the last two ribs.

Protective Coverings

The kidneys are protected by coverings that prevent massive blood loss from trauma. The outermost protective covering is pararenal fat that completely surrounds the three coverings of the kidneys. The next layer is the renal fascia, a membrane sheet that surrounds a layer of perirenal fat. This perirenal fat is actually a very dense layer of adipose tissue. It is very compact and surrounds the innermost covering of the kidney, the fibrous renal capsule. The fibrous renal capsule is a thin, resistant membrane that is contiguous with the kidney tissue itself.

Shape and Size

The kidneys are bean-shaped organs with an indentation on their medial surfaces. The indented area, called the hilum, is the entry site for the renal artery, lymphatics, and nerves and is also the exit site for the renal vein, ureters, lymphatics, and nerves. The average kidney is 10 to 12 cm long, 5 to 6 cm wide, and 3 to 4 cm thick. Its average weight is about 160 to 180 g.

Gross Anatomy

The cortex is the outer one-third of kidney tissue (Fig. 43-1). It is composed of the glomeruli of all the nephrons and the convoluted portions of the distal and proximal tubules. The cortex extends into the medulla between structures called pyramids. These extensions are the renal columns. The cortex itself extends inward from the renal capsule to the base of the pyramids.

The medulla is the inner portion of the kidney. It contains the loops of Henle, the vasa recta, and the collecting ducts. These loops and ducts are arranged in triangles or pyramids. The tips of the pyramids are called papillae. Groups of papillae merge to form

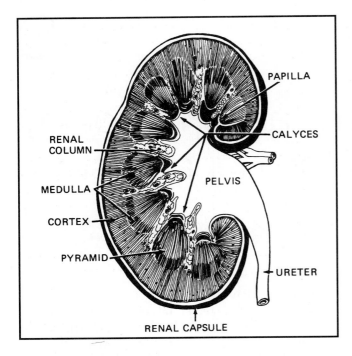

Figure 43-1. Gross anatomy of the kidney.

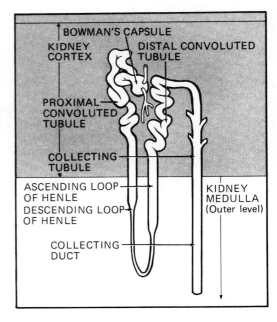

Figure 43-2. Cortical nephron.

into a single papilla that enters the calyx, which collects urine flow from the collecting ducts. Calyces channel the urine into the renal pelvis. Eventually, the urine flows from the renal pelvis into the ureter.

The number of calyces varies from 8 to 16 per kidney. Therefore, there is no symmetry in renal anatomy.

Nephron

The nephron is the functional unit of the kidney. Each kidney has more than a million nephrons. Up to 75% of the kidney's nephrons can be destroyed before the remaining nephrons are unable to compensate. While compensation is occurring, the functioning nephrons filter a higher solute load. Because of this increased workload, the functioning nephrons hypertrophy. There are two types of nephrons: cortical and juxtamedullary.

Cortical nephrons (Fig. 43-2) have glomeruli that lie close to the cortical surface and include thin, short segments of the loops of Henle. The loops of Henle do enter the medulla but do not go past the outer medulla. As the loops of Henle in the cortical nephrons are short and do not extend into the inner medulla, they do not participate in the concentration of urine. About 70% of the kidneys' nephrons

are cortical nephrons with short or nonexistent loops of Henle.

The juxtamedullary nephrons (Fig. 43-3) are found in the inner one-third of the cortex. They have long loops of Henle that dip deep into the medulla and are surrounded by the peritubular network, the vasa recta. These nephrons have a great

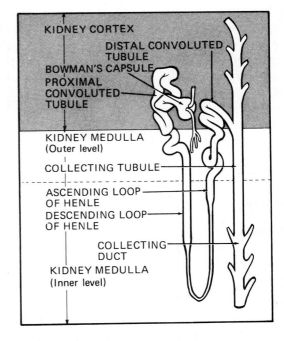

Figure 43-3. Juxtaglomerular nephron.

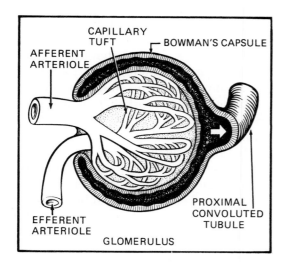

Figure 43-4. Schematic view of the glomerulus.

capacity to retain sodium and concentrate urine because of the long loops of Henle.

In hypovolemic and hypotensive patients, a large portion of the renal blood flow is shunted from the cortical nephrons to the juxtamedullary nephrons to maintain urine formation.

Structural Anatomy

The nephron, the functional unit of the kidney, is composed of the glomerulus, the proximal convoluted tubule, the loop of Henle, the distal convoluted tubule, and the collecting ducts.

The glomerulus is a network of capillaries (Fig. 43-4) that are spherical in shape and are formed by the afferent arterioles dividing into between two and eight subdivisions. These subdivisions branch to form as many as 50 capillary loops. The glomerulus is enclosed by an epithelium-lined membrane called Bowman's capsule. The efferent arteriole carries the blood out of the glomerulus.

The proximal convoluted tubule is about 14 mm in length. It receives the contents of the glomerulus. The lumen of the tubule contains tiny thread-like projections that help resorb the glomerular filtrate. The brush border increases the resorptive surface area per unit length of the tubule. The proximal convoluted tubule ends in the medulla of the kidney and becomes the descending limb of the loop of Henle.

The loop of Henle has three distinct portions: a thick descending limb, a thin segment that is the actual loop, and a thick ascending limb. The loops of Henle in the cortical nephron reach just to the inside of the kidney medulla. The loops of Henle in the juxtamedullary nephron reach almost to the tips

of the pyramids (the papillae) and then start ascending to become the ascending limb of the loop of Henle. The peritubular capillary network surrounds the loop portion of the juxtamedullary nephron. As the long loop of Henle dips deep into the medulla, it is surrounded by the vasa recta. Thirty percent of the nephrons in each kidney are juxtamedullary nephrons.

The distal convoluted tubule begins where the ascending limb of the loop of Henle starts twisting. The distal convoluted tubule closely passes its own glomerulus and may even touch it. The distal convoluted tubule continues without convolutions to become the collecting tubule.

The collecting tubule extends to become the collecting duct, which empties into a common collecting duct; it, in turn, empties into the renal pelvis.

Juxtaglomerular Apparatus

All nephrons have a juxtaglomerular apparatus (JGA) containing three specific components. As the distal convoluted tubule passes between the afferent and efferent arterioles, it encounters specialized cells (Fig. 43-5), the macula densa, that are tightly packed together.

There are also specialized cells, juxtaglomerular cells, on the outside of the afferent and efferent arterioles near their entry point into the glomerulus. These cells secrete granules of inactive renin.

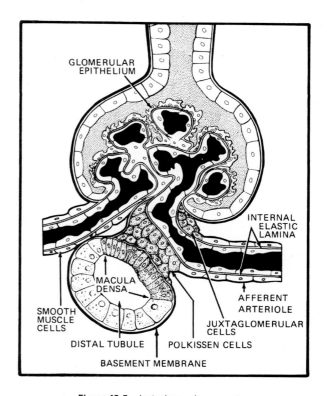

Figure 43-5. Juxtaglomerular apparatus.

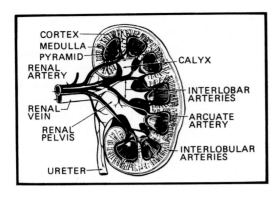

Figure 43-6. Vascular system of the kidney.

The area where the distal convoluted tubule passes by or touches the efferent arterioles is the third component of the JGA.

Vascular System

One renal artery arises from the aorta to supply both kidneys (Fig. 43-6). The renal artery enters the kidney at the hilum and bifurcates immediately at the kidney pelvis.

After this first splitting at the kidney pelvis, the renal arteries develop many branches called interlobar arteries. These arteries, as their name implies, travel between lobes of the renal parenchyma inside the renal columns toward the point where the cortex and medulla meet.

At the interface of the cortex and medulla, the interlobar arteries branch to form the arcuate arteries. These arteries form arcs between the lobes of the parenchyma.

From each arcuate artery, multiple intralobular arteries spread into the cortex. These intralobular arteries form short muscular afferent arterioles that supply the glomeruli. Efferent arterioles drain the blood from the glomerulus and flow through the peritubular capillary network that surrounds the cortical portions of the tubules. The small amount of remaining arterial blood flows into straight capillary loops called vasa recta, which extend down into the medulla to provide arterial blood to the lower parts of the thin segments of the loop of Henle before looping upward to enter the intralobular veins. From the intralobular veins, the blood enters the arcuate veins, the interlobar veins, the renal veins, and the inferior vena cava.

Nerve Supply

The sympathetic nervous system controls the constriction of renal arteries. These nerves follow the same course as the arterioles in order to maintain the vasoactive tone of the arterioles. The parasympathetic nervous system innervates the kidney through the vagus nerve fibers arising from the celiac plexus.

Ureter, Urinary Bladder, and Urethra

As the urine leaves the kidney pelvis, it enters the ureter. The ureter, approximately 10 in. in length, moves the urine along by peristaltic action to the urinary bladder, a hollow, muscular organ. It has a normal capacity of 250 to 500 mL. At the bottom of the bladder is the urethra. It is about 6 to 8 in. long in men and 1.0 to 1.25 in. long in women (Fig. 43-7).

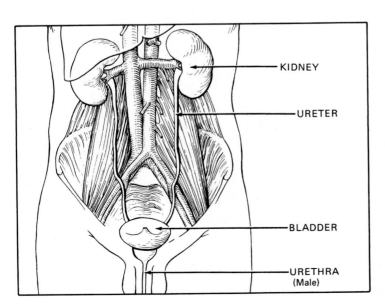

Figure 43-7. Ureter, urinary bladder, and urethra.

PHYSIOLOGY

Physiologic processes of the kidney include the formation of urine, the regulation of body water and electrolytes, the excretion of metabolic waste products, the regulation of acid-base balance and blood pressure, and the secretion of erythropoietin.

Formation of Urine

Three processes are involved in the formation of urine: glomerular filtration, tubular reabsorption, and tubular secretion.

Glomerular Filtration

The kidneys receive 20% to 25% of the cardiac output. Ninety-five percent of this quantity of blood will go through the glomerulus, where some solutes will be filtered out. An autoregulatory system exists to protect the glomerulus. The afferent and efferent renal arterioles constrict or dilate in response to systemic blood pressure. If systemic blood pressure increases, the afferent arteriole will constrict. This effectively reduces the pressure of the blood entering the glomerulus. In the same way, if systemic blood pressure decreases, the afferent arteriole will dilate to allow more blood to enter the glomerulus.

When the afferent arteriole constricts to reduce the pressure of blood in the glomerulus, the efferent arteriole relaxes (dilates) to allow the blood to leave more rapidly. This helps to control glomerular pressure. Conversely, when systemic pressure drops, the afferent arteriole dilates to let more blood into the glomerulus and the efferent arteriole constricts to help maintain the glomerular pressure. Below a mean arterial blood pressure of about 60 mm Hg, this autoregulatory system fails and the glomerulus suffers the effects of hypotension.

Glomerular filtration is influenced by two factors: filtration pressure and glomerular permeability.

Filtration pressure is determined in part by the anatomic blood flow through the nephron. Each nephron is actually perfused by two capillary beds (Fig. 43-8). The glomerular capillary bed is perfused by the afferent arteriole with an average hydrostatic pressure of about 60 mm Hg. The peritubular capillary bed is perfused by the efferent arteriole, which resists blood flow. Because of this, the glomerular capillary bed has a high pressure (which may be termed glomerular hydrostatic pressure). The peritubular capillary bed has a low pressure of about 13 mm Hg.

The high pressure in the glomerulus tends to filter fluid out of the glomerulus and into Bowman's capsule. At the same time and following the same principles, the low pressure in the peritubular capillary bed tends to draw fluid from the interstitial spaces into the peritubular capillaries. The high pressures in

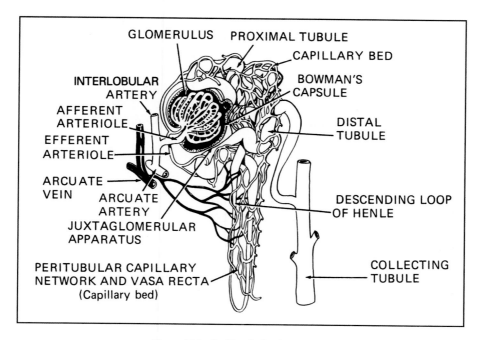

Figure 43-8. Capillary beds of a nephron.

the glomerulus cause a rapid filtration of fluid. The low pressure of the capillary bed of the peritubular system facilitates rapid uptake of the excreted tubular fluids by the peritubular capillaries. This diminishes backleak and increases net reabsorption.

Blood is brought into the glomerulus by the afferent arteriole. The pressure is close to 60 mm Hg, so fluid is forced from the glomerular capillaries into Bowman's capsule. This fluid is now called the glomerular ultrafiltrate. The fluid is called an ultrafiltrate because protein-sized (and larger) molecules cannot filter out of the glomerular capillaries. Those proteins remain in the blood entering the peritubular capillaries from the efferent arteriole. The retained protein molecules cause an increase in the plasma osmotic pressure, which, in turn, causes the rapid reabsorption of fluid from the peritubular interstitial spaces.

Glomerular permeability is the second influence on glomerular filtration. The glomerular membrane is different from other capillary membranes in the body. It has three layers: the endothelial layer of the capillary, a basement membrane, and a layer of epithelial cells on the other surface of the capillary (Fig. 43-9). In spite of three layers, the glomerular membrane is 100 to 1000 times more permeable than the usual capillary. The endothelial cells lining the glomerular capillary are full of thousands of tiny holes called fenestrae. Outside the capillary endothelium is a basement membrane similar to a mesh of fibers. The epithelial cells of the outer layer do not touch each other. The space between the cells is called a slit pore. Any particle >7 nm cannot penetrate the slit pore.

Composition of Glomerular Ultrafiltrate. Normally, the ultrafiltrate is free of protein and red blood cells (RBCs), as they are too large to pass through the slit pores. The semipermeable membrane of the glomerular capillary allows water, nutrients, electrolytes, and wastes to filter into Bowman's capsule.

Glomerular Filtration Rate. In the healthy kidney, the average glomerular filtration rate (GFR) is 125 mL/min. The total quantity of glomerular filtrate per day is about 180 L. More than 99% of this filtrate is reabsorbed in the tubules. The equation for calculating the GFR is the urine concentration of a substance times the urine flow rate divided by the plasma concentration of the same substance. The substance must be freely filtered and not affected by the tubules (Fig. 43-10). The normal adult urine volume is 1 to 2 L/day.

Factors Affecting the GFR. Any change in the glomerular hydrostatic pressure will alter the GFR. The most common cause of change in the hydrostatic pressure is a change in the systemic blood pressure. A change in systemic blood pressure changes the actual flow of blood into the glomerulus. Alterations in the afferent and efferent arteriole tone (constriction-dilatation) will also affect the glomerular pressure and hence the GFR.

Any alteration in the composition of the plasma, such as an increase in oncotic pressure (the osmotic pressure due to the presence of colloids in a solution), will alter the GFR. Such conditions as hyperproteinemia, hypoproteinemia, hypovolemia, or hypervolemia will also alter the composition of plasma because of alterations in the extracellular fluid (ECF) and intracellular fluid. Thus, these states will alter the GFR.

The GFR will automatically be altered by any abnormality of structure, presence of disease, or ingestion of nephrotoxic substances.

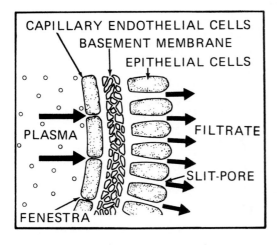

Figure 43-9. Three layers of the glomerular membrane.

$$GFR = \frac{(U_x \cdot V)}{P_x}$$

$$GFR = \frac{\text{URINE CONCENTRATION OF A FREELY FILTERED SUBSTANCE} \times \text{URINE FLOW RATE}}{\text{PLASMA CONCENTRATION OF SUBSTANCE IN } U_x}$$

Figure 43-10. Equation for calculating the glomerular filtration rate.

Tubular Absorption and Secretion

The glomeruli filter a total of 180 L/day; normal urine output is 1 to 2 L/day. The tubular function of the nephron is responsible (in part) for determining urinary output.

The nephron uses two processes, absorption and secretion, to convert this 180 L of ultrafiltrate to 1 to 2 L of urine. These processes may be active or passive and are influenced by hormones, electrochemical gradients, and Starling's law. The following definitions are useful in understanding renal function.

1. Diffusion is the movement of solutes from an area of high concentration to an area of low concentration.
2. Osmosis is the movement of water from an area of high water concentration to an area of low water concentration.
3. Absorption, as discussed here, is the movement of solutes and water from the tubule into the peritubular network (i.e., from the filtrate back into the bloodstream).
4. Secretion, as discussed here, is the movement of solutes and water from the peritubular network into the tubule (i.e., from the bloodstream back into the filtrate).
5. Passive transport is the movement of solutes by diffusion following concentration gradients and electrical gradients.
6. Active transport is the movement of any substance against an electrical or concentration gradient. Active transport requires energy, usually supplied by adenosine triphosphate (ATP).

A mnemonic may help unravel the maze of the movement of solutes in the various tubules. Cations are carried by active transport (CAT = carried active transport); anions are passively transported (ANI = a negative ion). Na^+, K^+, and H^+ are the most common cations in the body; Cl^- and HCO_3^- are the most common anions.

As with most rules, there is always an exception. In the collecting duct, chloride (anion) is actively absorbed and the cations are passively absorbed. Table 43-1 traces the formation of urine, starting with the ultrafiltrate and ending with urine after passage through both convoluted tubules, the loop of Henle, and the collecting ducts.

TABLE 43-1. URINE FORMATION[a–c]

Start	Proximal Convoluted Tubule	Loop of Henle (Three Parts)	Distal Convoluted Tubule	Collecting Duct	Finish
Ultrafiltrate	60%–80% of ultra-filtrate absorbed	**I. Descending Limb** H_2O absorbed (highly permeable to H_2O) Ultrafiltrate fluid becomes increasingly hypertonic	**Absorbed** HCO_3^- H_2O if ADH is present Na^+ actively if aldosterone is present	**Absorbed** Na^+ H_2O if ADH is present	Urine flows into renal pelvis, ureters, bladder
	Absorbed Na^+ Cl^- Glucose Amino acids All K^+ HCO_3^- H_2O passively absorbed	**II. Thin segment loop** Permeable to H_2O	**Secreted** K^+ H^+	**Secreted** H^+ K^+ NH_3	
	Secreted H^+ Urea Drugs Organic acids HCO_3^+ and H^+ (regulates acid-base balance) Ultrafiltrate isotonic to plasma	**III. Ascending limb** Cl^- absorbed actively; Na^+ absorbed Impermeable to H_2O Ultrafiltrate is hypotonic			

[a]Sulfates, nitrates, and phosphates are absorbed only in amounts sufficient to maintain the ECF concentration.
[b]All K^+ from the filtrate are absorbed in the proximal tubule.
[c]The K^+ secreted in the distal convoluted tubule equals about 12% of the K^+ in the original filtrate. Under certain circumstances, secretion may exceed the original filtered load.
ADH, antidiuretic hormone.

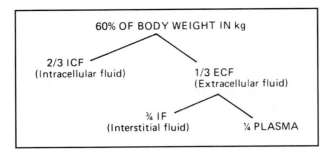

Figure 43-11. Distribution of water throughout the body.

The major function of the loop of Henle is to concentrate or dilute urine as necessary. This is accomplished by the countercurrent mechanism that maintains the hyperosmolar concentration in the renal medulla.

Regulation of Body Water

Throughout the discussion of body regulation, the terms *osmolarity* and *osmolality* will be used interchangeably. Osmolarity is the concentration of particles in solution. Osmolality is the amount of solvent in relation to the particles. The volume and concentration of body water content are maintained by the thirst-neurohypophyseal-renal axis. Approximately 60% of ideal body weight is water in men; the proportion is 50% to 55% in women. Figure 43-11 shows the distribution of water throughout the body. There are three mechanisms that help regulate body fluid: thirst, antidiuretic hormone, and the countercurrent mechanism of the kidney.

Thirst

Thirst is the major force in our awareness of a need for water. The thirst center is located in the hypothalamus. Intracellular dehydration causes the sensation of thirst. The most common cause of intracellular dehydration is an increase in osmolar concentration of the ECF. Increased sodium concentration of the ECF causes osmosis of fluid from the neuronal cells of the thirst center. Other important and frequent causes of thirst are excessive angiotensin II in the blood, hemorrhage, and low cardiac output.

The role of the thirst center is to maintain a conscious desire to drink the exact amount of fluid needed to maintain the body in a normal hydrated state or return a dehydrated state to the normal state of hydration.

Antidiuretic Hormone

Antidiuretic hormone (ADH) works closely with the thirst mechanism. The plasma protein and ECF sodium concentrations determine the osmolality of the ECF. Normal serum osmolality is 280 to 320 mOsm/L. Acid-base control mechanisms of the kidney adjust the negative ion in relation to the extracellular concentration (osmolality) to equal the positive ions in the body. ADH is synthesized in the supraoptic nuclei of the hypothalamus and then drips down the supraoptic-hypophyseal tracts to the posterior pituitary (neurohypophysis), where it is stored. The supraoptic area of the hypothalamus is so close to the thirst center that there is an integration of the thirst mechanism, osmolality detection, and ADH release.

The osmosodium receptors respond to changes in osmolality (sodium concentration) in the ECF. An increase in osmolality excites the osmoreceptors. They signal the neurohypophyseal tract that ADH is needed. The posterior pituitary (neurohypophysis) releases the ADH that it has stored. In the presence of ADH, the distal convoluted tubules and collecting ducts reabsorb water. The reabsorption of the water leaves a hypertonic urine. This cycle continues until the concentration of the ECF compartment and fluid homeostasis are returned to normal.

If osmolality of the ECF decreases, ADH release is inhibited because the osmoreceptors are not stimulated. Without ADH, the distal tubules and collecting ducts are impermeable to water. Urine will be very dilute because the water cannot be reabsorbed. The urine will continue to be diluted until the loss of water has raised the concentration of the ECF solutes to normal.

Countercurrent Mechanism

The countercurrent mechanism serves to concentrate urine and excrete excessive solutes. Excreting dilute urine is not a problem for the kidney unless there is a neurologic dysfunction, an endocrine dysfunction, or traumatic injury. These conditions may result in an inappropriate release and affect normal kidney function of ADH, aldosterone, and/or cortisol. Concentrating urine to excrete waste solutes is a complex interaction between the long loops of Henle, the peritubular capillaries, and the vasa recta.

The countercurrent multiplier mechanism functions constantly in a loop cycle, with fresh filtrate continuously entering the loop of Henle. At the entry to the loop, the filtrate has a concentration of 300 mOsm/L. The medulla increases this concentration so that, at the tips of the papillae in the pelvic

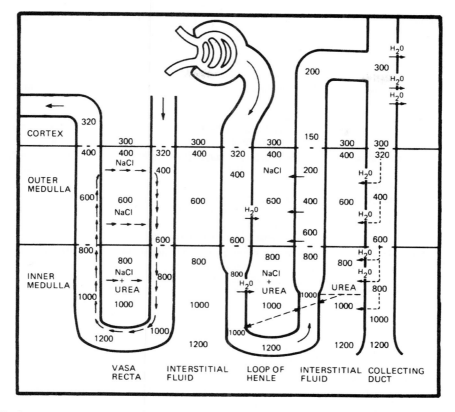

Figure 43-12. Countercurrent multiplier mechanism for maintaining medullary interstitial hyperosmolality and concentrating urine.

tip of the medulla, the concentration of the filtrate is 1200 to 1400 mOsm/L.

It is essential for the medullary interstitium to be hyperosmolar. There are four steps in concentrating the solutes to produce this hyperosmolality (Fig. 43-12).

In step 1, chloride ions are actively transported from the thick portion of the ascending limb of the loop of Henle into the upper medullary interstitial fluid. The active transport of chloride pulls sodium and some potassium, magnesium, and calcium also.

In step 2, the collecting ducts actively transport sodium into the medullary interstitial fluid. Chloride follows along passively. Steps 1 and 2 increase medullary interstitial fluid hyperosmolality by about 500 mOsm.

In step 3, the collecting duct yields urea to the lower medullary interstitial fluid if ADH is present. The hormone makes the collecting duct mildly permeable to urea and very permeable to water. Water leaves the collecting duct to enter the medullary interstitium, resulting in a high concentration of urea in the collecting duct. Urea, following concentration gradients, then diffuses out into the medullary interstitial fluid. This increases the medullary osmolarity by about another 200 to 400 mOsm.

In step 4, water osmosis occurs from the thin (descending) segment of the loop of Henle because of the high urea concentration in the lower medullary interstitial fluid. As the water moves from the loop of Henle, sodium ion concentration in the thin limb increases. Because of the high concentration, sodium and chloride diffuse passively out of the collecting duct into the lower medullary interstitium. This increases the osmolarity of the medullary interstitial fluid to between 1000 and 1200 mOsm.

Excess solutes concentrated in the medullary interstitium must not be allowed to reenter the bloodstream via the peritubular capillary network. This is prevented by sluggish blood flow in these capillaries and a very small amount of blood being present (<2% of the total renal blood supply), keeping ion movement to a minimum. Throughout the countercurrent multiplier activity, ion movement from the loop of Henle into the medullary interstitium has been by ionic secretion (ions moving from the tubule lumen) either actively or passively and by diffusion or osmosis.

TABLE 43-2. CATEGORIES OF DIURETICS

Category of Diuretic	Drug	Mechanism of Action	Side Effects
Loop diuretics	Furosemide Bumetanide Ethacrynic acid Torsemide	Inhibits sodium chloride reabsorption in thick ascending limb of loop of Henle	Hypovolemia, hypokalemia, hypochloremic alkalosis, hearing loss, hyponatremia
Osmotic diuretics	Mannitol	Inhibits sodium and water reabsorption by increasing the osmolality of the tubular fluid	Blurred vision, rhinitis, rebound hypervolemia, thirst, urinary retention, electrolyte imbalances
Thiazide diuretics	Hydrochlorothiazide Metolazone Chlorthalidone	Inhibits sodium reabsorption in proximal and distal tubules	Rash, hypokalemia, hyperglycemia, acute pancreatitis, thrombocytopenia
Potassium-sparing diuretics	Spironolactone Triamterene Amiloride	Inhibits aldosterone Promotes sodium excretion and potassium reabsorption in distal tubule causing a mild diuresis	Hyperkalemia, headache, hyponatremia, nausea, diarrhea, urticaria, menstrual disturbances, gynecomastia
Carbonic anhydrase inhibitors	Acetazolamide	Inhibits the enzyme carbonic anhydrase in the proximal tubule preventing bicarbonate and sodium reabsorption	Hyperchloremic acidosis, renal calculi, rash, nausea, vomiting, anorexia

The ion solutes present in the medullary interstitial fluid must move into the ascending limb of the loop of Henle so that they can be excreted with the urine. This is accomplished by the countercurrent exchange mechanism. The vasa recta are essentially straight tubes forming a long, slender, U-shaped blood vessel. Because both sides of the U are highly permeable, fluids and solutes readily exchange places in the high-concentration gradients of the lower medullary interstitium.

As the blood in the vasa recta flows back up the ascending loop of Henle, excess sodium and urea diffuse out of the blood in exchange for water diffusing into the blood. The blood leaves the medulla with almost the same osmolarity as when it entered the descending loop.

The fluid in the loop of Henle becomes more concentrated in the presence of ADH since water has diffused out. In the ascending thick limb of the loop of Henle and the diluting segment of the distal convoluted tubule, the osmolarity of the filtrate drops. In the distal convoluted tubules and the collecting ducts, the osmolarity depends on the presence of ADH and aldosterone. If these hormones are present, sodium and water will be absorbed and the tubule fluid will remain concentrated as it passes through the collecting ducts to the renal pelvis to enter the ureter. If the hormones are not present, water will be secreted and a more dilute urine will enter the ureter. Only juxtamedullary nephrons have long loops of Henle; they are responsible for concentrating and diluting the filtrate as urine is formed.

Many diuretics influence the reabsorption of sodium, potassium chloride, and water in the nephron. Table 43-2 presents categories of diuretics.

Excretion of Metabolic Waste Products

The metabolic waste products handled by the kidneys are estimated to be in excess of 200 different substances. These waste products are classified as threshold substances, nonthreshold substances, electrolytes, water, and other substances that may be reabsorbed or excreted by the kidneys according to individual fluctuating needs.

Threshold substances are those that are entirely reabsorbed by the kidneys unless the substances are present in excessive concentration in the blood. Glucose is the most common threshold substance. Amino acids are also threshold substances.

Nonthreshold substances are not reabsorbed by the kidney tubules. Creatinine is the most abundant nonthreshold substance. Urea is included in this category even though urea passively diffuses back into the kidney bloodstream. Proteins and acids of disease processes (lactic acid, ketones) are nonthreshold substances. Water and most electrolytes will be absorbed or secreted according to individual needs.

There are two commonly used tests to determine the efficiency of kidney function in handling waste products: blood urea nitrogen (BUN) and creatinine.

The BUN measures the level of urea, a nitrogen waste product of protein metabolism. The BUN is an unreliable test of renal function because the BUN level is affected by many factors. In the presence of liver disease, the BUN will remain low because the liver cannot synthesize urea at a normal rate. Conversely, with normal kidney function, dehydration, gastrointestinal bleeding, sepsis, trauma, drugs, diet, and changes in catabolism may elevate the BUN markedly, to as much as 50 mg/100 mL. Food in the digestive tract may also falsely elevate the BUN.

Serum creatinine is a more reliable index of kidney function. Creatinine is a waste product of muscle metabolism and is freely filtered. The nephron tubules neither reabsorb nor secrete creatinine. The normally functioning kidney filters creatinine from the blood at a rate equal to the GFR. As the amount of creatinine produced each day is constant and is proportional to the body's muscle mass, serial serum creatinines are valuable indices of kidney function except in septic patients and patients with muscle-wasting diseases.

Normally, a BUN-to-creatinine ratio of 10:1 is present in serum. A ratio of 20:1 or more is indicative of prerenal insufficiency (water and salt depletion), a high protein catabolism, or low renal perfusion pressures.

An elevation of both BUN and creatinine above the normal ratio indicates renal disease. In these patients, a creatinine clearance is usually performed. Creatinine clearance is probably the most reliable index of kidney function available. Normal creatinine clearance is 125 mL/min. Urine is collected for 12 or 24 h or for a specified period of time and a blood serum sample is drawn halfway through the urine collection. If the BUN, creatinine, and creatinine clearance tests are normal, the kidneys are functioning adequately in excreting metabolic waste products from the body.

Regulation of Acid-Base Balance

The body's acid-base balance is maintained by the lungs, blood buffers, and kidneys. The kidneys regulate acid-base balance by controlling the bicarbonate ion (HCO_3^-) and, in much lesser quantity, the hydrogen ion (H^+).

A normal diet contains some acids (phosphates and sulfates) that must be excreted. In addition, protein catabolism is markedly increased in the acutely ill. Protein catabolism adds to the acid load of the body. Products of protein catabolism are eliminated by the kidneys.

Four mechanisms provide for the excretion of acid and regulation of acid-base balance by the kidneys.

The first mechanism is direct excretion of hydrogen ions. Hydrogen ion is excreted in a very minute amount (<1 mEq of hydrogen ion per day) and has only a minor role in acid-base control. A passive secretion of hydrogen ion occurs in the proximal tubules. An active secretion of hydrogen ion occurs in the distal tubules.

The second mechanism is excretion of hydrogen with urine buffers. Nonvolatile acids are excreted in this process. The glomerulus filters these acids and bicarbonate. The phosphate acids filtered are an example of the process for excreting hydrogen ion with a urine buffer.

$$\underset{\substack{\text{carbonic}\\\text{acid}}}{H_2CO_3} + \underset{\substack{\text{bisodium}\\\text{phosphate}}}{Na_2HPO} \rightarrow \underset{\substack{\text{sodium}\\\text{bicarbonate}}}{NaHCO_3} + \underset{\substack{\text{sodium}\\\text{biphosphate}}}{NaH_2PO_4}$$

The carbonic acid combines with bisodium phosphate and yields sodium bicarbonate and sodium biphosphate. The sodium bicarbonate breaks down into sodium and bicarbonate and is reabsorbed as needed. The sodium biphosphate adds a hydrogen ion to become a molecule and is excreted in urine. The net result of the phosphate and sulfate wastes filtered by the glomerulus is the addition of a hydrogen ion per molecule excreted. Up to 20 mEq per day may be excreted with these buffers.

The third mechanism of acid-base control by the kidneys is excretion of acids by using ammonia (NH_3). Chemically, ammonia is produced in renal tubular cells and diffuses into tubular fluid, where carbonic acid combines with ammonia and actually produces two factors that benefit acid-base control.

$$\underset{\text{ammonia}}{NH_3} + \underset{\substack{\text{carbonic}\\\text{acid}}}{H_2CO_3} \rightarrow \underset{\substack{\text{ammonium}\\\text{ion}}}{NH_4} + \underset{\substack{\text{bicarbonate}\\\text{ion}}}{HCO_3}$$

Ammonium (ammonia with one additional hydrogen ion) combines with anions.

$$\underset{\substack{\text{ammonium}\\\text{bicarbonate}}}{2NH_4HCO_3} + \underset{\substack{\text{sodium}\\\text{sulfate}}}{Na_2SO_4} \leftrightarrow \underset{\substack{\text{sodium}\\\text{bicarbonate}}}{2NaHCO_3} + \underset{\substack{\text{ammonium}\\\text{sulfate}}}{(NH_4)_2SO_4}$$

The ammonium sulfate, which now has two hydrogen ions, is excreted in the urine. The sodium bicarbonate is available to buffer in the body as needed. Up to 50 mEq of acid per day may be excreted by using ammonia.

In the fourth mechanism, production and reabsorption of bicarbonate, new bicarbonate ion is manufactured in the distal convoluted tubule as needed. The formula is:

$$H_2O + CO_2 \overset{CA}{\leftrightarrow} H_2CO_3 \overset{CA}{\leftrightarrow} H^+ + HCO_3^-$$

water carbon dioxide — carbonic acid — hydrogen ion — bicarbonate ion

The process of forming a new bicarbonate can start in the distal tubule. Carbon dioxide results from dissolved carbon dioxide in the renal venous blood. The carbon dioxide combines with water present in the distal tubule to form carbonic acid. This is termed the hydration of carbon dioxide with the catalyst carbonic anhydrase (CA).

CA speeds up the chemical reaction without actually entering into the chemical reaction. The brush border of the proximal convoluted tubule contains a great deal of CA; the distal convoluted tubule does not. The formation of carbonic acid in the proximal tubule is very rapid. The carbonic acid produced ionizes more slowly in the distal tubule.

The carbonic acid ionizes into hydrogen ion and bicarbonate ion to buffer as needed. If the body is acidotic, the hydrogen ion is excreted in the urine. The bicarbonate is absorbed into the ECF along with sodium. If the body is in acid-base balance, the carbonic acid dissociates into water and carbon dioxide. The water joins the urine, and the carbon dioxide rapidly diffuses into the ECF.

In acidotic states, there is an increase in hydrogen ion secretion in the distal tubule that accompanies an increased excretion of acid buffers, phosphates, and sulfates. Ammonium formation is the predominant control mechanism. Because more acid is being excreted in the urine, urine pH may be as low as 4.4. In alkalotic states, there is a decrease in hydrogen ion secretion in the distal tubules. This is accompanied by an excess bicarbonate excretion in the urine, resulting in urine that is alkaline (pH >7).

Regulation of Blood Pressure

The kidneys participate in the regulation of blood pressure through four different mechanisms: by maintaining ECF volume and composition, by regulating aldosterone, through the renin-angiotensin mechanism, and by regulating prostaglandin synthesis.

Maintenance of ECF Fluid Volume and Composition

The autoregulatory system of the afferent and efferent arterioles responds to change in blood pressure to maintain consistent perfusion of the glomerulus. When this system fails, plasma flow may increase by two mechanisms. Vasoconstriction will maintain or elevate the blood pressure for a short period of time. If no more defense mechanisms exist, then only intravenous fluids (crystalloids or colloids) will alter the volume flow or composition of the plasma and the ECF. As the flow of plasma decreases, the patient becomes hypotensive, hypoxic, and hypoperfused. As the plasma flow deficit and the extracellular deficits are corrected, the patient becomes more closely normotensive.

Effect of Aldosterone on Blood Pressure

The main effect of aldosterone is to maintain normal sodium concentration in the ECF. Because sodium is the most abundant cation in the ECF, all other cations and anions will be present in varying ratios to the sodium. Aldosterone promotes reabsorption of sodium in both the distal convoluted tubule and the collecting ducts of the kidneys. Sodium will "drag along" water, bicarbonate, chloride, and other ions as it is reabsorbed. This mechanism helps to restore extracellular and intracellular fluid volumes, alter the composition of the compartments as needed, and subsequently, in a normal healthy kidney, maintain the blood pressure.

Renin-Angiotensin Mechanism

Any factor that decreases the GFR rate will activate the renin-angiotensin system. The most potent effect is upon systemic blood pressure.

Once activated, the JGA, located adjacent to the glomeruli, releases inactive renin. Factors triggering the release of inactive renin (e.g., decreased blood pressure and decreased sodium content in the distal tubule) reflect a diminished GFR. Once released, the inactive renin acts on angiotensinogen to split away the vasoactive peptide angiotensin I. Angiotensin I is split to angiotensin II in the presence of a converting enzyme found primarily in the lung and liver but also located in the kidney and all blood vessels.

Angiotensin II is a potent vasoconstricting agent. Angiotensin II in the circulatory system causes a severe constriction of peripheral arterioles and a milder constriction in the venous system. It also causes a constriction of renal arterioles. This results in the kidneys reabsorbing sodium and water and expanding the ECF volume.

Angiotensin II also stimulates the release of aldosterone to enhance sodium and water reabsorption, thus supporting an increase in circulating volume. This increase in sodium stimulates the thirst mechanism in an effort to reestablish circulating blood volume.

On rare occasions, some factors initiate the release of renin and the release is never turned off. The continuous presence of renin may maintain an active system known as malignant hypertension. The key to treating malignant hypertension is to cut off the release of renin.

Prostaglandins

It was once thought that prostaglandins were originally located in the seminal vesicles and produced by the prostate gland (thus their name). Prostaglandins are unsaturated fatty acids found in most cells but highly concentrated in the kidneys, brain, and gonads. Prostaglandins or their precursors are synthesized in the medullary interstitial cells and the collecting tubules of the kidneys. Prostaglandins promote a vasodilation of the renal medulla to maintain renal perfusion during severe or prolonged systemic hypoperfusion.

Red Blood Cell Synthesis and Maturation

Renal erythropoietic factor is an enzyme released by a hypoxic kidney as a result of decreased oxygen supply. After being released into the bloodstream, the

TABLE 43-3. BLOOD AND URINARY DIAGNOSTIC STUDIES FOR THE EVALUATION OF RENAL FUNCTION

Study	Significance
Blood	
Hematocrit/hemoglobin	Reflects bleeding or lack of erythropoietin
Creatinine	Reflects renal disease
BUN	Normal BUN-to-creatinine ratio is 10:1 Ratio in excess of 20:1, suspect dehydration, catabolic state Elevation in both BUN and creatinine results from decreased GFR
Electrolytes	
Arterial blood gases	
Clotting profile	
Osmolality	
Protein, albumin, glucose, cholesterol	
Urine	
Specific gravity (normal, 1.003–1.030)	<1.010, suspect DI, overhydration, or CHF
	>1.030, suspect proteinuria, glycosuria, radiographic contrast media, or severe dehydration
Creatinine clearance (24-h urine collection)	Estimates percentage of functioning nephrons
Culture and sensitivity	Presence or absence of infection
pH (normal, 4–8)	Alkaline urine seen with infection
Glucose	Present when renal threshold for glucose exceeded
Acetone	Present during starvation and DKA
Protein	Present in nephrotic syndrome and renal failure caused by myeloma proteins
Spot electrolytes (sodium, potassium, and chloride)	Assesses ability of renal tubules to conserve sodium and concentrate urine
Urinary sediment	
Casts	Protein that takes on the shape of the tubule in which it is formed
Hyaline casts	Present in large amounts in proteinuria
Erythrocyte casts	Diagnostic for active glomerulonephritis
Leukocyte casts	Diagnostic for infection
Granular casts	Result from degenerating erythrocyte or leukocyte casts
Fatty casts	Present in large amounts in lipoid nephrosis and nephrotic syndrome
Renal tubular casts	Present in acute renal failure
Renal epithelial cells	Present in large amounts during ATN and nephrotic injury
Erythrocytes	Present in large amounts in active glomerulonephritis, interstitial nephritis, infections
Bacteria	Presence determined by Gram stain
Leukocytes	Present in infection and interstitial nephritis
Crystals	Present in diseases of stone formation or following ethylene glycol intoxication
Eosinophils	Present during an allergic reaction in kidney

ATN, acute tubular necrosis; BUN, blood urea nitrogen; CHF, congestive heart failure; DI, diabetes insipidus; DKA, diabetic ketoacidosis; GFR, glomerular filtration rate.

TABLE 43-4. RADIOLOGIC STUDIES USED IN EVALUATING RENAL FUNCTION

Study	Significance
Abdominal radiograph	Determines position, shape, and size of kidney
IVP	Visualizes urinary tract to diagnose partial obstruction, renovascular hypertension, tumor, cysts, and congenital abnormalities
Renal scan	Determines renal perfusion, function, and presence of obstruction and masses
Retrograde pyelography	Determines presence of obstruction in upper region of urinary collecting system
Retrograde urethrography	Evaluates urethra
Cystoscopy	Detects bladder or urethral pathologic processes
Renal arteriography	Identifies tumors and status of renovascular disease
Ultrasonography	Identifies hydronephrosis and fluid collections
CT	Identifies tumors and other pathologic conditions that create variations in body density
MRI	Provides direct imaging in several planes conducive to detecting renal cystic disease, inflammatory processes, and renal cell carcinoma
Kidney biopsy	Determines cause and extent of lesions

CT, computed tomography; IVP, intravenous pyelogram; MRI, magnetic resonance imaging.

erythropoietic factor reacts with a glycoprotein to break away as erythropoietin. Erythropoietin circulates in the blood for about 24 h. During this time, it stimulates RBC production by the bone marrow. After 5 or more days, a maximum rate of RBC production is achieved. The life of the RBC is approximately 120 days.

Either the kidney itself or some other factor that is the precursor of erythropoietin synthesizes the erythropoietic factor by releasing an enzyme called renal erythropoietin factor. Bone marrow by itself does not respond to hypoxia by producing new RBCs.

Patients with chronic renal failure usually have hemoglobin of 5 and 6 g. The diseased kidneys are unable to respond to hypoxia and cannot produce erythropoietin factor. It is believed that possibly 10% of erythropoietin is formed in some place other than the kidney. Diagnostic studies used in evaluating renal function are presented in Tables 43-3 and 43-4.

This chapter has presented a review of the anatomy and physiology of the renal system with a focus on general features relevant to renal concepts that might be addressed in clinical practice.

44

Renal Regulation of Electrolytes

EDITORS' NOTE

This chapter contains information from the PCCN section on electrolyte imbalances. You will find more detail in this chapter than the exam requires. However, understanding this detail is helpful in answering the questions presented on the exam. Expect several questions from this chapter on the exam.

The kidneys play a major role in the regulation of electrolyte homeostasis. Dysfunction of the normal physiologic processes of the kidney can result in abnormalities in both fluid and electrolyte balance. Within 1 h of cessation of kidney function, physiologic deterioration begins because of a lack of electrolyte regulation. Electrolytes are in a precarious balance in the acutely ill patient. Continuous monitoring is essential to recognize imbalances early, prevent generalized deterioration, and help the kidneys to reestablish homeostasis as prompt recognition of altered renal status and institution of indicated interventions can prevent the progression of renal and nephron damage.

The electrolytes of major concern are sodium, potassium, calcium, phosphate, magnesium, and chloride. Electrolyte imbalances are a result of (1) excessive ingestion or reabsorption of an electrolyte or (2) the lack of ingestion or excessive excretion of an electrolyte. Most body fluid imbalances are caused by a dysfunction in the regulation of electrolytes and water by the kidney.

SODIUM

Sodium Regulation

Sodium (Na^+) is the most prevalent cation in the body's extracellular fluid compartment. It directly influences the fluid (water) load of the body and exists in the body in combination with an anion, usually chloride. Sodium is important in maintaining extracellular fluid osmotic pressure, serum osmolarity, and acid-base balance. Intracellularly, it plays a major role in chemical pathways. Sodium also controls muscle contraction. The normal serum sodium level ranges between 135 and 145 mEq/L. To maintain this level, sodium is reabsorbed from four parts of the kidney. Most of the filtered sodium is reabsorbed in the proximal convoluted tubules; lesser amounts are reabsorbed in the loop of Henle, the distal convoluted tubule, and the collecting ducts. Reabsorption of sodium increases with a decreased glomerular filtration rate (GFR), as seen with hypoperfusion states (shock, myocardial infarction).

Aldosterone has the greatest influence on sodium excretion. Aldosterone is a mineralocorticoid secreted by the adrenal cortex. It is the most potent natural inhibitor of sodium excretion. Aldosterone production and release is stimulated by high potassium levels, steroids (adrenocorticotropic hormone [ACTH]), and angiotensin II. Aldosterone acts on the distal convoluted tubule and the collecting duct to promote reabsorption of sodium and excretion of potassium. Without aldosterone present, the distal tubule and collecting ducts cannot closely regulate the amount of sodium reabsorbed. The increased reabsorption of sodium in the presence of aldosterone also results in the reabsorption of water.

Diuretic therapy is usually thought of in relation to potassium. However, the loop diuretics (furosemide [Lasix], ethacrynic acid [Edecrin], and bumetanide [Bumex]) block the chloride pump in the thick portion of the ascending limb of the loop of Henle. When chloride reabsorption is blocked, sodium cannot diffuse out of the ascending limb. Other factors that can increase the excretion of sodium include an increased GFR, decreased aldosterone secretion, and increased antidiuretic hormone (ADH) levels.

Hypernatremia

A serum sodium level above 145 mEq/L is termed hypernatremia. Most cases of hypernatremia are not due to Na^+ disturbances but due to fluid disturbances. Hypernatremia may be seen with dehydration. Treatment is centered on giving fluid, not removing sodium. If a pure water loss or decreased intake is causing the hypernatremia, the hematocrit will be elevated, serum chloride will be above 106 mEq/L, urine specific gravity will be greater than 1.025, and urine sodium levels will be low. Hypernatremia may also be associated with fluid volume excess with a gain of both sodium and water but a relatively greater gain of sodium. Hypernatremia is a significant electrolyte disturbance because of the neurologic and endocrine disturbances that result. Hypernatremia may cause some depression of cardiac function.

Etiology

With the exception of disturbances in vascular fluid levels, any condition leading to polyuria with conservation of sodium results in hypernatremic dehydration. The most common cause is the lack of or insufficient ADH secretion (e.g., diabetes insipidus). Increased insensible water loss (e.g., from severe burn injuries) and hypertonic enteral feedings may lead to hypernatremia. Potassium depletion (from vomiting, diarrhea, or nasogastric suction) and uncontrolled diabetes mellitus with osmotic diuresis secondary to hyperglycemia may also lead to a hypernatremia.

The comatose patient is at high risk for hypernatremia because the thirst mechanism cannot be recognized or expressed. Excessive administration of osmotic diuretics and sodium bicarbonate (in treating lactic acidosis) may also cause an iatrogenic hypernatremia. Overuse of high sodium-containing laxatives and antacids may also precipitate hypernatremia. Hypernatremia may also be seen with renal dysfunction. If the kidneys are too damaged to filter and excrete sodium, sodium and fluid retention may result.

Clinical Presentation

Hypernatremia generally occurs with dehydration. Signs include dry, sticky mucous membranes, thirst, oliguria, fever, tachycardia, and agitation. The patient may demonstrate behavior changes, hypotension, decreased cardiac output, convulsion, or coma; death may result. As long as renal function is intact, hypernatremia rarely produces increased mortality. Patients with hypernatremia associated with an excess of sodium and fluid volume present with edema, increased blood pressure, dyspnea, and weight gain.

Treatment

Fluid administration with free water (nonelectrolyte solutions like D_5W) in a dehydrated patient is the key to diluting the sodium and halting the progression toward hypovolemic shock. Identification and treatment of the underlying cause is the key to successful treatment of hypernatremia with fluid retention. The challenge is to stabilize the patient's hypertension, prevent pulmonary edema, and maintain neurologic stability. Diuretics and limitation of fluid intake are indicated.

Hyponatremia

Hyponatremia is present when the serum sodium level is less than 130 mEq/L. Usually, the plasma chloride will be less than 98 mEq/L. The hematocrit may be decreased due to water excess.

Etiology

Hyponatremia is due to either (1) an excessive amount of water or (2) sodium depletion. Excessive amounts of water can build up in many situations. The patient who has undergone gastric or intestinal surgery, who has nasogastric suction in use, and is receiving intravenous D_5W may become hyponatremic in only 2 or 3 days. Repeated tap water enemas may result in hyponatremia. Occasionally, patients drink too much plain water.

The syndrome of inappropriate ADH (SIADH) release may precipitate hyponatremia. In this instance, the stimulus that activated ADH release is never turned off. The presence of ADH causes the kidneys to reabsorb water continuously, thus diluting the body's sodium levels. Water retention that dilutes serum sodium levels may also occur with congestive heart failure, cirrhosis of the liver, or nephrotic syndrome. A low cardiac output precipitates water retention by the kidneys.

Hypovolemic hyponatremia due to sodium depletion or loss is commonly caused by the overuse of the thiazide or loop diuretics and mannitol. Diarrhea, Addison's disease, gastric suction, hyperglycemia (with a glucose-induced diuresis), vomiting, and extreme diaphoresis without intravenous replacement of sodium may also cause hypovolemic hyponatremia. Most causes of hyponatremia are associated with a low plasma osmolality; however, hypertonic hyponatremia due to hyperglycemia or intravenous administration of mannitol can occur.

Clinical Presentation. The clinical presentation of hyponatremia depends on its magnitude, rapidity of onset, and cause. In general, the faster the serum sodium drops and the lower the serum sodium level, the more likely that symptoms will be severe.

Hyponatremia with Water Retention

In hyponatremia with water excess, signs of water intoxication are usually present. They include apathy, coma, confusion, headache, generalized weakness, hyporeflexia, convulsions, and death. Increased blood pressure and edema are usually present.

Hyponatremia with Dehydration

If the hyponatremia is associated with decreased extracellular fluid, the symptoms are essentially the same as for heat prostration. Apprehension and anxiety are followed by a feeling of impending doom. The patient is weak, confused, or stuporous, and may have abdominal cramps and nausea. Mucous membranes are dry. Azotemia develops and progresses to oliguria. In severe cases, vasomotor collapse occurs, with hypotension, tachycardia, and shock.

An interesting clinical presentation exists in cases of hyponatremia associated with dehydration. As dehydration progresses, fluid moves from the extracellular to the intracellular compartment. A finger pressed over the sternum will result in a fingerprint. This "fingerprinting of the sternum" indicates that much extracellular fluid has been excreted and plasma fluid has moved into the intracellular spaces from the vascular system. Without appropriate intervention, the patient may die very quickly. In less severe cases, symptoms may include lassitude, apathy, headache, anorexia, nausea, vomiting, diarrhea, muscle spasms, and cramps.

Treatment

The goals of treatment of hyponatremia are aimed at reestablishing normal serum sodium levels and correcting the underlying cause. Acute or severe hyponatremia (plasma Na$^+$ level <110 to 115 mmol/L) often presents with altered mental status and/or seizures and requires rapid correction with hypertonic saline to raise the plasma Na$^+$ level by 1 to 2 mmol/L/h for the first 3 to 4 h or until the seizures subside. The plasma Na$^+$ concentration should not be raised by more than 12 mmol/L during the first 24 h. Fluid restriction or low-dose diuretic therapy is the treatment of choice if the hyponatremia is due to excess vascular fluid. Diuretics, if used, are given cautiously to avoid cerebral injury. Cerebral injury can occur from the overly rapid expansion of brain cells due to water removal. In instances other than SIADH, replacement of sodium with normal or hypertonic saline may also be indicated. Close monitoring of all body systems, along with monitoring of serial serum sodium levels, is essential during this period.

In SIADH, the treatment is to restrict water intake while attempting to help the kidneys excrete water normally. In susceptible SIADH patients, the administration of hypertonic saline may induce congestive heart failure.

POTASSIUM

Potassium Regulation

Potassium (K$^+$) is the most prevalent intracellular cation in the body. The normal serum potassium level is 3.5 to 5.0 mEq/L. Potassium maintains osmolarity and electrical neutrality inside the cell and helps maintain acid-base balance. Intracellular homeostasis is needed for converting carbohydrates into energy and for reassembling amino acids into proteins. Transmission of nerve impulses is dependent on potassium. The muscles of the heart, lungs, intestines, and skeleton cannot function normally without potassium.

All of the potassium filtered by the glomeruli is reabsorbed in the proximal convoluted tubule. Potassium that is excreted is secreted from the interstitial medullary space into the distal convoluted tubules. It amounts to about 10% to 12% of the original potassium volume of the ultrafiltrate in the proximal convoluted tubules. The amount of potassium excreted depends largely on the volume of urine. About 85% of the potassium is excreted in the urine and about 15% in the intestines. Even in hypokalemia (decreased potassium), a large urine volume will contain potassium, further compounding the problems. Sodium and potassium will compete with each other for reabsorption. The normal ratio of potassium to sodium ion reabsorption is 1:35.

Sodium and potassium are intimately related, and factors that affect sodium reabsorption and excretion also affect the potassium level. Potassium levels are commonly raised by intravenous fluids containing potassium chloride. Although the kidneys act readily to conserve sodium, potassium is poorly conserved, especially in patients who are acutely ill.

Factors that enhance the excretion of potassium include an elevated intracellular potassium level, which may be caused by an acute metabolic or respiratory alkalosis that forces potassium into the cells and hydrogen out of the cells. Diuretics and other factors resulting in high-volume flow rates in the distal convoluted tubule result in increased excretion of potassium. Aldosterone functions as a feedback mechanism on the distal convoluted tubule and collecting ducts to reabsorb sodium and excrete potassium when the potassium level in the extracellular fluid is increased. The enhancement of sodium reabsorption may force potassium excretion.

Potassium maintains an extracellular-to-intracellular fluid gradient. This gradient is affected by the adrenal steroids, hyponatremia, glycogen formation, testosterone, and pH changes. The most significant of these influences is the pH. Serum potassium moves inversely to the pH. If the pH falls, potassium concentration increases. If the pH rises, potassium concentration decreases, in part because of the ionic charge of potassium and hydrogen. Serum potassium must be evaluated with the arterial blood gases (ABGs) to avoid compounding problems of potassium therapy. Metabolic alkalosis is often associated with hypokalemia and occurs as a result of redistribution of potassium as well as excessive renal potassium loss.

Hyperkalemia

Hyperkalemia is a potassium level greater than 5.5 mEq/L. It is due to an inability of the kidney tubules to excrete potassium ions. Tubular damage or increased potassium load that exceeds the kidney's ability to handle the quantity of potassium results in hyperkalemia.

Etiology

Hyperkalemia may be due to acute or chronic renal disease, low cardiac output states, acidosis, sodium depletion, or large muscle mass injury. Any factor that destroys cells (e.g., burns, trauma, or crush injuries) will release the intracellular potassium, causing hyperkalemia. Excessive ingestion of potassium chloride (found in antacids and salt substitutes), adrenal cortical insufficiency, and the hemolysis of banked blood may also cause hyperkalemia.

Clinical Presentation

The membrane potential is related to the ratio of intracellular and extracellular potassium concentration, and hyperkalemia partially depolarizes the cell membrane. Prolonged depolarization impairs membrane excitability and is manifest as muscle weakness. Generalized muscle irritability or flaccidity, which may be severe enough to be a flaccid paralysis, and numbness of extremities are present. There may be abdominal cramping, nausea, and diarrhea. Generally, the patient is apathetic and may be confused.

The most serious effect of hyperkalemia is cardiac toxicity, which does not often correlate well with the plasma potassium concentration. The earliest changes in the electrocardiographic (ECG) tracing show a tall, peaked, or tent-shaped T wave with potassium levels of 5.5 to 7.5 mEq/L. In marked hyperkalemia (potassium of 7.5 to 9 mEq/L), there is a flattening and widening of the P wave, a prolonged PR interval, and usually depression of the ST segment. In severely advanced hyperkalemia (potassium of 8 to 9 meq/L and often more than 10 mEq/L), the P waves disappear and intraventricular conduction disturbances occur, producing intraventricular and supraventricular dysrhythmias progressing to ventricular tachycardia, ventricular standstill, or fibrillation and death.

Treatment

A serum potassium level above 5.5 mEq/L requires immediate intervention. Treatment is initiated to prevent increasing bradycardia and cardiac arrest. The objective of treatment is to reduce the serum potassium to a safe level as rapidly as possible. Cardiac monitoring is essential.

Intravenous 10% glucose with regular insulin will temporarily drive potassium into the cell. Intravenous sodium bicarbonate will buffer cellular hydrogen and allow potassium to move intracellularly. Calcium chloride will oppose the cardiotoxic effects of hyperkalemia. However, calcium therapy is contraindicated in patients on digoxin. Kayexalate is given orally or as an enema to rid the body of potassium. Kayexalate forces a one-for-one exchange of sodium for potassium in the intestinal cell wall; however, the patient must be monitored for sodium retention. Sorbitol is used to induce an osmotic diarrhea through semiliquid stools. Sodium bicarbonate can be administered when acidosis and hyperkalemia are present together. Albuterol (nebulized) can shift potassium intracellularly.

These measures are all emergency procedures to provide time to ascertain the cause of the hyperkalemia. If the cause is physiologic or if the hyperkalemia is refractory, dialysis is indicated. If the cause is overingestion of potassium, emergency measures may be sufficient and the patient may need only additional conservative treatment, close monitoring, and instruction on how to prevent recurrences.

Hypokalemia

Hypokalemia is a serum potassium level of less than 3.5 mEq/L. It can result from one or more of the following: decreased net intake, shift into cells, or increased net loss.

Etiology

Hypokalemia may be due to alkalosis, which stimulates hydrogen ion retention and potassium ion secretion in the distal convoluted tubules of the kidney. Diuretic therapy without potassium replacement, endocrine dysfunction (increased ACTH, thyroid storm), and renal dysfunction (tubular acidosis) may all cause hypokalemia.

High potassium losses, gastric and intestinal surgery, nasogastric suctioning, diarrhea, prolonged vomiting, and intestinal diseases predispose the patient to hypokalemia unless replacement therapy is maintained.

Clinical Presentation

The clinical signs and symptoms of hypokalemia vary greatly between individual patients; their severity depends on the degree of hypokalemia, with symptoms usually not occurring unless the potassium level is less than 3 mmol/L. Hypokalemia has many of the same signs as hyperkalemia. There is a general malaise and muscle weakness, which may progress to a flaccid paralysis. Anorexia, nausea, and vomiting may accompany a paralytic ileus. Mental status may range from drowsiness to coma. Hypotension may be present and may lead to cardiac arrest. If the patient is on digitalis, signs of digitalis toxicity may be present because hypokalemia potentiates the effect of digitalis.

Cardiac dysrhythmias are most commonly atrial unless the hypokalemia is profound; in which case, premature ventricular beats are seen. Other ventricular dysrhythmias are rare unless digitalis toxicity is present. Electrocardiographic tracings most commonly show a prominent U wave. Depression or flattening of the ST segment or inversion of the T wave may be apparent. An inverted T wave may fuse with the U wave, giving the appearance of a prolonged QT interval. There is a generalized cardiac irritability in hypokalemic states.

Weakness of the muscles results in shallow respirations that may progress to apnea. In hypokalemia, death may occur due to respiratory arrest.

Treatment

Emergency treatment of severe hypokalemia is the slow intravenous administration of potassium chloride (approximately 10 to 20 mEq/h) while the patient's ECG patterns are monitored for dysrhythmias due to hyperkalemia. Monitoring of symptoms, serum potassium levels, and ABGs is imperative to prevent an iatrogenic hyperkalemia.

Nonemergency treatment is to replace potassium with intravenous fluids containing potassium chloride or with oral potassium supplements. Oral supplements should be diluted to prevent gastrointestinal irritation and facilitate absorption. The patient is monitored for adequate intake and output, cardiac status, potassium levels, and signs of alkalosis or impending digitalis toxicity.

CALCIUM

Calcium Regulation

The normal serum calcium (Ca^{2+}) concentration is 8.5 to 10.5 mg/dL. Calcium, with phosphorus, makes bones and teeth rigid and strong. Calcium is integral to determining the strength and thickness of cell membranes. Calcium exerts a quieting action on nerve cells, thus maintaining normal transmission of nerve impulses. Calcium also activates specific enzymes of the blood-clotting process and those involved in the contraction of the myocardium.

Ninety-eight percent of calcium filtered by the kidneys is reabsorbed along the same pathways as sodium. There are four major factors influencing calcium reabsorption: parathyroid hormone (PTH), vitamin D, corticosteroids, and diuretics.

Parathyroid Hormone

If the serum PTH level is increased, there is increased reabsorption of ionized calcium from renal tubules. Reciprocally, the PTH increases phosphate excretion as well as calcium absorption from the gastrointestinal tract. PTH will mobilize calcium from the bones when the kidneys cannot or do not reabsorb sufficient calcium.

Vitamin D

Vitamin D must be present in an activated form to promote the absorption of calcium from the small intestine. Vitamin D is ingested in food, especially milk. The vitamin must then be activated by ultraviolet (sun) light, which changes a chemical in the skin. This vitamin is additionally changed in the liver. Finally, the kidneys convert the vitamin to 1,25-dihydroxycholecalciferol, which is also known as activated vitamin D. The activated vitamin D promotes absorption of calcium from the small intestine. The PTH stimulates this activation process, since a low serum level of calcium precludes an increase of calcium absorption in the kidney without PTH.

Corticosteroids

Corticosteroids are suspected of interfering with the activation of vitamin D, possibly in the liver, and decreasing the amount of calcium absorbed from the small intestine.

Diuretics

Diuretics can cause increased excretion of calcium and other electrolytes. If a loss of fluid volume results in a decreased volume of total body fluid, there will be a decreased GFR, resulting in reduced calcium excretion.

Hypercalcemia

Etiology

Hypercalcemia exists when the serum calcium level is above 10.5 mg/dL. Increased renal reabsorption of calcium may cause hypercalcemia. It may also be the result of increased intestinal absorption of calcium due to excessive dietary calcium intake or excessive vitamin D ingestion.

Hyperparathyroidism caused by parathyroid adenoma will lead to hypercalcemia by increasing the release of calcium from bone and by continuously stimulating the kidneys to reabsorb calcium. This also occurs in carcinoma of the parathyroid glands. Milk-alkali syndrome can occur in patients with peptic ulcer disease who have been treated for a prolonged period with milk and alkaline antacids, particularly calcium carbonate.

Multiple myeloma and metastatic carcinoma of the bone cause hypercalcemia secondary to the release of calcium from bone into the serum. Prolonged bed rest or immobilization potentiates the movement of calcium from the bones, teeth, and intestines. This process is more conspicuous in patients with Paget's disease. Frequently, the calcium is deposited in joints, in muscle tissue close to joints, and in the kidneys as calcium stones.

Drugs, especially thiazide diuretics, inhibit calcium excretion, thus causing hypercalcemia in susceptible patients. Renal tubular acidosis, thyrotoxicosis, and hypophosphatemia may all cause hypercalcemia in those who are susceptible.

Clinical Presentation

Neurologic changes include subtle personality changes in early and mild hypercalcemia; this progresses to lethargy, confusion, and coma as the severity of the hypercalcemia increases. Neuromuscular changes progress from weakness and hypotonicity to flaccidity.

The renal system may be affected by the formation of calcium calculi with varying amounts of urine output; depending on their location, such calculi may cause thigh or flank pain. Polyuria and polydipsia are often present because the increased calcium inhibits the action of ADH on the distal tubules and the collecting ducts.

Gastrointestinal symptoms include anorexia, nausea, vomiting, and constipation. Hypercalcemia stimulates the secretion of gastric acid and may lead to peptic ulcers. The hypotonicity caused by hypercalcemia results in decreased intestinal motility and constipation.

Cardiac changes are less common in hypercalcemia than in hyperkalemia. The earliest ECG change is a shortening of the QT interval due to shortening of the ST segment. Digitalis and calcium are synergistic. Sudden death in hypercalcemia is often attributed to ventricular fibrillation stemming from this synergism.

An ocular abnormality known as band keratopathy may occur as a result of the deposition of calcium crystals in the cornea. Calcium is deposited at the lateral borders of the cornea in the shape of parentheses. If the calcification is extensive, calcium will be deposited in semilunar bands across the cornea, connecting the parentheses. This band keratopathy may be seen by the naked eye.

Treatment

The objective of treatment of hypercalcemia is to reduce the serum calcium level. Normal saline intravenous solutions and diuretics will increase the GFR and thus the excretion of calcium provided that there are no obstructive calculi. These treatments require accurate monitoring of intake and output.

Contemporary management includes the use of intravenous bisphosphonates such as pamidronate, furosemide plus fluid administration, or calcitonin. Neurologic and cardiac monitoring is essential in assessing the efficacy of treatment. Some underlying conditions (such as multiple myeloma) will tend to make hypercalcemia refractory to treatment. In such cases, the goal of therapy becomes keeping the calcium level as low as possible.

Hypocalcemia

Etiology

Hypocalcemia is a clinical condition in which the serum calcium level is below 8.5 mg/dL. Hypocalcemia usually develops from an excessive loss of calcium as a result of, for example, diarrhea, use of diuretics, malabsorption syndromes, or hypoparathyroidism. Chronic renal failure is probably the most common cause of hypocalcemia. If calcium is lost in peritoneal dialysis or hemodialysis, hyperphosphatemia may occur. This enhances a peripheral deposition of calcium. Calcium deposits prevent calcium from being available to raise serum levels. Furthermore, the patient with chronic renal failure is unable to absorb calcium from the intestines secondary to a lack of activated vitamin D. Alkalosis can cause hypocalcemia because the calcium becomes bound to albumin and thus remains inactive in the serum.

Chronic malabsorption syndromes may cause hypocalcemia. These syndromes are found following gastrectomies, in diseases of the small bowel, in patients with a high-fat diet (fat impairs calcium absorption), and in those with a magnesium deficiency (magnesium inhibits PTH).

Malignancies may also cause hypocalcemia. These include osteoblastic metastases (whereby calcium is used for abnormal bone synthesis) and medullary carcinoma of the thyroid (causing an increased secretion of thyrocalcitonin, which in turn stimulates osteoblasts and prevents calcium from entering the serum).

Hypoparathyroidism of any cause results in hypocalcemia since the secretion of PTH is decreased. The most common causes are surgical removal of the parathyroid glands, adenoma of the parathyroid glands, depleted magnesium levels (inhibits PTH), and idiopathic hypoparathyroidism.

A vitamin D–deficient state (or state of nonactivated vitamin D) is often seen in chronic renal failure, liver failure, and rickets. Without activated vitamin D, calcium is not absorbed from the intestines. Acute pancreatitis causes a precipitation of calcium in the inflamed pancreas and in intra-abdominal lipids.

In hyperphosphatemia, phosphates and calcium bind together and precipitate in tissues. This is commonly found in chronic renal failure as a result of decreased excretion of phosphates. Increased oral intake of phosphates rarely causes hyperphosphatemia if renal function is normal.

Clinical Presentation

Neuromuscular irritability is the overwhelming symptom present and is the most dangerous. Muscle tremors and cramps are present in mild hypocalcemia. As the calcium level drops, tetany and generalized tonic-clonic seizures occur. Neuromuscular irritability causes labored, shallow respirations. Wheezing will be present if bronchospasm has occurred. Bronchospasm may lead to laryngospasm and tetany of the respiratory muscles, resulting in respiratory arrest. It is important to monitor neurologic status by testing Chvostek's and Trousseau's signs.

To test for Chvostek's sign, tap your finger over the supramandibular portion of the parotid gland, which is located in the subcutaneous tissue of the cheek. If the upper lip twitches on the side of stimulation, the test is positive.

To test for Trousseau's sign, apply a blood pressure cuff to the arm and inflate it until a carpopedal spasm occurs. If no spasm appears in 3 min, the test is negative. To test this result, remove the blood pressure cuff and have the patient hyperventilate (>30 breaths per min). The respiratory alkalosis that develops may produce a carpopedal spasm. This indicates a positive test.

Neuromuscular irritability frequently causes a decreased cardiac contractility, leading to a cardiac arrest. The earliest ECG change is a lengthening of the QT interval due to a lengthening of the ST segment. Significant dysrhythmias due to hypocalcemia are extremely rare. Neuromuscular irritability may also cause biliary colic and paralytic ileus.

An alteration in blood clotting may be seen in hypocalcemia. Since calcium is necessary for normal blood clotting, hypocalcemia is often accompanied by bleeding dyscrasias.

Treatment

The aim of treatment of hypocalcemia is to raise the calcium level to normal as rapidly as possible so as to halt or prevent tetany.

In cases of tetany or impending tetany, intravenous 10% calcium gluconate or calcium chloride is administered. The patient must be on a cardiac monitor because a rapid infusion may enhance digitalis toxicity and also because hypocalcemic patients are often also hyperkalemic. Vitamin D supplements are administered if a deficiency is present.

The efficacy of treatment is evaluated by monitoring serum calcium, phosphate, and potassium levels along with the ECG and neurologic status (using Chvostek's and Trousseau's signs).

PHOSPHATE

The normal serum level of phosphate (PO_4) is 3.0 to 4.5 mg/dL. The phosphate ion is found in bones and is a major factor in the intracellular production of adenosine triphospate (ATP) (energy). Phosphate combines with proteins and lipids to form important intracellular molecules. Intracellular phosphate ions may react with deoxyribonucleic acid (DNA) and ribonucleic acid (RNA) molecules. Phosphate acts as a buffering agent for urine, is responsible for bone growth, promotes the phagocytic action of white blood cells (WBCs), and is important in platelet structure and function.

Phosphate Regulation

Phosphate levels are influenced by two major factors: PTH secretion (increases renal excretion of phosphate ions) and calcium concentration. Calcium and phosphate have a reciprocal relationship. If calcium levels increase, phosphate levels decrease; conversely, if calcium levels decrease, phosphate levels increase.

Reabsorption of phosphates occurs actively in the proximal convoluted tubule in the presence of sodium. Without sodium, phosphates will not be reabsorbed.

Excretion of phosphates is regulated by PTH and the GFR. The PTH inhibits reabsorption of phosphates in the proximal tubule, so phosphates will be excreted. With a decrease in the GFR, phosphate excretion will decrease; with an increase in the GFR, phosphates excretion will increase.

Hyperphosphatemia

Etiology

A serum phosphate level above 4.5 mg/dL constitutes hyperphosphatemia. An inability to excrete phosphates or excessive ingestion of phosphates are the two pathologic processes of hyperphosphatemia. The inability to excrete phosphates may be due to a decreased GFR or to renal failure.

Excessive ingestion of phosphates may be due to the routine use (or abuse) of phosphate-containing laxatives and enemas or the use of cytotoxic agents for the treatment of leukemias and lymphomas.

Hypoparathyroidism causes hyperphosphatemia secondary to the effects of PTH on the kidney. Occasionally, overadministration of intravenous or oral phosphates will induce hyperphosphatemia.

Clinical Presentation

The clinical presentation of hyperphosphatemia is the same as that of hypocalcemia. Elevated phosphate levels enhance the movement of calcium into bone. If seizures occur, they are due to hypocalcemia caused by hyperphosphatemia. Remember that calcium and phosphate have a reciprocal relationship.

Metastatic calcification occurs when calcium and phosphates combine chemically to form calcium phosphate, which then precipitates in arteries, soft tissue, and joints.

Treatment

The objective of therapy for hyperphosphatemia is to decrease the serum phosphate level. In urgent situations, this is accomplished by giving aluminum hydroxide gels or calcium antacids that combine with phosphate, thus limiting the amount of phosphate available for absorption in the intestines. Long-term management of hyperphosphatemia includes the use of oral phosphate binders such as calcium carbonate or calcium acetate, sevelamer, or lanthanum.

Hypophosphatemia

Etiology

Hypophosphatemia is a serum phosphate level below 3 mg/dL. Any factor that increases the cellular uptake to form sugar phosphates will decrease serum levels of phosphate. For example, prolonged intense hyperventilation can depress serum phosphate by inducing respiratory alkalosis. Sepsis and diabetic ketoacidosis also contribute to hypophosphatemia. Decreased phosphate absorption from the intestines (malabsorption syndromes), severe diarrhea, loss of proximal convoluted tubular function with renal phosphate wasting as seen in Fanconi's syndrome, rickets, and conditions that are vitamin D resistant may also cause hypophosphatemia.

Chronic alcoholism results in a dietary deficiency of phosphates and may interfere with the absorption of any phosphates present. Abuse (including overuse) of phosphate-binding agents such as Maalox or Amphojel causes hypophosphatemia, as does hyperparathyroidism (causing renal phosphaturia).

Long-term hyperalimentation may contribute to hypophosphatemia if phosphates are not included in the solution in adequate amounts. Use of hyperalimentation solutions with a high glucose content requires phosphates. This is no longer a common etiology.

Clinical Presentation

Complaints of general malaise, anorexia, and vague muscle weakness may be of chronic or acute onset. With chronic onset, muscle wasting is apparent. With acute onset, rhabdomyolysis (a diffuse muscle-wasting necrosis) is due to a depletion of intracellular ATP and a concurrent decrease in all ATP-mediated processes. Hypercalcemia and hypercalciuria, with associated symptoms, are indicators of acute phosphate depletion due to hyperparathyroidism (PTH increases serum calcium by removing it from bone and decreases serum phosphate by excretion in the urine).

Hypoxia occurs because of a deficit in the red blood cell (RBC) phosphate content necessary for the formation of 2,3-diphosphoglycerate (2,3-DPG). With a decrease in 2,3-DPG, a decrease in the dissociation of oxygen from hemoglobin is seen and tissue hypoxia results.

Complicating hypophosphatemia may be osteomalacia, severe metabolic acidosis, and insulin resistance resulting in hyperglycemia. This syndrome is rare and is usually seen in chronic alcoholism. It is a severe intravascular hemolysis caused by phosphate depletion, which results in a decrease of 2,3-DPG in RBCs.

Treatment

The objective of therapy for hypophosphatemia is to replace the phosphates, first by intravenous administration and then orally. Use of phosphate-binding gels is discontinued and then treatment of the underlying cause of hypophosphatemia is begun.

MAGNESIUM

The normal serum level of magnesium (Mg^{2+}) is 1.5 to 2.5 mEq/L. The magnesium ion is the second major intracellular cation. Magnesium acts as a coenzyme in the metabolism of carbohydrates and proteins. It regulates neuromuscular excitability and phosphate levels. It is stored in bone, muscle, and soft tissue.

Magnesium Regulation

Renal reabsorption of magnesium is essentially the same as for calcium. The presence of sodium directly affects reabsorption in the proximal tubules. Without sodium, there is no reabsorption of magnesium. Parathyroid hormone appears to have a minimal effect on reabsorption. Reabsorption processes of calcium and magnesium are mutually suppressive.

Hypermagnesemia

Etiology

Hypermagnesemia is a serum magnesium level above 2.5 mEq/L. This is extremely rare. Reabsorption is similar to the calcium process. Absorption of excessive sodium (for any reason) in the renal tubules may "drag" an excessive amount of magnesium back into the blood.

Chronic renal disease and untreated diabetic acidosis are the usual causes. Addison's disease, hyperparathyroidism, excessive magnesium administration, and overuse of magnesium-containing antacids are other causes of hypermagnesemia.

Clinical Presentation

Lethargy, coma, depressed respirations, hyporeflexia, and hypotension are the usual symptoms. All the symptoms of hyperkalemia may be present. The ECG changes consist first of prolonged PR intervals followed by widening of the QRS complex as the magnesium concentration rises. Death usually occurs with a concentration of 6 mEq/L or more.

Treatment

Attempts to lower magnesium levels by hemodialysis with a hypomagnesium dialysate have been successful.

Hypomagnesemia

Etiology

A magnesium level below 1.5 mEq/L is a state of hypomagnesemia. Any inhibition of absorption of magnesium from the gastrointestinal tract or of reabsorption from the renal system may account for hypomagnesemia. Severe malabsorption syndromes, acute pancreatitis, chronic alcoholism, primary aldosteronism, diabetic ketoacidosis, diuretic therapy, and renal disease are the usual causes.

Clinical Presentation

Neuromuscular and central nervous system hyperirritability characterize hypomagnesemia. Muscle tremors, delirium, convulsion, and coma are seen. Positive Chvostek's and Trousseau's signs, tachycardia, increased blood pressure, depressed ST segments, and prolonged QT intervals are also seen. Hypomagnesemia may result in digitalis-induced dysrhythmias.

Treatment

The objective of treatment for hypomagnesemia is simply to provide sufficient magnesium to raise the serum level. Low magnesium levels have been implicated in the development of ventricular dysrhythmias and have been treated more aggressively in recent years. Usually 1 to 2 g of magnesium can be given by intravenous administration.

CHLORIDE

Chloride Regulation

The normal serum chloride (Cl) level is 98 to 106 mg/dL. Chloride is reabsorbed by the kidney at all of the sites for sodium reabsorption. Chloride moves freely with the gastric and intestinal fluids and is reabsorbed accordingly.

Anion Gap

Excretion of chloride is influenced by the acid-base balance. In acidosis, chloride is excreted, while bicarbonate is reabsorbed. In alkalosis, chloride is reabsorbed, while bicarbonate is excreted. Chloride can be used in combination with bicarbonate and sodium to obtain an estimated "anion gap." Although an anion gap never really exists, since cations and anions must be in balance to maintain electrochemical neutrality, an anion gap appears to be present if only sodium, bicarbonate, and chloride are measured. A normal anion gap is less than 15 mEq and is obtained by subtracting bicarbonate and chloride from sodium. For example, a patient with a sodium of 140, bicarbonate of 25, and chloride of 100 would have an anion gap of 15 (140 − [100 + 25] = 15).

The value of computing an anion gap is simple. If an anion gap exceeds 15, a specific type of metabolic acidosis exists. If the anion gap exceeds 15, either a lactic, keto-, or chronic renal failure acidosis exists. The anion gap appears to increase because bicarbonate to buffer the acidosis is lost without a simultaneous increase in chloride. In lactic, keto-, and chronic renal failure acidosis, anions other than chloride increase to offset the loss of bicarbonate.

Hyperchloremia

Etiology

Hyperchloremia is a serum chloride level above 106 mg/dL. An excessive ingestion of chloride or an excessive kidney reabsorption of chloride ions are the pathophysiologic changes in hyperchloremia.

Clinical Presentation

The symptoms are the same as (or very similar to) those of hypernatremia.

Treatment

The objectives of treatment for hyperchloremia are to reduce the chloride level, which is most often achieved by the treatment of metabolic acidosis.

Hypochloremia

Etiology

Hypochloremia is a serum chloride below 98 mg/dL. Chloride ions are lost through excessive vomiting or gastric suction without replacement of electrolytes. This causes a physiologic metabolic alkalosis. The bicarbonate ion and chloride ion normally balance each other in kidney function.

Clinical Presentation

Symptoms of hypochloremia include changes in the sensorium, possible neuromuscular irritability, and usually slow, shallow respirations.

Treatment

The objective of treatment for hypochloremia is to replace the lost chloride ions either orally or intravenously and to treat the metabolic alkalosis so as to reestablish an acid-base balance.

45

Diagnosis and Treatment of Renal Failure

EDITORS' NOTE

The content of this chapter is designed to address PCCN exam questions on acute renal failure (e.g., acute tubular necrosis) and chronic renal failure. Expect several questions on the exam regarding material covered in this chapter.

ACUTE RENAL FAILURE

Acute renal failure (ARF) is a sudden loss of renal function with a decreased glomerular filtration rate (GFR) that may or may not produce oliguria or anuria with a concurrent increase in plasma creatinine and blood urea nitrogen (BUN). Oliguria is present if less than 400 mL of urine is produced per day. This is an obligatory water loss; that is, the minimum amount of urine needed to rid the body of its daily wastes. Of significance, however, is that ARF can develop without the development of oliguria; therefore, astute monitoring and assessment of patients with altered renal function are important. Acute renal failure is a common complication of acute illness. The incidence of ARF occurs in up to 25% of acutely ill patients, with a mortality rate ranging from 40% to 70%. Mortality rates vary depending on the amount of renal nephron damage, extent and duration of the ARF, and development of organ system dysfunction occurring as a result of ARF.

Pathophysiology

ARF can be classified as prerenal, intrarenal, or postrenal.

Prerenal ARF is defined as a decreased renal perfusion secondary to renal hypoperfusion, often due to decreased cardiac output. Prerenal ARF contributes to 30% to 60% of all cases of ARF. Decreased renal perfusion causes a decrease in renal artery pressure, leading to a reduced afferent arteriolar pressure. Afferent arteriolar pressures of less than 100 mm Hg may decrease the GFR, resulting in oliguria and/or anuria. Hypovolemia is the most common cause of ARF in the acutely ill patient.

Intrarenal ARF is caused by disease or injuries of the nephron from the glomerulus to the collecting duct. The most common cause of intrarenal failure is acute tubular necrosis (ATN). Consequently, these intrarenal conditions can be cortical or medullary in nature.

Cortical conditions involve swelling of the renal capillaries and cellular proliferation. Infectious, vascular, and/or immunologic processes cause edema and some resultant cellular debris that obstructs the glomeruli, resulting in a fall in urine output.

Medullary involvement specifically affects the tubular portions of the nephron, causing necrosis. The extent of medullary damage differs depending on the cause of the necrosis: nephrotoxic injury or ischemic injury. Nephrotoxic injury affects the epithelial cells, which can regenerate after the nephrotoxic injury is resolved. Ischemic injury extends to the tubular basement membrane and may involve peritubular capillaries and other parts of the nephron. Ischemic injury is more serious, since the tubular basement membrane cannot regenerate. Ischemic injury occurs when the mean arterial pressure falls below 60 mm Hg for more than 40 min secondary to massive hemorrhage or shock.

Postrenal ARF usually indicates an intrarenal or extrarenal obstruction at or below the level of the collecting ducts. The obstruction may be partial or complete. If the obstruction is complete, the blockage and subsequent backup of urine flow involves both kidneys. Eventually, urine output is decreased as a result of decreased glomerular filtration. Postrenal ARF is much less frequently encountered (1% to 10% of hospital-acquired ARF), and it is almost always amenable to treatment.

Etiology

Prerenal failure has a number of causes. One major cause is hemorrhage resulting in hypovolemia with fluid and electrolyte imbalance. Other causes include excessive use of diuretics and decreased glomerular perfusion after an acute myocardial infarction or congestive heart failure. Occasionally, following anesthesia and surgery, increased renovascular resistance and/or the hepatorenal syndrome occurs. Sepsis progressing to septic shock results in vasodilation and a resultant hypovolemia. Embolism or thrombosis may cause a bilateral renovascular obstruction, resulting in decreased or no perfusion to the kidneys. Other causes include burns, dehydration, and gastrointestinal fluid loss.

The causes of intrarenal failure can be fairly well categorized as either cortical or medullary. Table 45-1 summarizes the multiple causes of cortical and medullary intrarenal failure.

Causes of postrenal ARF are obstructive in nature and include prostatic hypertrophy; bladder, pelvic, or retroperitoneal tumors; renal calculi; ureteral blockage (after surgery or instrumentation); urethral obstruction; bladder infections; and a neurogenic bladder.

Phases

There are four phases in the cycle of ARF: onset, oliguric, diuretic, and recovery.

Onset or Initial Phase

The onset or initial phase precedes the actual necrotic injury and is associated with decreased cardiac output, renal blood flow, and GFR. If mean arterial blood pressure falls below 60 mm Hg for more than 40 min, the risk of ARF is high. A consistent

TABLE 45-1. CAUSES OF INTRARENAL FAILURE

Cortical Nephron Failure	Medullary Nephron Failure
Infections	**Nephrotoxic causes**
Poststreptococcal glomerulonephritis	Heavy metals
Acute pyelonephritis	Pesticides
Goodpasture's syndrome	Fungicides
Systemic lupus erythematosus	Hemoglobinuria
Malignant hypertension	Myoglobinuria
	Hypercalcemia
	Antibiotics
	Aminoglycosides
	Cephalosporins
	Tetracyclines
	Penicillins
	Amphotericin
	Ischemic causes
	Crush injuries
	Burns
	Sepsis
	Cardiogenic shock
	Postsurgical hypotension
	Hemorrhage with multiple trauma

increase in cardiac output will produce a consistent increase in renal blood flow and protect the patient from ARF.

Oliguric Phase

The oliguric phase reflects obstruction of tubules from edema, tubular casts, and cellular debris. Damage to the tubules makes absorption and secretion of solutes variable. If the obstruction and damage are severe enough, a backleak of filtrate through the epithelium may occur, returning the filtrate into the circulation.

During the oliguric phase, laboratory reports will indicate rising levels of urea, creatinine, and potassium. Serum and urine osmolality are increased. Hypervolemia and electrolyte imbalances caused by retention of the metabolic waste products are the greatest dangers to the patient. This phase lasts 8 to 14 days.

Diuretic Phase

The diuretic phase indicates the beginning of the return of tubular function. It lasts about 10 days. The greatest danger to the patient in this phase is excessive loss of water and electrolytes. Extreme diuresis is due to the osmotic diuretic effect produced by the elevated BUN and the inability of the tubules to conserve sodium and water, resulting in an output of 3000 mL or more of urine per 24 h. Hypokalemia is usually present.

Recovery Phase

The recovery phase begins when the diuresis is no longer excessive. There is a gradual improvement in kidney function, which may continue for 3 to 12 months. The end result may be a permanent reduction in the GFR, which may or may not be sufficient to maintain adequate renal function without dialysis. Acute renal failure may progress to chronic renal failure, but this is uncommon unless the patient has an underlying kidney disease or is advanced in age.

Clinical Presentation

Oliguria may or may not be present in ARF. Fifty percent of ARF patients and many ATN patients are anuric. Therefore, urine volume alone is not an adequate guide to renal function. Progressive azotemia (an excess of urea or other nitrogenous bodies in the blood) occurs as a result of decreased GFR in spite of apparently adequate urine output. Acute renal failure should be diagnosed before uremic signs are present. Table 45-2 summarizes the clinical presentation of uremia.

Diagnosis

Diagnosing ARF or ATN may be difficult, especially in the nonoliguric patient. Factors that must be considered in a diagnosis include urinary volume, urinary sediment, BUN levels, serial serum creatinines, creatinine clearance, arterial blood gases, trauma, and postsurgical status.

Urinary Volume

Normal urinary output is about 0.5 mL/kg/h. In prerenal failure, urine volume is decreased. In ATN, daily urine output may be constant or may gradually increase or decrease. Complete anuria suggests obstruction or cortical necrosis. It may occur in acute glomerulonephritis and complete postrenal obstruction but is very rare otherwise. Different degrees of obstruction are suggested by large, irregular daily urine volumes. Partial obstruction can cause progressive azotemia, even though there may be normal or increased urine volume.

Laboratory Data

In prerenal failure, urinary sodium (Na^+) is less than 20 mEq/L as the kidneys attempt to conserve sodium and water. Urinary osmolality, which reflects the concentrating ability of the kidney, is elevated. Urinary osmolality is usually greater than 500 mOsm (normal level is 300 to 900 mOsm). Specific gravity, a less sensitive indicator of concentrating power than osmolality, is also elevated. Specific gravity is greater than 1.020. There is minimal or no proteinuria and normal urinary sediment. The BUN increase is greater than the creatinine increase (20:1; normal ratio is 10:1). Normal serum creatinine is about 0.8 to 1.8 mg/dL and normal BUN is about 10 to 20 mg/dL. The fractional excretion of sodium (FeNa) is less than 1% in prerenal failure.

In cortical intrarenal failure, urinary sodium is less than 10 mEq/L. Specific gravity will vary with moderate to heavy proteinuria. Serum BUN and creatinine will be elevated (10 to 15:1). Hematuria is present with erythrocyte casts and leukocytes. In medullary intrarenal failure or ATN, urinary sodium is greater than 20 mEq/L, an abnormal sign when urine output is low. Normally, the kidneys conserve sodium in an attempt to maintain extravascular water. In ATN, when urine output is low, the expected conservation of sodium fails to occur, resulting in a normal urinary sodium level (40 to 220 mEq/L). Urinary osmolality decreases (<500 mOsm), reflecting the inability of the kidneys to concentrate the urine. Simultaneously, the specific gravity also decreases, usually between 1.008 and 1.012. Minimal to moderate proteinuria is present with an elevated serum BUN and creatinine. The FeNa is above 1% in

TABLE 45-2. UREMIC SIGNS OF ARF

Respiratory	Metabolic
Deep or rapid respiratory rate (metabolic acidosis)	Electrolyte imbalance
Bilateral rales	
Pulmonary edema	
Cardiovascular	Integument
Tachycardia	Dry skin
Dysrhythmias	Uremic frost (excretion of urea)
Pericarditis	
Friction rub	Pruritus
	Increased susceptibility to infection
	Edema
Neurologic	Hematologic
Decreased level of consciousness	Anemias
Confusion	Uremic coagulopathies
Lethargy	Bruising
Stupor	
Gastrointestinal	
Nausea	
Vomiting	
Anorexia	
Constipation or diarrhea	
Abdominal distention	

ATN. Urinary sediment consists of numerous renal tubular epithelial cells, tubular casts, and a rare erythrocyte.

In postrenal failure there is scanty sediment as well as rare white cells, red cells, hyaline casts, and fine granular (>40 mEq/L) casts. Urinary sodium is elevated, specific gravity varies, and BUN and creatinine are elevated (10 to 15:1).

CHRONIC RENAL FAILURE

The final stage of renal failure or chronic kidney disease is called end-stage renal disease (ESRD). The kidneys no longer function and the patient needs dialysis or a kidney transplant. End-stage renal disease affects more than 2 of every 1000 people in the United States. Diabetes and high blood pressure are the two most common causes and account for most cases.

Many other diseases and conditions can damage the kidneys, including:

- Problems with the arteries leading to or inside the kidneys
- Birth defects of the kidneys (such as polycystic kidney disease)
- Some pain medications and other drugs
- Certain toxic chemicals
- Autoimmune disorders (such as systemic lupus erythematosus and scleroderma)
- Injury or trauma
- Glomerulonephritiss
- Kidney stones and infection
- Other kidney diseases

The 5-year survival rate for a patient undergoing chronic dialysis in the United States is approximately 35%. This is approximately 25% in patients with diabetes. The most common cause of death in the dialysis population is cardiovascular disease.

The Kidney Disease Outcomes Quality Initiative (K/DOQI) of the National Kidney Foundation (NKF) defines chronic kidney disease as either kidney damage or a decreased kidney GFR of less than 60 mL/min/ 1.73 m^2 for 3 or more months. The stages include:

- Stage 1: Kidney damage with normal or increased GFR (>90 mL/min/1.73 m^2)
- Stage 2: Mild reduction in GFR (60 to 89 mL/ min/1.73 m^2)
- Stage 3: Moderate reduction in GFR (30 to 59 mL/min/1.73 m^2)

- Stage 4: Severe reduction in GFR (15 to 29 mL/ min/1.73 m^2)
- Stage 5: Kidney failure (GFR <15 mL/min/ 1.73 m^2 or dialysis)

Patients with chronic kidney disease stages 1 to 3 (GFR >30 mL/min) are usually asymptomatic and do not experience clinically evident alterations in electrolyte balance or endocrine/metabolic derangements. Generally, clinical signs occur with chronic kidney disease stages 4 to 5 (GFR <30 mL/min). Uremic manifestations in patients with chronic kidney disease stage 5 are believed to be primarily secondary to an accumulation of toxins. Metabolic acidosis and electrolyte imbalances occur. In chronic kidney disease, the kidneys are unable to excrete the endogenous acid into the urine and conduct normal reabsorption of fluids and electrolytes.

Other signs of uremia in ESRD, many of which are more likely in patients who are inadequately dialyzed, include the following:

- Pericarditis: Can be complicated by cardiac tamponade, possibly resulting in death.
- Encephalopathy: Can progress to coma and death.
- Peripheral neuropathy
- Restless leg syndrome
- Gastrointestinal symptoms: Anorexia, nausea, vomiting, diarrhea
- Skin manifestations: Dry skin, pruritus, ecchymosis
- Fatigue, increased somnolence, failure to thrive
- Malnutrition
- Erectile dysfunction, decreased libido, amenorrhea
- Platelet dysfunction with tendency to bleeding

Controlling blood pressure is the key to delaying further kidney damage. Angiotensin-converting enzyme (ACE) inhibitors or angiotensin receptor blockers (ARBs) can be used. The goal is to keep blood pressure at or below 130/80 mm Hg. Avoidance of nephrotoxins, including IV radiocontrast, nonsteroidal anti-inflammatory agents, and aminoglycosides is also indicated. Management principles include treating anemia, using dietary phosphate binders for hyperphosphatemia, calcium supplements for hypocalcemia, managing volume overload with diuretics or ultrafiltration, and mitigating uremic manifestations with chronic renal replacement therapy. The general management of patient care problems and associated nursing implications are outlined below.

MANAGEMENT OF PATIENT CARE PROBLEMS

There are four major problems of patient care in renal failure: an increase in the products of catabolism, severe electrolyte imbalance with associated acidosis, fluid overload, and infection.

Increase in the Products of Catabolism

Protein catabolism increases in the acutely ill, stressed patient. A decrease in proteins available for catabolism will retard the rate of azotemia, decrease the incidence and severity of acidosis, and decrease the occurrence and levels of hyperkalemia in the serum. The patient's caloric requirements must be met mainly through an adequate intake of carbohydrates in the diet.

Serum Electrolyte Imbalance and Acidosis

Sodium intake is restricted unless there is a serum sodium deficit. No salt substitutes are used because of their potassium content. Careful management of fluids and sodium intake will prevent overhydration, congestive heart failure, hyponatremia, and water intoxication.

Hyperkalemia is a significant imbalance seen in ARF. It is further compounded as a result of catabolism associated with fever and also occurs as a result of decreased potassium excretion caused by volume depletion or drugs. Metabolic acidosis can also cause hyperkalemia. The fall of the pH forces hydrogen ions into the cells and potassium into the extracellular fluid.

Fluid Overload

It is essential to determine the patient's state of hydration and to continually monitor this state. Indicators of overhydration include weight gain, edema, anasarca, ascites, increased blood pressure, jugular vein distention (JVD), and dyspnea. Indicators for dehydration include weight loss, decreased blood pressure, poor skin turgor, no evidence of JVD, and decreased central venous pressure.

Fluids are restricted to amounts equal to urine output plus 400 mL for insensible fluid loss. It is important that accurate daily weights be taken using the same scales. It is also important to remember that 1000 mL of fluid weighs about 2.2 lb (1 kg).

Infection

Because proper kidney function affects all body systems, the chance of infection is greatly increased in patients with renal failure. The body defense systems do not function properly, and the patient is predisposed to urinary tract infections, septicemia, pneumonia, and wound or skin infections (due to the severe pruritus that some patients experience). Good nutritional intake by the patient and proper hygiene will help prevent infections. If fever develops, culture and sensitivities of blood, urine, sputum, or any wound should be performed to identify the invading organism. Once the organism is identified, appropriate antibiotic therapy is started with antibiotic doses adjusted to renal function.

DIALYSIS

As the patient develops systemic symptoms of renal failure, the need for dialysis is assessed. The purposes of dialysis are to (1) remove the by-products of protein metabolism, including urea, creatinine, and uric acid; (2) remove excess water; (3) maintain or restore the body's buffer system; and (4) maintain or restore the body's concentration of electrolytes. Dialysis is defined as the diffusion of dissolved particles from one fluid compartment to another across a semipermeable membrane. Three principles are utilized in dialysis: osmosis, diffusion, and filtration; this is achieved through peritoneal dialysis, hemodialysis, and continuous renal replacement therapies (CRRT).

Osmosis is the movement of fluid across a semipermeable membrane from a less concentrated solution to a more concentrated solution. Diffusion is the movement of particles (or solutes) across a semipermeable membrane from a more concentrated solution to a less concentrated solution. Filtration is the movement of particles or solutes across a semipermeable membrane through the utilization of hydrostatic pressure.

Peritoneal Dialysis

In peritoneal dialysis, the peritoneum is the semipermeable membrane. The peritoneum is a strong, smooth, colorless serous membrane that lines the abdominal cavity with a parietal layer and wraps the abdominal organs with a visceral layer (Fig. 45-1).

The dialysate is instilled into the abdominal cavity between these two layers of peritoneum through

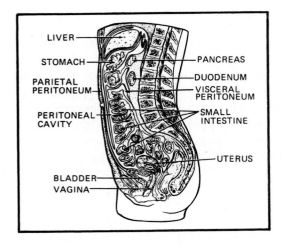

Figure 45-1. The peritoneal space (female).

a catheter. The visceral peritoneum is contiguous with the intestinal wall and the capillary beds of the intestines. The dialysate is instilled into the peritoneal space, bathing the intestines. Osmosis, diffusion, and filtration occur readily after "dwelling" in the abdomen.

Indications

There are a number of instances in which peritoneal dialysis may be used. In ARF, peritoneal dialysis may be used to treat the renal failure or to prevent uremia while ascertaining an underlying cause or while stabilizing a patient for surgery.

Patients with chronic renal failure who have had a recent infection may undergo peritoneal dialysis to prevent localization of the infection at the fistula site. Patients in whom there is no vascular access route for hemodialysis may undergo peritoneal dialysis until an access route is available.

Circulatory overload from renal impairment with congestive heart failure is amenable to peritoneal dialysis. Refractory hyperkalemia and metabolic acidosis and intoxication from dialyzable drugs and poisons are also indicators for peritoneal dialysis.

In chronic renal failure, peritoneal dialysis may postpone the need for chronic hemodialysis. In patients with diabetes, chronic hemodialysis may cause blindness associated with diabetic retinopathy. Patients awaiting renal transplantation may utilize peritoneal dialysis because it is less expensive than hemodialysis. Some patients undergo peritoneal dialysis instead of hemodialysis because of religious beliefs and the desire to avoid blood transfusions associated with hemodialysis emergencies.

The use of peritoneal dialysis in peritonitis is a controversial topic. Some nephrologists believe in adding antibiotics to the dialysate in addition to using oral or intravenous antibiotics. The rationale is to bathe the infected area itself with antibiotics. Other nephrologists believe that peritonitis is a justification for stopping peritoneal dialysis. The rationale here is to treat the patient with intravenous antibiotics to prevent septic shock from developing or to prevent weakening (to the actual point of rupture) of an inflamed, infected visceral peritoneum and the contiguous intestinal wall.

Contraindications

Any patient with blood-clotting dyscrasias should not undergo peritoneal dialysis until the blood-clotting problems have been resolved. Patients with fresh postoperative vascular prostheses, such as a fresh femoral-popliteal bypass, are not candidates for peritoneal dialysis because the procedure may result in graft failure at the site of anastomosis, leading to exsanguination.

Patients who have had recent peritoneal surgery or those with postoperative abdominal drains are not candidates for peritoneal dialysis. The peritoneum may not be strong enough to hold the dialysate without rupture or tearing of the peritoneum, and abdominal drains preclude any dwell time since the dialysate would flow out of the drains.

Abdominal adhesions or any other condition where a danger of puncturing viscera exists is a contraindication to peritoneal dialysis. Pregnant women should not undergo peritoneal dialysis because of the increased risk of fetal distress.

Advantages

Peritoneal dialysis can be performed at the bedside. The expensive, elaborate equipment and highly skilled personnel utilized for hemodialysis are not needed in peritoneal dialysis. Because it takes more time to effectively remove metabolic wastes and restore electrolyte and fluid balance, it is less stressful for pediatric and elderly patients and can be initiated quickly. There is no need for systemic anticoagulation.

Disadvantages

Peritoneal dialysis is slower to rid the body of waste products than hemodialysis. Exchanges of 2000 mL performed every 3 h achieve approximately the same solute clearance as a 4-h hemodialysis treatment performed every other day. Prolonged peritoneal dialysis results in a protein depletion and may cause ascites, poor wound healing, and decreased resistance to infection. Peritonitis, usually resulting from staphylococci or Gram-negative organisms, may develop with repeated treatments.

Dialysate

The concentration of the dialysate solution is selected by the physician. The more concentrated the solute concentration, the greater the osmotic forces exerted to remove fluid and waste products. Osmotic forces are determined by the concentration of glucose in the dialysate, usually ranging from 1.5% to 4.25%. During the administration of 4.25% dialysate, the serum glucose must be monitored because glucose can diffuse into the serum.

The temperature of the dialysate influences the effectiveness of peritoneal dialysis; urea clearance is 35% greater at body temperature (98.6°F) than at room temperature (75°F). Body-temperature dialysate will also enhance patient comfort.

The volume of the dialysate influences effectiveness. An exchange volume of 3 L of dialysate in 1 h almost doubles the urea clearance achieved with 1 L/h. Most adults are comfortable with 2 L per exchange, and a few can tolerate 3 L.

The physician will order the amount of heparin to be added to the dialysate to prevent fibrin or blood from clotting the catheter. The amount of potassium chloride added depends on the patient's serum potassium level, state of digitalization, and arterial blood gases.

Some physicians add lidocaine, usually 50 mg/2 L of dialysate, for generalized abdominal discomfort. Some physicians also add antibiotics if peritonitis is present or suspected.

Procedure and Nursing Care

To help obtain the patient's cooperation, the nurse should explain the procedure, making the patient aware of the discomforts of the procedure, limited mobility during it, and its duration. The patient is weighed before the procedure and then either daily or after the last exchange.

The patient should void or be catheterized immediately before the physician inserts the peritoneal dialysis catheter. Using strict sterile technique at the bedside, the physician inserts the catheter at the midline of the abdomen between the umbilicus and the symphysis pubis. Once the catheter is in place, 2 L of warmed dialysate is infused and drained as soon as it is instilled to ensure patency of the catheter. Outflow should drain in a steady stream.

When catheter patency is confirmed, the warmed dialysate is infused, allowed to dwell in the abdomen, usually for 20 to 45 min, and then allowed to drain via gravity as completely as possible. One exchange usually takes about an hour. Turning the patient side-to-side may enhance the drainage of dialysate.

At the end of the dwell time, the dialysate is assessed for color. Normally, it is a clear pale yellow. If the drainage is cloudy, suspect infection or peritonitis. If it is brownish, suspect bowel perforation. Blood-tinged dialysate during the first four exchanges is normal. However, if after four exchanges the dialysate is still bloody, discontinue and notify the physician. The patient may have abdominal bleeding or a uremic coagulopathy.

Periodic cultures of the dialysate drainage are obtained to assess for infection, and the tip of the catheter is cultured when it is removed.

Monitoring vital signs every 15 min during the first hour and then every 1 to 2 h is the usual procedure if the vital signs are stable. The outflow period is the most likely time for abnormal or changing vital signs. Signs of impending shock, fluid overload, and pulmonary edema will be most apparent in this outflow period.

One of the most important aspects of peritoneal dialysis is the intake-output record maintained by the nurse. Hospital policies vary as to the format for recording peritoneal dialysis intake and output. Information needed includes the time the exchange was started, the number of the exchange, the amount of fluid infused, the dwell time, the amount of fluid drained, and the fluid balance.

Fluid balance is crucial. If 2000 mL is instilled and only 1750 mL drains out, the patient's fluid balance is +250 mL. If the next exchange instills 2000 mL and drains 1900 mL, the patient's fluid balance for the exchange is +100 mL. The present balance is now +350 mL. Assume that the third exchange is with a 4.5% dialysate (hypertonic solution). The amount instilled was 2000 mL, and the output drainage was 2275 mL. The patient's balance for this exchange is −275 mL. The patient gave back more fluid than was instilled in this exchange. However, in the continuous fluid balance columns, the patient is still at a fluid balance of +75 mL. Intake-output records are maintained for each exchange and overall for total exchanges.

Complications

Infection is among the most common complications of peritoneal dialysis. Insertion of the catheter under sterile technique and closed sterile instillation and drainage of dialysate will help reduce infection. Daily sterile changes of the dressing over the tube insertion site helps decrease the chance of infection. Perhaps the most effective way to prevent infection is to keep the procedure time to 36 h or less.

Volume depletion occurs if the dialysis is too effective and removes several hundred milliliters of fluid per exchange. This will result in hypotension. Water removal may cause hypernatremia if the 4.25% glucose dialysate is used. Nursing intervention includes monitoring for signs of increasing sodium retention.

Volume overload may occur during peritoneal dialysis. When the patient is severely hyponatremic, sodium and water move into the third space. As third spacing resolves by sodium and water returning to the intravascular bed, cardiovascular overload may occur. Shortening the dwell time and repositioning the patient may help. If not, the patient may need hemodialysis.

Hyperglycemia may be severe if hypertonic fluid is used in a diabetic patient. Hyperosmolar coma and death have occurred. If hyperglycemia develops, the dialysis is discontinued until the blood sugar is controlled. Suspect hyperglycemia if the patient complains of thirst or if the patient's level of consciousness deteriorates.

Metabolic alkalosis may occur if dialysis is continued for a long time. Dialysate fluid contains sodium lactate or acetate (45 mEq/L), which is converted to sodium bicarbonate in the body.

Digitalis intoxication is a serious complication in patients taking digoxin in renal failure. It is a result of lowering the serum potassium and at the same time correcting hypocalcemia, hyponatremia, and acidosis. The dose of digitalis is usually reduced in uremic patients. Serum levels of cardiac glycosides are not affected by routine dialysis. Disequilibrium syndrome occurs more often in hemodialysis, and it is covered in the discussion of hemodialysis below.

Respiratory insufficiency may occur as the 2 L of dialysate is infused into the abdomen and pushes the abdominal viscera against the diaphragm, resulting in decreased depth of respirations. There is also an increased risk for atelectasis and pneumonia.

Severe pain at the end of inflow or outflow must be assessed. The pain may be caused by the temperature of the dialysate, incomplete draining of the previous exchange, early development of peritonitis, or instillation of too much dialysate.

Hemodialysis

Hemodialysis is a process of removing metabolic waste products of the body by the use of extracorporeal circulation. The patient's blood is transferred by tubing from the patient to a machine that functions like a kidney to filter out waste products and then returns the filtered blood to the patient by another tube. Hemodialysis uses the same principles of osmosis, diffusion, and filtration that are used in peritoneal dialysis.

Indications

Hemodialysis has the same indications as peritoneal dialysis. Other reasons for performing hemodialysis include ARF due to trauma or infection, chronic renal failure no longer controlled by medication and diet, when rapid removal of toxins, poisons, and drugs is essential, and when peritoneal dialysis is contraindicated.

Contraindications

Labile cardiovascular states that would deteriorate with rapid changes in extravascular fluid volume are the major contraindications to hemodialysis.

In the past, patients who could not tolerate systemic heparinization could not be hemodialyzed. Today, however, the heparin is infused into the dialysis machine to keep blood anticoagulated within the machine. Before the blood is returned to the patient, protamine is infused to neutralize the heparin. This process is called regional heparinization (Fig. 45-2).

For the patient without a condition that would be worsened by heparin, intermittent heparinization is used. In these cases, 2000 to 5000 units of heparin is infused at the start of hemodialysis and 1000 to 2000 units of heparin is added for each hour that the patient is on the machine. These patients must be monitored closely for signs of bleeding.

There are three ways to access a patient's blood for hemodialysis: an arteriovenous (AV) shunt, single- or double-lumen catheters, and an AV fistula. The AV shunt (Fig. 45-3) consists of two Silastic catheters; one is inserted into an artery and the other is inserted into a nearby vein. Blood is channeled from the artery to the dialysis machine and back to the vein. Part of the shunt lies subcutaneously and part lies outside the skin.

When the patient is not undergoing hemodialysis, blood flows directly from the artery through the shunt and into the vein. Shunts are inserted under local anesthesia. The favored sites are the arm, wrist, legs, and ankles. In the upper extremity, the preferred vessels are from the radial artery to the cephalic vein. In the lower extremity, the preferred vessels are from the posterior tibial artery to the great saphenous vein.

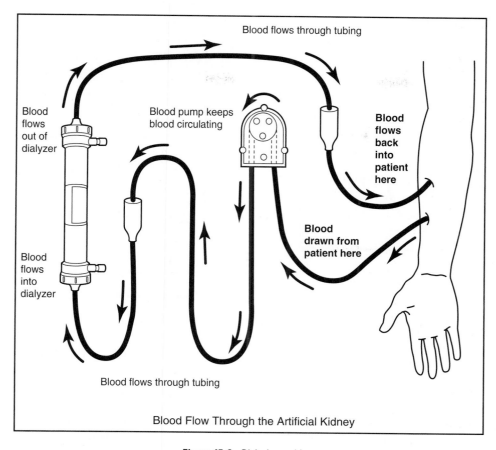

Figure 45-2. Dialysis machine.

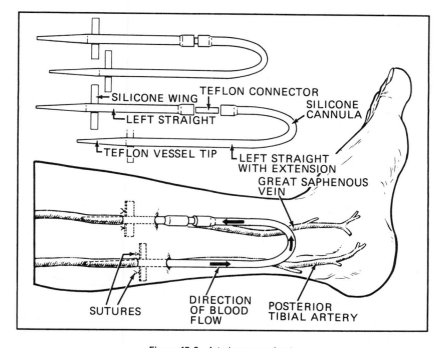

Figure 45-3. Arteriovenous shunt.

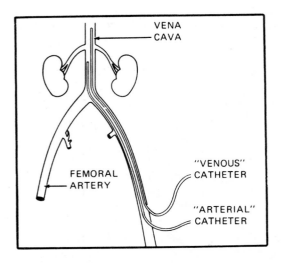

Figure 45-4. Dialysis catheters.

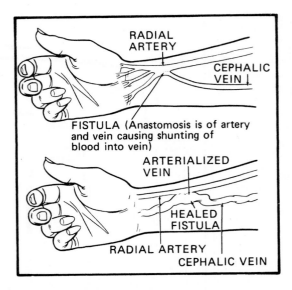

Figure 45-5. Anastomosis to form an arteriovenous fistula.

Dialysis catheters (Fig. 45-4) are short-term shunts. They can be placed in the femoral or subclavian vein. With femoral access, one or two cannulas may be placed in the femoral vein. During dialysis, one catheter is used to channel blood to the dialysis machine and the other is used to channel blood from the dialysis machine back to the patient. One bifurcated catheter can also be used. Peripheral pulses must frequently be assessed in the cannulized extremity. The patient must be maintained on bed rest. Assessment for signs of bleeding or hematoma formation is done frequently. If the catheter(s) is to remain after dialysis, low-dose heparin is utilized to maintain catheter patency.

Subclavian access also provides immediate short- or long-term access. One bifurcated catheter is utilized with heparin irrigations to maintain catheter patency between dialysis treatments. Patient activity is not restricted with subclavian access. However, the patient must be monitored for signs of a pneumothorax.

Fistulas have a longer life span than do AV shunts and tend to preserve the blood vessels in which they are placed. Fistulas are less restrictive than other forms of vascular access and, therefore, offer greater freedom to the patient. The fistula can be formed by the patient's vessels or by a graft (Fig. 45-5). Examples of graft materials are bovine carotid, woven Dacron, and umbilical vein. If grafts are used, they are tunneled under the skin in a U shape (Fig. 45-6). The surgical procedure involves anastomosis of the artery directly to the vein, most often utilizing a side-to-side technique. Fistulas must mature over a 10- to 14-day period. During this time, the vein adapts to the high pressure of the arterial blood by dilatation and thickening of

the venous wall. When the fistula matures, the vein will be able to withstand the insertion of a large-bore needle (14 to 16 gauge). The insertion of needles in the arterial and venous arms of the fistula permits attachments to the dialysis machine.

Complications associated with the AV fistula are infection, clotting, venous hypertension, and steal syndrome. Infection at the fistula site has direct access to systemic circulation and can precipitate septicemia. Localized infections present as reddened, tender,

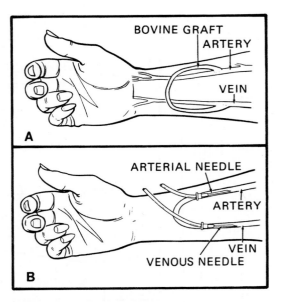

Figure 45-6. (A) A graft in place and **(B)** placement of needles in a graft for hemodialysis.

warm areas over the fistula, particularly at the anastomosis or needle puncture sites. Clotting sometimes causes severe pain and numbness in the affected arm; this can be confirmed by the absence of the bruit and thrill at the fistula site.

In venous hypertension, there is too much blood in the extremity distal to the fistula. This may cause ulcerations and may necessitate a fistula revision. In the steal syndrome, there is insufficient blood flow to the extremity because of excessive diversion of arterial blood to the vein at the anastomosis. Symptoms include coldness and poor function of the extremity. In severe cases, gangrene with necrosis of the extremity tips may develop. The steal syndrome is corrected by revising the fistula.

Once an access site is available, an evaluation of the patient's most recent electrolytes is made to determine what adjustments in the dialysate bath are to be made. An accurate predialysis weight of the patient is determined daily. By weighing the patient postdialysis, it is possible to calculate exactly how much fluid was removed or added.

Nursing Care

Infection is prevented by cleaning the shunt site daily using sterile technique and also by cleaning the fistula site until the incision is healed. If the shunt or fistula becomes infected, culture and sensitivity tests are done to identify the infecting organism. Once the organism is identified, intravenous antibiotics are started. If the shunt or fistula remains infected, it is removed and a new shunt or fistula is created.

The prevention of thrombosis is always a challenge. Anything that decreases blood flow increases the chance of thrombosis. Some examples are hypotension, hypovolemia, tourniquets, blood pressure cuffs, tight clothing and jewelry, heavy handbags and packages, and dehydration.

If the shunt is patent, one can see bright red blood flowing freely through it and it feels warm to the touch. There should not be any layering of the blood components (cells at the bottom, clear serum at the top). Proximal to the insertion site, one should feel a thrill (the turbulence of the arterial blood). With a stethoscope, one should hear a bruit (arterial blood turbulence). If either the thrill or bruit is absent, notify the physician immediately.

If the shunt becomes clotted, the physician may insert a catheter to remove the clot. After patency has been established, routine use of heparin will maintain patency.

To prevent hemorrhage due to shunt disconnection, clamps are attached to the dressing to ensure immediate availability. If the catheter becomes unconnected, the arterial cannula is clamped first to control excessive blood loss from the arterial system, and then the venous cannula is clamped.

The precautions taken for shunts are also taken for fistulas. A thrill and bruit should be present. The arm with a fistula is not used for intravenous fluids, blood pressure monitoring, venipuncture, or injections. The fistula is cleansed daily using sterile technique. Bleeding, skin discoloration, or drainage is reported to the physician.

Complications

Problems associated with hemodialysis occur most often during the initial stages or during a procedure lasting more than 4 h. Hypotension is caused by dehydration, sepsis, or blood loss. The patient may already be hypotensive or may rapidly become hypotensive when dialysis is initiated. This is treated by reducing the blood flow, discontinuing ultrafiltration (fluid removal), and giving fluids. If the patient does not respond to this method of treatment, dialysis is discontinued.

Cardiac dysrhythmias may be caused by potassium intoxication, but usually no specific electrolyte derangement can be identified. In some instances, dysrhythmias may be related to the development of transient myocardial ischemia as evidenced by premature ventricular contractions. Treatment consists of decreasing the blood flow and using appropriate medication as indicated. The dialysis procedure must be stopped if the dysrhythmia is severe or does not respond to treatment. Congestive heart failure in most instances is secondary to fluid overload, which can be reversed by ultrafiltration.

Disequilibrium syndrome may occur in reaction to the slowed clearance of urea from the cerebrospinal fluid during dialysis. Fluid shifts that occur to restore equilibrium result in cerebral swelling. Symptoms include headache, nausea, vomiting, restlessness progressing to disorientation, twitching, and seizures. Treatment focuses on prevention.

Air embolism may occur through an arterial or venous site as a result of a leak in the dialysis tubing, a loose connection, or the disconnection of dialysis tubing. With arterial air embolism, air travels the arterial system to a point distal to the entry site. In the head, the emboli enter the small vessels of the brain. Seizures may occur, followed by rapid brain cell damage. Death will ensue if critical areas of the brain are destroyed.

Venous emboli migrate back to the lungs and may cause pulmonary emboli. In the sitting patient with dialysis access in the lower extremities, air enters the venous system of the leg and travels to the inferior vena cava, then up through the right atrium to the superior vena cava, and finally to the head. In this case, the symptoms are the same as for arterial emboli in the brain.

If the patient is lying flat when air is introduced, the air enters the right atrium and moves into the right ventricle. Essentially, the air is trapped in the right ventricle and cannot be propelled from the heart. Blood cannot enter the pulmonary system. The lack of pulmonary blood return to the left atrium quickly stops the pumping of blood into the systemic circulation.

Symptoms of air embolism include deep respirations, coughing, cyanosis, unconsciousness, and cessation of breathing. Auscultation over the heart reveals a "mill wheel" sound during both phases of contraction. This is the sound of air turbulence in the heart.

Once air embolism has occurred, rapid corrective action is imperative. There are several important differences in the resuscitation of a patient with an air embolism as compared with the usual cardiopulmonary resuscitation. The patient must be placed in Trendelenburg's position and turned on the left side. Once resuscitated, the patient must be kept in the Trendelenburg's left-side position until the air is absorbed. This will prevent movement of the air into the cerebral tissues and heart and promote movement toward the feet (air will be higher than fluid). The absorption time will vary, but it usually takes from days to weeks; the mortality rate is extremely high.

Continuous Renal Replacement Therapy

Continuous renal replacement therapy (CRRT) is indicated when the treatment of ARF requires renal support or replacement therapy when there is an acute fall in GFR and has developed or is at risk for developing clinically significant solute imbalance/toxicity or volume overload. These therapies are being used with increasing frequency in acute care for the management of ARF. Advantages of using CRRT compared with hemodialysis are that CRRT is usually better tolerated hemodynamically, it facilitates gradual correction of metabolic and electrolyte abnormalities, it is highly effective in removing fluid, and it is technically simple to perform. To promote removal of urea and diffusible substrates,

CRRT utilizes the properties of convective transport driven by the circuitous movement of blood from the patient through a highly permeable filter. CRRT is an inexpensive and efficient method of treating fluid and electrolyte problems in the acute care setting.

Indications

The principal indication for CRRT is the treatment of patients with acute oliguric renal failure. Because fluid volume alteration and electrolyte removal is a slow process, CRRT is especially beneficial in treating acute volume overload in patients with unstable cardiovascular systems unresponsive to diuretic therapy, as occurs in acute pulmonary edema, congestive heart failure, postcardiac surgery, and recent myocardial infarction.

CRRT is also indicated in patients who require large quantities of parenteral fluid, as in hyperalimentation, intravenous antibiotic administration, and the continuous administration of vasopressors. CRRT is also considered when other forms of dialysis are contraindicated, and it may also be used to treat hyperkalemia, azotemia, and drug or poison intoxication.

Contraindications

Contraindications to CRRT are an inability to tolerate anticoagulation and a hematocrit greater than 45%. Both of these problems precipitate clotting in the hemofilter. Lack of vascular access is also a contraindication of CRRT.

Advantages

CRRT has distinct advantages over hemodialysis. It allows the elimination of large amounts of fluid without the osmolar changes associated with hemodialysis, thus maintaining extracellular fluid status. During hemodialysis, rapid water removal causes the extracellular fluid to become hypotonic in relation to the hypertonic environment of the cell. Extracellular fluid is drawn into the cell, creating a depleted or hypovolemic state. The slow, consistent process of CRRT maintains osmolality and cardiovascular stability. Another problem occurring with hemodialysis but absent with CRRT is the reduction in the platelet and white blood cell count as the patient's blood comes into contact with cuprophane, cellulose acetate, or regenerated cellulose membrane. CRRT can be managed by the progressive care nurse at the bedside rather than by hemodialysis staff.

Disadvantages

The main disadvantage of CRRT is its limited ability to remove waste products and excess solutes with minimal volume replacement.

Hemofiltration Process

Three modes of CRRT are readily available in the acute care setting: slow continuous ultrafiltration (SCUF), continuous arteriovenous hemofiltration (CAVH), and continuous arteriovenous hemodialysis (CAVHD) (Table 45-3). All three modes use the same equipment: a highly porous hemofilter, arterial and venous blood lines, and a fluid-collection device (Fig. 45-7). CRRT is dependent on the rate of blood flow, which is determined by the mean arterial blood pressure (MAP). An MAP of at least 60 mm Hg is needed to maintain the system.

Cannulation of a large artery and vein is performed by the physician, usually at the femoral site. A hemofilter and blood lines are primed with heparinized saline. Blood flow begins at the arterial site and passes through the blood line to the hemofilter. The hemofilter separates plasma water and certain solutes from the blood and passes the ultrafiltrate to a graduated measuring device. Blood, minus the ultrafiltrate, is then returned through the venous blood line to the venous site.

Slow Continuous Ultrafiltration. Slow continuous ultrafiltration (SCUF), the removal of molecules dissolved in plasma, is based on the principle of convection. Some elements in the plasma water are conveyed across the semipermeable hemofilter as a result of the differences in hydrostatic pressure. Albumin and protein-bound substances are retained in the plasma and returned to the patient. SCUF removes filterable solutes in proportion to plasma water: large amounts of plasma water removed result in large amounts of filterable solutes removed (ultrafiltration). SCUF, therefore, does not alter the concentration of solutes in the blood.

Continuous Arteriovenous Hemofiltration. Continuous arteriovenous hemofiltration (CAVH) uses the principles of convection and replacement. The concentration of the ultrafiltrate is lowered by replacing the ultrafiltrate with a solution free of unwanted solutes (e.g., potassium-free lactated Ringer's solution). The infusion rate of this replacement fluid is determined by the ultrafiltration rate, intake, output, and desired fluid removal. CAVH can filter up to 20 L/24 h. An infusion pump placed on the arterial blood line may be used to increase the rate of ultrafiltrate production.

Continuous Arteriovenous Hemodialysis. Continuous arteriovenous hemodialysis (CAVHD) uses the principles of convection and diffusion. It provides more solute (urea, creatinine) clearance; therefore, it is used in uremic patients with high catabolic rates (acidosis, hyperkalemia). Urea clearance is

TABLE 45-3. CONTINUOUS RENAL REPLACEMENT THERAPIES

Type of Therapy	Abbreviation	Description
Continuous arteriovenous hemofiltration	CAVH	Uses the principles of convection to promote slow continuous removal by hemofiltration of solute and fluids through a permeable membrane filter using an extracorporeal pump that is dependent on the patient's blood pressure
Continuous venovenous hemofiltration	CVVH	Uses the principles of convection to promote slow continuous removal of solute and fluids through a permeable membrane filter that is driven by an external extracorporeal pump
Continuous venovenous hemodialysis	CVVHD	Uses the principles of diffusion with limited convection to promote slow continuous removal of solute and fluid facilitated by the addition of dialysate which promotes diffusion of solutes
Continuous venovenous hemodiafiltration	CVVHDF	Uses the principles of diffusion and convection to promote slow continuous removal of solute and fluids

Source: Adapted from Rempher J. "Variations of Continuous Renal Replacement Therapy," by J. Rempher, 2003, *AACN Advanced Critical Care, 14*(4), pp. 512–519. With permission.

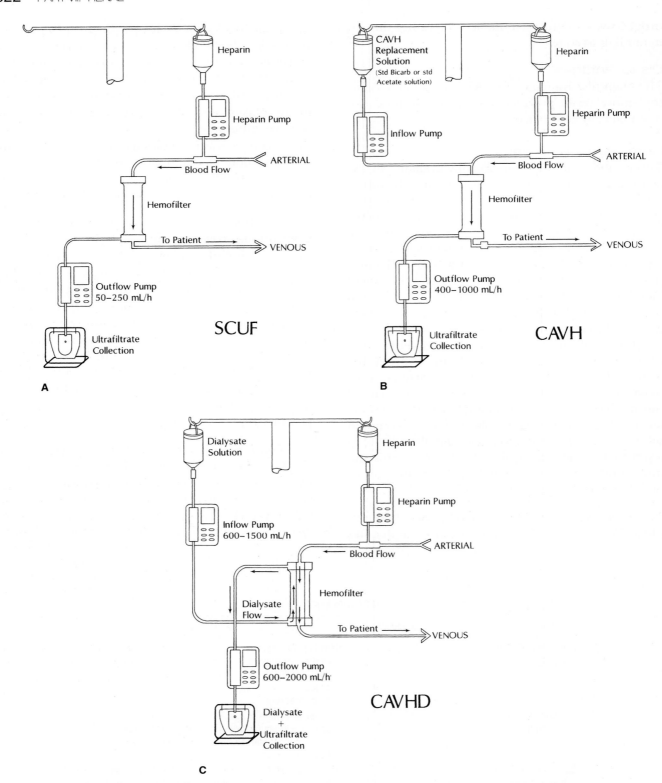

Figure 45-7. Modes of continuous renal replacement therapy (CRRT). **(A)** Slow continuous ultrafiltration (SCUF). **(B)** Continuous arteriovenous hemofiltration (CAVH). **(C)** Continuous arteriovenous hemodialysis (CAVHD).

approximately twice that of CAVH. A peritoneal dialysate solution is used to create a diffusion gradient, enhancing the removal of urea and creatinine into the dialysate solution and out of the hemofilter into the ultrafiltrate. The higher the glucose concentration in the dialysate solution (1.5, 2.5, and 4.25%), the greater the solute and fluid removal.

Nursing Care

Access sites are cleansed and inspected daily for signs of infection. Patency of the system can be assessed by inspection and palpation. Both the arterial and venous blood lines should be warm and a thrill palpable. Signs that the system is no longer patent include a decrease in the production of ultrafiltrate, a darkened or streaked filter, and blood-tinged ultrafiltrate. Laboratory values, daily weights, and hourly records of intake and output are performed.

Complications

The insertion site is inspected frequently for signs of infection, infiltration, and bleeding. If any of these occur, the access will be changed and appropriate antibiotic therapy instituted. The tubing and catheter are kept free of kinks. A kinked catheter will decrease blood flow and greatly increase the risk of clotting as blood stagnates in the hemofilter.

Disconnection of the system from the hemofilter, blood lines, or access catheter may result in exsanguination. The system must be reconnected under sterile conditions. The circuit is clamped off to prevent air from entering the system. If air has entered the system, it is allowed to pass through the filter and must be removed through the blood infusion port (venous) so that it is not delivered to the patient.

The large doses of heparin required for CRRT place the patient at risk for bleeding. This danger can be minimized by monitoring clotting profiles.

Problems with the ultrafiltration rate may develop from problems with the patient or circuit. If the patient is hypovolemic or hypotensive, the force that pushes the blood through the circuit will be reduced. This will decrease the amount of ultrafiltrate generated. It also contributes to clot formation in the hemofilter, resulting in slower filtration and less ultrafiltrate production. To minimize these complications, the filter is always kept below the level of the patient's

heart and the collecting system low enough to the floor that the ultrafiltrate moves with the assistance of gravity.

BIBLIOGRAPHY

Angus, D., Belloma, R., & Star, R. Acute dialysis quality initiative. Selection of patients for acute extracorporeal renal support in general and CRRT in particular. Available at: http://www.ccm.upmc.edu/adqi/ADQIg2.pdf Accessed 8/12/2010.

Arora, P. Chronic renal failure http://emedicine.medscape.com/article/238798-overview. Accessed 9/22/2010.

Brunton, L. L., Lazo, J. S., Parker, L. K., Murri, N., Blumenthal, D. K., Knollmann, B. C. Diuretics. In *Goodman & Gilman's the pharmacological basis of therapeutics*. Online. Accessed 8/10/2010.

Dirkes, S., & Hodge, K. (2007). Continuous renal replacement therapy in the adult intensive care unit: History and current trends. *Critical Care Nurses, 27,* 61–80.

Gunnerson, K. J., & Kellum, J. A. (2003). Acid-base and electrolyte analysis in critically ill patients: Are we ready for the new millennium? *Current Opinions in Crit Care, 9,* 468–473.

Harrison's Online. Acute renal failure. Accessed 8/10/2010.

Harrison's Online. Dialysis in the treatment of renal failure. Accessed 8/10/2010.

Harrison's Online. Fluid and electrolyte disturbances. Accessed 8/10/2010.

Hinkle, C. (2010). Renal system. In M. Chulay, S.M. Burns (Eds.), *AACN essentials of progressive care nursing.* (pp. 323–336) New York, NY: McGraw-Hill.

Martin, R. I. (2005). Continuous renal replacement therapies. In J. D. Lynn-McHale, D. J. Wiegand, & K. K. Carlson (Eds.), *AACN procedure manual for critical care* (5th ed.) (pp. 937–960). St. Louis, MO: Mosby.

McGraw-Hill's Access Medicine Online. Acute renal failure. Accessed 8/2/2010.

Molzhan, A., & Butera, E. (Eds.) (2007). *Contemporary nephrology nursing: Principles and practice* (2nd ed.). Pittman, NJ: American Nephrology Nursing Association.

Salinitri, F., Berlie, H., & Desai, H. (2009). Pharmacotherapeutic blood pressure management in chronic kidney disease. *American Association of Nurses Advances in Critical Care, 20*(3), 205–213.

Tonelli, M., Manns, B., Wiebe, N., et al. (2007). Continuous renal replacement therapy in adult patients with acute renal failure: Systematic review and economic evaluation. Technologic Report No. 88. Ottawa: Canadian Agency for Drugs and Technologies in Health. Available at: http://www.cadth.ca/media/pdf/338_CRRT_Report_tr_e.pdf. Accessed 8/22/2010.

Renal Practice Exam

1. A 64-year-old woman is in your unit with the diagnosis of possible sepsis secondary to a urinary tract infection. Over the past 2 days, she was aggressively treated with normal saline fluid boluses, antibiotics, and dobutamine. She has gained 10 kg. Based on the information below, what has happened in terms of her electrolytes?

Na	121
K	4.9
Cl	94
HCO_3	25

(A) Not enough chloride has been given.
(B) She has received too much fluid.
(C) She has become dehydrated.
(D) She needs more sodium in her IV fluids.

2. A 78-year-old man is in your unit with a diagnosis of congestive heart failure (CHF). He has received increasing amounts of furosemide (Lasix) over the past 3 days because of his low urine output. Based on the information below, the physician believes that a contraction alkalosis has developed. Do the following electrolytes agree with this observation?

Na	144
K	4.3
Cl	90
HCO_3	39

(A) Yes, based on the increased sodium level.
(B) Yes, based on the decreased chloride and increased bicarbonate levels.
(C) No, based on the high potassium.
(D) No, because the key electrolyte, magnesium, is not given.

3. The right kidney is slightly lower than the left. What is the reason for this difference?
(A) The right kidney is larger because of the presence of more nephric structures.

(B) The left kidney is displaced upward by the spleen.
(C) The right kidney is displaced downward by the liver.
(D) The left kidney is drawn upward by the diaphragm.

4. Fluid is forced from the glomerulus forming an ultrafiltrate. Into which compartment is the fluid forced?
(A) Bowman's capsule
(B) Proximal tubule
(C) Collecting ducts
(D) Distal tubule

5. Glomerular filtration is affected by all of the following factors. Which has the most significant effect on glomerular filtration rate?
(A) Osmotic pressure of the blood
(B) Hydrostatic pressure of the blood
(C) Dilation of the afferent arteriole
(D) Constriction of the efferent arteriole

6. Which of the following corresponds most closely to the range of normal serum potassium values?
(A) 1 to 2 mEq/L
(B) 2 to 3 mEq/L
(C) 3.5 to 5.0 mEq/L
(D) 5.0 to 6.5 mEq/L

7. Which of the following corresponds most closely to the range of normal serum calcium levels?
(A) 1 to 3 mg/dL
(B) 4.5 to 6.5 mg/dL
(C) 6 to 8 mg/dL
(D) 8.5 to 10.5 mg/dL

8. An 81-year-old man has been on your unit for 45 days because of complications from a ruptured bowel. The physician suspects that the man may have nutritional impairment despite total parenteral nutrition. Laboratory tests reveal the following serum electrolyte information:

Na^+	141 mEq/L
K^+	3.9 mEq/L
Cl^-	102 mEq/L
HCO_3^-	25 mEq/L
Ca^{2+}	8.9 mg/dL
Mg^{2+}	4.3 mg/dL

   Which of the preceding laboratory values is/are abnormal?
   (A) Mg^{2+}
   (B) Ca^{2+}
   (C) Cl^- and Na^+
   (D) K^+ and HCO_3^-

9. Which of the following corresponds most closely to the range of normal phosphate levels?
   (A) 3.0 to 4.5 mg/dL
   (B) 4.5 to 6.5 mg/dL
   (C) 6 to 8 mg/dL
   (D) 8.5 to 10.5 mg/dL

10. Creatinine level is a valuable indicator of glomerular filtration rate for which reason?
   (A) Once filtered in the glomerulus, creatinine is not reabsorbed in the tubular system.
   (B) Creatinine enters the glomerulus only when glomerular filtration pressures exceed 60 mm Hg.
   (C) Creatinine filtration is unaffected by renal disease.
   (D) Creatinine is formed in the glomerulus and decreases only in filtration, causing creatinine levels to change.

11. What is the effect of antidiuretic hormone (ADH) on renal function?
   (A) It inhibits water reabsorption in the distal tubules and collecting ducts.
   (B) It increases water reabsorption in the distal tubules and collecting ducts.
   (C) It increases fluid excretion from the glomerulus.
   (D) It blocks the effect of loop diuretics, such as furosemide (Lasix).

12. A 46-year-old man is in your unit following an episode of respiratory failure after radiation therapy for lung cancer. On day 3 of his stay, his urine output decreases to 20 mL/h. The physician asks you to call him if the patient's BUN (blood urea nitrogen)/creatinine ratio becomes abnormal. You have the following laboratory data:

Serum BUN	64
Serum creatinine	2
Urine Na^+	76

   Based on this information, is the BUN/creatinine ratio abnormal and should you contact the physician?
   (A) The BUN/creatinine level is normal; do not call the physician.
   (B) The BUN/creatinine level is low; call the physician.
   (C) The BUN/creatinine level is high; call the physician.
   (D) BUN/creatinine ratios cannot be calculated without urinary creatinine and BUN values.

13. Which of the following corresponds most closely to the range of normal serum creatinine levels?
   (A) 0.8 to 1.8
   (B) 2 to 2.9
   (C) 3.2 to 4.0
   (D) 4.5 to 5.0

14. Which of the following corresponds most closely to the range of normal serum BUN levels?
   (A) 10 to 20 mg/dL
   (B) 20 to 30 mg/dL
   (C) 30 to 40 mg/dL
   (D) 40 to 50 mg/dL

15. The presence of oliguria, a BUN/creatinine ratio greater than normal suggests that which condition has developed?
   (A) Prerenal failure
   (B) Renal failure
   (C) Postrenal failure
   (D) Acute tubular necrosis

16. A 34-year-old man with chronic renal failure has a hemoglobin level of 7.4 g/dL and a hematocrit of 23%. His blood pressure is 160/92 mm Hg and his heart rate is 98. What is the most likely explanation for his hemoglobin and hematocrit values?
   (A) The values are abnormally elevated because of hemoconcentration.
   (B) The values are abnormally low because of a reduced cardiac output.
   (C) The values are normal.
   (D) The values are abnormally low because of loss of erythropoietin.

17. What is the primary action of aldosterone?
    (A) Inhibits sodium excretion
    (B) Promotes sodium excretion
    (C) Blocks water reabsorption
    (D) Stimulates vasoconstriction

18. What is the primary cause of hypernatremia?
    (A) Vascular water deficits
    (B) Excessive vascular free water
    (C) Excessive serum sodium levels
    (D) Loss of serum chloride

19. Which of the following is NOT a common sign of hypernatremia?
    (A) Tachycardia
    (B) Dry mucous membranes
    (C) Poor skin turgor
    (D) Distended neck veins

20. Administration of which of the following is a typical treatment for hypernatremia?
    (A) Diuretics and fluid restriction
    (B) Nonelectrolyte (free water) solutions
    (C) Normal saline
    (D) Potassium salts

21. Hyponatremia is most often caused by which of the following?
    (A) Excessive sodium levels
    (B) Decreased sodium levels
    (C) Excessive vascular volume
    (D) Decreased vascular volume

22. The most dangerous symptoms of hyponatremia center on which organ system?
    (A) Central nervous system
    (B) Cardiac system
    (C) Renal system
    (D) Respiratory system

23. Treatment of severe hyponatremia (<120 mEq/L) consists of administration of which of the following?
    (A) Diuretics
    (B) Nonelectrolyte (free water) solutions
    (C) Normal saline
    (D) Potassium salts

24. Hypokalemia is associated with which acid-base disturbance?
    (A) Metabolic acidosis
    (B) Metabolic alkalosis
    (C) Respiratory acidosis
    (D) Systemic acidosis

25. Which of the following electrocardiographic (ECG) changes is NOT associated with hyperkalemia?

    (A) Peaked T waves
    (B) Depressed P waves
    (C) Premature ventricular contractions (PVCs)
    (D) Widening QRS complex

26. Which of the following is NOT recommended for the treatment of hyperkalemia?
    (A) Sodium polystyrene sulfonate (Kayexalate)
    (B) Glucose/insulin infusion
    (C) Dialysis
    (D) Ammonium chloride

27. Hypokalemia is associated with which of the following ECG changes?
    (A) Peaked T waves
    (B) Depressed P waves
    (C) PVCs
    (D) Prolonged QT interval

28. The concentration of which electrolyte is inversely related to that of calcium?
    (A) Sodium
    (B) Potassium
    (C) Phosphate
    (D) Magnesium

29. Which mechanism is calcium NOT involved in regulating?
    (A) Coagulation
    (B) Formation of bone
    (C) Transmission of electrical impulses
    (D) Absorption of vitamin D

30. A 51-year-old man with a history of alcoholism has marked muscle irritability. The following laboratory data are available:

Na^+	135 mEq/L
K^+	4.8 mEq/L
Ca^{2+}	3.7 mg/dL
Mg^{2+}	1.8 mg/dL

    Which of the following electrolytes is most likely to be the source of the muscle hyperirritability?
    (A) Sodium
    (B) Calcium
    (C) Potassium
    (D) Magnesium

31. Chvostek's sign is tested by which maneuver?
    (A) Tapping the flexor tendon over the knee
    (B) Tapping the supramandibular area
    (C) Stroking the sole of the foot
    (D) Measuring clotting times after venipuncture

32. Trousseau's sign is a test for which electrolyte deficiency?
    (A) Hypophosphatemia
    (B) Hypercalcemia
    (C) Hypocalcemia
    (D) Hypokalemia

33. Which organ or organ system is involved in the regulation of phosphate elimination?
    (A) Liver
    (B) Respiratory system
    (C) Renal system
    (D) Spleen

34. A 75-year-old woman is admitted to your unit with pneumonia and malnutrition. Her chief complaint is weakness and inability to perform her normal "chores." She states that she has not eaten well for the past several months. The following information is available:

Na^+	150 mEq/L
K^+	3.6 mEq/L
Cl^-	110 mEq/L
Mg^{2+}	2.1 mg/dL
Ca^{2+}	9.2 mg/dL
PO_{43}^-	2.3 mg/dL

    Which of the preceding levels is a likely source of her weakness?
    (A) Low phosphate
    (B) High sodium and chloride
    (C) Low magnesium
    (D) High calcium

35. Which of the following does NOT have phosphate as a component?
    (A) Adenosine triphosphate (ATP)
    (B) Adenosine diphosphate (ADP)
    (C) 2,3-Diphosphodiglyceride (2,3-DPG)
    (D) Parathyroid hormone (PTH)

36. Hypomagnesemia is manifested clinically by which of the following symptoms?
    (A) Muscle irritability
    (B) Muscle fatigue
    (C) Nausea
    (D) Positive Turner's sign

37. A 61-year-old man admitted with the diagnosis of chronic obstructive pulmonary disease (COPD) has the following set of laboratory data for arterial blood gases and electrolytes:

PO_2	63 mm Hg
PCO_2	71 mm Hg
pH	7.37
HCO_3^-	39 mEq/L
Na^+	146 mEq/L
Cl^-	87 mEq/L

    The COPD-induced blood gas changes have altered the electrolytes as well. Based on the preceding information, which electrolyte change occurred because of the PCO_2 elevation?
    (A) Decrease in pH
    (B) Chloride increased
    (C) Sodium increased
    (D) Increased HCO_3^-

38. Elevated chloride levels are associated with which condition?
    (A) Alkalosis
    (B) Acidosis
    (C) Hyponatremia
    (D) Hypercalcemia

39. Left ventricular failure will cause which effect on the BUN/creatinine ratio?
    (A) It will cause the ratio to rise. (BUN rises faster than creatinine.)
    (B) It will cause the ratio to fall. (BUN rises more slowly than creatinine.)
    (C) It will have no effect on the ratio but will elevate creatinine levels.
    (D) It will reverse the ratio.

40. A 71-year-old woman is admitted to your unit from a nursing home. At the time of admission she seemed confused, although she is currently alert and oriented. She has had a "cold" for the past several days. Her laboratory data are as follows:

Na^+	155
K^+	3.6
Cl^-	122
HCO_3^-	24

    What is the most likely reason for the abnormal sodium level?
    (A) Excess total sodium
    (B) Decreased total potassium
    (C) Dehydration
    (D) Fluid excess

41. During the care of a patient undergoing peritoneal dialysis, the infusate has not completely drained. Which method would be acceptable to help facilitate drainage?
    (A) Applying continuous low-pressure suction
    (B) Turning the patient from side to side
    (C) Manipulating the peritoneal catheter
    (D) Applying manual pressure to the abdomen

PART VII

Renal Practice Exam

Practice Fill-Ins

1. _____
2. _____
3. _____
4. _____
5. _____
6. _____
7. _____
8. _____
9. _____
10. _____
11. _____

12. _____
13. _____
14. _____
15. _____
16. _____
17. _____
18. _____
19. _____
20. _____
21. _____
22. _____

23. _____
24. _____
25. _____
26. _____
27. _____
28. _____
29. _____
30. _____
31. _____
32. _____
33. _____

34. _____
35. _____
36. _____
37. _____
38. _____
39. _____
40. _____
41. _____

PART VII

Answers

1. B	12. C	23. A	34. A
2. B	13. A	24. B	35. D
3. C	14. A	25. C	36. A
4. B	15. A	26. D	37. D
5. B	16. D	27. D	38. A
6. C	17. A	28. C	39. A
7. D	18. A	29. D	40. C
8. A	19. D	30. B	41. B
9. A	20. B	31. B	
10. A	21. B	32. C	
11. B	22. A	33. C	

VIII

MULTIORGAN PROBLEMS

....

Thomas S. Ahrens

46

Sepsis and Multiorgan Syndrome

EDITORS' NOTE

Sepsis and multiorgan dysfunction syndrome (MODS) are key parts of the PCCN exam. This chapter, along with chapters on burns and toxic ingestions, make up as much as 10% of the PCCN exam (20 questions). The present chapter addresses the areas of sepsis and MODS, which may account for anywhere from 5 to 15 questions on the PCCN exam. Because of the relevance of sepsis and MODS to acute and critical care, this is a valuable area to learn about. Understanding these two major concepts involves becoming familiar with relatively complex cellular activities. However, the in-depth physiology will not likely be on the exam. It is better to focus on identifying sepsis and the key treatments.

In this chapter, a brief summary of these complex activities is given in an attempt to maintain a simplified approach that covers essential PCCN content. Try to understand the major terms and the general sequence of events occurring in sepsis. If you understand the major therapies and symptoms of sepsis, you will probably be adequately prepared for the exam.

"Our arsenals for fighting off bacteria are so powerful, and involve so many different defense mechanisms, that we are more in danger from them than from the invaders. We live in the midst of explosive devices; we are mined!"

This statement from Lewis Thomas is a good introduction to understanding sepsis: how the body responds to an infection and how this response changes helps to clarify the septic process. Also, a major aid to the understanding, identification, and treatment of sepsis is provided by the Surviving Sepsis Campaign guidelines (www.survivingsepsis.org). This campaign, part of an international effort to improve treatment and outcomes in sepsis, will serve as a guide to the treatment recommendations outlined here. Since the campaign was launched in 2004, it is likely that its guidelines will be used for the PCCN exam as well.

SEPSIS

Sepsis is one of the leading causes of increased morbidity and mortality in critical care. It is still a confusing entity for clinicians in that it is a difficult condition to identify, it is difficult to predict who is at risk, and it is even more difficult to treat. Sepsis can present in a mild or severe (septic shock) form, with mortalities ranging anywhere from 20% to 80% depending on the number of organs affected. Part of the problem with sepsis is identifying when it is present and why it occurs. In this chapter, potential causes of sepsis are presented along with physical symptoms and responses. Current concepts in treating sepsis are discussed, as well as controversies over the management of the septic patient.

Etiology

Sepsis is defined as the systemic response to infection. It is not only the direct result of an infection but also reflects an inflammatory response produced by the immune system. Sepsis can originate from any antigen, bacterial, viral, or fungal, although by far the most common sources are bacterial. The most significant infections seen in critical care are usually Gram-negative bacterial infections (e.g., *Pseudomonas aeruginosa*, *Klebsiella*, *Serratia*, and *Escherichia coli*), although Gram-positive infections (e.g., *Staphylococcus aureus*) are also responsible for sepsis.

The antigen eventually causing sepsis must take hold in tissues and start to grow in order to produce an infectious process. For example, an antigen can exist on the skin (colonization) or even in the blood but will not produce an infection until it resides and grows in normal tissue or the bloodstream. Normally, most infections are controlled by the immune system and further progression does not take place. However, in sepsis, the initial infection progresses to a more advanced state. The urinary and respiratory systems are the most common sites for initial infections.

Septic Cascade

From the initial infection, an extension of the infectious response occurs. The extension involves a series of events, primarily an inflammatory response sequence as well as a direct physiologic response to the infection. The extension can be viewed as a cascade of events that probably becomes self-perpetuating after a certain point. Several events occur that characterize the septic process and subsequent inflammatory response.

The exact sequence of events in sepsis is unclear, although one potential scenario is as follows (Fig. 46-1). The antigen (e.g., bacteria) is recognized by a monocyte, which immediately releases inflammatory mediators. The mediators include factors such as interleukin-1 (IL-1), IL-6, tumor necrosis factor alpha (TNF-α), and tissue factor. These mediators set off a series of responses. The main actions of these responses are to:

1. Initiate the coagulation cascade to form a clot and seal the antigen in a localized area.
2. Inhibit the body's ability to lyse the clot, at least temporarily until the antigen is destroyed.
3. Change the endothelial lining to become more permeable, allowing activated neutrophils to enter the area to destroy the antigen.

For example, the complement system (particularly C3a and C5a) is activated to stimulate neutrophil activity. In addition, platelet activation and aggregation are promoted; perhaps as an attempt to isolate the infection. The neutrophil or other macrophage (e.g., monocytes) will initiate a sequence of events also designed to control the antigen. The major immunologic responses are discussed below.

Arachidonic Acid Sequence

In response to the infection, macrophage (neutrophil and monocyte) activity (polymorphonuclear leukocytes [PMNs]) in the area increases. The PMNs attempt to control the infection through a variety of processes, including the release of highly destructive molecules such as oxygen free radicals. Another method used by the PMNs involves the breakdown of arachidonic acid. As arachidonic acid is generated, it is further degraded. The degradation of arachidonic acid takes place by either the cyclooxygenase or lipooxygenase pathway (Fig. 46-2). From the cyclooxygenase pathway, two important by-products, thromboxane A_2 and prostacyclin (a prostaglandin), are generated. From the lipooxygenase pathway, various leukotrienes (e.g., leukotrienes B_4, C_4, D_4, and E_4) are released.

Both leukotrienes and thromboxane A_2 generate a series of reactions, including an increased tendency for platelet aggregation, increased capillary permeability, and vasoconstriction. Prostacyclin (the precursor to specific prostaglandins) produces essentially the opposite responses; that is, a decreased tendency for platelet aggregation, decreased capillary permeability, and vasodilatation.

Downregulation of the Immune/Inflammatory Response

An important aspect of the immune/inflammatory response is the body's ability to neutralize toxic products produced by the immune system. The ability of components of the immune system to control infection is based on the generation of substances that destroy virtually any substance with which they come into contact, including normal cells. For example, oxygen radicals, once released, will damage or destroy any cell with which they come into contact. The body will attempt to produce neutralizing substances, such as peroxidases for oxygen radicals, to avoid injury to normal tissues. One theory of sepsis holds that the downregulation of the immune system malfunctions and allows normal tissue to be damaged by the immune responses.

T-Cell Response

The macrophage also stimulates T-cell activity by alerting the T cell to the presence of an ingested antigen through markers on its cell surface. The T cell senses these markers and promotes the formation of IL-2. From IL-2, specific interferons as well as granulocyte-macrophage colony-stimulating factor are released. IL-2 is an active cardiovascular modifier. With release of IL-2, the systemic vascular resistance (SVR) decreases and cardiac output increases.

Tumor Necrosis Factor

Tumor necrosis factor (TNF) is thought to be produced in response to a substance such as endotoxin. This factor stimulates platelet aggregation, increased

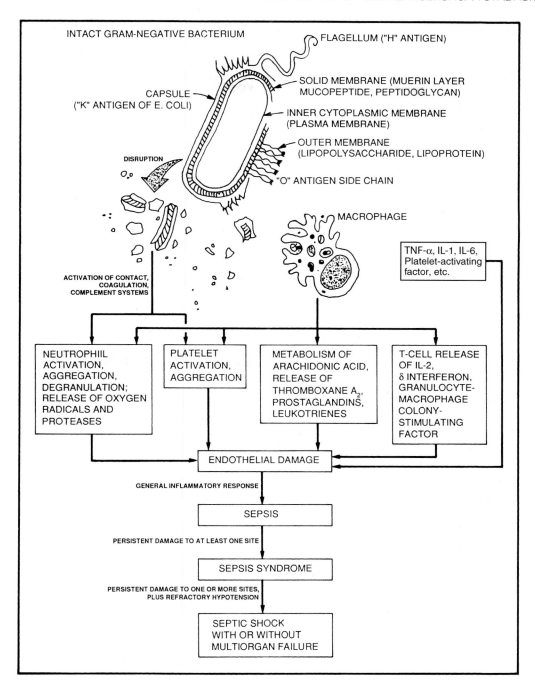

Figure 46-1. The septic response.

capillary permeability, neutrophil activation, and the release of IL-1, IL-6, and IL-8. It may have a role in mediating the central response to sepsis, although the exact mechanism for this is unclear. Tumor necrosis factor is also a pyrogenic (fever-producing) substance.

In addition to these responses, the body generates increased quantities of endorphins (releases endogenous opiates). These opiates produces

vasodilation (a reduction in SVR) and changes in capillary permeability.

Effect of Immune Response on Endothelial Cells

All of the activities described above are designed to help control the growth of antigens. If properly

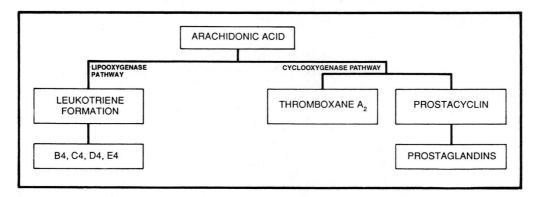

Figure 46-2. Arachidonic acid sequence.

released, the immune/inflammatory response does not injure normal tissue. However, if the response is not controlled, normal cells can be injured. The most likely cells to be at risk of such injury are the endothelial cells of the blood vessels. If this endothelial layer is damaged, every organ is threatened, since control of vascular fluid and the supply of oxygen and nutrients may be disrupted.

The immune response is initially a local response. Under normal circumstances, these responses control antigen growth. Keep in mind, however, that all of these processes, which are designed to control antigen growth, can also damage endothelial cells.

If the immune response spreads beyond a local level, either because the infection is too great to be controlled or because downregulation fails to occur, the immune response may spread systematically. It is such systemic spread that is probably the first major indicator of a septic process. This process is called the systemic inflammatory response syndrome (SIRS) and is marked by tachycardia, tachypnea, fever, and increased numbers of white blood cells.

Role of Activated Protein C

Protein C is a component of many natural body actions; for example, it is one of the three natural anticoagulant systems in the body. However, it can play a major role in sepsis through other actions. When it is activated, protein C (activated protein C [APC]) inhibits clot formation; allows natural fibrinolysis to occur; and interferes with endothelial cell changes (e.g., permeability), neutrophil attraction, and apoptosis (programmed cell death). Protein C levels are deficient in sepsis, likely at a crucial stage. By replenishing APC, the effects of APC are restored,

possibly explaining its positive impact on outcome in septic patients.

Extensions of Sepsis

As the septic process manifests itself, at least one organ will be affected. If the inflammatory response spreads to more than one organ, multiorgan dysfunction syndrome (MODS) is likely to occur. In addition, if the systemic spread produces hypotension, septic shock is likely to occur. Survival from septic shock depends on many factors, a reduced survival being associated with advanced age (>65 years), immunosuppression, or undernourishment.

Clinical Presentation

Sepsis likely occurs in phases, with the initial phase being marked by signs of SIRS (Table 46-1). Hemodynamically, the patient presents with low cardiac output and reduced levels of $ScvO_2$. Blood lactate will rise as tissue hypoxia develops. Sepsis is

TABLE 46-1. CRITERIA FOR SEPSIS

Infection
Inflammatory response to microorganisms
Invasion of normally sterile tissues
SIRS
Two or more of the following:
Core temperature >38°C or <36°C (>100.4°F or <96.8°F)
Elevated heart rate (>90 beats per min)
Respiratory rate >20 breaths per min or $Paco_2$ <32 mm Hg or mechanical ventilation for acute respiratory process
WBC count >12,000/mm³ or <4000/mm³ or >10% immature neutrophils

SIRS, systemic inflammatory response syndrome; WBC, white blood cell.

difficult to identify and a biomarker to identify sepsis is desperately needed.

The physical signs of sepsis are generated by several mechanisms. For example, several substances, such as TNF, are directly pyrogenic. Temperature elevation is common in sepsis, although hypothermia can exist. Fever is a reflection of the responses of the immune system to the initial infection and the subsequent inflammatory responses.

The patient generally is tachycardic as a result of an increased cardiac output which is secondary to a decrease in SVR. This effect is somewhat contradictory since sepsis has been demonstrated to produce myocardial depression. The increase in cardiac output is probably a consequence of an increased end-diastolic volume since ejection fraction is usually reduced.

The patient may have pulmonary symptoms reflective of increased extravascular lung water secondary to increased capillary permeability (as is seen in the acute respiratory distress syndrome). If pulmonary symptoms are present, they may result in refractory hypoxemia (PaO_2 unresponsive to oxygen therapy), generalized crackles heard on auscultation, shortness of breath, and increased production of secretions.

As the septic process continues, any organ system can be affected. For example, a change in level of consciousness may reflect central nervous system involvement or acute renal or hepatic failure. Physical signs of these organ systems failures are the same as if the organ had failed for other reasons. Specific signs of individual organ failure can be found in chapters addressing each organ. If the septic process is severe and involves multiple organs, MODS can result.

Treatment

Treatment of sepsis currently is designed to treat the infectious process, control undesirable immune responses, and provide support to any organ system in failure.

Therapies for Sepsis

According to the guidelines of the Surviving Sepsis Campaign, there are few effective treatments for sepsis. Those that do exist should be given immediately. Several organizations have emphasized the need for treatment within hours (concept of "bundles"). All therapies should be given within 24 h of recognition of sepsis. The best treatment for sepsis would be to avoid infections and, if an infection exists, to provide appropriate antibiotic support.

Cultures are necessary to identify the infectious agent. If this is unknown, broad antibiotic coverage is given. This treatment frequently employs two or three types of antibiotics; for example, Gram-positive coverage (such as a penicillin or cephalosporin), Gram-negative coverage (such as an aminoglycoside; e.g., gentamicin), and broad Gram-negative and Gram-positive coverage (e.g., imipenem). The PCCN exam generally does not require that you know the specific type of antibiotic.

Treatments for Sepsis (Table 46-2)

Goal-Directed Therapy. Research has shown that fluids, inotropes, vasopressors, and blood transfusions have better outcomes if given to improve the $ScVO_2$ level. Fluids are given, usually at a rate of about 20 mL/kg until the $ScVO_2$ is about 70%.

To monitor the $ScVO_2$ level, triple-lumen catheters are required, preferably fiber-optic catheters, to continuously monitor $ScVO_2$ levels.

The administration of dobutamine (or other inotropes) is titrated to achieve an optimal $ScVO_2$. If the blood pressure falls and is not maintained by fluids and inotropes, vasopressors may be used. The vasopressor generally utilized is either norepinephrine (Levophed), dopamine (Intropin), or phenylephrine (Neosynephrine). Vasopressin has been shown to have a positive effect on blood pressure in septic patients. It may be the preferred agent.

Activated Protein C. If the patient is at high risk of death (e.g., double-organ failure, need for vasopressors, or APACHE II score of >25), APC has been shown to improve survival. The only side effect is bleeding, with the risk of bleeding approximately 5%. If bleeding occurs, the drug should be stopped. Most of the actions of the drug will be cleared in 30 to 120 min. This drug will only be administered in ICUs and will not likely be on the exam.

Steroids. Steroid use in sepsis is currently restricted to administration only if the patient is hemodynamically unstable after fluid and vasopressor administration. This drug will only be administered in ICUs and will not likely be on the exam.

Glycemic Control. Maintaining glucose levels below 150 mg/dL has been suggested to have a positive impact on outcome in the septic patient. However, the most recent research calls into question the use of tight glycemic control. At this point, primarily keeping the blood glucose levels below 150 mg/dL is the key target.

TABLE 46-2. TREATMENTS FOR SEPSIS

Fluid resuscitation	20 mL/kg of normal saline	Used if lactate >4 mmol/L (36 mg/dL): Goals: Achieve Scvo₂ of ≥70% and (CVP) of 8–12 mm Hg
Recombinant human activated protein C (Drotrecogin alpha or Xigris)	24 µ/kg/h	Used only with high risk of death (two or more organ failures, APACHE II >25, need for vasopressors)
Steroids; e.g., hydrocortisone	200–300 mg/day for 7 days in 3 or 4 divided doses or by continuous infusion	
Optional: Add fludrocortisone to this regimen	50 mcg orally once a day	
Glycemic control	Glucose <150 mg/dL	Continuous infusion insulin and glucose or feeding (enteral preferred) Monitoring: Initially, q30–60 min After stabilization, q4h
Vasopressors: Dopamine for hypotension Norepinephrine for dopamine-refractory shock	1–20 mcg/kg/min	
Vasopressin	1–20 mcg/min 0.01–0.4 units/min	
Dobutamine for low cardiac output state	1–20 mcg/kg/min	

APACHE, acute physiology, age, and chronic health evaluation; CVP, central venous pressure; Scvo₂, central venous oxygen saturation.

Sepsis is a difficult clinical entity to understand and treat. Symptoms are inconsistent and not clear enough to differentiate sepsis from other conditions. Although our understanding of the events that occur in sepsis is improving, treatments are limited in helping improve outcomes. There is great promise for better therapies over the next several years, but the current approach is centered on supportive rather than on curative treatment.

SEPTIC SHOCK

Septic shock is a continuation of the septic process. In this situation, however, hypotension develops and is resistant to most therapies. Aggressive fluid resuscitation, inotropic support, and vasopressor application may be required to improve the Scvo₂. Unfortunately, little works at this point. The only therapy likely to reverse the tissue effects of sepsis is APC. However, even this novel therapy has limited effect if given late.

In septic shock, the likelihood of ameliorating symptoms is limited. Mortality from septic shock is high because of the lack of definitive treatment for the original septic problem.

Septic shock usually presents with hypotension secondary to a markedly reduced SVR. The Scvo₂ is elevated because of microcapillary obstruction and poor oxygen utilization at the tissue level. Cell stunning, specifically mitochondrial dysfunction, is likely one of the many mechanisms for poor utilization of oxygen. Clinically, the patient presents with a reduced blood pressure (mean arterial presssure [MAP] <65 mm Hg), tachycardia, tachypnea, warm skin (due to peripheral vasodilatation), and reduced urine output. It was originally thought that septic shock progressed to a terminal phase in which the cardiac output fell and the SVR increased, although recent evidence suggests that this stage does not necessarily occur prior to death from septic shock.

MULTIORGAN DYSFUNCTION SYNDROME

As organs fail in sepsis, the term *multiorgan dysfunction* is sometimes used. There is no real treatment for this condition other than the treatment of each organ.

Treatment for MODS is supportive of the organs failing, in conjunction with use of any of the therapies described above. It is important to remember that support of an organ is not curative. Consequently, supporting a patient on mechanical ventilation for respiratory failure secondary to sepsis may not improve survival. Perhaps all that is gained is a prolongation of life for several days until the systemic response causes other organs to fail.

Communication with the family is critical. Since survival is poor at this point, it is of paramount importance to understand whether the treatments are aligned with the patient's wishes. Family communication can be led by the nurse and critical care physician and should take place early and throughout this dangerous period.

47

Toxic Emergencies

EDITORS' NOTE

The PCCN exam will probably include only one to four questions on toxicology. These are likely to center on the immediate critical care setting, although knowledge of emergency department care may be useful. This section provides a brief but intense review of the area of toxicology. The information provided may be more than you will need; however, because this area is new to the PCCN exam, it may be best to overprepare. The other option is not to study this area in any depth and take the risk of missing these few questions; the choice is yours. Once again, do not focus on minor details but try to understand the major concepts in assessing and managing the patient with an acute overdose.

Toxic emergencies are grouped in four categories: poisonings, overdoses, drug abuse, and alcoholism. It is difficult to know the exact number of toxic ingestions that occur. Reports from poison control centers capture only a portion of toxic ingestions or exposures each year.

STATISTICS

- Of the more than two million poisonings that were reported in the United States in 2002, the majority involved children younger than 6 years and are classified as unintentional.
- Most fatalities from poisoning occur in adults and are classified as intentional.
- Over 19,000 deaths were reported to the national vital statistics for the year 2000.

- According to the Centers for Disease Control and Prevention (CDC), carbon monoxide is the number one cause of unintentional fatalities in the United States, with most deaths occurring in the winter months.
- Approximately one-half of all poisonings involving teens are classified as suicide attempts.
- In 2000, over 100,000 toxic exposures or poisonings required hospitalization.
- Poisonings account for 5% to 10% of all emergency visits and more than 5% of adult intensive care admissions.
- Acetaminophen toxicity accounts for 42% of acute liver failures in the United States.
- Every year, 20,000 people die from alcohol-related causes. This does *not* include alcohol-related automobile accidents or alcohol-induced liver disease.

A poison is defined as any substance that, when introduced into an organism, acts chemically on the tissue to produce serious injury or death. There are four routes of entry: ingestion, inhalation, injection, and surface absorption.

Poisonings most commonly involve household products such as petroleum-based agents, cleaning agents, and cosmetics. Medications are the next most frequent and most lethal source, followed by toxic plants and contaminated food. Toxic effects of ingested substances can be delayed or immediate. Delayed effects are dependent on the rate of absorption and metabolism from the gastrointestinal tract. Since most absorption occurs in the small intestine, toxins may remain in the stomach for up to several hours if a large amount of food is present. Medications or other substances that slow gastrointestinal motility may interfere. Some medications or toxins are more rapidly absorbed than others. Immediate effects of a toxin can be seen with the ingestion of corrosive substances such as strong acids or alkalis or with highly toxic and rapidly absorbed toxins such as organophosphates (pesticides) or cyanide.

TOP 12 AGENTS ASSOCIATED WITH THE HIGHEST MORTALITY RATES

1. Antidepressants
2. Analgesics (acetaminophen, aspirin)
3. Street drugs
4. Cardiovascular drugs
5. Alcohol
6. Gases and fumes (carbon monoxide)
7. Asthma therapies
8. Industrial chemicals
9. Pesticides
10. Household cleaning products
11. Anticonvulsant medications
12. Foods, plants, and insects

ASSESSMENT

Assessment begins with the taking of a history. This should include the five Ws: (1) who (patient age and previous medical history, including allergies and current therapies); (2) what (inquire about the suspected agent[s] or toxin[s] to which the patient has had access, then obtain management information from local poison control center); (3) when (determine the approximate time of ingestion, corroborating with others in contact with the patient); (4) where (it is important to know the surroundings or circumstances in order to prepare for complications, as in the case of an overdose that takes place in a running car in a garage or in a tub full of water); and (5) why (assess the patient's psychiatric stability to account for inaccuracies in the history or the intent of the patient to deliberately mislead). These questions are important tools in assessment because many initial intake histories are incorrect with respect to agent, time, and/or amount.

Patient Assessment

In dealing with a suspected toxic ingestion or exposure, it is important to refer to the local poison control center as a guide to identification of the toxin or drug, what associated symptoms to expect, and information on management of toxic exposures. Because many overdose situations involve multiple drugs or substances, it is important to identify those substances that are most likely to produce severe or life-threatening effects. The examination should include vital signs, with a temperature and respiratory rate. Cardiopulmonary stabilization and anticipation of possible deterioration should also occur during initial assessment. Cardiac monitoring, pulse oximetry, and use of a large-bore intravenous line should be initiated.

Respiratory Assessment

Respiratory rate and depth can be affected by a number of agents. Check for airway patency. An increased rate and depth can be attributed to sympathomimetics such as cocaine, amphetamines, or caffeine. An abnormal rate and pattern may be your first clue to an acid-base disorder. Tachypnea may result in primary alkalosis from salicylates or as a compensation for a dangerous metabolic acidosis, which can occur from ethylene glycol, methanol, or other agents. Assessment of lung sounds, noting the presence of crackles or wheezes, is an important part of serial assessment in patients who may have aspirated or are experiencing congestive heart failure.

Cardiovascular Assessment

Evidence of cardiac dysrhythmias, hypotension, or hypertension requires advanced cardiac life support as well as intensive care observation. Continuous cardiac monitoring is required, since life-threatening dysrhythmias can occur rapidly with such agents as tricyclics, beta blockers, or cardiac glycosides.

Neurologic Assessment

A depressed level of consciousness is a major complication in the overdose patient. Describe the patient's responses to stimuli; reflexes—presence or absence and type; as well as disturbances in vital signs. Other causes of decreased level of consciousness (e.g., trauma, diabetes, anoxia, sepsis) should be investigated. The Glasgow Coma Scale is helpful and is commonly used in neurologic assessment.

Seizures are best managed by treating the underlying cause (e.g., hypoxia, hypoglycemia, or hyponatremia). Diazepam, phenytoin, and phenobarbital can be effective in controlling seizures from nonspecific causes or until underlying causes can be determined. Seizures may be a clue to drug withdrawal; they may be seen after administration of naloxone to a comatose patient who is narcotic-dependent or after the administration of flumazenil if the patient is dependent on a benzodiazepine or tricyclic antidepressant.

Gastrointestinal Assessment

Common symptoms associated with gastrointestinal poisoning center around the loss of gastrointestinal fluids and subsequent hypovolemia. Electrolyte imbalances can occur as well. Blood loss can result from irritation of the gastric mucosa or from a Mallory-Weiss tear of the esophagus during protracted vomiting. Gastrointestinal decontamination may be a consideration in the treatment of toxic ingestions. Refer to your hospital policy and procedure manual and poison control center for information in preferred methods of decontamination for the specific toxin involved.

Hepatic and Renal Assessment

Laboratory studies are essential to assess potential damage to hepatic and renal systems. Liver function tests (e.g., serum glutamic pyruvic transaminase [SGPT], serum glutamic oxaloacetic transaminase [SGOT], and alkaline phosphatase) are useful in assessing hepatic function.

In assessment of the renal system, urine output, the presence of myoglobinuria or hematuria, as well as laboratory studies (blood urea nitrogen, creatinine) are significant in determining renal failure.

Assessment of Skin and Mucous Membranes

Such assessment can provide important clues as to the causative agent. Observe for burns or erosion of oral mucosa as well as cutaneous bullous lesions. Unexplained puncture wounds and/or contusions may be indicative of snake bites, drug abuse, or trauma.

TREATMENT

The goals in treatment for a known or suspected toxic ingestion are to remove the agent(s), detoxify the patient, and prevent absorption of the suspected agent(s).

Removal of Toxic Agents

Decontamination of Skin and Eyes
For patients with dermal exposures, prompt removal of clothing and thorough washing of the patient with mild soap and copious amounts of water are required. Emergency care providers should use protective equipment to prevent contamination by the offending agent. In patients with eye exposures, immediate eye irrigation with normal saline should be done until the ocular pH is 7.4.

Emesis
Syrup of ipecac is no longer routinely used or recommended to induce vomiting. Refer to the hospital's policy and procedure and the recommendations from the local poison control center.

Gastric Lavage
Gastric lavage is another method for removal of toxins. It involves the insertion of a large-bore orogastric tube and the instillation and removal of large amounts of water through the tube in order to empty the stomach when a recent ingestion is suspected.

Because gastric lavage is an invasive procedure, it is associated with certain risks and complications. Risks versus benefits should be determined before this procedure is performed. It is important to refer to the poison control management and your hospital's policy and procedural manual for contraindications to using gastric lavage. Airway protection is essential if this procedure is used.

Cathartics
Cathartics are used to decrease the transit time for any unabsorbed toxin, thereby minimizing absorption in the bowel. Sorbitol is a common cathartic and is an ingredient in most of the activated charcoal preparations used for patients who have ingested toxic substances. Although the use of cathartics is based primarily on empiric and anecdotal evidence, most toxicologists agree with their use as a means of decreasing gastrointestinal transit time for toxins.

Detoxification and Prevention of Absorption
Activated Charcoal. The dry, powder form of activated charcoal is an inert fine black powder. It is tasteless and odorless, and has a gritty consistency. Activated charcoal is also available as an aqueous slurry or in a suspension of 20% activated charcoal in 70% sorbitol. It can be given either orally or through a lavage tube. The charcoal slurry tends to be thick and gritty and is not very palatable when administered orally. Whenever lavage is required, it is advantageous to instill the activated charcoal prior to removal of the lavage tube. Activated charcoal is thought to be a safe,

inert, nontoxic material. No harmful effects have been shown from exposure of the skin; however, aspiration can be harmful. Although activated charcoal is useful in absorbing many toxins, there are agents that it does not appear to absorb. Refer to the poison control management to determine the recommended use. It is important to remember that activated charcoal absorbs not only toxins but also therapeutic medications. If the toxin requires giving multiple doses of charcoal, activated charcoal *without* a cathartic (sorbitol) should be considered for the additional doses.

Enhanced Elimination

Enhanced elimination of certain drugs may be implemented by making use of certain pharmacokinetic parameters that affect drug excretion. These include forced diuresis (with or without ion trapping), multiple-dose charcoal, dialysis, hemoperfusion, and plasmapheresis.

Forced Diuresis

This method involves enhanced elimination of the agent through urinary excretion. Normally, excretion takes place through glomerular filtration, active tubular secretion, and tubular reabsorption. This method deals with inhibiting tubular reabsorption only by diluting the concentration gradient between the blood and the urine. This will lessen the time during which the agent is exposed to the absorptive sites in the distal tubules.

Ion-Trapping Methods

Ion-trapping methods cause a solution to become more alkaline or acidic, so that the substance is trapped in the kidney and excretion is enhanced. Weak acids are more ionized in an alkaline solution, and weak bases are more ionized in an acidic solution.

TABLE 47-1. COMMON DRUGS AND ANTIDOTES

Drug/Toxin	Antidote/Dose	Comment
Acetaminophen: also found in combination with other over-the-counter or prescription medications	*N*-acetylcysteine oral or intravenous	Symptoms may not appear until 4–6 h after ingestion
Beta blockers; e.g., atenolol, metoprolol, labetalol	Glucagon: 1–5 mg IV for bradycardia and hypotension	Aggressive cardiac and pulmonary support
Benzodiazepines; e.g., diazepam, clorazepate, alprazolam	Flumazenil: follow pharmacy recommendations	Observe for withdrawal seizures in chronic users
Cardiac glycosides; e.g., digoxin	Digibind	Used in severe dysrhythmias or with digitoxicity with a K^+ >5–6
Carbon monoxide; e.g., car fumes, fumes from faulty heating systems	Oxygen: 100% reduces half-life of CO to 1.5 h	Hyperbaric chamber at 3 stm reduces half-life of CO to 23 min
Ethylene glycol, methanol; e.g., antifreeze	Ethyl alcohol in conjunction with dialysis	Competes for alcohol dehydrogenase; prevents formation of formic acid and oxalates. Death occurs from severe acidosis
Narcotics/opiates; e.g., morphine, codeine, propoxyphene, heroin	Naloxone 0.01 mg/kg IV	Frequent repeated doses may be needed, may precipitate acute withdrawal, so should be reserved for severe respiratory depression
Tricyclic antidepressants; e.g., amitriptyline, protriptyline, doxepin	Sodium bicabonate	Protein binding of tricyclics occurs in an alkalotic pH
Warfarin	Vitamin K	Promotes hepatic biosynthesis of prothrombin

IV, intravenous; CO, carbon monoxide.

If a difference in pH occurs across a membrane, ion trapping will occur. Alkaline diuresis is more commonly used and can be achieved by the administration of sodium bicarbonate in intravenous fluids. Usually, sodium bicarbonate (2 to 3 ampules) is added to each liter of intravenous fluids to achieve a urinary pH of 7.5 or greater. Refer to your hospital's policy and procedures for specific recommendations. This method is useful for agents that produce metabolic acidosis (salicylates), and careful monitoring of electrolytes is essential in using alkaline diuresis.

Multidose Charcoal

Multiple doses of activated charcoal appear to be effective in enhancing the elimination of drugs that undergo enterohepatic or enterogastric circulation. Activated charcoal without sorbitol should be considered for additional doses. Poison control management can provide guidance when the use of multiple doses of charcoal is being considered.

Extracorporeal Methods of Elimination

Hemodialysis. Hemodialysis can be useful in further clearance of certain substances from the body. It is usually reserved for the patient who has not responded to more conservative and conventional methods.

Antidotes

Certain drugs and toxins have specific antidotes that counteract their harmful effects (Table 47-1). It is best to use an antidote if available, although reversal of certain drugs can precipitate withdrawal symptoms and seizures. Poison control management can help to identify those toxins that have specific antidotes.

The national number for Poison Control Centers is 1-800-222-1222, available 24 h a day, 7 days a week.

Illegal/Street Drugs

Because of increasing access to and use of illegal drugs, it is important to question the patient and/or family and friends about the patient's recreational use of such substances. A urine drug toxicology screen is necessary to identify patients who have such drugs in their systems (Table 47-2).

TABLE 47-2. COMMON STREET DRUGS

Drug Name(s)	Drug Class	Route of Ingestion	Effects
Heroin (H, horse, monkey, smack)	Opioid/narcotic	Injected, snorted, smoked	CNS depression
Cocaine + heroin (speedball)	Sympathetic stimulant/opioid	Injected, snorted, smoked	CNS depression CNS and cardiac stimulation
Cocaine (blow, coke, dust, flake girl, snow)	Sympathetic stimulant	Injected, snorted	CNS and cardiac stimulation
Crack: cocaine in rock form (freebase, rock)	Sympathetic stimulant	Smoked	CNS and cardiac stimulation, vasoconstriction (CVA or MI)
Methamphetamine (crank, crystal, ice, meth, speed)	Sympathetic stimulant	Injected, smoked	CNS and cardiac stimulation
MDMA (Adam, ecstasy, X-TC, hug-drug, love-drug)	Sympathetic stimulant	Ingested, snorted, inserted rectally	CNS and cardiac stimulation
LSD (acid, dragon, red/green dragon, blotters, Zen, microdots, windowpane)	Hallucinogen	Ingested	No specific physical effects; injury or death results from paranoid or violent behavior
PCP (angel dust, crystal, supergrass, ozone, rocket fuel, whack)	Hallucinogen, sedative, paralytic	Ingested, snorted, smoked	CNS and respiratory depression, hypertension, seizures
Rohypnol (roofies; commonly called the date-rape drug)	Sedative/hypnotic	Ingested (often with alcohol)	CNS and cardiac depression, amnesia

CNS, central nervous system; CVA, cerebrovascular accident; LSD, lysergic acid diethylamide; MDMA, methylenedioxymethamphetamine; MI, myocardial infarction; PCP, phencyclidine.

TABLE 47-3. BIOLOGIC AGENTS

Agent	Route of Exposure	Symptoms	Treatment
Anthrax (bacteria)	Cutaneous contact, inhalation, ingestion	Blister-like lesions, respiratory distress, severe GI distress	Ciprofloxacin, doxycycline, penicillin, steroids
Brucella (bacteria)	Ingestion, inhalation	Acute febrile illness, respiratory symptoms without obvious signs of pneumonia	Doxycycline with streptomycin or rifampin
Pneumonic plague (bacteria)	Inhalation, inoculation (flea bites)	Severe and rapidly progressive respiratory and GI symptoms	Ciprofloxacin, doxycycline, tetracycline
Smallpox (virus)	Inhalation, cutaneous contact	Severe febrile illness, maculopapular rash	Vaccination within 3–4 days of exposure may decrease severity. Use of cidofovir is only experimental
Viral encephalitis: various forms	Inhalation	Fever, malaise, seizures	Symptomatic treatment, supportive care

GI, gastrointestinal.

TABLE 47-4. BIOLOGIC TOXINS

Agent	Route of Exposure	Symptoms	Treatment
Botulinum toxin (neurotoxin)	Ingested	Blurred vision, dry mouth, descending flaccid paralysis	Trivalent equine antitoxin from the CDC, symptomatic treatment, supportive care
Ricin (toxin extracted from castor bean)	Ingested, inhaled	Vomiting, diarrhea, rapidly progressive pulmonary edema	Symptomatic treatment, supportive care
Enterotoxin B (*Staphylococcus aureus*)	Ingested, inhaled	Severe GI symptoms, fever, nonproductive cough	

CDC, Centers for Disease Control and Prevention; GI, gastrointestinal.

TABLE 47-5. CHEMICAL AGENTS

Name	Route of Exposure	Symptoms	Treatment
Sarin, Soman (organophosphates/nerve agents)	Cutaneous contact, inhalation, ingestion	Severe cholinergic effects (lancination, salivation, sweating, pulmonary edema)	Decontamination, anticholinergics (atropine), anticonvulsants
Hydrogen, sulfur mustard (vesicant)	Cutaneous contact, inhalation, ingestion	Intense itching of skin; delayed, painless blister eruption with resulting deep burns; pulmonary edema; severe GI distress	Decontaminate with copious amounts of water, symptomatic treatment
Lewisite (vesicant)	Cutaneous contact, inhaled, ingested	Burns on contact, rapid pulmonary edema, severe GI distress	Initial decontamination with talcum powder or flour to absorb chemical, symptomatic treatment

GI, gastrointestinal.

TABLE 47-6. PULMONARY/ASPHYXIATION AGENTS

Name	Route of Ingestion	Symptoms	Treatment
Ammonia (pulmonary)	Cutaneous contact, inhalation, ingestion	Irritation and burning, respiratory distress, tracheal burns, GI distress	Symptomatic treatment; consider bronchodilators and steroids
Chlorine (pulmonary)	Cutaneous contact, inhalation, ingestion	Corrosive effects, respiratory distress, severe GI distress	Symptomatic treatment
Cyanide (cellular asphyxiation)	Cutaneous contact, inhalation, ingestion	Rapid onset of respiratory distress, nausea/vomiting	Decontamination with copious washing, cyanide antidote kit containing amyl nitrite, sodium nitrite, sodium thiosulfate

GI, gastrointestinal.

AGENTS/TOXINS OF TERRORISM

It is unlikely that many health-care facilities will treat patients with exposures to these agents or toxins, due to actual and increasing threats of terrorist events; however, it is important to have a basic awareness of the agents that have either been used in the past or that have the potential for current or future use in terrorist attacks (Tables 47-3 to 47-6).

In the event of mass casualty events, whether through acts of individuals or acts of nature, it is important to be able to access your facility's disaster management plan to determine your role in such an event.

Airway Obstruction

UPPER AIRWAY OBSTRUCTION

Upper airway obstruction is among the highest priority emergencies a critical care clinician can encounter. The prompt recognition and treatment of a partially or fully obstructed airway can mean the difference between life and death for the patient. Multiple conditions may be responsible for acute compromise of the upper airway (superior to the primary carina), all of which require prompt diagnosis followed by definitive therapy to reestablish airflow.

Identifying Characteristics

Upper airway obstruction may present either as an obvious life-threatening emergency or in a more subtle fashion depending on the degree of occlusion as well as its cause. The classic finding in a patient with a partial airway obstruction at or above the larynx is a high-pitched crowing or harsh whistle with inspiration, termed stridor. In contrast, an intrathoracic obstruction in the trachea is signaled by expiratory stridor due to the natural narrowing of the airway with expiration. Clinically, the obstructed patient may also present with dyspnea, clutching of the throat ("choking sign"), facial swelling, neck vein prominence, pallor or cyanosis, coughing, wheezing, sore throat, altered voice or phonation, dysphagia (difficulty swallowing secretions, which can lead to drooling), or accessory muscle contraction. Foreign-body aspiration is frequently accompanied by paroxysmal coughing. With complete obstruction, the patient is unable to breathe, cough, or speak and rapidly deteriorates to a state of unconsciousness.

Etiology

The underlying causes of upper airway obstruction are varied. As one might expect, foreign-body aspiration is first among these. Infectious processes such as epiglottitis, retropharyngeal abscess, laryngeal diphtheria, Ludwig's angina (a progressive submaxillary cellulitis that involves the neck and floor of the mouth, frequently following dental disease), tonsillitis, pharyngitis, mononucleosis, and otitis can all cause asphyxiation by obstruction. More commonly, the infection may actually erode a blood vessel, causing massive hemorrhage, or a purulent pocket may rupture. Noninfectious laryngeal edema may result from trauma, inhalation of noxious gases, burns, or anaphylactic shock (caused by inhalants, bee stings, drugs, contrast media, blood products), or it may follow removal of an endotracheal tube. Neck surgery, trauma, diagnostic procedures (carotid angiography), or erosion of a blood vessel by the invasion of cancerous or infectious cells may result in retropharyngeal hemorrhage.

Treatment

In cases of severe upper airway obstruction, a mixture of helium and oxygen may be administered to provide temporary support pending a definitive diagnosis and treatment plan. Severe or complete obstruction requires immediate airway control. Following institution of the head-tilt and jaw-thrust maneuver to minimize the soft tissue contribution to obstruction, the larynx and oropharynx must be inspected and any obstructive material (blood, vomitus, foreign matter) removed via suctioning. If adequate ventilation is not then achieved with a bag-valve-mask device driven by 100% oxygen, an airway must be emergently established with the placement of an endotracheal tube or by a tracheostomy or cricothyrotomy.

NEAR-DROWNING

An estimated 9000 lives are lost from drowning each year. Additionally, there are 75,000 near-drowning victims annually. Near-drowning is defined as a submersion injury after which the patient survives for at least 24 h. Drowning, on the other hand, is defined as a submersion injury that causes death within 24 h.

Identifying Characteristics

Although each near-drowning victim presents somewhat differently depending on his or her previous state of health, quantity, and type (fresh, salt, chlorinated, polluted) of water aspirated, length of time submerged, and the temperature of the water, there is a predictable sequence of events that occurs during the submersion injury. Initially, the victim begins to cough and gasp as water enters the mouth and nose, which results in a variable amount of water being swallowed. Simultaneously, as water is aspirated into the larynx, laryngospasm develops, which helps to protect the airway from further aspiration of water. Subsequently, the laryngospasm causes asphyxia, which causes the victim to lose consciousness. Hypoxemia then leads to the development of metabolic acidosis. If the victim dies during the laryngospasm phase, it may be called a "dry" drowning, or suffocation, because a large quantity of water was not aspirated. However, it is estimated that only 10% to 15% of drowning cases are dry drownings. For the other 85% to 90% of victims who aspirate at some point during the submersion injury, the loss of consciousness is thought to cause relaxation of the laryngeal muscles, which allows aspiration of water. However, it is also thought that the hypercarbic or hypoxic drives stimulate inhalation or aspiration of water, thus resulting in a "wet" drowning.

Earlier, it was believed that the inhalation of salt water, with its increased concentration of electrolytes and, thus, the ability to draw fluid into the lungs, resulted in an electrolyte imbalance and pulmonary edema. Freshwater, on the other hand, was thought to produce hemodilution and hemolysis from the hypotonic fluids. It is now believed that most near-drowning victims do not aspirate sufficient quantities of water to produce these changes. It is thought that it is the amount of aspirated water and not the type of water that results in pulmonary changes during the submersion injury. The aspiration of water decreases pulmonary compliance. Whether surfactant is washed out of the alveoli with freshwater aspiration or is denatured by salt water entering the alveoli, an intrapulmonary shunt develops, and hypoxia occurs. Therefore, the focus of attention with submersion injuries should be the management of hypoxia.

The other inherent problem with submersion injuries is hypothermia. A danger of hypothermia is the development of lethal cardiac dysrhythmias that may result in cardiac arrest. However, hypothermia may be beneficial if it occurs before the development of hypoxia. It is thought to be neuroprotective, as evidenced by those who have survived ice-water submersions for longer than 30 min, especially children.

Treatment

Patient care for the victim of near-drowning includes early endotracheal intubation with the administration of 100% oxygen at 5 to 10 cm positive end-expiratory pressure (PEEP). Early intubation may also protect the airway from the aspiration of gastric contents, which is likely with submersion injuries. In cold-water submersion injuries, cardiac dysrhythmias should be anticipated and aggressively managed. Standard resuscitation protocols should be used in the management of cardiac arrest. Because the metabolic acidosis may be severe, the administration of sodium bicarbonate may be warranted. After resuscitation, monitoring for the development of bronchospasm is necessary, and the treatment of bronchospasm, if it develops, must be aggressive. Hemodynamic monitoring may be necessary in the management of pulmonary edema.

Burns

EDITORS' NOTE

This chapter contains a large amount of information that is likely to be addressed only superficially on the PCCN exam. Do not be concerned if you do not understand or remember everything in this chapter. Try to remember major assessment categories and therapeutic maneuvers. This approach should prepare you for the few questions relating to burns on the PCCN exam.

Burn care is one of the new areas on the PCCN exam. Questions on the PCCN exam are likely to center on immediate postburn care, which is the focus of this chapter. It is possible that you will find from two to four questions on burns on the exam.

Burns are among the most devastating injuries that a nurse can encounter. They can affect multiple organ systems, beyond what appears to be the area involved. Unfortunately, burns are relatively common and are the third leading cause of accidental death in adults.

Burns can be the result of thermal, chemical, electrical, or inhalation injury. According to the American Burn Association, more than 2.5 million people in the United States experience thermal injury each year. Approximately 100,000 of those are hospitalized, and 12,000 will die. Burn mortality has improved: a 70% total body surface area (TBSA) burn today has the same 50% mortality that a 30% TBSA burn had in 1970. The best rate of survival exists for persons between 5 and 34 years of age. The very young and very old have the worst prognosis. The median age for a burn victim is 22 years. Because of the loss of body image and self-esteem,

burns can leave both physical and emotional scars that prevent a person from returning to or becoming a productive member of society. Burns typically require a prolonged rehabilitation phase. The medical and societal costs of burns are truly great.

The common variable in all burn injuries is skin damage. The skin is our largest organ system. It is composed of two layers, the epidermis and dermis. The epidermis is the outer, thinner layer. The dermis is a deeper, thicker layer that contains the hair follicles, sweat glands, sebaceous glands, and sensory fibers (Fig. 49-1).

The skin is our first defense against infection and injury. It protects us from the environment, prevents loss of body fluids, regulates body temperature, and provides sensory contact with the environment through pain, touch, pressure, and temperature.

Burns are classified by the extent of TBSA affected and the depth of skin damage. The extent of a burn is a product of the temperature generated by the heat source and the exposure time. The center of the burn wound has the most contact with the heat source. The cells have been coagulated and are necrotic. This area is referred to as the zone of coagulation. Lying next to the zone of coagulation is the zone of stasis. This area has cells that have been injured but are not necrotic. If proper resuscitation occurs, these cells will survive; however, they will usually become necrotic within 24 to 48 h and extend the severity of the burn. The outermost area of the burn wound is the zone of hyperemia. These cells have suffered the least injury and usually recover in 7 to 10 days. The "rule of nines" formula is used to estimate the TBSA involved (Fig. 49-2), but this method gives only a gross estimate. A more exact measure of TBSA involvement can be calculated with the use of more detailed charts (e.g., Lund and Browder); however, the charts must be available for use and are not

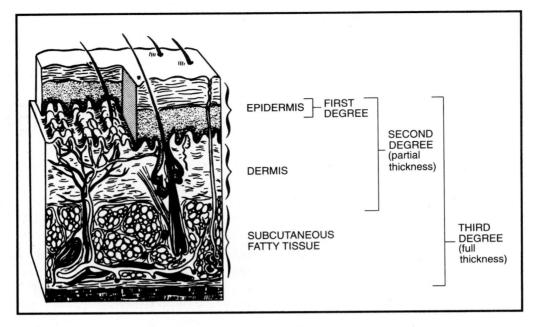

Figure 49-1. Anatomy of the skin. The depth of injury determines whether a burn will heal or require skin grafting. (From Kravitz, M. [1988]. Thermal injuries. In Cardona, V. D., Hurn, B. J., Mason, P. J. B., Scanlon, A. M., and Veise-Berry, S. W. [Eds.]. *Trauma nursing* [p. 709]. Philadelphia: Saunders. With permission.)

easily committed to memory. The TBSA can also be estimated with the use of the victim's palm, which is equal to 1% of the TBSA. This is a useful method with scattered or irregular patterns of burns. The extent of TBSA involved is used to calculate the patient's fluid replacement needs.

CLASSIFICATION

The depth of the burn will determine to what degree or whether any skin grafting is needed. Variable destruction of skin can occur. Formerly, burns were classified as first-, second-, or third-degree. More recently, burns have been subdivided into partial- and full-thickness wounds (Fig. 49-1). The partial-thickness wounds are further divided into superficial and deep wounds.

First-degree burns damage the epidermis, or superficial layer of the skin. The wounds appear pink, dry (no blistering), and slightly edematous; they are painful. Clinically, first-degree burns are of little importance and are not typically considered in fluid replacement.

Second-degree, or partial-thickness, burns destroy the epidermis and varying degrees of the dermis. The wounds appear blistered and are painful, and blanching will be detected.

Third-degree, or full-thickness, burns destroy both the epidermis and dermal layers of the skin. These burns may extend into the subcutaneous tissue to muscle and may even reach bone. The wounds appear dry, hard, and leathery, and no blanching is detected as a result of destruction of the capillary bed. A common misconception is that the wound is painless since the nerve endings are destroyed. However, the patients may experience deep somatic pain from ischemia or inflammation. Wound edges may also be hypersensitive in making the transition from third-degree to less severely burned areas.

INITIAL MANAGEMENT

The initial management of a burn victim is to stop the burning process. This is usually accomplished before the patient receives hospital care, but, depending on the type of burn, irrigation may still be necessary once the patient reaches the hospital. All clothing must be removed, including jewelry, which can retain heat, have a tourniquet-like effect on limbs, and cause neurovascular compromise. As with all trauma patients, attention must then be given to airway management, assistance with breathing, and support of circulation as needed. The possibility of other injuries must also be assessed, with

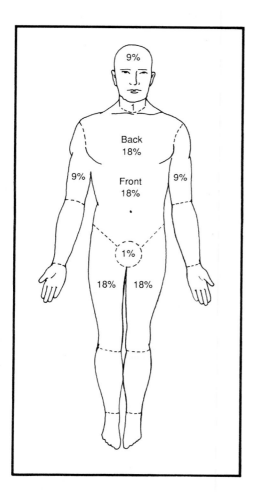

Figure 49-2. The rule of nines. (Adapted from Rue, L. W., III, & Cioffi, W. [1991]. Resuscitation of thermally injured patients. *Critical Care Nursing Clinics of North America, 3*[2], 183. With permission.)

management as appropriate. Since victims of major burns are often intubated at the scene or in the emergency department, a history must be obtained from witnesses, rescue personnel, and/or family members.

BURN SHOCK

Burn shock has both a cellular and a hypovolemic component. Burns of less than 20% TBSA have primarily a local response, whereas major burns of greater than 20% to 25% TBSA have a systemic response. The greater the percentage of burn, the greater the systemic response.

Initially, burn patients experience a rise in capillary hydrostatic pressure and an increase in capillary permeability. Rapid fluid shifts occur, with fluid moving from the intravascular space to the interstitium, causing edema formation within the wound and a decrease in circulating blood volume. The cardiac output can decrease as much as 50% in the first hour if adequate resuscitation is not initiated. Catecholamine release may further compromise cardiac output by causing the heart to pump against increased systemic vascular resistance. The greatest fluid shifts occur during the first 6 to 8 h postburn. Adequate and rapid fluid replacement is required to prevent hypovolemic shock. As a result of decreased cardiac output, the systemic vascular resistance increases in an attempt to preserve some organ perfusion and protect the blood pressure. This increase in systemic vascular resistance, however, further depresses cardiac output. Myocardial depressant factors may also play a role in lowering cardiac output, but attempts to isolate them have been inconclusive.

Fluid requirements are based on the percentage of TBSA burned. The clinician must keep in mind that this is only an estimate, and the patient's response to therapy must be closely monitored to assist with fluid replacement and adjust fluid rates accordingly. Many formulas exist to calculate fluid replacement (Table 49-1). The most frequently used calculation is the Parkland formula, which is 4 mL/kg/% TBSA of lactated Ringer's solution. Most agree that colloids are not to be used during the first 24 h since the degree of capillary leakage is so severe that the large colloid molecules will also pass through the capillaries. Fifty percent of the calculated fluid requirement is given in the first 8 h postburn; the remaining 50% is given over the last 16 h. It may be necessary for the critical care nurse to catch up on fluid requirements that have not been adequately met early in the patient's care. Remember that fluid replacement is based on the first 24 h after injury, not after hospital admission. The nurse must inquire about prior fluid administration and time of injury and also obtain an accurate weight. Clinical indicators of adequate fluid resuscitation are maintenance of a stable blood pressure with a urine output of 0.5 to 1.0 mL/kg/h. Invasive hemodynamic monitoring is usually required only in high-risk patients who have underlying cardiopulmonary disorders or those who are not responding as predicted. Patients who may require higher than expected fluid requirements are those with inhalation injury, underlying dehydration preburn, or electrical burns. The most common reason for low urine output and low blood pressure is inadequate fluid resuscitation. However, if invasive hemodynamic monitoring indicates that fluid volume is adequate, inotropic agents may be necessary. Because of

TABLE 49-1. FORMULAS FOR FLUID REPLACEMENT/RESUSCITATION

Name of Resuscitation Regime	FIRST 24 H			SECOND 24 H		
	Electrolyte	Colloid	Glucose in Water	Electrolyte	Colloid	Glucose in Water
Burn budget of F.D. Moore	1000–4000 mL lactated Ringer's solution and 1200 mL 0.5N saline	7.5% of body weight	1500–5000 mL	1000–4000 mL lactated Ringer's solution and 1200 mL 0.5N saline	2.5% of body weight	1500–5000 mL
Evans	Normal saline, 1 mL/kg/% burn	1 mL/kg/% burn	2000 mL	One-half of first 24-h requirement	One-half of first 24-h requirement	2000 mL
Brooke	Lactated Ringer's solution, 1.5 mL/kg/% burn	0.5 mL/kg/% burn	2000 mL	One-half to three-fourths of first 24-h requirement	One-half to three-fourths of first 24-h requirement	2000 mL
Parkland	Lactated Ringer's solution, 4 mL/kg/% burn				20%–60% of calculated plasma volume	
Hypertonic sodium solution	Volume to maintain urine output at 30 mL/h (fluid contains 250 mEq Na/L)			One-third of salt solution orally, up to 3500 mL limit		
Modified Brooke	Lactated Ringer's solution, 2 mL/kg/% burn				0.3–0.5 mL/kg/% burn	Goal: maintain adequate urinary output
Burnett Burn Center	Isotonic or hypertonic alkaline sodium solution/% burn/kg			D_5 1/4 NS maintenance	Colloid 0.5 mL/% burn/kg	D_5W (% burn) (TBSAm^2)

Source: Hudak C, Gallo B, Berg J. *Critical care nursing: A holistic approach* (5th ed.) by C. Hudak, B. Gallo, & J. Berg, 1990, Philadelphia: Lippincott, p. 766. With permission.

the large amount of catecholamine released postburn, larger than normal doses of inotropic agents may be necessary since some downregulation of the receptors may occur.

Capillary integrity returns to normal by 24 to 36 h postburn, resulting in decreased loss of fluid and protein into the wounds. If fluid resuscitation has been adequate, cardiac output will return to normal and then proceed to a hyperdynamic level, at which cardiac output is above normal. At this point, the goal of fluid therapy changes compared with the first 24 h and is now meant to maintain organ perfusion. Inadequate fluid resuscitation can lead to acute tubular necrosis, stress ulcers, and conversion of partial-thickness wounds to full-thickness wounds. Colloids may now be given to help replace the plasma volume deficit. Approximately 10% of red blood cell mass is decreased after thermal injury. Most is lost as a result of direct destruction by heat but other causes may include hemorrhage, wound stasis, and increased fragility of the red blood cells. Because of the large sodium load given in the first 24 h, patients usually have a whole-body excess of sodium. Fluid management is aimed at helping the patient excrete the large sodium and water load obtained during initial resuscitation. Rapid sodium shifts should be avoided since cerebral edema may result. The patient's weight

and serum sodium level are used to guide fluid replacement.

Overresuscitation should be avoided, as it can have serious consequences, such as pulmonary edema or excessive wound edema, inhibiting perfusion either locally or distally to the wound. Decreased local wound perfusion can cause conversion of wounds from partial to full thickness. Decreased perfusion distally can lead to neurovascular compromise of extremities.

Current research is looking into alternatives in fluid resuscitation. One possibility is the use of high-osmolar solutions such as hypertonic lactate saline, 7.5% sodium chloride, or 6% dextran 70. In theory, high-osmolar solutions will cause a rapid shift of fluid from the intracellular compartment to the intravascular space, expanding plasma volume. This improvement in cardiovascular performance, however, may be only transient. The potential risks of high-osmolar solutions are cellular dehydration and hypernatremia.

The ability of hypertonic solutions to produce less wound edema may be advantageous, particularly in patients with inhalation injuries, circumferential full-thickness burns of extremities, and intracranial injuries. Serum sodium levels must be monitored closely since serum sodium exceeding 160 mEq/L is associated with oliguria and mental status changes.

FLUID REMOBILIZATION PHASE

Fluid remobilization or diuresis usually begins 48 to 72 h postburn and lasts 1 to 3 days. Fluid shifts from the interstitial space into the intravascular compartment, causing a great increase in blood volume. As a result, urine volume will increase. Caution should be used with fluid volume replacement since giving large amounts during this phase may lead to fluid overload. The nurse must assess the patient for signs of volume overload such as venous distention, crackles, and frothy sputum. Patients with impaired renal or cardiovascular function are at high risk during this time since they may be less likely to handle the large fluid shifts. Most patients return to preburn weight by postinjury day 10. Remember that loss of skin integrity will increase water loss by evaporation.

OTHER INITIAL MANAGEMENT

Patients with a greater than 15% TBSA burn should have a nasogastric tube inserted and hooked to low continuous suction. These patients are prone to paralytic ileus. Gastric prophylaxis should be initiated since burn patients are prone to stress ulcers.

Pain relief is an essential treatment for burn victims. Typically, narcotics are given intravenously in small doses until pain relief is achieved. Because of the unpredictability of circulation and absorption, intramuscular and subcutaneous routes should not be utilized.

Edema formation related to initial fluid shifts occurs both locally at the wound sites and systemically in burns of greater than 20% TBSA. Edema formation may cause neurovascular compromise to the extremities; therefore, frequent assessments are necessary to evaluate pulses, skin color, capillary refill, and sensation. Arterial circulation is at greatest risk on circumferential burns. The Doppler flow probe may be the best way to evaluate compromise. Elevating extremities may help decrease some of the edema formation. An escharotomy may be required to restore arterial circulation, prevent ischemia and necrosis, and allow for further swelling. Eschar, which forms from full-thickness burns, is tight, leathery, and nondistensible and does not have pain fibers. The escharotomy can be performed at the bedside, utilizing a sterile field and scapel (Fig. 49-3). Care should be taken to avoid major nerves, vessels, and tendons. The incision should extend through the length of the eschar, over joints, and down to the subcutaneous fat. The incision is placed laterally or

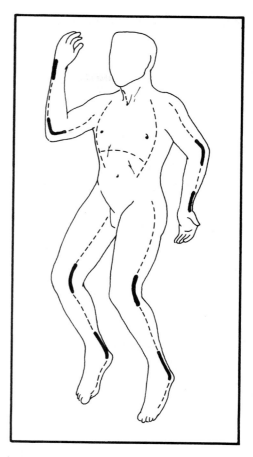

Figure 49-3. Preferred sites of escharotomy incisions. (Redrawn from Rue L. W., III, & Cioffi, W. [1991]. Resuscitation of thermally injured patients. *Critical Care Nursing Clinics of North America, 3*[2], 181-189. With permission.)

medially on the extremity. If a single incision does not restore circulation, bilateral incisions will be required.

Circumferential burns can also cause problems when they occur on the chest. Adequacy of ventilation must be assessed continually. Ventilatory excursion may be restricted, requiring a chest escharotomy. Bilateral incisions should be made down the anterior axillary line. If burns are extensive, the incision may be extended onto the abdomen. The incisions are then connected by a transverse incision along the costal margin.

WOUND MANAGEMENT

Treatment of other life-threatening conditions takes priority over burn wound management. Initially, the burn wound should be covered with clean sheets. Ice is never used to treat burns because of the susceptibility to hypothermia or frostbite. If transfer to a burn center is anticipated, it is not necessary to debride or apply topical antimicrobial agents within the first 24 h.

Besides hypovolemia, the major threat to the patient is sepsis of the burn wound. The incidence of infection varies with burn size, patient's age and current health, and type of bacteria. None of the topical antimicrobials sterilizes the wound, but they do control bacterial proliferation and provide the best control over bacterial growth. The most common topical antimicrobial agents are mafenide acetate (Sulfamylon), silver sulfadiazine (Silvadene), or 0.5% silver nitrate soaks. The nonviable eschar is an ideal environment for bacterial growth. Systemic antibiotics have little control over this bacterial growth since they are unable to reach the injured tissue. Systemic antibiotics are reserved for severe wound infections.

Once a patient is hemodynamically stable, wound care begins. All burned areas are cleansed once or twice daily with normal saline or an antimicrobial liquid detergent. Loose and necrotic tissue is gently removed, with care taken not to damage viable tissue or cause excessive bleeding. Large blisters (>2 cm in diameter) are debrided. Once the wounds are cleansed, a topical antimicrobial agent is applied. One of two methods is utilized depending on the philosophy of the burn center. The open method applies the antimicrobial agent sterilely and leaves the wound open to the air. Advantages of this method are that it allows for constant wound assessment, eliminates painful dressing changes, and may limit bacterial proliferation. The closed method also applies an antimicrobial agent, but then covers the wound with a gauze dressing. Advantages include less heat loss and faster eschar separation.

The common recommendation is that if a burn wound will not heal in 10 to 14 days, excision should be undertaken to improve functional and cosmetic results, decrease length of hospital stay, and reduce cost of care. Superficial partial-thickness burns, if protected from infection, usually heal in 7 to 10 days, with a functional and cosmetic result that cannot be improved upon by excision and grafting. Deep partial-thickness burns will require 10 to 21 days to heal. After healing, hypertrophic scar formation often results. The amount of scar is proportional to the time required for healing. Full-thickness burns have no surviving skin appendages and so require excision and grafting to achieve definitive closure.

Excision of burn tissue is usually done by a tangential technique. Blood loss associated with this procedure can be large, with some estimates at 9% of circulating blood volume per percentage of body surface excised. The endpoint of excision is the presence of uniformly dense capillary bleeding from the entire bed of the burn wound. Since approximately 20% of burn wound debridements induce bacteremia, systemic antibiotics are administered prophylactically in the perioperative period. Patients with burns of greater than 50% TBSA will require staging of successive operations to achieve complete burn excision and coverage. The use of meshed autografts, or a biological dressing or skin substitute followed by autograft, or, more recently, the application of cultured epidermal autografts, permits timely closure of even massive burn wounds that have been excised.

INHALATION INJURY

With any burn situation, the clinician must consider the possibility of an inhalation injury, since 80% of all fire victims die of smoke inhalation. Death at the scene of a fire is almost always a result of smoke inhalation. The degree of thermal injury, however, is not an indication of the presence or absence of inhalation injury. Inhalation injury can occur from direct thermal injury or inhalation of carbon monoxide or other toxic gases that result from incomplete combustion.

Patients at risk for smoke inhalation are those with a history of being in a closed space where fire was present and/or flame burned of the face, neck, and chest. Early recognition and intervention is critical to the patient's survival. Suspect smoke inhalation if you observe singed nasal hairs; mucosal burns of the nose, lips, mouth, or throat; carbonaceous or sooty material in sputum; or hoarseness. If inhalation injury is suspected, the patient should be intubated immediately. Airway edema can occur rapidly, making it impossible to insert an endotracheal tube.

Direct thermal damage occurs usually just to the upper respiratory tract. Heat is dissipated by the upper respiratory tract in the nasal pharynx and upper airways. Cellular damage occurs, leading to tissue swelling and edema. Airway obstruction can result. Direct thermal injury below the glottis is rare but may occur with steam exposure. Pulmonary edema develops in 5% to 30% of inhalation injury patients. The lower respiratory tract injury is most often the result of inhalation of noxious gases. Destruction of surfactant can occur, resulting in a high incidence of acute respiratory distress syndrome.

Carbon monoxide is a product of incomplete hydrocarbon combustion. It has a 200 times greater affinity for hemoglobin than oxygen. As a result, carbon monoxide attaches to hemoglobin, displacing oxygen and making less oxygen available to the cells. The oxyhemoglobin dissociation curve shifts to the left, so the oxygen on the hemoglobin is not readily given up to the cells. Carbon monoxide also attacks the cytochrome oxidase system, which affects mitochondrial activity and thus further decreases cellular oxygenation. The result can be massive tissue hypoxia. A pulse oximeter (SpO_2) will provide an inaccurate assessment of hemoglobin oxygen saturation. The pulse oximeter sees oxyhemoglobin and carboxyhemoglobin as the same, so the (SpO_2) reading will be falsely elevated. Carboxyhemoglobin levels should be drawn on admission to the emergency department and repeated every 4 h until the level returns to normal.

Treatment of inhalation injuries includes first the maintenance of a patent airway. Prophylactic intubation carries little risk when compared to the danger of complete airway obstruction. The greatest risk of laryngeal and upper airway edema is 12 to 36 h postinjury. Oxygen therapy should be instituted early. Carbon monoxide elimination can be decreased from 4 h to 45 min with an inspired oxygen concentration of 100%. Hyperbaric oxygen therapy can shorten the time even more. Ventilatory support with positive end-expiratory pressure and continuous positive airway pressure will be required since the patient often experiences decreased lung compliance and atelectasis. Following airway edema and pulmonary edema, the third stage of an inhalation injury is bronchopneumonia. Bronchopneumonia occurs 3 to 10 days postexposure in 15% to 60% of the patients and carries a mortality rate of 50% to 80%. A high incidence of sepsis is associated with the development of bronchopneumonia. Antibiotics should be given for documented infections.

ELECTRICAL BURNS

Electrical burns result from electrical energy being converted to heat. Electrical injuries are divided into high-voltage (>1000 V) or low-voltage injuries. In the United States, alternating current (AC) is more common, with direct current (DC) found predominately in industry. AC is more dangerous than DC.

The point of contact will receive the greatest heat. Electricity will travel through the body in the path of least resistance. Nerves offer the least resistance, followed by blood vessels, then muscle, with bone offering the most resistance. Electrical burns can be difficult, at best, to assess. The skin may appear intact except for entrance and exit wounds, while the underlying tissues may be injured to the point of necrosis.

Electrical burns can cause vascular disruption, resulting in hemorrhage and/or thrombus formation. Underlying edema and swelling can cause compartment syndrome. Breakdown of muscle can cause myoglobin to be released into the circulation (rhabdomyolysis). Myoglobinuria is suspected if pink to dark red pigment is noted in the urine. If not excreted, myoglobin can precipitate in the renal tubules and cause renal failure. Myoglobinuria is treated by keeping urine output up with crystalloids, mannitol, and the administration of sodium bicarbonate since myoglobin is excreted better in alkaline urine.

Because it is difficult to estimate the extent of the burn, fluids are generally given to maintain a urine output of 75 to 100 mL/h. If the urine is clear, fluids can be given to maintain a urine output of 30 to 50 mL/h. Peripheral pulses, skin color, capillary refill, and sensation are assessed hourly to monitor for compartment syndrome. Fasciotomies may be necessary if vascular compromise occurs.

A 12-lead electrocardiogram (ECG) is obtained on admission, followed by continuous ECG monitoring since dysrhythmias may develop. Wound care is the same as with thermal burns.

CHEMICAL BURNS

Chemical burns result from direct contact with agents such as acids, alkalis, and/or petroleum-based products. The severity of chemical injury is related to the agent, concentration, volume, and duration of contact. Alkaline chemicals cause the most serious burns. Treatment consists of removing saturated clothing, brushing any powder from the skin, and irrigating with large amounts of water or normal saline. Irrigation should be continued until the patient experiences a decrease in pain in the wound. Alkaline substances require longer irrigation than acids. It may be necessary to contact a regional poison control center to determine the best methods to neutralize the chemicals. Personnel caring for patients exposed to chemical agents must always wear protective clothing in the form of a gown, gloves, goggles, and mask to avoid contact with the chemical.

Petroleum burns (gasoline or diesel fuel) can often produce full-thickness burns that initially appear to involve only a partial thickness. Systemic toxicity may appear with evidence of pulmonary, hepatic, or renal failure. Care must be taken not to ignite the gasoline or diesel fuel. Tar or asphalt burns should be cooled with water but will require a petroleum product like mineral oil to dissolve the substance.

Hydrofluoric acid burns can be life threatening since inhalation of this acid can cause pulmonary edema. The activity of fluoride in soft tissue combines with calcium or magnesium to produce an insoluble salt. Copious irrigation may be followed with a local injection of 5% to 10% calcium gluconate. Relief of pain following injection is immediate.

BIBLIOGRAPHY

Ahrens, T., & Tuggle, D. (2004). Surviving severe sepsis: Early recognition and treatment. *Critical Care Nurse Oct*(Suppl), 2–15.

Angus, D. C., & Abraham, E. (2005). Intensive insulin therapy in critical illness. *American Journal of Respiratory and Critical Care Medicine, 172*(11), 1358–1359.

Bernard, G. R., Margolis, B. D., Shanies, H. M., Ely, E. W., Wheeler, A. P., Levy, H., . . . Wright, T. J. (2004). Extended Evaluation of Recombinant Human Activated Protein C United States Investigators. Extended evaluation of recombinant human activated protein C United States Trial (ENHANCE US): A single-arm, phase 3B, multi-center study of drotrecogin alfa (activated) in severe sepsis. *Chest, 125*(6), 2206–2216.

Barclay, L., & Murata, P. (2005). Acetaminophen may be the leading cause of acute liver failure. *Hepatolog, 42,* 1252–1254, 1364–1372.

Centers for Disease Control: National Center for Injury Prevention and Control (2004). Poisonings: Fact sheet. http://www.cdc.gov/nicpc/factsheets/poisonings.htm Accessed 12/5/2005.

Hollenberg, S. M., Ahrens, T. S., Annane, D., Astiz, M. E., Chalfin, D. B., Dasta, J. F., . . . Zanotti-Cavazzoni, S. (2004). Practice parameters for hemodynamic support of sepsis in adult patients: 2004 update. *Critical Care Medicine, 32*(9), 1928–1948.

Mackenzie, A. F. (2005). Activated protein C: Do more survive? *Intensive Care Medicine, 31*(12), 1624–1626.

McKinley, M. G. (2005). Alcohol withdrawal syndrome. *Critical Care Nurse 25,* 40–48.

Missouri Department of Health and Senior Services: Center for Emergency Response and Terrorism. (June 2004). *Biological, Chemical and Radiological Terrorism: Basic Information for Medical Professionals.*

Mokhlesi, B., Garimella, P. S., Joffe, A., Velho, V. (2004). Street drug abuse leading to critical illness. *Intensive Care Medicine, 30,* 1526–1536.

Mokhlesi, B., Leiken, J. B., Murray, P., Corbridge, T. C. (2003a). Part I: General approach to the intoxicated patient. *Chest, 123,* 577–592.

Mokhlesi, B., Leiken, J. B., Murray, P., Corbridge, T. C. (2003b). Adult toxicology in critical care: Part II. Specific poisonings. *Chest, 123,* 897–922.

Rivers, E. P., McIntyre, L., Morro, D. C., Rivers, K. K. (2005). Early and innovative interventions for severe sepsis and septic shock: Taking advantage of a window of opportunity. *Canadian Medical Association Journal, 173*(9), 1054–1065.

Zimmerman, J. (2003). Poisonings and overdoses in the intensive care unit: General and specific management issues. *Critical Care Medicine, 31,* 2794–2801.

Multisystem Organ Dysfunction Practice Exam

1. A blood culture report returns for a 73-year-old man who is on your unit for possible sepsis. The report states that he has *Escherichia coli* (a Gram-negative bacterium) in the blood. He is currently receiving gentamicin, imipenem, and cefoxitin. Based on the report, which drug is likely to have the best effect?
(A) Cefoxitin.
(B) Imipenem.
(C) Gentamicin.
(D) They all work about the same.

2. Activated protein C is of potential benefit in treating which of the following?
(A) Sepsis and acute renal failure
(B) Sepsis and acute respiratory distress syndrome (ARDS)
(C) Acute renal failure and ARDS
(D) All of the above

3. Which of the following organs is/are likely to be affected in multisystem organ dysfunction?
(A) Liver and kidney
(B) Liver and lungs
(C) Kidney and lungs
(D) All of the above

4. A 19-year-old woman is admitted to your unit after an argument with her parents. Her parents state that they found her in her room with an empty bottle of acetaminophen (Tylenol) on her nightstand. Which of the following is the initial treatment for an overdose of acetaminophen?
(A) Ipecac
(B) Charcoal and intravenous *N*-acetylcysteine
(C) Dialysis
(D) Lavage and oral *N*-acetylcysteine

5. A 20-year-old man is admitted to your unit following a suicide attempt after a breakup with his girlfriend. He ingested an unknown drug or drugs. He is currently combative with a reduced level of consciousness. A large-bore nasogastric tube has been inserted in an attempt to lavage his stomach. Which of the following nursing actions should be initiated at this point?
(A) Protection against aspiration
(B) Intubation and mechanical ventilation
(C) Sedation to reduce the combativeness
(D) All of the above

Questions 6 and 7 refer to the following scenario:

A 47-year-old man is admitted to the hospital following complaint of an infection he developed after stepping on a nail that penetrated his boot. He now has a cellulitis of his right lower leg. During his stay on your unit, his level of consciousness has changed. He is now arousable only by deep stimuli. The laboratory results and vital signs data are:

Blood pressure	88/54 mm Hg
Pulse	126
Respiratory rate	24
Temperature	39°C
HCO_3^-	18
White blood cells	31,000
BUN	38
ALT	433
Hemoglobin	13
Creatinine	2.6
AST	512
Alkaline phosphatase	199

6. Based on this information, which condition is likely to be developing?
   (A) Guillain-Barré syndrome
   (B) ARDS
   (C) Sepsis and multisystem organ dysfunction syndrome (MODS)
   (D) Amyotrophic lateral sclerosis

7. Treatment for this condition is most likely to include which of the following?
   (A) Increased intravenous fluids
   (B) Plasmapheresis
   (C) Dopamine
   (D) Beta blockers, such as propranolol or esmolol

8. Which of the following are the most characteristic responses of the cardiovascular system to sepsis?
   (A) Increased ejection fraction and increased cardiac output
   (B) Increased ejection fraction and reduced systemic vascular resistance
   (C) Increased cardiac output and reduced systemic vascular resistance
   (D) All of the above

9. A 54-year-old woman is in your unit with acute hepatic failure from hepatitis C. She is under evaluation for a liver transplant and for management of a persistent fever (temperature >39°C). She has become hypotensive (84/50 mm Hg) and tachycardic (130 beats per minute). Based on this information, which condition explains her current clinical status?
   (A) Portal hypertension
   (B) Left ventricular failure
   (C) Hypovolemia secondary to loss of plasma proteins
   (D) Sepsis

Questions 10 and 11 refer to the following scenario:

A 19-year-old soldier is brought to your hospital from a foreign country for treatment of an unidentifiable source of inflammation. He is restless, responsive only to deep pain, and appears to be uncomfortable. His urine output has been 400 mL for the past 24 h. The following physical and laboratory information is available:

Blood pressure	100/54 mm Hg
Pulse	133
Respiratory rate	38
Temperature	39.5°C
White blood cells	19,300

Red blood cells	3,500,300
Hb	11
Hct	32
Na^+	155
K^+	3.9
Cl^-	111
HCO_3^-	26

10. Based on this information, the physician prescribes a fluid bolus with 500 mL of D_5W. Which of the following findings support this order?
    (A) K^+ of 3.9 and Na^+ level of 155
    (B) Red blood cell count of 3,500,300 and clinical picture of systemic inflammation
    (C) Na^+ level of 155, urinary Na^+ of 9, and clinical picture of sepsis
    (D) All of the above

11. Given an unknown source of inflammation, which of the following therapies would most likely be prescribed?
    (A) Aminoglycosides (e.g., gentamicin) and anti-inflammatory agents (e.g., methylprednisolone)
    (B) Aminoglycosides and cephalosporins (e.g., cefoxitin)
    (C) Anti-inflammatory agents and cephalosporins
    (D) All of the above

12. A 38-year-old woman is on your unit with a fever of unknown origin. She has developed acute shortness of breath. Her mental status is confused and she is restless. Her vital signs and laboratory data are:

Blood pressure	136/82 mm Hg
Pulse	127
Respiratory rate	34
Temperature	38.8°C
PaO_2	65
$PaCO_2$	34
pH	7.31
HCO_3^-	17

One of your fellow nurses states that in systemic inflammatory responses, as in this patient's case, oxygen consumption and energy requirements are increased. Another nurse says that this is not always true, that only in some instances are energy requirements increased. Which data suggest that this patient has increased energy expenditure and oxygen consumption?
    (A) Respiratory rate of 34 and PaO_2 of 65
    (B) Respiratory rate of 34 and temperature of 38.8°C

(C) PaO$_2$ of 65 and temperature of 38.8°C

(D) All of the above

13. Which of the following are the two most common sources of infection in the hospital patient population?

(A) Urinary tract infection and respiratory system infection.

(B) Urinary tract infection and central nervous system infection.

(C) Respiratory system infection and central nervous system infection.

(D) They are all equal in the incidence of infections.

Multisystem Organ Dysfunction Practice Exam

Practice Fill-Ins

1. _____   5. _____   9. _____   13. _____
2. _____   6. _____   10. _____
3. _____   7. _____   11. _____
4. _____   8. _____   12. _____

PART VIII

Answers

1. __C__	5. __A__	9. __D__	13. __A__
2. __B__	6. __C__	10. __C__	
3. __D__	7. __A__	11. __B__	
4. __B__	8. __C__	12. __B__	

IX

SYNERGY

....

Ruth M. Kleinpell

Professional Caring and Ethical Practice

EDITORS' NOTE

Professional Caring and Ethical Practice make up approximately 20% of the PCCN exam. These questions address the content areas of professional caring, ethical practice, and components of the Synergy Model, which serves as the organizing framework for the PCCN exam. The Synergy Model states that the needs or characteristics of patients and families influence and drive the characteristics or competencies of nurses. Components of Professional Caring and Ethical Practice outlined in the blueprint for the PCCN exam relate to the nursing characteristics of the model, which include advocacy/moral agency, caring practices, collaboration, systems thinking, response to diversity, clinical inquiry, and facilitation of learning. The PCCN exam questions cover application of the Synergy Model, not its terminology or model components.

This chapter contains information related to Professional Caring and Ethical Practice and the application of content to clinical care.

PROFESSIONALISM IN NURSING

Professional Caring and Ethical Practice

Professional nursing practice focuses on providing excellent clinical care as well as promoting the best outcomes for patients. The goal of professional nursing practice is to provide patient-centered care, focusing on the cultural and ethnic diversity of patients and their significant others. The hallmarks of professional nursing practice include a philosophy of clinical care emphasizing quality, safety, multidisciplinary collaboration, and professional accountability, behaviors, and actions.

Professional nursing practice incorporates the use of clinical judgment skills including clinical reasoning and critical thinking, serving as an advocate to present the concerns of the patient and family, and demonstrating caring practices to provide for physical and psychosocial needs. In addition, promoting a healing environment, incorporating evidence-based practices, and instituting interventions to promote best patient outcomes are incorporated in providing professional nursing care.

An important aspect of progressive care nursing is helping the patient and family to manage their responses to acute illness. These include:

- Stress
- Crisis
- Fear/anxiety
- Loneliness
- Powerlessness
- Anger
- Depression
- Denial
- Death and dying

Additional concepts of focus for professional nursing practice include patient- and family-centered care. Knowledge and recognition of anxiety and stress, promoting coping strategies, and meeting the needs of families of acutely ill hospitalized patients are essential aspects of nursing care. It is important to recognize that each family system is unique and varies by culture, values, religion, previous experience with crisis, health beliefs, and communication styles. The recognition and acknowledgment of diversity in patients and families requires that the nurse appreciate and incorporate differences while providing care. Additional areas of diversity include:

- Ethnicity
- Race
- Spiritual beliefs
- Family configuration
- Socioeconomic status
- Age
- Values
- Alternative medicine

In addressing family needs, a focus on the unique viewpoints and needs of families is essential. Research on the needs of families during acute illness has identified that the need for information, honest answers, reassurance, and hope are important areas that should be addressed by nursing care. Additional family needs include having questions answered, knowing the prognosis, knowing the treatment, being near the patient, and having support available.

Several ethical principles guide nursing care, including the principles of respect, autonomy, beneficence, nonmaleficence, and justice. Respect for persons focuses on treating patients and families as autonomous agents, and remembering that patients with diminished autonomy are entitled to protection. *Autonomy* is the duty to maximize the individual's right to make his or her own decisions. *Beneficence* promotes doing no harm and maximizing possible benefits and minimizing possible harms in providing patient care. The Hippocratic Oath's "Do no harm" admonition has long been a fundamental principle of medical ethics. The principle of *nonmaleficence* identifies the duty to cause no harm. *Justice* is the duty to treat all patients fairly, distributing the risks and benefits of treatment equally. An awareness of ethical principles is important, as they have significant impact on nursing care. Some specific examples of managing ethical issues in progressive care nursing include:

- Code versus no-code decision
- Technology versus cost
- Resource allocation and triage decisions
- Informed consent
- Advanced directives and end-of-life care
- Withholding treatment
- Quality of life issues

Several strategies for promoting optimal nursing care related to ethics include:

- Recognizing that values and beliefs vary not only among different cultures but also within cultures.
- Viewing values and beliefs from different cultures within historical, health-care, cultural, spiritual, and religious contexts.
- Being aware of cultural values and biases.
- Being cognizant of possible ethical issues in providing care to acutely ill patients.
- Identifying and promoting discussion of ethical issues or dilemmas with members of the health-care team, the patient, and family.
- Promoting appropriate care for the acutely ill including identification of the need for palliative care.

SYNERGY MODEL

The Synergy Model serves as the organizing framework for the PCCN exam. The Synergy Model was developed in the 1990s by an American Association of Critical-Care Nurses (AACN) task force to construct an organizing framework that promotes recognition of the value of nursing practice in focusing on the relationship between the nurse and the patient. The model outlines that the needs or characteristics of patients and families influence and drive the characteristics or competencies of nurses. According to the Synergy Model, synergy results when the needs and characteristics of a patient, clinical unit, or system are matched by a nurse's competencies. The Synergy Model identifies eight patient needs or characteristics and eight nursing competencies. When these patient needs and nursing competencies are aligned, patient outcomes are optimized.

The eight patient characteristics that are evaluated by nurses include:

- **Stability:** The ability to maintain a steady state, including physiologic, psychologic, emotional, and family or social stability.
- **Complexity:** The intricate interconnectedness of two or more systems (e.g., body, family, and social systems).
- **Predictability:** The characteristic that allows one to expect a certain trajectory of illness.
- **Vulnerability:** A susceptibility to stressor that may affect patient outcomes adversely.
- **Resiliency:** The capacity to return to a restorative level of functioning using compensatory and coping mechanisms.

- **Participation in decision making:** The extent to which the patient and the patient's family engage in decision making.
- **Participation in care:** The extent to which the patient or family engages in aspects of care.
- **Resource availability:** The resources that the patient/clinical unit/system can bring to a situation.

Patients and families vacillate along these eight continuums over time and influence how a nurse would approach and care for the patient. The Synergy Model outlines eight nursing competencies to respond to patient needs in order to enhance outcomes. These dimensions of nursing practice span the continuum from competent to expert and include:

- **Clinical judgment:** Clinical reasoning, which includes clinical decision making, critical thinking, and a global grasp of the situation, coupled with nursing skills acquired by integrating formal and experiential knowledge.
- **Clinical inquiry:** The ongoing process of questioning and evaluating practice and providing informed practice.
- **Caring practices:** The constellation of nursing activities that are responsive to the uniqueness of the patient and family and that create a compassionate and therapeutic environment with the aim of promoting comfort and healing and preventing unnecessary suffering.
- **Response to diversity:** The sensitivity to recognize, appreciate, and incorporate differences in the provision of care.
- **Advocacy:** Working on another's behalf and representing the concerns of the patient/family/colleagues/community and serving as a moral agent in identifying and helping to resolve ethical and clinical concerns within the clinical setting.
- **Facilitation of learning:** The ability to facilitate patient/staff/system learning.
- **Collaboration:** Working with others (patient, family, health-care providers, colleagues, community) in a way that promotes and encourages each person's contributions.
- **Systems thinking:** Appreciating the care environment from a perspective that recognizes the holistic interrelationships that exist within and across health-care systems.

Several assumptions regarding nurses, patients, and families guide the AACN Synergy Model for patient care:

- Patients are biologic, psychologic, social, and spiritual entities who present at a particular developmental stage. The whole patient (body, mind, and spirit) must be considered.
- The patient, family, and community all contribute to providing a context for the nurse-patient relationship.
- Patients can be described by a number of characteristics. All characteristics are connected and contribute to each other. Characteristics cannot be seen in isolation.
- Similarly, nurses can be described on a number of dimensions. The interrelated dimensions paint a profile of the nurse.
- A goal of nursing is to restore a patient to an optimal level of wellness as defined by the patient. Death can be an acceptable outcome, in which the goal of nursing care is to move a patient toward a peaceful death. Supporting patients and families during the dying process is also a focus of professional nursing practice.

The Synergy Model outlines that when patients' characteristics and nurses' competencies synergize, optimal patient outcomes are achieved. As the patient is the primary focus, optimal outcomes are defined as what patients themselves acknowledge as important. Three levels of outcomes are outlined: patient level, unit level, and system level. The Synergy Model helps to promote the measurement of nurse-sensitive outcomes. Based on the model, the outcome of a synergistic relationship is termed "safe passage," which includes helping the patient and family move toward greater self-awareness and self-understanding, competence, and health and/or a peaceful death.

In addition to serving as the organizing framework, the Synergy Model has also been used to describe nursing practice, serve as a framework for nursing interventions and nursing education, and guide advanced practice nursing care.

BIBLIOGRAPHY

American Association of Critical-Care Nurses. (2005). AACN standards for establishing and sustaining healthy work environments: A journey to excellence. *American Journal of Critical Care, 14*(3), 187–197.

American Association of Critical-Care Nurses. (2007). Protocols for Practice: Creating a Healing Environment (2nd ed.). Aliso Viejo, CA: AACN.

American Association of Critical-Care Nurses. The AACN Synergy Model of Patient Care. Available at http://www.aacn.org/certcorp/certcorp.nsf/vwdoc/SynModel Accessed 8/10/2010.

American Association of Colleges of Nursing. Hallmarks of the Professional Nursing Practice Environment. Available at: http://www.aacn.nche.edu/Publications/positions/hallmarks.htm Accessed 8/12/2010.

Benner. P. (2003). Enhancing patient advocacy and social ethics. *American Journal of Critical Care, 12*(4), 374–375.

Benner, P. (2004). Relational ethics of comfort, touch, and solace—Endangered arts? *American Journal of Critical Care, 13*(4), 346–349.

Brewer, B. B, Wojner-Alexandrov, A. W, Triola, N., Pacini C., Cline M., Rust J. E., Kerfoot K. (2007). AACN's synergy model's characteristics of patients: Psychometric analysis in a tertiary care health system. *American Journal of Critical Care, 16*, 158–167.

Briggs, L. A, Kirchhoff, K. T, Hammes, B. J, Song, M. K., Colvin, E. R. (2004). Patient-centered advance care planning in special patient populations: A pilot study. *Journal of Professional Nursing, 20*(1), 47–58.

Curley, M. A. Q. (2007). Synergy: The unique relationship between nurses and patients. Indianapolis, IN: Sigma Theta Tau International.

Gorman, L. M, & Sultan, D. F. (2008). *Psychosocial nursing for general patient care*. Philadelphia, PA: F. A. Davis.

Hardin, S., & Kaplow, R. (2005). Synergy for clinical excellence: The AACN synergy model for patient care. Boston, MA: Jones & Bartlett.

Hayes, C. (2000). The Synergy Model in practice. Strengthening nurses' moral agency. *Critical Care Nurse, 20*(5), 90–94.

Ludwick, R., & Silva M. Nursing around the world: Cultural values and ethical conflicts. Online Journal of Issues in Nursing. Available at: http://www.nursingworld.org/ojin/ethicol/ethics_4.htm Accessed 7/25/2010.

Nibert, A. T. (2005). Teaching clinical ethics using a case study family presence during cardiopulmonary resuscitation. *Critical Care Nurse, 25*(1), 38-44.

Reilly, T., Humbrecht, D. (2007). Fostering synergy: A nurse-managed remote telemetry model. *Critical Care Nurse, 27*, 22–33.

Sigma Theta Tau International. The State of Synergy. Excellence in Nursing Knowledge. Available at http://www.nursingknowledge.org/Portal/main.aspx?pageid=3507&ContentID=55889. Accessed 8/10/2010.

Tracy, M. F. (2010). Assessment of progressive care patients and families. In M. Chulay & S. Burns (Eds.). *AACN essentials of progressive care nursing* (pp. 3–15). New York, NY: McGraw-Hill.

Tracy, M. F. (2010). Assessment of progressive care patients and families. In M. Chulay & S. Burns (Eds.). *AACN essentials of progressive care nursing* (pp. 17–30). New York, NY: McGraw-Hill.

Synergy Practice Exam

1. Which of the following is among the most important needs of family members during critical illness?
   (A) To know the status of transfer plans
   (B) To be near the patient
   (C) To be kept informed
   (D) To participate in treatment decisions

2. Which ethical principle refers to maximizing possible benefits and minimizing possible harms in providing patient care?
   (A) Respect
   (B) Beneficence
   (C) Nonmaleficence
   (D) Autonomy

3. Which of the following categories of needs should take priority in caring for the critically ill patient?
   (A) The needs of the patient
   (B) The needs of the family
   (C) The needs of the nurse
   (D) The needs of the physician

4. Which of the following interventions would best help family members to cope with a patient's life-threatening illness?
   (A) Encouraging the family to participate in patient care
   (B) Requesting that a chaplain speak with the family
   (C) Encouraging the family to ask questions
   (D) Extending visiting hours

5. The family of a critically ill patient disagrees with the patient's advance directives and asks the nurse to inform the physician that full aggressive treatment should be given to the patient. Which of the following nursing interventions would be most appropriate?

   (A) Directly inform the physician of the family's request.
   (B) Inform the family that they will need to discuss this issue with the physician.
   (C) Arrange to have the family meet with the physician to discuss treatment options for the patient.
   (D) Inform the family that the patient's advance directives for comfort care must be honored.

6. Based on the premises of the Synergy Model, which of the following is not considered an acceptable outcome of patient care?
   (A) Death
   (B) Optimal wellness
   (C) Uncertain prognosis
   (D) Patient perceptions of a poor outcome

7. The Hippocratic Oath is a fundamental principle that focuses on what medical ethic?
   (A) Treat all patients with respect.
   (B) Do no harm.
   (C) Provide care to all patients regardless of their ability to pay.
   (D) Provide the best possible care to patients.

8. Which of the following interventions would ensure that a patient understands and has given informed consent for a test or procedure?
   (A) Asking the patient to explain the test/procedure
   (B) Giving the patient written instructions for the test/procedure
   (C) Verbally informing the patient about the test/procedure
   (D) Obtaining the patient's signature on the consent form

9. A patient says that she has not slept well during the night. What might be an indicated nursing action?
   (A) Inform the physician that the patient needs a sleeping pill.
   (B) Encourage the patient to stay awake during the day so that she will be able to sleep at night.
   (C) Allow the patient to rest during the day.
   (D) Limit caffeine intake for the patient during the day.

10. An elderly patient with advanced metastatic disease is placed on "do not resuscitate" status. The family asks to hold a Native American prayer service at the patient's bedside. The patient is in a two-bed room with another patient who is comatose. Which of the following is the best action for the nurse?
    (A) Inform the family that the prayer service cannot be conducted.
    (B) Allow the prayer service to be conducted, as the patient's roommate would not be aware of the event.
    (C) Arrange to transfer the patient to a single room to facilitate the family's request to hold the service.
    (D) Since it is near shift change, wait and let the next shift nurse decide.

11. Which of the following terms corresponds with serving as a moral agent?
    (A) Collaboration
    (B) Systems thinking
    (C) Clinical judgment
    (D) Advocacy

12. What ethical principle focuses on the duty to treat all patients fairly, distributing the risks and benefits of treatment equally?
    (A) Nonmaleficence
    (B) Autonomy
    (C) Respect
    (D) Justice

13. A patient who was hospitalized for revision of an arteriovenous fistula for dialysis says that he has been practicing yoga at home daily. He asks the nurse whether there is an area of the hospital where he can go to practice his yoga. Which of the following would be the best nursing action?
    (A) Inform the patient he cannot practice yoga while hospitalized.
    (B) Tell the patient that the doctor would need to issue an order to allow it.

(C) Consult with the health-care team to pursue options for the patient to practice yoga.
(D) Help the patient to perform yoga in his room.

14. What is the least likely response to a family's initial attempts to manage a critical illness?
    (A) Denial
    (B) Stress
    (C) Acceptance
    (D) Fear

15. What ethical principle identifies the duty to cause no harm?
    (A) Nonmaleficence
    (B) Beneficence
    (C) Veracity
    (D) Autonomy

The next question relates to the following situation: The nurse for an elderly patient who sustained a recent stroke with expressive aphasia was able to communicate with the patient in writing; this patient expressed his desire to return to his assisted-living facility and receive further treatment there. The nurse contacted the social service department to pursue placement in the facility after discharge.

16. In doing so, the nurse is exhibiting which of the following competencies?
    (A) Caring practices
    (B) Moral agency
    (C) Advocacy
    (D) Systems thinking

17. A patient has just returned from physical therapy when a family member comes to visit. The patient appears tired. What would be the most appropriate nursing action?
    (A) Inform the family member that the patient needs to rest.
    (B) Ask the patient whether she wants to have a visitor now.
    (C) Make the patient comfortable in bed while she visits with her family member.
    (D) Ask the family member if he can come back to visit in an hour.

18. When the night shift nurse questions the routine nursing care of instilling saline during endotracheal suctioning, she is demonstrating which of the following nurse characteristics?
    (A) Resistance
    (B) Systems thinking
    (C) Clinical inquiry
    (D) Advocacy

SYNERGY PRACTICE EXAM **577**

19. The modification of visiting hours to accommodate an out-of-town relative is an example of what type of nursing action?
    (A) Seeking clinical inquiry
    (B) Meeting family needs
    (C) Promoting resource availability
    (D) Reducing patient vulnerability

20. During patient care rounds, the attending physician asks the physical therapist and nurse for input on the best ways to encourage a patient to increase his mobility. The physician is facilitating which clinical competency?
    (A) Facilitator of learning
    (B) Clinical inquiry
    (C) Collaboration
    (D) Advocacy

21. The Synergy Model holds that caring practices represent the constellation of nursing activities that are responsive to the uniqueness of the patient. Which of the following represents a caring practice?
    (A) Honesty
    (B) Presence
    (C) Truthfulness
    (D) Openness

22. A woman patient admitted with acute respiratory failure has become progressively worse.

Her husband asks that their 9-year-old son be allowed to visit. Which of the following would be the best action by the nurse?
    (A) Explain to the husband that visitation is limited to adults.
    (B) Suggest to the husband that the child might be frightened by the hospital environment and that the husband take a picture of the patient instead.
    (C) Allow the son to visit at midnight, when activity on the unit is slow.
    (D) Arrange for a patient-care conference with the husband and members of the health-care team to discuss possible options.

23. A new attending physician is routinely rude to the nursing staff and often refuses to answer their questions. What would be an appropriate nursing action?
    (A) Inform the physician that his actions are inappropriate.
    (B) Point out the offensive behavior to him the next time it occurs.
    (C) Report the physician to the hospital administrator.
    (D) Ask that the physician attend the next multidisciplinary unit meeting and discuss the unit's philosophy of professional communication.

Synergy Practice Exam

Practice Fill-Ins

1. _____

2. _____

3. _____

4. _____

5. _____

6. _____

7. _____

8. _____

9. _____

10. _____

11. _____

12. _____

13. _____

14. _____

15. _____

16. _____

17. _____

18. _____

19. _____

20. _____

21. _____

22. _____

23. _____

PART IX

Synergy Practice Exam

PART IX

Answers

1. C	7. B	13. C	19. B
2. B	8. A	14. C	20. C
3. A	9. C	15. A	21. B
4. C	10. C	16. C	22. D
5. C	11. D	17. B	23. D
6. D	12. D	18. C	

X

BEHAVIOR

....

Linda Nattkemper York
Robin Gutman
Sharon Ryback

Behavioral and Psychologic Factors in Critical Care

EDITORS' NOTE

This is a new chapter for the PCCN exam. You can expect to see 4% of the total exam's questions from this area (about six questions). There are eight sections in this chapter, so about one question from each section could be anticipated.

These sections are presented in a very brief format, designed to acquaint you with basic fundamentals. The section is not designed to be comprehensive, but to help you understand key components that could be addressed on the PCCN exam.

This chapter includes the following content areas:

1. Abuse and neglect
2. Antisocial personality disorder (aggression/violence)
3. Delirium and dementia
4. Depression
5. Developmental delays
6. Geriatric failure to thrive
7. Substance dependence (withdrawal, chronic alcohol or drug dependence, drug-seeking behavior)
8. Suicidal behavior

ABUSE AND NEGLECT

Although the precise prevalence of abuse is not known because of underreporting, it is estimated that one-half of Americans have experienced violence in their families. Current surveys report that 40% to 50% of abuse victims are men. Abuse and neglect is found in all religious, cultural, educational, and socioeconomic backgrounds. Table 51-1 lists categories of abuse and neglect.

Assessment

The concern that a patient may have suffered abuse or neglect must always be discussed in private. Use an empathetic, professional, and nonjudgmental manner. It is most effective to ask open-ended questions in honest and direct language that patient will understand. Be aware of your response to patient's disclosure avoiding any display shock, horror, disapproval, or anger toward the perpetrator or situation.

Intervention

1. Establishing a rapport of trust and assuring confidentiality is essential.
2. If patient is a victim of violence, consider placing patient on a "protective" status in accordance with hospital policy and the patient's wishes.
   a. Ensure that *all* staff caring for the patient are aware of and observe protective status.
3. Plan care with consideration to type of violence. For example, if a female patient is raped, avoid male care staff.
4. Always approach a traumatized patient from the front to reduce startling.
5. Refer patient to psychiatry for observed symptoms of depression, suicidal ideation, anxiety, and symptoms of acute stress or posttraumatic stress disorder (PTSD).

TABLE 51-1. CATEGORIES OF ABUSE AND NEGLECT

Types with Examples	Symptoms/Observations
Physical: Infliction of physical pain or bodily harm. Biting, burning restraining, slapping, pushing, throwing.	1. Injuries inconsistent with stated cause or reason for hospitalization 2. Fractures and bruising at variable stages of healing 3. Explanation of injury is vague, minimized, or avoided. "Accident prone" 4. Somatic or stress related conditions, headaches, backaches, and dizziness 5. Changes in behavior, anxiety, withdrawal, overly solicitous, when perpetrator in room 6. Depression 7. Comments on "problems" with spouse/family member
Sexual: Any form of sexual contact or exposure without consent or when victim is unable to consent. It is estimated that 1 in 4 women and 1 in 6 men are sexually abused in childhood.	1. Bruising/injury to genitalia 2. Depression, anxiety/panic attacks 3. Symptoms of acute stress or PTSD: startle, numbing, avoidance, nightmares, insomnia hypervigilance, irritability, anger 4. Fear and anxiety of care procedure 5. Fear of gender of perpetrator
Emotional: Infliction of emotional/mental anguish. Threats, humiliation, intimidation, withholding of affection, controlling, and isolation.	1. Low self-esteem 2. Depression/anxiety 3. Timidity, nervousness around abuser 4. Complacency /helplessness 5. Poor eye contact
Neglect: Failure to provide for physical, developmental, or educational needs.	1. Evidence of starvation or malnutrition 2. Poor hygiene, dirty clothes 3. Lack of medical, dental 4. Ill-fitting clothing/shoes 5. Lacks knowledge of use of routine things; i.e., how to use remote control of TV
Economic: Illegal or improper exploitation of money and/or resources of for personal gain or withholding financial support.	1. Evidence of starvation or malnutrition 2. Patient not given needed medications 3. Bills not paid resulting in utilitiesturned off or foreclosure of home 4. Patient hinting at or complaint that another is controlling their funds/assets

PTSD, posttraumatic stress disorder.

6. Know your state's reporting requirements and report elder, child, and adolescent abuse or neglect to the appropriate protective authority. Reporting abuse or neglect in good faith is immune from prosecution.

ANTISOCIAL PERSONALITY DISORDER

In general, a person with a personality disorder (PD) exhibits an ongoing pattern of maladaptive personality traits that are both persistent and rigid. The disorder occurs in approximately 10% of the population but can be erroneously attributed to people who are ethnically or culturally different from healthcare professionals. As nursing professionals, it is important to acknowledge that many people with personality disorders have suffered prolonged abuse and/or neglect in childhood or throughout their lives. The problematic behaviors they manifest helped them adapt to and survive an abnormal situation and represent their best effort in meeting their needs.

Antisocial personality disorder (ASPD) is characterized by a persistent disregard for, and violation of, the rights of others. Deceit and manipulation are central features of this disorder. Because these antisocial behaviors are commonly observed in children and adolescents, this disorder is diagnosed only if antisocial behaviors are present by 18 years of age. Prior to 15 years, this pattern is identified as a conduct disorder. Individuals with this disorder are at increased risk of dying prematurely by violent means. About 80% to 85% of incarcerated criminals have ASPD.

Antisocial behavior that occurs exclusively during the course of schizophrenia or a manic episode does not constitute ASPD. It is also important to recognize that some antisocial behaviors may indeed be survival strategies for a person from a low socioeconomic or urban setting.

Diagnostic Criteria

Three or more of the following are required:

1. Failure to conform to social norms with respect to lawful behaviors as indicated by repeatedly performing acts that are grounds for arrest
2. Deceitfulness, as indicated by repeatedly lying, use of aliases, or conning others for personal profit or pleasure
3. Impulsivity or failure to plan ahead
4. Irritability and aggressiveness, as indicated by repeated physical fights or assaults
5. Reckless disregard for safety of self or others
6. Consistent irresponsibility, as indicated by repeated failure to sustain consistent work behavior or honor financial obligations

7. Lack of remorse, as indicated by being indifferent to or rationalizing having hurt, mistreated, or stolen from another

Assessment

One of the earliest indicators of a patient's having ASPD is when the nursing staff disagrees on how to address the patient's problematic behaviors. Because of the manipulative and deceitful nature of this disorder, unsuspecting nursing staff may become sympathetic to the patient's special request, unreasonable expectations, or stated needs. These patients will often times seek to break or bend established hospital policies and rules. When these patients do not get their wish, they can become verbally or physically aggressive.

Intervention

1. Confirm vital information with collateral sources whenever possible.
2. Communicate frequently as a care team to ensure that all staff approach problematic behaviors in a consistent manner.
3. The greatest predictor of violence is a history of past violence.
   a. This is of even greater concern if the violence was recent.
   b. Maintain a demeanor of respect, concern, and professionalism. Research indicates that patients are more likely to become assaultive in response to perceived disrespect or rejection by staff.
   c. Always verbally prepare the patient and explain any necessary care procedures, especially with a victim of violence to reduce startling or misunderstanding.
   d. Negotiate a compromise with patient if possible.
   e. If compromise is not possible, set a clear time limit when care will be done (e.g., "This needs to be done now or in 20 minutes. Your choice.")
4. Avoid power struggles with the patient. Focus on what is required.
5. If patient is a victim of violence, ensure that all nursing staff observe the structure of protective status.
6. Excessive irritability, negativity, or anxiety may indicate the patient is also struggling with comorbid mood disorder. A victim of violence may have acute stress disorder or PTSD. Consider psychiatric consultation.
7. If the patient becomes verbally or physically aggressive, step outside of the patient's reach for your own safety, and get assistance.
8. Avoid disclosing any personal information. These patients can be very charming and seductive but lack the capacity to truly consider others.

DELIRIUM AND DEMENTIA

Possibly the best resource for understanding delirium in the intensive care unit is from Vanderbilt University. They have created a web site specifically for helping clinicians learn about delirium in the ICU (www.icudelirium.org). The information in this section can be used in addition to their excellent web site.

Definitions

Delirium is an acute disturbance of consciousness with inattention. There may be changes in cognition and fluctuates over time. Dementia is characterized by an alert patient and tends to be chronic.

Based on research from Vanderbilt University, three subtypes of delirium are present: hyperactive, hypoactive, and mixed. Most clinicians associate the hyperactive form with dementia but all types can be encountered in a clinical setting.

Delirium is a serious condition associated with worse patient outcomes. Delirium can be thought of as an organ dysfunction, much like hypotension or a low PaO_2/FIO_2 ratio.

Why delirium develops is not clear. There are several potential anatomic and physical causes of delirium but the PCCN exam is more likely to focus on risk factors. Many critically ill patients are at risk for developing delirium. Most patients on mechanical ventilation will experience delirium, yet are often not recognized. ICU delirium has been shown to increase costs and mortality,

Evaluation

One validated test for delirium is the confusion assessment method for the ICU (CAM-ICU). Because a primary feature of delirium is inattention in an arousable patient, the CAM-ICU aids clinicians in the assessment of inattention.

Treatment

One of the causes of inability to keep attention is too much sedation. The use of sedation scores, such as the Richmond Agitation and Sedation Scale (RASS) can be useful in avoiding oversedation. For example, in the RASS, a patient should be maintained on sedation at a score of approximately 0 to −2. This would mean the patient opens his or her eyes with voice simulation in <10 s. Any physical stimulation required for the patient to open his or her eyes is likely to represent too deep of sedation. Subsequently, in evaluating a patient for an inability to keep attention should focus on removing any known causes. Any physiologic causes of inattention should also be addressed.

Help the patient remained properly oriented by techniques such as providing nonverbal music, any assistance with visual and hearing aids, and orient the patient as much as possible. As nursing routines allow, maintain consistency in staff and routines. Encourage familiar objects and allow normal television viewing if possible.

In addition, keep the environment conducive to rest. For example, keep lights off at night and on during the day and control excess staff and other ICU noise. Help the patient to remain active as much as possible.

Of course, any clinical disturbances should be corrected; for example, hypotension, hypoperfusion, and hypoxia. Any correctable clinical problem that could lead to inattentiveness should be addressed as soon as possible. Pharmacologically, haloperidol 2 to 5 mg IVP or IM every 6 h could be used to address delirium, although addressing the cause is a better solution. One side effect is prolongation of the QT with possible development of torsade de pointes (ventricular tachycardia).

DEPRESSION

Depression is a mood disorder involving the body, thoughts, and behavior. It affects the way one eats and sleeps, the way one feels about the self, and the way one thinks about once pleasurable activities. At any given time, 10 million Americans suffer from this disabling disorder, which can appear at any age. One in five adults experience depression at some point in their lives. About 5% of children and adolescents also suffer from this disorder, and is twice as common in females as in males.

It is estimated that 25% to 33% of medically ill patients have coexisting depression. Unfortunately,

TABLE 51-2. MEDICAL CONDITIONS AND MEDICATIONS THAT MIMIC DEPRESSION

Medical Conditions that Mimic Depression	Medications that Mimic Depression
Anemia	Central nervous system depressants
Hepatitis	Benzodiazepines
Mononucleosis	Beta blockers
Hypothyroidism	Calcium channel blockers
Chronic pain/fatigue	Estrogen
syndromes	Fluoroquinolone antibiotics
	Statins
	Isotretinoin
	Narcotics
	Acyclovir

depression is often unrecognized and untreated in the medically ill person; in part because the symptoms are attributed to their primary illness. Left untreated, depression complicates care and compounds the pain and suffering of medical illness (Table 51-2).

Diagnostic Criteria

Diagnostic criteria for depressive disorder would include five or more of the following symptoms nearly every day for most waking hours over the same 2-week period. These symptoms are a change in the person's previous function and are the cause of significant distress or impairment in these areas of function.

1. Depressed, sad mood
2. Irritable mood in children and adolescents
3. Anhedonia: decreased interest or pleasure in almost all activities
4. Significant weight gain or loss (>5% change over 1 month)
5. Changes in sleep pattern
6. Increase or decrease in motor activity
7. Anergia: fatigue, loss of energy, feeling "slowed down"
8. Feelings of worthlessness, inappropriate guilt
9. Decreased concentration or indecision
10. Recurrent thoughts of death or suicidal ideation

Assessment

It is not unusual for a critically ill person to appear depressed during the acute or early recovery stage of an illness. This is described as a, "situational depression." As the person recovers and health improves, the depressive symptoms will also improve. If these symptoms persist in spite of improved health, the person is exhibiting depression and may benefit from treatment.

Intervention

1. If a person has an established history of depression, ensure that the prior medication regime is resumed as soon as possible.
2. Request a psychiatric consultation as soon as it is identified that the person is exhibiting symptoms of depression.
3. Safety of the person is the priority.
   a. Ask the patient if he or she is thinking of harming self or ending life.
   b. This will not increase a person's risk of self-harm and may save their life.
   c. If suicidal, place person on continuous observation until psychiatric evaluation indicates it is no longer necessary.
4. Other supportive services may help including the person's community support network, hospital chaplain, psychiatric clinical nurse specialist (CNS), and social work if person has many social or financial stressors.

DEVELOPMENTAL DELAYS

A developmental delay is defined as any significant lag in a person's physical, cognitive, behavioral, emotional, or social development in comparison with norms. According to the Centers for Disease Control and Prevention, "Developmental disabilities are a diverse group of severe chronic conditions that are due to mental and/or physical impairments . . . resulting in problems with major life activities such as language, mobility, learning, self-help, and independent living." Although these terms are frequently used interchangeably, it is the disabling condition that is the cause of the observed developmental delay. Intellectual disabilities or forms of mental retardation account for the majority of developmental disorders. Mental retardation is present before 18 years of age and has many causes including infection, injury, genetic condition, and birth injury (Table 51-3).

Assessment

It is essential for nurses to be familiar with the nature of an intellectual disability because there are often

TABLE 51-3. CATEGORIES OF MENTAL RETARDATION WITH ASSOCIATED IQ SCORES AND LEVELS OF FUNCTION

Category	IQ Score	Level of Function
Mild accounts for 85% Intermittent Support	50–75	1. Usually independent 2. School is up to grade level 3. Will understand and learn with little support
Moderate accounts for 10% Limited Support	35–55	1. Self-care and work with moderate supervision 2. Language skills acquired in childhood 3. Additional support to learn health management skills
Severe accounts for 3%–4% Extensive Support	20–40	1. May master basic self-care and communication skills 2. Group home supportive living 3. Will need health-care regimes provided
Profound accounts for 1%–2% Pervasive Support	20–25	1. May master basic self-care with training 2. Require ongoing structure and supervision 3. Care provided by others

coexisting medical conditions. Examples of this are Down's syndrome and cardiac anomaly. Since mental retardation exists on a continuum, it is also important to identify the degree of intellectual disability and adjust care accordingly. Family, caregivers, or residential staff will likely be the best resources for this information. Gather as much information as possible about unique means of communication for pain, thirst, toileting, and so on.

Interventions

1. Previously independent patient may need additional support and reinforcement while critically ill.
2. New environment may be stressful since patient has limited adaptive skills.
3. Integrate words, communication, and techniques used by care providers into plan of care.
4. Use consistent care providers when possible.
5. Have care providers bring comfort measure, items, pictures, and so on.
6. Recognize the patients with mental retardation are also vulnerable to mental illness but may have difficulty describing their feelings.
7. If patient is aggressive or self-injurious, consider psychiatry consult.

a. While antipsychotic medications are controversial, these can be effective for psychotic disorders when other alternatives have failed.

b. Prozac has shown some benefit in self-injury.

GERIATRIC FAILURE TO THRIVE

Failure to thrive is a diagnosis that indicates a decline in health often associated with weight loss of greater than 5% of baseline, lack of appetite, poor nutrition, inactivity, often accompanied by dehydration, depressive symptoms, impaired immune function, and low cholesterol levels. (National Institute of Medicine guidelines)

The definition of geriatric failure to thrive (GFTT) includes four syndromes which include (1) impaired physical functioning, (2) malnutrition, (3) depression, and (4) cognitive impairment. In older adults, GFTT is distinguished by an inability to maintain body weight, a decline in functional capacity, and a decline in social and cognitive skills. This syndrome is not part of normal aging and warrants a careful medical workup to treat factors uncovered that may reverse this syndrome.

Assessment

Early recognition is the key to treating any reversible factors in GFTT. A comprehensive medical assessment including a thorough history and physical examination, labs, and diagnostic tests may uncover cancer, chronic obstructive pulmonary disease (COPD), congestive heart failure (CHF), renal and hepatic diseases, rheumatologic diseases, diabetes, stroke, anemia, immune deficiencies, postoperative complications, chronic infections, poorly controlled diabetes, intestinal motility and malabsorption disorders, pressure ulcers, and tuberculosis. A medication review of all prescribed and over-the-counter (OTC) medications, side effects from medications, possible drug interactions, and medicines that may impair appetite and induce weight loss should be initiated. Screen for cognitive status, dementia, delirium, depression, substance abuse, and alcoholism. A full nutritional assessment, screening for protein malnutrition in dementia, dental and denture assessment, speech and swallowing assessment are valuable. Assess the degree of disability which may be measured by the instrumental activities of daily living (IADLs) and activities of daily living (ADLs). Assessment of time by caregivers to feed dependent patients should be measured. An environmental assessment of the patient's home may uncover barriers to independent functioning. Be alert for complaints from the patient and family regarding the decline of the patient "for no apparent reason."

Intervention

A multidisciplinary approach with physician, mental health professional, dietician, speech therapist, social worker, and physical therapist is recommended.

Target treatment to any identifiable problems uncovered in the assessment for the four syndromes:

1. **Impaired physical functioning:** Physical therapy, occupational therapy, modify the environment for maximum safety, strength training.
2. **Malnutrition:** Treat oral pathology, increase feedings, offer nutritional supplements. Serial weight measurements, dietician to evaluate diet and caloric intake.
3. **Depression:** Medication, psychotherapy, exercise, activity therapy, spiritual support, emotional support.
4. **Cognitive Impairment:** Treat dementia and depression, treat malnutrition and infection, optimize living situation. Minimize social isolation—patient may have impaired hearing and vision that impedes communication.

Use of orexigenic agents (agents that improve appetite and muscle mass). Many of these have dramatic side effects for the elderly population warrant clinical trials of these medications in the elderly. Mirtazapine (Remeron) has been widely used. Antipsychotics used for dementia often cause weight gain.

SUBSTANCE ABUSE/DEPENDENCE

Many patients arrive in the ICU with conditions directly or indirectly related to their substance use/dependence. Prolonged substance use affects brain functioning and therefore behavior. Adequate assessment and intervention can shorten their ICU stay and enhance survival.

Ethyl alcohol (ETOH) is the most commonly abused substance. Table 51-4 lists commonly abused drugs.

Assessment

All patients should be assessed for use of substances on admission or as soon as feasible. There are many tools for assessment, some brief, others very detailed.

TABLE 51-4. COMMONLY ABUSED DRUGS

Drug Category and Name	Intoxication Effects/Potential Health Consequences
Depressants	
Barbiturates	
Amytal (amobarbital), Nembutal (pentobarbital), Seconal (secobarbital), phenobarbital, Fiorinal (combination of butalbital, aspirin, and caffeine)	For barbiturates and benzodiazepines taken in greater than prescribed dose, feelings of euphoria and intoxication similar to ETOH/physical dependence and withdrawal syndrome
Benzodiazepines	
Ativan (larazepam), Librium (chlordiazepoxide), Xanax alparzolam), Valium (diazepam)	
Flunitrazepam, rohypnol	Associated with sexual assaults/amnesia, sedation
Gamma-hydroxybutyric acid	Both sedative and euphoric effects/slowed breathing and heart rate
Dissociative Anesthetics	
Ketamine	Increased heart rate and blood pressure, impaired motor function, memory loss/delirium, respiratory depression and arrest
PCP	Aggression, panic, hallucinations, violence/mood and cognitive alterations
Hallucinogens	
LSD	Altered states of perception and feeling/flashbacks
Opioids and Morphine Derivatives	
Codeine, fentanyl, morphine, heroin, oxycodone, hydrocodone	Pain relief, euphoria, drowsiness, constipation, confusion, sedation, respiratory depression, arrest death, tolerance, physical dependence, withdrawal syndrome
Stimulants	
Amphetamines	
Dextroamphetamine, methamphetamine	Increased heart rate, blood pressure, and energy, euphoria/paranoia, weight loss, anxiety, insomnia, irregular heart rate, depression
Cocaine and crack	Increased heart rate, blood pressure, euphoria/chest pain, MI, CVA, seizures, paranoia
Methlylenedioxymethamphetamine (MDMA, ecstasy)	Both hallucinogenic and stimulant effects, increased tactile sensitivity and empathic feelings/hyperthermia, hypertension, dehydration, renal failure
Other	
Inhalants/solvents	Euphoria, stimulation/memory impairment, loss of motor control, muscle weakness, sudden death
Dextromethorphan (in cough and cold medicines)	Distorted visual perceptions, euphoria/impaired motor function and memory
Marijuana	Euphoria, relaxation, slowed thinking and reaction time/impaired memory and learning, anxiety, panic attacks, paranoia, withdrawal syndrome

CVA, cerebrovascular accident; ETOH, ethyl alcohol; LSD, lysergic acid diethylamide; MI, mycardial infarction; PCP, phencyclidine.

In an ICU setting a few brief questions can reveal patient problematic alcohol use.

> "On average, how many alcohol drinks per week do you have?"
> "On a typical day, how many alcohol drinks do you have?"

> "How many times in past year have you had x or more drinks in a day?" (x = 5 drinks for men and 4 drinks for women)
> "When was your last drink?"

Risk factors for withdrawal include—previous history of withdrawal, older age patients, poor health and nutritional deficits, comorbid medical conditions, psychiatric disorder.

In addition to alcohol, all patients should be assessed for drug use. Urine drug screens are helpful tools in addition to asking patient directly. In addition to specific drugs inquire about duration, frequency, amount, and date of last use. This information is essential in assessing for intoxication effects and likelihood of withdrawal from depressants and opioids.

Intervention

Alcohol

- Withdrawal is progressive, unless treated.
- Early stages can begin as soon as 3 h after last drink and can occur up to 7 days after last drink.
- Peak for withdrawal is at 48 to 72 h after last drink.
- Early signs and symptoms include anxiety, irritability, problems sleeping, decreased appetite, nausea, elevated heart rate and blood pressure, hand tremors, sweating.
- Severe withdrawal including delirium tremens (DTs): In addition to previous symptoms, patients experience disorientation to time, place, person, situation and hypersensitivity to light and noise. Perceptual disturbances include hallucinations, usually visual and tactile. Fluctuating levels of consciousness from lethargy to agitation.
- Withdrawal seizures: Majority occur within first 48 h, with peak at 24 h; can occur with or without delirium, usually generalized tonic-clonic.
- Treatment: Adequate hydration (either PO or IV); correction of electrolyte imbalances; multivitamins, thiamine and folate; monitor vital signs.
- Medications for withdrawal: Benzodiazepines including chlordiazepoxide, diazepam, or lorazepam; phenobarbital can also be used.
- Nursing interventions (see section on Delirium above).

Depressants

- Signs and symptoms of intoxication and withdrawal are similar to those of alcohol.
- Seizures can occur with or without other signs and symptoms of withdrawal and should always be considered if person is benzodiazepine dependent.

- Patients who take benzodiazepines for anxiety or panic attacks may have those symptoms emerge during withdrawal.

Dissociative Anesthetics and Hallucinogens

- Treatment consists of providing safety to patients who may be agitated, violent, or at risk of harming themselves or others. Symptomatic treatment of altered vital signs.

Opioids and Morphine Derivatives

- For known or suspected overdoses, naloxone (Narcan) will reverse excessive sedation.
- Unlike alcohol and benzodiazepine/barbiturate withdrawal, opioid withdrawal is seldom life threatening.
- Withdrawal symptoms from heroin and most short-acting opioids begin within 8 to 12 h after last use and peak at 48 to 72 h.
- Withdrawal from long-acting opioids such as methadone begins within 24 to 36 h after last use and peaks at 72 to 96 h.
- Withdrawal symptoms—autonomic instability includes elevated heart rate and blood pressure, sweating, chills, hot/cold flashes, elevated temperature.
- Other withdrawal symptoms—anxiety, restlessness; irritability; insomnia; muscle aches, bone pain; nausea, vomiting and diarrhea; cravings.
- Medications—withdrawal is usually managed in one of three ways—methadone, clonidine with or without benzodiazepines, or buprenorphine. Opioids given for pain management or other medical reasons will also diminish withdrawal symptoms.
- Methadone—prevents withdrawal by binding to mu-opioid receptors displacing shorter acting opioids. Dosage varies depending on amount and duration of use, but should rarely exceed 40 mg total daily dose. Given in bid or tid dosing. Withdrawal can usually be completed in 3 to 5 days. Safe for use during pregnancy.
- Clonidine—address autonomic instability symptoms. Benzodiazepines can be added to address restlessness, irritability, insomnia, and to provide some relief from cravings. Clonidine should be held if patient's blood pressure <90/60.
- Buprenorphine/naloxone (Suboxone)—partial mu-opioid agonist. Patients receiving

prescribed opioids in ICU setting should not be treated with this medication for withdrawal.

- Nursing Interventions—tell patients that goal of medications is to diminish withdrawal symptoms, not to remove them completely; help patients differentiate withdrawal symptoms from those of other medical problems; patients' subjective experience of withdrawal will be more intense than objective symptoms.

Stimulants

- Symptomatic treatment of altered vital signs, seizures, altered mental states.
- Providing for safety as patient behavior indicates.
- Profound dysphoria—often accompanies withdrawal and can lead to suicide attempts or completed suicide. Assess patient for suicidal ideation, provide for safety, obtain psychiatric consultation.

Inhalants/Solvents

- Many different substances in the category from adhesives such as airplane glue; aerosols such as spray paint and computer keyboard cleaner; cleaning agents such as spot removers.
- Important to know which substance patient is using as ingredients may require differing treatments.
- Symptomatic treatment of neurotoxic effects on cognition, motor, and sensory involvement.

Dextromethorphan

- See Dissociative Anesthetics section above.

Marijuana

- Withdrawal syndrome consists of irritability, sleep disturbances, anxiety, restlessness.
- Symptomatic treatment for symptoms which persist.

Drug-Seeking Behavior

- Term often applied to patients seeking pain relief. Complex set of behaviors in which patient is viewed by staff in negative, blaming manner.
- Assessment is very important and should include:
  - Is pain being undertreated?
  - Which behaviors of patient are being labeled drug seeking?

- Are there other ways to explain this behavior?
- What is patient level of functioning and quality of life? Adequate pain relief will improve functioning and quality of life for patients.
- Look for patterns of behavior, not isolated incidences.

SUICIDAL BEHAVIOR

Patients may present to ICU as a result of an attempted suicide or may have suicidal thoughts upon or during their admission. Suicide affects all demographic groups. In 2006, 33,000 persons committed suicide, making it the 11th leading cause of death. Risk factors include persons 15 to 24 years of age and those older than 65 years. White males and Native Americans have the highest rate of completed suicide. Substance use and psychiatric disorders increase likelihood of suicide. For every 25 persons who attempt, 1 person completes suicide.

Assessment

Nurses may be reluctant to address the issue of suicide with patients because they may be concerned it will cause a patient to become suicidal. This is a myth. The topic needs to be openly acknowledged and discussed with patients. Patients who make direct threats such as, "I want to kill myself" or indirect statements such as, "I wish I were dead" need to be taken seriously and assessed. Asking questions such as, "Do you have thoughts of wanting to hurt yourself?" and "Do you have thoughts of wanting to hurt others?" provides important information. If the patient gives an affirmative response to either question, further assessment is necessary. Inquire about previous suicide attempts and what plans patient has for acting on suicidal thoughts.

Interventions

Providing for safety is primary concern for suicidal patients. An ICU setting provides many means and opportunities for intentional self-harm. Some possible means can be controlled such as not leaving medications accessible to patients. Other means such as IV and oxygen tubing and monitoring wires must be in close proximity to patients. Therefore, close observation is essential. If a patient is actively trying to harm self, then one-to-one with a sitter may be appropriate. Restraints should be used only when other less restrictive interventions have failed. A psychiatric consultation should be initiated.

BIBLIOGRAPHY

Abuse and Neglect

American Psychiatric Association. (2000). *Diagnostic and statistical manual of mental disorders,*TR (4th ed.) (pp. 467–470). Washington, DC: APA.

Responding to child sexual abuse. (2004). *American Acadamey of Childhood and Adolescent Psychiatry,*(28)July, 1–2.

Varcarolis, E. M. (2000). *Psychiatric nursing clinical guide: assessment tools and diagnosis* (pp. 405–420). Philadelphia, PA: Saunders.

Varcarolis, EM. (2002). *Foundations of psychiatric nursing: a clinical approach* (4th ed.) (pp. 689–699). Philadelphia, PA: Saunders.

Antisocial Personality Disorder

American Psychiatric Association. (2000). *Diagnostic and statistical manual of mental disorders,*TR (4th ed.) (pp. 701–706). Washington, DC: APA.

Chou, K. R., Lu, R. B., & Chang, M. (2001). Assaultive behavior by psychiatric in-patients and its related factors. *Journal of Nursing Research, 9*(5), 139–151.

Gutmann, R. (2009). *An approach to the aggressive patient.* Lecture for First Year Psychiatry Residents, July 28.

Varcarolis, E. M. (2000). *Psychiatric nursing clinical guide: assessment tools and diagnosis* (pp. 100–106). Philadelphia, PA: Saunders.

Delirium and Dementia

Pun B. T., Ely E. W. (2007). The importance of diagnosing and managing ICU delirium. *Chest, 132*(2), 124–136. www.icudelirium.org.

Sona, C. (2009). Assessing delirium in the ICU. *Critical Care Nurse, 29,* 103–105.

Depression

American Psychiatric Association. (2000). *Diagnostic and statistical manual of mental disorders,*TR (4th ed.) (p. 349). Washington, DC: APA.

The Cleveland Clinic, Health Information Center, No. 28, 2004.

Stuart, S. (1995). *Principles and practice of psychiatric nursing* (pp. 414–431). St. Louis, MO: Mosby.

Varcarolis, E. M. (2000). *Psychiatric nursing clinical guide: assessment tools and diagnosi* (p. 163). Philadelphia, PA: Saunders.

Developmental Delays

American Psychiatric Association. (2000). *Diagnostic and statistical manual of mental disorders,*TR (4th ed.) (pp. 41–50). Washington, DC: APA.

Murphy, C. C., Boyle, C., Schendel, D., et al. (1998). Epidemiology of mental retardation in children. *Mental Retardation and Developmental Disability Research Reviews, 4,* 6–13.

Ricketts, R. W., et al. (1993). Fluoxetine treatment of severe self-injury in young adults with mental retardation. *Journal of the American Acadamey of Childhood and Adolescent Psychiatry, 32*(4), 865–869.

Tervo, R. (2003). Identifying patterns of developmental delays can help diagnose neurodevelopment disorders: A pediatric perspective. *Clinical Pediatrics, 12*(July), 1–5.

Failure to Thrive

Blazer, D. G. (2000). Psychiatry and the oldest old. *American Journal of Psychiatry, 157,* 1919.

Golden, A. G., Daiello, L. A., Silverman, M. A., et al. (2003). University of Miami division of clinical pharmacology therapeutic rounds: Medications used to treat anorexia in the frail elderly. *Americal Journal of Therapy, 10,* 292.

Robertson, R. G., & Montagnini, M. (2004). Geriatric failure to thrive. *American Family Physician, 70,* 343.

Rocchiccioli, J. T., & Sanford, J. T. (2009). Revisiting geriatric failure to thrive. *Journal of Gerontologic Nursing, 35*(1), 18.

Suicidal Behavior

McCaffery, M. (1999). *Pain: Clinical manual* (2nd ed.). St. Louis, MO: Mosby.

McIntosh, J. L. (2009). USA Suicide:2006 Final Data. American Association of Suicidology. Available at: http://www.suicidology.org/c/document_library/get_file?folderId=228&name=DLFE-142.pdf Accessed 2/7/2010.

US Department of Health and Human Services. (2006). *Detoxification and substance abuse treatment: A treatment improvement protocol, TIP 45.* Rockville, MD: U.S. Department of Health and Human Services.

US Department of Health and Human Services. (2008). *Substance abuse and suicide prevention: Evidence and implications.* Rockville, MD: U.S. Department of Health and Human Services.

Behavior Practice Exam

1. Which of the following is the most effective nursing intervention when caring for suicidal patients?
   (A) Close observation
   (B) Four-point restraints
   (C) Removing all potential harmful objects from environment
   (D) Asking family to watch the patient

2. Which of the following patients with alcohol abuse problems would be most likely to experience withdrawal?
   (A) A 76-year-old woman with history depression and liver disease
   (B) A 30-year-old man who is dependent on heroin
   (C) A 45-year-old man with gastric ulcers and anxiety disorder
   (D) A 50-year-old woman with congestive heart failure and diabetes

3. Your patient's last drink was Tuesday at 2200. When would the patient be most likely to experience withdrawal symptoms?
   (A) Wednesday morning
   (B) Friday morning
   (C) Saturday evening
   (D) Sunday evening

4. A patient is admitted with diagnosis of alcohol dependence. Which of the following would indicate the patient is likely experiencing withdrawal?
   (A) B/P 94/66, HR 100, tremors, hot dry skin
   (B) B/P 156/94, HR 108, moist damp skin, restlessness
   (C) B/P 120/74, HR 84, tremors, nausea, vomiting
   (D) B/P 170/102, HR 72, headache, nausea, vomiting

5. Which of the following is most important in providing care for patients experiencing benzodiazepine withdrawal? The nurse should observe for:
   (A) Paranoia
   (B) Hallucinations
   (C) Seizures
   (D) Irregular heart beat

6. In planning care for patients experiencing opioid withdrawal, which of the following understandings should the nurse consider?
   (A) Patients are at a high risk for seizures.
   (B) Patients often experience visual and tactile hallucinations.
   (C) Medications are ineffective in treating symptoms.
   (D) Medications are used to diminish, not to alleviate symptoms completely.

7. Your patient has been requesting increases in dose of opioid pain medications. Staff are concerned that the patient is "drug-seeking." Which of the following would be most important in planning care for this patient?
   (A) Assess for adequacy of pain relief.
   (B) Recommend the doctor change pain medications.
   (C) Request pain management consultation.
   (D) Recommend the doctor increase opioid dose.

8. Which is the key feature of delirium?
   (A) Fatigue
   (B) Anxiety
   (C) Inability to sleep
   (D) Inattention

9. The behaviors associated with "ICU psychosis" are manifestations of which form of delirium?
   (A) Hyperactive
   (B) Hypoactive

(C) Mixed
(D) Subclinical

10. The Confusion Assessment Method for the ICU (CAM-ICU) tool is a measure for which condition?
    (A) Dementia
    (B) Delirium
    (C) Psychosis
    (D) Alcohol and barbiturate withdrawal

11. The RASS (Richmond Agitation and Sedation Score) is a measure for which condition?
    (A) Delirium
    (B) Neuromuscular paralysis
    (C) Dementia
    (D) Adequacy of sedation

12. Which of the following is a pharmacologic treatment for delirium?
    (A) Haloperidol
    (B) Midazolam
    (C) Fentanyl
    (D) Selenium

13. Which of the following is a potentially serious side effect of haloperidol?
    (A) Delirium
    (B) Prolonged QT interval
    (C) Decreased level of consciousness
    (D) Agitation

14. The definition of geriatric failure to thrive includes which of the following?
    (A) Difficulty swallowing
    (B) Passive/aggressive behavior

(C) Heart failure
(D) Cognitive impairment

15. Which of the following medical conditions can mimic depression?
    (A) Anemia
    (B) Heart failure
    (C) Hyperthyroidism
    (D) Steroid abuse

16. Your patient is to undergo a cardiac catherization in the morning. He tells you, "I don't think I'll be able to sleep tonight" but refuses the ordered sleeping medication. Which of the following should the nurse suggest to enhance sleep?
    (A) Counting sheep
    (B) Watching television
    (C) Imagery
    (D) Playing a solitaire card game

17. Your patient with pneumonia has a past medical history of type 2 diabetes and hypertension. During the day she is alert, oriented, and cooperative. In the late evening and early morning, she is confused and pulls at her oxygen and IV lines. Your initial response is:
    (A) Administer haloperidol per the PRN order.
    (B) Place the patient in soft wrist restraints.
    (C) Optimize sleep-wake cycles by controlling lighting and noise.
    (D) Assign an unlicensed assistive personnel (sitter or aide) to observe the patient constantly.

Behavior Practice Exam

Practice Fill-Ins

1. _____	6. _____	11. _____	16. _____
2. _____	7. _____	12. _____	17. _____
3. _____	8. _____	13. _____	
4. _____	9. _____	14. _____	
5. _____	10. _____	15. _____	

PART X

Answers

1. __A__	6. __D__	11. __D__	16. __C__
2. __A__	7. __A__	12. __A__	17. __C__
3. __B__	8. __D__	13. __B__	
4. __B__	9. __A__	14. __D__	
5. __C__	10. __B__	15. __A__	

Page numbers followed by *f* or *t* denote figures or tables, respectively.